Handbook
of
Biochemistry
and
Molecular Biology

CRC Handbook
of
Biochemistry
and
Molecular Biology

3rd Edition

Lipids, Carbohydrates, Steroids

Editor

Gerald D. Fasman, Ph.D.
Rosenfield Professor of Biochemistry
Graduate Department of Biochemistry
Brandeis University
Waltham, Massachusetts

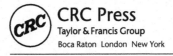

CRC Press
Taylor & Francis Group
Boca Raton London New York

CRC Press is an imprint of the
Taylor & Francis Group, an **informa** business

CRC Press
Taylor & Francis Group
6000 Broken Sound Parkway NW, Suite 300
Boca Raton, FL 33487-2742

Reissued 2019 by CRC Press

A Library of Congress record exists under LC control number:

Publisher's Note
The publisher has gone to great lengths to ensure the quality of this reprint but points out that some imperfections in the original copies may be apparent.

Disclaimer
The publisher has made every effort to trace copyright holders and welcomes correspondence from those they have been unable to contact.

ISBN 13: 978-0-367-20931-5 (hbk)
ISBN 13: 978-0-367-20933-9 (pbk)
ISBN 13: 978-0-429-26421-4 (ebk)

Visit the Taylor & Francis Web site at http://www.taylorandfrancis.com and the
CRC Press Web site at http://www.crcpress.com

Handbook
of
Biochemistry
and
Molecular Biology

3rd Edition

Lipids, Carbohydrates, Steroids

Editor
Gerald D. Fasman, Ph. D.
Rosenfield Professor of Biochemistry
Graduate Department of Biochemistry
Brandeis University
Waltham, Massachusetts

The following is a list of the four major sections of the *Handbook*, each consisting of one or more volumes

Proteins — Amino Acids, Peptides, Polypeptides, and Proteins

Nucleic, Acids — Purines, Pyrimidines, Nucleotides, Oligonucleotides, tRNA, DNA, RNA

Lipids, Carbohydrates, Steroids

Physical and Chemical Data, Miscellaneous — Ion Exchange, Chromatography, Buffers, Miscellaneous, e.g., Vitamins

CONTRIBUTORS

R. G. Ackman
Environment Canada
Fisheries and Marine Research and
Development Directorate
Halifax Laboratory
Halifax, Nova Scotia
Canada

Waldo E. Cohn
Senior Biochemist, Biology Division
Oak Ridge National Laboratory
Oak Ridge, Tennessee 37830

Isidore Danishefsky
Professor, Department of Biochemistry
New York Medical College
New York, New York 10029

Glyn Dawson
Associate Professor, Department of
Pediatrics
The University of Chicago
Chicago, Illinois 60637

Sen-itiroh Hakamori
Fred Hutchinson Cancer
Research Center 2D-08
Seattle, Washington 98104

Ineo Ishizuka
Department of Biochemistry
Faculty of Medicine
Tokyo University
Tokyo
Japan

Akira Kobata
Chairman, Department of Biochemistry
Kobe University School of Medicine
Ikuta-ku, Kobe
Japan

Fred A. Kummerow
Burnsides Research Laboratory
University of Illinois
Urbana, Illinois 61801

Su-Chen Li
Department of Biochemistry
Tulane University
New Orleans, Louisiana 70112

Yu-Teh Li
Department of Biochemistry
Tulane University
New Orleans, Louisiana 70112

Irving Listowski
Department of Biochemistry
Albert Einstein College of Medicine
Yeshiva University
New York, New York 10461

Donald L. MacDonald
Department of Biochemistry and Biophysics
Oregon State University
Corvallis, Oregon 97331

George G. Maher
Research Chemist
Northern Utilization Research and
Development Division
Agricultural Research Service
U.S. Department of Agriculture
Peoria, Illinois 61604

Hiroshi Nikaido
Department of Bacteriology and Immunology
University of California
Berkeley, California 94720

Rudolf A. Raff
Department of Biology
Massachusetts Institute of Technology
Cambridge, Massachusetts 02319

CONTRIBUTORS (continued)

V. S. R. Rao
  Molecular Biophysics Unit
  Indian Institute of Science
  Bangalore
  India

F. Edward Roberts
  Merck Sharp & Dohme Research
    Laboratories
  Merck & Company, Inc.
  Rahway, New Jersey 07065

Robert W. Wheat
  Department of Microbiology and
    Immunology
  Duke University Medical Center
  Durham, North Carolina 27706

Thomas R. Windholz
  Merck Sharp & Dohme Research
    Laboratories
  Merck & Company, Inc.
  Rahway, New Jersey 07065

PREFACE

The rapid pace at which new data is currently accumulated in science presents one of the significant problems of today — the problem of rapid retrieval of information. The fields of biochemistry and molecular biology are two areas in which the information explosion is manifest. Such data is of interest in the disciplines of medicine, modern biology, genetics, immunology, biophysics, etc., to name but a few related areas. It was this need which first prompted CRC Press, with Dr. Herbert A. Sober as Editor, to publish the first two editions of a modern *Handbook of Biochemistry*, which made available unique, in depth compilations of critically evaluated data to graduate students, post-doctoral fellows, and research workers in selected areas of biochemistry.

This third edition of the *Handbook* demonstrates the wealth of new information which has become available since 1970. The title has been changed to include molecular biology; as the fields of biochemistry and molecular biology exist today, it becomes more difficult to differentiate between them. As a result of this philosophy, this edition has been greatly expanded. Also, previous data has been revised and obsolete material has been eliminated. As before, however, all areas of interest have not been covered in this edition. Elementary data, readily available elsewhere, has not been included. We have attempted to stress the areas of today's principal research frontiers and consequently certain areas of important biochemical interest are relatively neglected, but hopefully not totally ignored.

This third edition is over double the size of the second edition. Tables used from the second edition without change are so marked, but their number is small. Most of the tables from the second edition have been extensively revised, and over half of the data is new material. In addition, a far more extensive index has been compiled to facilitate the use of the Handbook. To make more facile use of the Handbook because of the increased size, it has been divided into four sections. Each section will have one or more volumes. The four sections are titled:

Proteins – Amino Acids, Peptides, Polypeptides, and Proteins
Nucleic Acids – Purines, Pyrimidines, Nucleotides, Oligonucleotides, tRNA, DNA, RNA
Lipids, Carbohydrates, Steroids
Physical and Chemical Data, Miscellaneous – Ion Exchange, Chromatography, Buffers, Miscellaneous, e.g., Vitamins

By means of this division of the data, we can continuously update the *Handbook* by publishing new data as they become available.

The Editor wishes to thank the numerous contributors, Dr. Herbert A. Sober, who assisted the Editor generously, and the Advisory Board for their counsel and cooperation. Without their efforts this edition would not have been possible. Special acknowledgments are due to the editorial staff of CRC Press, Inc., particularly Ms. Susan Cubar Benovich, Ms. Sandy Pearlman, and Mrs. Gayle Tavens, for their perspicacity and invaluable assistance in the editing of the manuscript. The editor alone, however, is responsible for the scope and the organization of the tables.

We invite comments and criticisms regarding format and selection of subject matter, as well as specific suggestions for new data (and their sources) which might be included in subsequent editions. We hope that errors and omissions in the data that appear in the Handbook will be brought to the attention of the Editor and the publisher.

Gerald D. Fasman
Editor
August 1975

PREFACE TO LIPIDS, CARBOHYDRATES, STEROIDS

This volume contains the complete section of the *Handbook of Biochemistry and Molecular Biology* with data pertaining to Lipids, Carbohydrates, and Steroids.

The subsection of Carbohydrates contains information on monosaccharides, disaccharides, oligosaccharides, phosphate esters, amino sugars, glycolipids, and glycohydrolases. X-Ray and optical activity data are also included.

The subsection on Lipids lists data on fatty acids (physical and chemical data, densities, specific volumes, temperature coefficients, refractive indices), alkyl monoesters of carboxylic and diesters of dicarboxylic acids, triglycerides, and long chain aliphatic acids. Information on fats and oils, chromatographic separation, physical data such as NMR, proton chemical shifts, and mass spectra are included.

The subsection on Steroids contains information on adrogens, bile acids, corticoids, estrogens, progestagens, and sterols.

Although far from complete, this volume will hopefully be of assistance to researchers in these areas.

Gerald D. Fasman
Editor
September 1975

THE EDITOR

Gerald D. Fasman, Ph.D., is the Rosenfield Professor of Biochemistry, Graduate Department of Chemistry, Brandeis University, Waltham, Massachusetts.

Dr. Fasman graduated from the University of Alberta in 1948 with a B.S. Honors Degree in Chemistry, and he received his Ph.D. in Organic Chemistry in 1952 from the California Institute of Technology, Pasadena, California. Dr. Fasman did postdoctoral studies at Cambridge University, England, Eidg. Technische Hochschule, Zurich, Switzerland, and the Weizmann Institute of Science, Rehovoth, Israel. Prior to moving to Brandeis University, he spent several years at the Children's Cancer Research Foundation at the Harvard Medical School. He has been an Established Investigator of the American Heart Association, a National Science Foundation Senior Postdoctoral Fellow in Japan, and recently was a John Simon Guggenheim Fellow.

Dr. Fasman is a member of the American Chemical Society, a Fellow of the American Association for the Advancement of Science, Sigma Xi, The Biophysical Society, American Society of Biological Chemists, The Chemical Society (London), the New York Academy of Science, and a Fellow of the American Institute of Chemists. He has published 180 research papers.

The Editor and CRC Press, Inc. would like to dedicate this third edition to the memory of Eva K. and Herbert A. Sober. Their pioneering work on the development of the Handbook is acknowledged with sincere appreciation.

TABLE OF CONTENTS

Nomenclature

BIOCHEMICAL NOMENCLATURE

This synopsis of the recommendations of the IUPAC-IUB Commission on Biochemical Nomenclature (CBN) was prepared by Waldo E. Cohn, Director, NAS-NRC Office of Biochemical Nomenclature (OBN, located at Biology Division, Oak Ridge National Laboratory, Oak Ridge, TN 37830), from whom reprints of the CBN publications listed below and on which the synopsis is based are available.

The synopsis is divided into three sections: Abbreviations, symbols, and trivial names. Each section contains material drawn from the documents (A1 to C1, inclusive) listed below, which deal with the subjects named.

Additions consonant with the CBN Recommendations have been made by OBN throughout the synopsis.

RULES AND RECOMMENDATIONS AFFECTING BIOCHEMICAL NOMENCLATURE AND PLACES OF PUBLICATION (AS OF FEBRUARY 1975)

I. IUPAC-IUB Commission on Biochemical Nomenclature
    A1. Abbreviations and Symbols [General; Section 5 replaced by A6]
    A2. Abbreviated Designation of Amino-acid Derivatives and Peptides (1965) [Revised 1971; Expands Section 2 of A1]
    A3. Synthetic Modifications of Natural Peptides (1966) [Revised 1972]
    A4. Synthetic Polypeptides (Polymerized Amino Acids) (1967) [Revised 1971]
    A5. A One-letter Notation for Amino-acid Sequences (1968)
    A6. Nucleic Acids, Polynucleotides, and their Constituents (1970)

    B1. (Nomenclature of Vitamins, Coenzymes, and Related Compounds)
         a.   Miscellaneous [A, B's, C, D's, tocols, niacins; see B2 and B3]
         b.   Quinones with Isoprenoid Side-chains: E, K, Q [Revised 1973]
         c.   Folic Acid and Related Compounds
         d.   Corrinoids: B-12's [Revised 1973]
    B2. Vitamins B-6 and Related Compounds [Revised 1973]
    B3. Tocopherols (1973)

    C1. Nomenclature of Lipids (1967) [Amended 1970; see also II, 2]
    C2. ,Nomenclature of α-Amino Acids (1974) [See also II, 5]

    D1. Conformation of Polypeptide Chains (1970) [See also III, 2]

    E1. Enzyme Nomenclature (1972)[a] [Elsevier (in paperback); Replaces 1965 edition.]
    E2. Multiple Forms of Enzymes (1971) [Chapter 3 of E1]
    E3. Nomenclature of Iron-sulfur Proteins (1973) [Chapter 6.5 of E1]
    E4. Nomenclature of Peptide Hormones (1974)

II. Documents Jointly Authored by CBN and CNOC [See III]
    1.   Nomenclature of Cyclitols (1968) [Revised 1973]
    2.   Nomenclature of Steroids (1968) [Amended 1971; Revised 1972]
    3.   Nomenclature of Carbohydrates-I (1969)
    4.   Nomenclature of Carotenoids (1972) [Revised 1975]
    5.   Nomenclature of α-Amino Acids (1974) [Listed under I, C2 in the following table]

III. IUPAC Commission on the Nomenclature of Organic Chemistry (CNOC)
    1.   Section A (Hydrocarbons), Section B (Heterocyclics): *J. Am. Chem. Soc.*, 82, 5545;[a] Section C (Groups containing N, Hal, S, Se/Te): *Pure Appl. Chem.*, 11, Nos. 1–2[a] [A, B, and C Revised 1969:[a] Butterworth's, London (1971)]
    2.   Section E (Stereochemistry):[b] *J. Org. Chem.*, 35, 2489 (1970); *Biochim. Biophys. Acta*, 208, 1 (1970); *Eur. J. Biochem.*, 18, 151 (1970) [See also I, D1]

[a] No reprints available from OBN; order from publisher.
[b] Reprints available from OBN (in addition to all in IA to ID and II).

RULES AND RECOMMENDATIONS AFFECTING BIOCHEMICAL NOMENCLATURE
AND PLACES OF PUBLICATION (AS OF FEBRUARY 1975)(continued)

IV.   Physiochemical Quantities and Units (IUPAC)[a] *J. Am. Chem. Soc.*, 82, 5517 (1960) [Revised 1970: *Pure Appl. Chem.*, 21, 1 (1970)]

V.   Nomenclature of Inorganic Chemistry (IUPAC) *J. Am. Chem. Soc.*, 82, 5523[a] [Revised 1971: *Pure Appl. Chem.*, 28, No. 1 (1971)][a]

VI.   Drugs and Related Compounds or Preparations
   1.   U.S. Adopted Names (USAN) No. 10 (1972) and Supplement [U.S. Pharmacopeial Convention, Inc., 12601 Twinbrook Parkway, Rockville, Md.]
   2.   International Nonproprietary Names (INN) [WHO, Geneva]

CBN RECOMMENDATIONS APPEAR IN THE FOLLOWING PLACES[a]

	Arch. Biochem. Biophys.	Biochem. J.	Biochemistry	Biochim. Biophys. Acta	Eur. J. Biochem.	J. Biol. Chem.	Pure Appl. Chem.[b]	Biochimie (Bull. Soc.)[c]	Molek. Biol.[d]	Z. Phys. Chem.[e]
A1[f]	136,1	101,1	5,1445		1,259	241,527		50,3	1,872	348,245
A2(Revised)	150,1(R)	126,773(R)	11,1726(R)	263,205(R)	27,201(R)	247,977(R)	40,(R)	49,121*	2,282*	348,256*
A3(Revised)	121,6*	104,17*	6,362*	133,1*	1,379*	242,555*	31,649(R)	49,325*	2,466*	348,262*
A4(Revised)[g]	151,597(R)	127,753(R)	11,942(R)	278,211(R)	26,301(R)	247,323(R)	33,439(R)	51,205*	5,492(R)	349,1013*
A5	125(3),i	113,1	7,2703	168,6	5,151	243,3557	31,641	50,1577	3,473	350,793
A6[h]	145,425	120,449	9,4022	247,1	15,203	245,5171	40,		6,167	351,1055
B1*	118,505	102,15		107,1(a–c)	2,1	241,2987		49,331		348,266
B1b(Revised)	165,1(R)	147,15(R)		387,397(R)	53,15(R)		38,439			
B1d(Revised)	161(2),iii(R)	147,1(R)	13,1555(R)		45,7(R)					
B2(Revised)	162,1(R)	137,417(R)	13,1056(R)	354,155(R)	40,325(R)	245,4229*	33,447(R)			351,1165*
B3(Revised)	165,6(R)	147,11(R)			46,217(R)					
C1[f]	123,409	105,897	6,3287	152,1	2,127	242,4845		50,1363	2,784	350,279
Amendments		116(5)		202,404	12,1	245,1511				
C2			14,449		53,1					
D1[i]	145,405	121,577	9,3471	229,1	17,193	245,6489			7,289	
E2	147,1	126,769	10,4825	258,1	24,1	246,6127		54,123		353,852
E3	160,355	135,5	12,3582	310,295	35,1	248,5907				
E4		151,1	14,2559			250,3215				
II,1(Revised)	128,269*	112,17*	8,2227	165,1*	5,1*	243,5809(R)	37,285(R)	51,3*		350,523*
II,2[f]	136,13	113,5	10,4994	164,453	10,1		31,285(R)	51,819		351,663
Amendments	147,4	127,613	10,3983	248,387	25,2					
II,3		125,673	10,4827	244,223	21,455	247,613				
II,4		127,741	14,1803	286,217	25,397	247,2633				
Amendments		151,507								

[a] Reprints available from OBN.
[b] No reprints available from OBN; order from publisher.
[c] In French.
[d] In Russian.
[e] In German.

[f] Also in other journals.
[g] Also in Biopolymers, 11, 321.
[h] J. Mol. Biol. 55, 299.
[i] J. Mol. Biol. 52, 1.

* First, unrevised version.
(R) = revised version.

ABBREVIATIONS

Abbreviations are distinguished from **symbols** as follows (taken from Reference A1):

    a. **Symbols,** for monomeric units in macromolecules, are used to make up abbreviated structural formulas (e.g., Gly-Val-Thr for the tripeptide glycylvalylthreonine) and can be made fairly systematic.

    b. **Abbreviations** for semi-systematic or trivial names (e.g., ATP for adenosine triphosphate; FAD for flavinadenine dinucleotide) are generally formed of three or four capital letters, chosen for brevity rather than for system. It is the indiscriminate coining and use of such abbreviations that has aroused objections to the use of abbreviations in general.

[Abbreviations are thus distinguished from symbols in that they (a) are for semi-systematic or trivial names, (b) are brief rather than systematic, (c) are usually formed from three or four capital letters, and (d) are not used — as are symbols — as units of larger structures. ATP, FAD, etc., are abbreviations. Gly, Ser, Ado, Glc, etc., are symbols (as are Na, K, Ca, O, S, etc.); they are sometimes useful as abbreviations in figures, tables, etc., where space is limited, but are usually not permitted in text. The use of abbreviations is permitted when necessary but is never required.]

    1. Nucleotides (N = A, C, G, I, O, T, U, X, ψ — see One-letter Symbols)

NMP	Nucleoside 5'-phosphate
NDP	Nucleoside 5'-di(or pyro)phosphate
NTP	Nucleoside 5'-triphosphate

Prefix d indicates deoxy.

    2. Coenzymes, vitamins

CoA(or CoASH)	Coenzyme A
CoASAc	Acetyl Coenzyme A
DPN[a]	Diphosphopyridine nucleotide
FAD	Flavin-adenine dinucleotide
FMN	Riboflavin 5'-phosphate
GSH	Glutathione
GSSG	Oxidized glutathione
NAD[b]	Nicotinamide-adenine dinucleotide (cozymase, Coenzyme I, diphosphopyridine nucleotide)
NADP[b]	Nicotinamide-adenine dinucleotide phosphate (Coenzyme II, triphosphopyridine nucleotide)
NMN	Nicotinamide mononucleotide
TPN[c]	Triphosphopyridine nucleotide

    3. Miscellaneous

ACTH	Adrenocorticotropin, adrenocorticotropic hormone, or corticotropin
CM-cellulose	*O*-(Carboxymethyl)cellulose
DEAE-cellulose	*O*-(Diethylaminoethyl)cellulose
DDT	1,1,1-Trichloro-2,2-bis(*p*-chlorophenyl)ethane
EDTA	Ethylenediaminetetraacetate
Hb,HbCO,HbO$_2$	Hemoglobin, carbon monoxide hemoglobin, oxyhemoglobin
P$_i$	Inorganic orthophosphate

[a]Replaced by NAD (also DPN$^+$ by NAD$^+$, DPNH by NADH).
[b]Generic term; oxidized and reduced forms are NAD$^+$, NADH (NADP$^+$, NADPH).
[c]Replaced by NADP (also TPN$^+$ by NADP$^+$, TPNH by NADPH).

PP$_i$	Inorganic pyrophosphate
TEAE-cellulose	O-(Triethylaminoethyl)cellulose
Tris	Tris(hydroxymethyl)aminomethan (2-amino-2-hydroxymethylpropane-1,3-diol)

4. Nucleic Acids

DNA, RNA	Deoxyribonucleic acid, ribonucleic acid (or -nucleate)
hnRNA	Heterogeneous RNA
mtDNA	Mitochondrial DNA
cRNA	Complementary RNA
mRNA	Messenger RNA
nRNA	Nuclear RNA
rRNA	Ribosomal RNA
tRNA	Transfer RNA (generic term; sRNA should not be used for this or any other purpose)
tRNA^{Ala}	Alanine tRNA; tRNA$_1^{Ala}$, tRNA$_2^{Ala}$: isoacceptor alanine tRNA's
AA-tRNA	Aminoacyl-tRNA; aminoacylated tRNA; "charged" tRNA (generic term)
Ala-tRNA or Ala-tRNA^{Ala}	Alanyl-tRNA
tRNA^{Met}	Methionine tRNA (not enzymically formylatable)
tRNA^{fMet} or tRNA$_f^{Met}$	Methionine tRNA, enzymically formylatable to . . .
fMet-tRNA	Formylmethionyl-tRNA (small f, to distinguish from fluorine F)

SYMBOLS

Symbols are distinguished from abbreviations in that they are designed to represent specific parts of larger molecules, just as the symbols for the elements are used in depicting molecules, and are thus rather systematic in construction and use. Symbols are not designed to be used as abbreviations and should not be used as such in text, but they may often serve this purpose when space is limited (as in a figure or table). Symbols are always written with a single capital letter, all subsequent letters being lower-case (e.g., Ca, Cl, Me, Ac, Gly, Rib, Ado), regardless of their position in a sequence, a sentence, or as a superscript or subscript.

Some abbreviations expressed in symbols as examples of the use of symbols:

Dimethylsulfoxide	Me$_2$SO [a]
Tetranitromethane	$(NO_2)_4$C [b]
Guanidine hydrochloride	Gdn · HCl [c]
Guanidinium chloride	GdmCl
Cetyltrimethylammonium bromide	CtMe$_3$NBr [d]
Ethyl methanesulfonate	MeSO$_3$Et
Methylnitronitrosoguanidine	MeN$_2$O$_2$Gdn
-nitrosourea	-Nur [e]
-nitrosamine	-Nam [f]
-fluorene	-Fln
Aminofluorene	NH$_2$Fln
Acetylaminofluorene	AcNHFln [g]
Acetoxyacetylaminofluorene	Ac(AcO)NFln
N-Acetylneuraminic acid	AcNeu [h]

[a] Replaces DMSO.
[b] Replaces TNM.
[c] Replaces Gu, Gd, and G.
[d] Replaces CTAB (similarly for other ammonium compounds).
[e] Replaces NU.
[f] Replaces NA.
[g] Replaces AAF.
[h] Not NANA.

I. Phosphorylated Compounds (Reference A1)

-PO$_3$H$_2$ (or its ions)	-P(or P-) ("p" in Nucleic Acids)
-PO$_2$H-(or its ion)	-P-(hyphen in Nucleic Acids)
-PO$_2$H-PO$_3$H$_2$ (or ions)	-P-P or -PP or PP- (cf. PP$_i$ in Abbreviations)

Examples:[a]

Glucose 6-phosphate	Glucose-6-P (or Glc-6-p; see II below).
Phosphenolpyruvate (pyruvenol phosphate)	P-enolPyruvate or enolPyruvate-P or e Prv-P[b]
Fructose 1,6-bisphosphate (not di)	Fructose-1,6-P$_2$ (or Fru-1,6-P$_2$; see II below).
Creatine phosphate	Creatine-P
Phosphocreatine	P-Creatine

[a]Note that symbols are hyphenated even where names are not.
[b]Recommended by OBN.

II. Carbohydrates (Reference A1)

Sugars[a]

Fructose	Fru	Arabinose	Ara [c]
Galactose	Gal	Lyxose	Lyx
Glucose	Glc [b]	Ribose	Rib [d]
Mannose	Man	Xylose	Xyl

Prefix d indicates 2-deoxy; 3-d, etc., indicates 3-deoxy, etc.

[a]Always one capital, two small letters (i.e., never glc or GLC).
[b]To distinguish from Glu = glutamic acid; G is permitted only where confusion is minimal, and in the special case of UDPG (uridinediphosphoglucose).
[c]Becomes ara or a when used as a modifier, as before C e.g., araC or aC.
[d]Never R (= purine nucleoside; see Nucleic Acids).

Derivatives

Using glucose, Glc, as an example		Using ribose, Rib, as an example	
Gluconic acid	GlcA	Ribulose	Rbu
Glucuronic acid	GlcU	Ribitol	Rbo
Glucosamine	GlcN	Ribityl	Rby
N-Acetylglucosamine	GlcNAc		
but N-Acetylneuraminic acid	AcNeu (not NANA)		

Configuration

p,f	pyranose, furanose (suffixes)	used without hyphenation (see examples). D may be omitted.
D,L	(prefixes)	

Sequence and direction

→	glycoside link, pointing *away from* hemiacetal carbon.
–	glycoside link, assumes hemiacetal carbon at left.
(1 → 4), etc.	glycoside link, from hemiacetal carbon (C-1) to C-4, etc.
(1 – 4), etc.	glycoside link, assumes hemiacetal carbon (C-1) at left, etc.

Examples

Maltose, Glcp(α1−4)Glc
Lactose, Galp(β1−4)Glc
Stachyose, Galp(α1−6)Galp(α1−6)Galp(α1−2)βFruƒ

A branched chain tetrasaccharide:

Glc(β1−3)Gal(β1−4)Glc
(2
↑
1)αFuc

Inulin[a]

Fruƒ2−1[Fruƒ2)ₓ₋ᵧ·3Glcp1   (1Fruƒ2)ᵧ·1Glcp

Xylan[a]

βXylp1−(4βXylp1)ₓ−4βXylp-(4βXylp1)ᵧ·βXylp
3
↑
1
βXyl1−(4βXylp1)ᵧ

[a]From Carbohydrate Rules [*J. Org. Chem.*, 28, 281 (1963)].

TRIVIAL NAMES

I. Lipids (except Carotenoids and Steroids) (Reference C1)
A. Generic Terms (Reference C1)

1. **Phosphoglyceride** − Any derivative of glycerophosphoric acid (glycerol-*P* or Gro-*P*) that contains at least one *O*-acyl, *O*-alkyl, or *O*-alk-1-en-1-yl group attached to glycerol.

2. **X phosphoglyceride** − If X is the other ester component of a phosphoglyceride (e.g., if X = choline, name is glycerophosphocholine (Symbol: Gro-*P*-choline).

3. **Phosphatidic acid** − Both alcoholic OH groups of glycerophosphoric acid are esterified by fatty acids. (Symbol: Ptd-OH.)

4. **Lecithin** − Permitted, but not recommended, for 1,2-diacyl-*sn*-glycero-3-phosphocholines (see 5).

5. **3-*sn*-phosphatidylcholine** − Recommended for lecithin (see 4) (Symbol: Ptd-choline or Ptd-Cho).

6. **Tri(di)acylglycerol** − Replaces tri(di)glyceride (Figure 2).

7. **Phospholipid** − Any lipid containing a radical of H_3PO_4 (Figures 1, 3, 4, 6, 7).

8. **Phosphoinositide** − Any lipid containing inositol and H_3PO_4 radicals, phosphatidyl inositol, etc.

9. **"Long chain base"** − Used in this table to refer to sphinganine (see 20 below) and its homologues, stereoisomers, and hydroxy or unsaturated derivatives of these.

10. **Sphingolipid** − Any lipid containing a "long chain base" (see 9).

11. **Glycosphingolipid** − Any lipid containing a "9" and one or more sugars.

12. **Ceramide** − Any *N*-acyl "9" (Symbol: Cer).

13. **Cerebroside** – Any monoglycosyl ceramide (see 12).

14. **Gangliodise** – Any cerebroside (see 13) containing neuraminic acid (see 16). AcNeu); (see 16).

15. **Sphingomyelin** – A ceramide 1-phosphocholine (see 12).

16. **Neuraminic acid** – 5-Amino-3,5-dideoxy-D-*glycero*-D-*galacto*-nonulosonic acid; (radicals = neuraminosyl[a], neuraminosyl[b]) (Figure 8) (Symbol: Neu).

17. **Sialic acid** – *N*-Acylneuraminic acids, their esters, and other derivatives of the alcoholic hydroxyl groups (radicals = sialoyl,[a] sialosyl[b]) (Symbol: AcNeu for the *N*-acetyl derivative.)

[a]If OH is deleted from carboxyl group.
[b]If OH is deleted from anomeric carbon of cyclic structure.

B. Stereospecific Nomenclature of Lipids (Reference C1)

18. (a) Substitution for H of alcoholic-OH of X by "group"; name is *group X*. (b) Esterification of alcoholic-OH of X by "acidate", the anion of "acidic acid", name is *X acidate*.

19. Glycerol derivatives may be numbered "stereospecifically," the C atom at top in that Fischer projection having the secondary hydroxyl to the left being C-1 (Figure 5). Such numbering takes the prefix *sn* (for *s*tereospecifically *n*umbered), which immediately precedes the "glycero" term. It is replaced by *rac* (which precedes the *full* name) if the product is an equal mixture of both antipodes, or by *X* (same position) if the configuration is unknown or unspecified.

Examples:

The older terms

L-α-Glycerophosphoric acid;   }   are replaced by   *sn*-Glycerol 3-(dihydrogen phosphate);
D-Glycerol 1-phosphate   *sn*-Glycero-3-phosphoric acid (Figure 1)

1-Alk-enyl-2-acyl-*sn*-glycerophosphoric ester
O-(1-acyl- *sn*-glycero-3-phospho)ethanolamine
diacyl-*sn*-glycero-3-phospho-1'-*sn*-glycerol
= 3-*sn*-phosphatidyl-1'-*sn*-glycerol (Figure 7).

20. Sphingolipids may be named as sphinganine [2D-aminoöctadecane-1,3D-diol, or D-erythro-2-amino-octadecane-1,3-diol, or (2S, 3R)-2-aminoöctadecane 1,3-diol] derivatives. The name implies identical configurations in the *D/L* system, not the *R,S* system, unless the contrary is specified in *D/L* terms. *D* and *L* refer to right or left position of functional groups written in the Fischer projection, vertically, with C–1 at the top; they follow the number of the substituted C atom and are replaced by *X* when configuration is unknown, or *rac* (before the name) for racemic mixtures.

Examples:

Old, nonrecommended terms	Recommended equivalents
"Phytosphingosine"	4D-Hydroxysphinganine
Sphingosine	4-Sphingenine ^{1} ^{8}CH$_3$(CH$_2$)$_{12}$CH = ^{4}CH-CHOH-CHNH$_2$-^{1}CH$_2$OH
"cis"-sphingosine	*cis*-4-Sphingenine
C-2 Epimer of sphinganine	2L-Sphinganine 2L-CH$_3$(CH$_2$)$_{12}$CH$_2$-CH$_2$CHOH-CHNH$_2$-CH$_2$OH
	4X-Hydroxy-2X,3X-eicosasphinganine
	4X-Hydroxy-19-methyl-2X,3X-eicosasphinganine

CH₂OH ... (Figure structures)

FIGURE 1. *sn*-Glycerol 3-phosphate (cf. Figure 6).

FIGURE 2. (*S*)-1,2-Diacylglycerol or 1,2-diacyl-*sn*-glycerol.

FIGURE 4. 1,3-Diacyl-2-*sn*-phosphatidylcholine.

FIGURE 3. (*R*)-Phosphatidic acid or 3-*sn*-phosphatidic acid or 1,2-diacyl-*sn*-glycerol 3-phosphate.

FIGURE 5. Glycerol (*sn* numbering to right).

FIGURE 6. *sn*-Glycerol 1-phosphate (cf. Figure 1).

FIGURE 7. 3-*sn*-Phosphatidyl-1'-*sn*-glycerol.

FIGURE 8. Neuraminic acid (Neu): 5-Amino-3,5-dideoxy-D-*glycero*-D-galacto-nonulosonic acid.

C. Miscellaneous Symbols

Glycerol	Gro
Glyceraldehyde	Gra
Glycerone (dihydroxy acetone)	Grn
Glyceric acid (glycerate)	Gri
Phosphatidyl	Ptd
Neuraminic acid	Neu (Also, AcNeu for the *N*-acetyl derivative)
-ethanolamide	Etn (OEtn for ester)*

NOMENCLATURE OF LABELED COMPOUNDS

The statement below was adopted by the IUB Commission of Editors of Biochemical Journals* (CEBJ) and appears, in the same or in similar form, in the Instructions to Authors of their journals. This system originated with the Chemical Society (London) and was subsequently adopted by the American Chemical Society (Handbook for Authors, 1967). It was adopted by CEBJ in 1971 and is the only system currently permitted in the pages of their journals.

ISOTOPICALLY LABELED COMPOUNDS

The symbol for the isotope introduced is placed in *square* brackets directly attached to the front of the name (word), as in $[^{14}C]$ urea. When more than one position in a substance is labeled by means of the same isotope and the positions are not indicated (as below), the number of labeled positions is added as a right-hand subscript, as in $[^{14}C_2]$ glycollic acid. The symbol "U" indicates uniform and "G" general labeling, e.g., $[U^{-14}C]$ glucose (where the ^{14}C is uniformly distributed among all six positions) and $[G^{-14}C]$ glucose (where the ^{14}C is distributed among all six positions, but not necessarily uniformly); in the latter case it is often sufficient to write simply "$[^{14}C]$ glucose."

The isotopic prefix precedes that part of the name to which it refers, as in sodium $[^{14}C]$ formate, iodo$[^{14}C_2]$ acetic acid, 1-amino$[^{14}C]$ methylcyclopentanol $(H_2N-^{14}CH_2-C_5H_8-OH)$, α-naphth$[^{14}C]$ oic acid $(C_{10}H-^{14}CO_2H)$, 2-acetamido-7-$[^{131}I]$ iodofluorene, fructose 1,6-$[1^{-32}P]$ diphosphate, D-$[^{14}C]$ glucose, 2H-$[2^{-2}H]$ pyran, S-$[8^{-14}C]$ adenosyl$[^{35}S]$ methionine. Terms such as "^{131}I-labeled albumin" should not be contracted to "$[^{131}I]$ albumin" (since native albumin does not contain iodine), and "^{14}C-labeled amino acids" should similarly not be written as "$[^{14}C]$ amino acids" (since there is no carbon in the amino group).

When isotopes of more than one element are introduced, their symbols are arranged in alphabetical order, including ^2H and ^3H for deuterium and tritium, respectively.

When not sufficiently distinguished by the foregoing means, the positions of isotopic labeling are indicated by Arabic numerals, Greek letters, or prefixes (as appropriate), placed within the square brackets and before the symbol of the element concerned, to which they are attached by a hyphen; examples are $[1^{-2}H]$ ethanol $(CH_3-C^2H_2-OH)$, $[1^{-14}C]$ aniline, L-$[2^{-14}C]$ leucine (or L-$[\alpha^{-14}C]$-leucine), $[carboxy^{-14}C]$ leucine, $[Me$-$^{14}C]$ isoleucine, $[2,3^{-14}C]$ maleic anhydride, $[6,7^{-14}C]$ xanthopterin, $[3,4^{-13}C,^{35}S]$-methionine, $[2^{-13}C; 1^{-14}C]$ acetaldehyde, $[3^{-14}C; 2,3^{-2}H; ^{15}N]$ serine.

The same rules apply when the labeled compound is designated by a standard abbreviation or symbol, other than the atomic symbol, e.g. $[\gamma^{-32}P]$ ATP.

For simple molecules, however, it is often sufficient to indicate the labeling by writing the chemical formulae, e.g. $^{14}CO_2$, $H_2^{18}O$, ^2H_2O (not D_2O), $H_2^{35}SO_4$, with the prefix superscripts attached to the proper atomic symbols in the formulae. The square brackets are not to be used in these circumstances, nor when the isotopic symbol is attached to a word that is not a chemical name, abbreviation or symbol (e.g. ^{131}I-labeled).

*CEBJ consists of the Editors-in-Chief of the following journals: *Archives of Biochemistry and Biophysics, Biochemical Journal, Biochemistry, Biochimica et Biophysica Acta, Biochimie, European Journal of Biochemistry, Hoppe-Seyler's Zeitschrift für Physiologische Chemie, Journal of Biochemistry, Journal of Biological Chemistry, Journal of Molecular Biology, and Molekulyarnaya Biologiya;* corresponding members include *Proceedings of the National Academy of Sciences* (U.S.A.) and approximately 40 others.

THE CITATION OF BIBLIOGRAPHIC REFERENCES IN BIOCHEMICAL JOURNALS RECOMMENDATIONS (1971)*

IUB Commission of Editors of Biochemical Journals (CEBJ)

These Recommendations were reviewed by the Commission in August 1972, when it was decided to publish them.

PREAMBLE

Two basic systems for the citation of references are used at present. The so-called Harvard System (where names of authors and the date are cited in the text, and the reference list is in alphabetical order) and the Numbering System (where numbers, but not necessarily names of authors, are cited in the text, and the reference list is in order of citation in the text). Several ways of quoting references in the list are in current use.

The Commission is of the opinion, arrived at as a result of much consultation between many senior editors, that it is unlikely that all journals would accept a recommendation to use either the Harvard or the Numbering System to the exclusion of the other. It believes, however, that most biochemists will accept the need for, and indeed welcome, a substantial degree of unification of practices, there being no strong case for the individuality of each journal on this issue. Accordingly, the Commission makes the following Recommendations to all biochemical journals; the reasons for some of them are given. The Recommendations deal first with the way in which references should be cited in the list; the proposal is suitable for journals adopting either the Harvard or the Numbering System. Secondly, there are Recommendations about the way in which each of these systems is used. Thirdly, abbreviations for titles of journals and a few other points are considered. Implementation of the Recommendations would mean that any very small differences between journals in their practices would be of the type that can be attended to at the redactory stage of preparation for press. The Commission recognizes that it cannot deal with a number of smaller problems concerning citations that arise from time to time.

RECOMMENDATIONS

1. Citations of References in the List of References Should Be as Follows
Braun, A., Brown, B. & LeBrun, C. (1971) *Journal*, 11, 111–113.
Notes: (a) This form can be used by both systems.

(b) Journals using the Numbering System should arrange the references in numerical order beside the number (which can be italicized or in brackets according to the house custom of the journal).

(c) Journals using the Harvard System should arrange the references in alphabetical order, whatever the language, except in certain situations (see Recommendation 4a below).

(d) This recommendation incorporates the following points:
    i.   Initials after surnames (full first names are not given in the list).
    ii.   The use of the symbol "&" is recommended if at all possible because of its widespread usage and the fact that it is independent of the language. No comma before "&."

*From IUB Commission of Editors of Biochemical Journals (CEBJ), *J. Biol. Chem.*, 248(21), 7279–7280 (1973). With permission.

iii. Year in parentheses (this follows immediately after the authors' names because it is essential to the Harvard System).

iv. Journal title (abbreviated). This can be in italics according to house practice (see Recommendation 7 below concerning journal title abbreviations).

v. Volume number. This can be in heavy type or italics according to house practice.

vi. A few journals do not have volume numbers in which case the page numbers should follow immediately after the abbreviated journal title.

If it is necessary to quote both a volume and a part number, the reference should read: Brown, B. (1971) *Journal*, 11, pt 1, 121–123.

vii. First and last pages should be given. The Commission decided to make this Recommendation mainly on the basis of evidence that the additional information provided by quoting the last page was being required increasingly in many types of library and information retrieval services. Citation of the last page (as well as the first) has been requested for some time by the secondary and abstracting journals. Citation of both first and last pages is also an aid in the prevention of errors.

viii. The number of stops and commas is kept as small as possible.

(e) Authors' names and the abbreviated name of the journal when repeated in the next reference should be spelled out in full; ibid. and similar terms should not be used.

(f) Recommendations of the IUPAC-IUB Commission on Biochemical Nomenclature (CBN) and similar documents should be referred to as: Commission on Biochemical Nomenclature (1970) followed by a journal reference.

(g) Junior should be abbreviated to "Jr," not "jun."

2. Numbering System in the Text

The use of authors' names is permissible as authors wish; only the initial letter of the name should be in capital type. Numbers can be inserted in parentheses or as superscripts according to house custom. The printing of references at the foot of the page on which they are first quoted is considered to be helpful with the Numbering System but is not part of the Recommendation because the extra cost is generally considered to be prohibitive.

3. Harvard System in the Text

For multi-author papers, it is recommended that:

a. Not more than two authors to be named either on the first or any subsequent occasion;

b. et al. should be used for three or more authors on every occasion;

c. Each name to have the initial letter in capital type only.

Examples (Harvard System style):

Braun et al. (1969) did some work that was confirmed by LeBrun (1970).

These results (Braun et al., 1969; LeBrun, 1970) have been discussed by Brown & Braun (1971). The same Recommendation (without the year) applies when authors are quoted in the text in the Numbering System.

4. Harvard System in the List of References

a. A special problem arises in the list when there are several papers by, e.g., Green et al. in the same or over several years. While the list could be in strict alphabetical order of the full reference, the reader will find no clue in the text to the alphabetical status of the names of the second and subsequent authors (see Recommendations 3a and 3b). It is therefore recommended that all the papers by Green et al. (that is by Green and more than one co-author) should be arranged, irrespective of the names of the other authors, in chronological order (over many years if necessary) and designate tham a, b, c, etc.

Examples:

Green, G. (1970) etc.
Green, G. & Brown, B. (1971) etc.
Green, G. & White, W. (1969) etc.
Green, G., White, W. & Black, B. (1968a) etc.   sequence governed by order or date of
                                                                  publication, as far as can be ascertained.
Green, G., Brown, B. & Black, B. (1968b) etc.
Green, G., White, W., Black, B. & Brown, B. (1969) etc.
Green, G., Black, B. & Brown, B. (1970) etc.

b. Names beginning with "Mc" should be listed under "Mc" and not under "Mac," to decide alphabetical order.

c. Names beginning with "De," "Van," or "von," etc. should be arranged under D or V/v, etc.

5. Reference to Books

These should appear in text like any reference to a journal paper. The reference in the list should read: Brown, B. & Braun, A. (1971) in *Book Title* (LeBrun, C., ed.), pp. 1–20, Publisher, Town.

Notes:
a. If a volume number has to be quoted, this would appear before the pp. as, e.g., "vol. 2," with the number in Arabic numerals (even when Roman numerals are printed on the cover of the book).

b. Where an author wishes to refer to a specific page within a book reference, this should be given in the text.

Example (in text): ". . . discussed on p. 21 of Braun et al.(1971)."

6. Other Forms of References

a. *In the press.* It is recommended that (i) this should mean that the paper has been finally accepted by a journal, (ii) it is quoted in the text (both systems) just as any other paper, (iii) the year quoted should be the best estimate revised if necessary at proof stage, and (iv) the full citation in the list to read: Braun, A. & Brown, B. (1971) *Journal*, in the press.

b. *Submitted for publication* should be used in a typescript only when it is reasonable to expect that it will be possible to alter the quotation to a final form at a stage before publication; if such alteration cannot be made then the name of the journal involved should be stated.

c. The use of *in preparation* and *private communication* should not be allowed because they have no real value.

d. *Personal communication* and *unpublished work* should be permitted in the text only, i.e., not in the list of references. Editors may require to see written evidence of the former.

7. Abbreviations for Journal Titles

Most biochemical journals use the *Chemical Abstract** system but a few use the World List, 4th Edition. The Commission noted that the latest information available (International List of Periodical Title Word Abbreviations prepared for the UNISIST/ ICSU-AB Working Group on Bibliographical Descriptions) suggests that the abbreviations that will be recommended finally by ICSU will be very similar to those now used by *Chemical Abstracts*.

Believing that complete uniformity on this issue is highly desirable now and estimating that it may be a few more years before ICSU finally reports, the Commission recommends that all biochemical journals should now use the *Chemical Abstracts* (American Chemical Society) system. The Commission believes that any changes that will be required when ICSU eventually issues recommendations on this point will be comparatively minor ones.

8. Implementation of these Recommendations

The Commission at its meeting in Menton, May 7 to 8, 1971, has taken the view that the degree of uniformity envisaged in the Recommendations is highly desirable and therefore further recommends to all biochemical journals that the changes required should be made as soon as possible. The Commission recognizes that all journals will have to make some changes (in most cases these are minor) from their present established practices to implement these Recommendations in full. It considers that the possible objections of difficulties even for a commercial publisher with an established "house style" are outweighed by the advantage that conformity of style in the citation of references will prove to the authors, editors, and readers upon whom all journals depend for their existence.

*The journal-title abbreviations in *Biological Abstracts* are essentially the same in *Chemical Abstracts*. A *List of Serials with Title Abbreviations* is available from BioSciences Information Service of Biological Abstracts, 2100 Arch Street, Philadelphia, PA 19103.

IUPAC TENTATIVE RULES FOR THE NOMENCLATURE OF ORGANIC CHEMISTRY SECTION E. FUNDAMENTAL STEREOCHEMISTRY*

International Union of Pure and Applied Chemistry

INTRODUCTION

This Section of the IUPAC Rules for Nomenclature of Organic Chemistry differs from previous Sections in that it is here necessary to legislate for words that describe concepts as well as for names of compounds.

At the present time, concepts in stereochemistry (that is, chemistry in three-dimensional space) are in the process of rapid expansion, not merely in organic chemistry, but also in biochemistry, inorganic chemistry, and macromolecular chemistry. The aspects of interest for one area of chemistry often differ from those for another, even in respect to the same phenomenon. This rapid evolution and the variety of interests have led to development of specialized vocabularies and definitions that sometimes differ from one group of specialists to another, sometimes even within one area of chemistry.

The Commission on the Nomenclature of Organic Chemistry does not, however, consider it practical to cover all aspects of stereochemistry in this Section E. Instead, it has two objects in view: To prescribe, for basic concepts, terms that may provide a common language in all areas of stereochemistry; and to define the ways in which these terms may, so far as necessary, be incorporated into the names of individual compounds. The Commission recognizes that specialized nomenclatures are required for local fields; in some cases, such as carbohydrates, amino acids, peptides and proteins, and steroids, international rules already exist; for other fields, study is in progress by specialists in Commissions or Subcommittees; and further problems doubtless await identification. The Commission believes that consultations will be needed in many cases between different groups within IUPAC and IUB if the needs of the specialists are to be met without confusion and contradiction between the various groups.

The Rules in this Section deal only with Fundamental Stereochemistry, that is, the main principles. Many of these Rules do little more than codify existing practice, often of long standing; however, others extend old principles to wider fields, and yet others deal with nomenclature that is still subject to controversy.

Rule E-0

The stereochemistry of a compound is denoted by an affix or affixes to the name that does not prescribe the stereochemistry; such affixes, being additional, do not change the name or the numbering of the compound. Thus, enantiomers, diastereoisomers, and *cis–trans* isomers receive names that are distinguished only by means of different stereochemical affixes. The only exceptions are those trivial names that have stereo-chemical implications (for example, fumaric acid, cholesterol).

Note: In some cases (see Rules E-2.23 and E-3.1) stereochemical relations may be used to decide between alternative numberings that are otherwise permissible.

E-1. Types of Isomerism

E-1.1. The following nonstereochemical terms are relevant to the stereochemical nomenclature given in the Rules that follow.

*From *IUPAC Inf. Bull. Append. Tentative Nomencl. Sym. Units Stand.*, No. 35, August 1974, pp. 36–80. With permission.

(a) The term structure may be used in connection with any aspect of the organization of matter.

Hence: structural (adjectival)

(b) Compounds that have identical molecular formulas but differ in the nature or sequence of bonding of their atoms or in arrangement of their atoms in space are termed isomers.

Hence: isomeric (adjectival)
        isomerism (phenomenological)

Examples:

H_3C — O — CH_3 is an isomer of H_3C — CH_2 — OH

$$
\begin{array}{c}
H_3C \\ \diagdown \\ C = C \\ \diagup \\ H
\end{array}
\begin{array}{c}
CH_3 \\ \diagup \\ \\ \diagdown \\ H
\end{array}
\quad\text{is an isomer of}\quad
\begin{array}{c}
H \\ \diagdown \\ C = C \\ \diagup \\ H_3C
\end{array}
\begin{array}{c}
CH_3 \\ \diagup \\ \\ \diagdown \\ H
\end{array}
$$

(In this and other Rules a broken line denotes a bond projecting behind the plane of the paper, and a thickened line denotes a bond projecting in front of the plane of the paper. In such cases a line of normal thickness denotes a bond lying in the plane of the paper.)

(c) The constitution of a compound of given molecular formula defines the nature and sequence of bonding of the atoms. Isomers differing in constitution are termed constitutional isomers.

Hence: constitutionally isomeric (adjectival)
        constitutional isomerism (phenomenological)

Example:

H_3C–O–CH_3 is a constitutional isomer of H_3C–CH_2–OH.

Note: Use of the term "structural" with the above connotation is abandoned as insufficiently specific.

E-1.2. Isomers are termed stereoisomers when they differ only in the arrangement of their atoms in space.

Hence: stereoisomeric (adjectival)
        stereoisomerism (phenomenological)

Examples:

$$
\begin{array}{c}
H_3C \\ \diagdown \\ C = C \\ \diagup \\ H
\end{array}
\begin{array}{c}
CH_3 \\ \diagup \\ \\ \diagdown \\ H
\end{array}
\quad\text{is a stereoisomer of}\quad
\begin{array}{c}
H_3C \\ \diagdown \\ C = C \\ \diagup \\ H
\end{array}
\begin{array}{c}
H \\ \diagup \\ \\ \diagdown \\ CH_3
\end{array}
$$

$$
\begin{array}{c}
CHO \\ | \\ H \cdots C \\ \diagup\quad\diagdown \\ HO\quad CH_2OH
\end{array}
\quad\text{is a stereoisomer of}\quad
\begin{array}{c}
CHO \\ | \\ HO \cdots C \\ \diagup\quad\diagdown \\ H\quad CH_2OH
\end{array}
$$

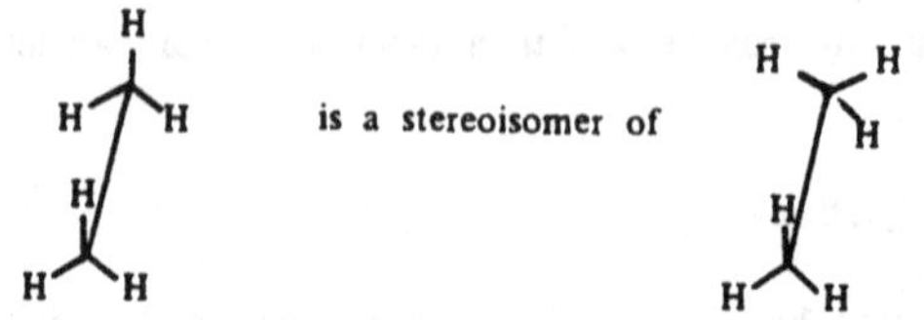

$$\text{(structure)} \quad \text{is a stereoisomer of} \quad \text{(structure)}$$

E-1.3. Stereoisomers are termed *cis–trans* isomers when they differ only in the positions of atoms relative to a specified plane in cases where these atoms are, or are considered as if they were, parts of a rigid structure.

Hence: *cis–trans* isomeric (adjectival)
      cis–trans isomerism (phenomenological)

Examples:

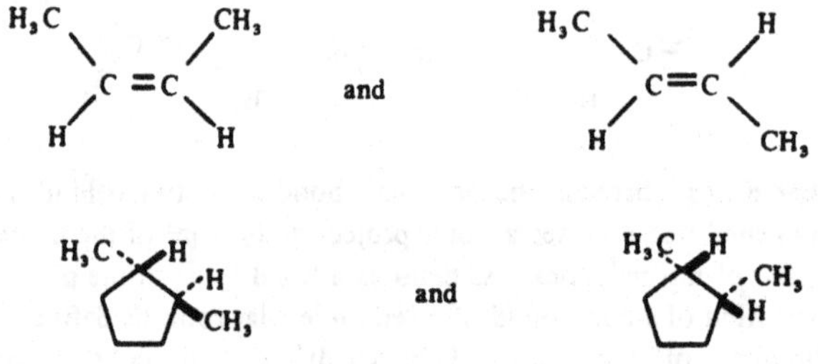

$$\text{(structure)} \quad \text{and} \quad \text{(structure)}$$

$$\text{(structure)} \quad \text{and} \quad \text{(structure)}$$

E-1.4. Various views are current regarding the precise definition of the term "configuration." (a) Classical interpretation: The configuration of a molecule of defined constitution is the arrangement of its atoms in space without regard to arrangements that differ only as after rotation about one or more single bonds. (b) This definition is now usually limited so that no regard is paid also to rotation about π bonds or bonds of partial order between one and two. (c) A third view limits the definition further so that no regard is paid to rotation about bonds of any order, including double bonds.

Molecules differing in configuration are termed configurational isomers.

Hence: configurational isomerism

Notes: (1) Contrast conformation (Rule E-1.5). (2) The phrase "differ only as after rotation" is intended to make the definition independent of any difficulty of rotation, in particular independent of steric hindrance to rotation. (3) For a brief discussion of views (a) to (c), see Appendix 1. It is hoped that a definite consensus of opinion will be established before these Rules are made "Definitive."

Examples: The following pairs of compounds differ in configuration:

(i)
$$\text{(structure)} \qquad \text{(structure)}$$

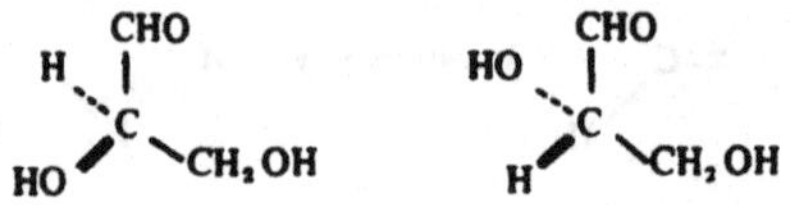

(ii)

(iii)

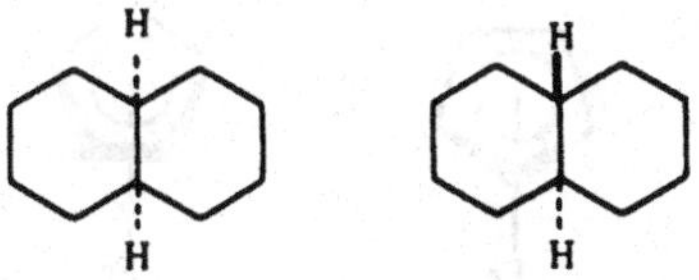

(iv)

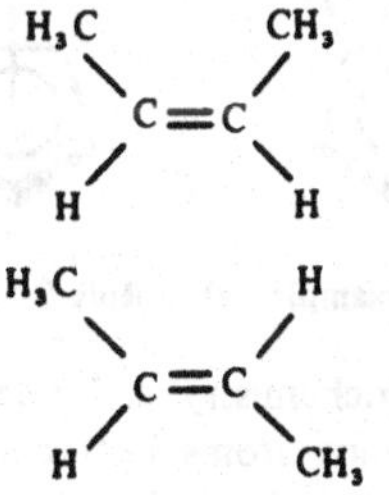

These isomers (iv) are configurational in view (a)
or (b) but are conformational (see Rule E-1.5)
in view (c)

E-1.5. Various views are current regarding the precise definition of the term "conformation." (a) Classical interpretation: The conformations of a molecule of defined configuration are the various arrangements of its atoms in space that differ only as after rotation about single bonds. (b) This is usually now extended to include rotation about π bonds or bonds of partial order between one and two. (c) A third view extends the definition further to include also, rotation about bonds of any order, including double bonds.

Molecules differing in conformation are termed conformational isomers.

Hence: conformational isomerism

Notes: All the Notes to Rule E-1.4 apply also to E-1.5.

Examples: Each of the following pairs of formulas represents a compound in the same configuration but in different conformations.

(a, b, c)

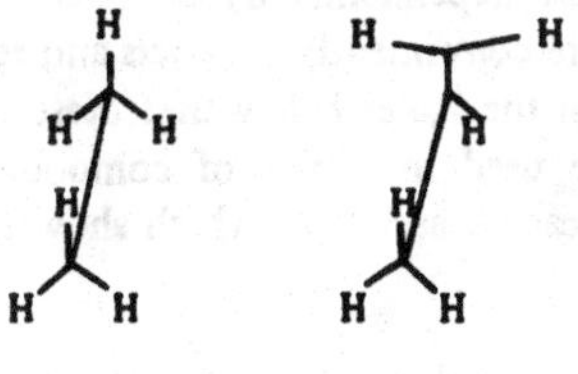

(a, b, c)

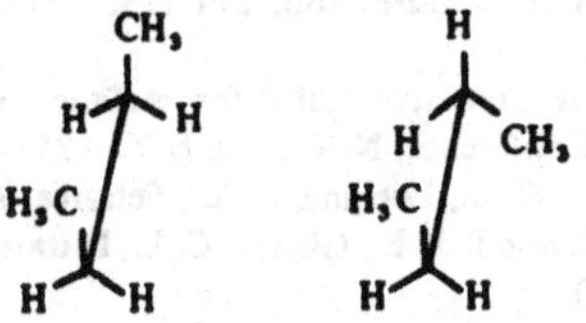

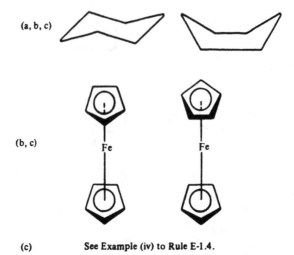

(a, b, c)

(b, c)

Fe   Fe

(c)   See Example (iv) to Rule E-1.4.

E-1.6. The terms relative stereochemistry and relative configuration are used with reference to the positions of various atoms in a compound relative to one another, especially, but not only, when the actual positions in space (absolute configuration) are unknown.

E-1.7. The terms absolute stereochemistry and absolute configuration are used with reference to the known actual positions of the atoms of a molecule in space.*

E-2. *cis—trans* Isomerism[†]

Preamble. The prefixes *cis* and *trans* have long been used for describing the relative positions of atoms or groups attached to nonterminal doubly bonded atoms of a chain or attached to a ring that is considered as planar. This practice has been codified for hydrocarbons by IUPAC.** There has, however, not been agreement on how to assign *cis* or *trans* at terminal double bonds of chains or at double bonds joining a chain to a ring. An obvious solution was to use *cis* and *trans* where doubly bonded atoms formed the backbone and were nonterminal and to enlist the sequence-rule preferences to decide other cases; however, since the two methods, when generally applied, do not always produce analogous results, it would then be necessary to use different symbols for the two procedures. A study of this combination showed that both types of symbols would often be required in one name and, moreover, it seemed wrong in principle to use two symbolisms for essentially the same phenomenon. Thus it seemed to the Commission wise to use only the sequence-rule system, since this alone was applicable to all cases. The same decision was taken independently by Chemical Abstracts Service who introduced Z and E to correspond more conveniently to *seqcis* and *seqtrans* of the sequence rule.

It is recommended in the Rules below that these designations Z and E based on the sequences rule shall be used in names of compounds, but Z and E do not always correspond to the classical *cis* and *trans* which show the steric relations of like or similar

---

*Determination of absolute configuration became possible through work by Bijvoet, J. M., Peerdeman, A. F., and van Bommel, A. J., *Nature,* 168, 271 (1951); cf. Bijvoet, J. M., *Proc. Kon. Ned. Akad. Wetensch.,* 52, 313 (1949).
[†]These Rules supersede the Tentative Rules for olefinic hydrocarbons published in the Comptes rendus of the 16th IUPAC Conference, New York, N.Y., 1951, pp. 102–103.
**Blackwood, J. E., Gladys, C. L., Loening, K. L., Petrarca, A. E., and Rush, J. E., *J. Amer. Chem. Soc.,* 90, 509 (1968); Blackwood, J. E., Gladys, C. L., Petrarca, A. E., Powell, W. H., and Rush, J. E., *J. Chem. Doc.,* 8, 30 (1968).

groups that are often the main point of interest. So the use of *Z* and *E* in names is not intended to hamper the use of *cis* and *trans* in discussions of steric relations of a generic type or of groups of particular interest in a specified case (see Rule E-2.1 and its Examples and Notes, also Rule E-5.11).

It is also not necessary to replace *cis* and *trans* for describing the stereochemistry of substituted monocycles (see Subsection E-3). For cyclic compounds the main problems are usually different from those around double bonds; for instance, steric relations of substitutents on rings can often be described either in terms of chirality (see Subsection E-5) or in terms of *cis–trans* relationships, and, further, there is usually no single relevant plane of reference in a hydrogenated polycycle. These matters are discussed in the Preambles to Subsections E-3 and E-4.

E-2.1. *Definition of cis–trans.* Atoms or groups are termed *cis* or *trans* to one another when they lie respectively on the same or on opposite sides of a reference plane identifiable as common among stereoisomers. The compounds in which such relations occur are termed *cis–trans* isomers. For compounds containing only doubly bonded atoms, the reference plane contains the doubly bonded atoms and is perpendicular to the plane containing these atoms and those directly attached to them. For cyclic compounds, the reference plane is that in which the ring skeleton lies or to which it approximates. When qualifying another word or a locant, *cis* or *trans* is followed by a hyphen. When added to a structural formula, *cis* may be abbreviated to *c*, and *trans* to *t* (see also Rule E-3.3).

Examples: (Rectangles here denote the reference planes and are considered to lie in the plane of the paper.)

The groups or atoms a,a are the pair selected for designation but are not necessarily identical; b,b are also not necessarily identical but must be different from a,a.

cis or *trans* according as a or b is taken as basis of comparison

Notes: The formulas above are drawn with the reference plane in the plane of the paper, but for doubly bonded compounds it is customary to draw the formulas so that this plane is perpendicular to that of the paper; atoms attached directly to the doubly bonded atoms then lie in the plane of the paper and the formulas appear as, for instance

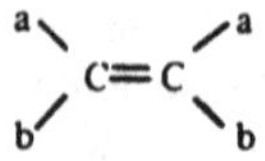

cis

Cyclic structures, however, are customarily drawn with the ring atoms in the plane of the paper, as above. However, care is needed for complex cases, such as

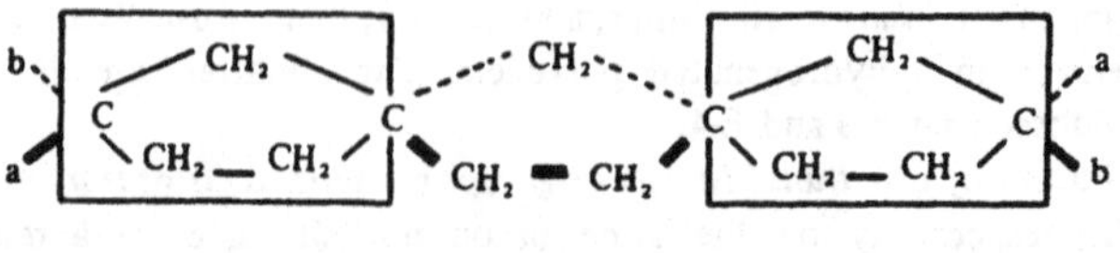

The central five-membered ring lies (approximately) in a plane perpendicular to the plane of the paper. The two a groups are *trans* to one another; so are the b groups; the outer cyclopentane rings are *cis* to one another with respect to the plane of the central ring. *cis* or *trans* (or *Z* or *E*; see Rule E-2.21) may also be used in cases involving a partial bond order when a limiting structure is of sufficient importance to impose rigidity around the bond of partial order. An example is

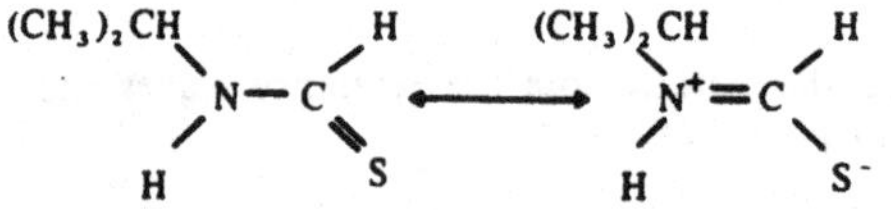

trans (or E)

E-2.2. *cis-trans Isomerism around Double Bonds.*

E-2.21. In names of compounds steric relations around one or more double bonds are designated by affixes *Z* and/or *E*, assigned as follows. The sequence-rule-preferred* atom or group attached to one of a doubly bonded pair of atoms is compared with the sequence-rule-preferred atom or group attached to the other of that doubly bonded pair of atoms; if the selected pair are on the same side of the reference plane (see Rule 2.1) an italic capital letter *Z* prefix is used; if the selected pair are on opposite sides an italic capital letter *E* prefix is used.[†] These prefixes, placed in parentheses and followed by a hyphen, normally precede the whole name; if the molecule contains several double bonds, then each prefix is immediately preceded by the lower or less primed locant of the relevant double bond.

Examples:

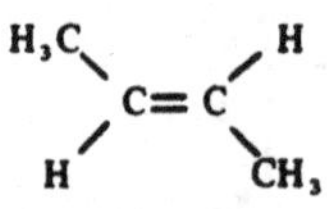

(*E*)-2-Butene

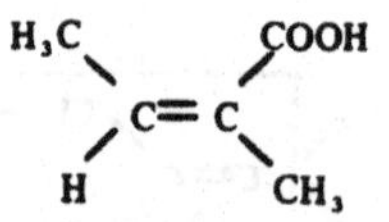

(*Z*)-2-Methyl-2-butenoic acid** *or* (*Z*)-2-methylisocrotonic acid (see Exceptions below)

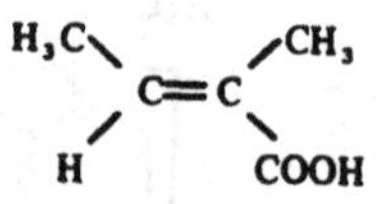

(*E*)-2-Methyl-2-butenoic acid[††] *or* (*E*)-2-Methylcrotonic acid (see Exceptions below)

*For sequence-rule preferences see Appendix 2.
[†]These prefixes may be rationalized as from the German *zusammen* (together) and *entgegen* (opposite).
**The name angelic acid is abandoned because it has been associated with the designation *trans* with reference to the methyl groups.
[††]The name tiglic acid is abandoned because it has been associated with the designation *cis* with reference to the methyl groups.

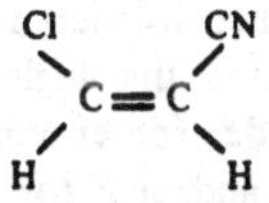

(*Z*)-3-Chloroacrylonitrile

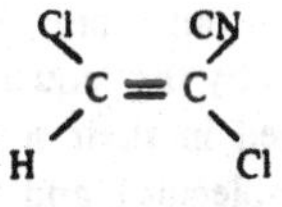

(*E*)-2,3-Dichloroacrylonitrile

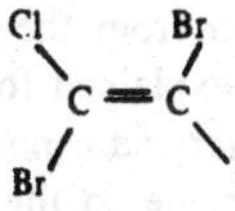

(*Z*)-1,2-Dibromo-1-chloro-2-iodoethylene
(By the sequence rule, Br is preferred to Cl, but I to Br)

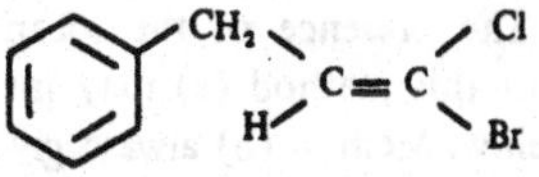

(*E*)-(3-Bromo-3-chloroallyl)benzene

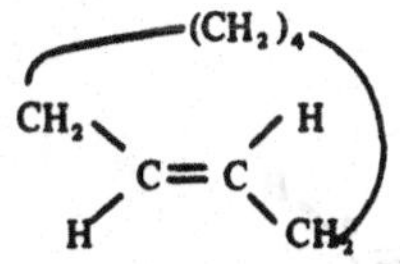

(*E*)-Cyclooctene

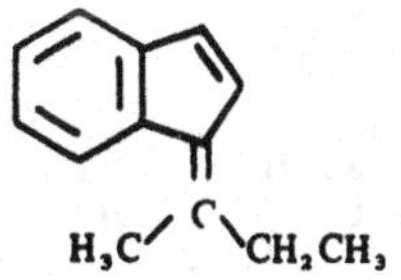

(*E*)-1-*sec*-Butylideneindene

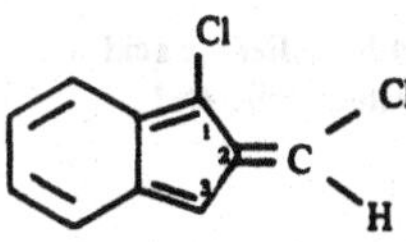

(*Z*)-1-Chloro-2-ethylidene-2*H*-indene

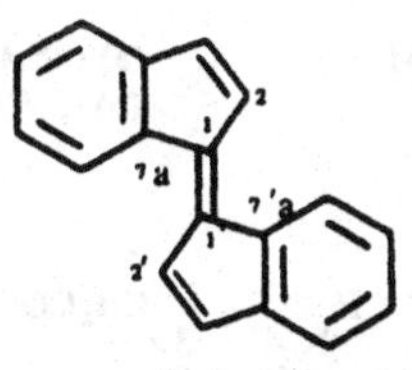

(*E*)-1,1′-Biindenylidene

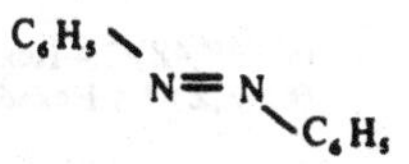

(*E*)-Azobenzene

Exceptions to Rule E-2.21. The following are examples of accepted trivial names in which the stereochemistry is prescribed by the name and is not cited by a prefix.

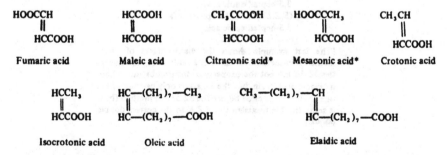

Fumaric acid	Maleic acid	Citraconic acid*	Mesaconic acid*	Crotonic acid
HOOCCH ‖ HCCOOH	HCCOOH ‖ HCCOOH	CH_3CCOOH ‖ HCCOOH	$HOOCCCH_3$ ‖ HCCOOH	CH_3CH ‖ HCCOOH

Isocrotonic acid	Oleic acid	Elaidic acid
$HCCH_3$ ‖ HCCOOH	HC—$(CH_2)_7$—CH_3 ‖ HC—$(CH_2)_7$—COOH	CH_3—$(CH_2)_7$—CH ‖ HC—$(CH_2)_7$—COOH

E-2.22 (*Alternative to Part of E-2.21*). (a) When more than one series of locants starting from unity is required to designate the double bonds in a molecule, or when the name consists of two words, the *Z* and *E* prefixes together with their appropriate locants may be placed before that part of the name where ambiguity is most effectively removed.

(b) [Alternative to (a)] When several *Z* or *E* prefixes are required they are arranged in

*Systematic names are recommended for derivatives of these compounds formed by substitution on carbon.

order as follows: Of the four atoms or groups attached to each doubly bonded pair of atoms, that one preferred by the sequence rule is selected; the single atoms or groups thus selected are then arranged in their sequence rule order (determined in respect of their position in the whole molecule), and the prefixes *Z* and/or *E* for the respective double bonds are placed in that order, but *without* their locants.

Note: In method (a) the final choice is left to an author or editor because of the variety of cases met and because the problems are not always the same in different languages. The presence of the locants usually eases translation from the name to a formula, but this method (a) may involve the logical difficulty explained for the third example below. Method (b) always gives a single unambiguous order and is not subject to the logical difficulty just mentioned, but translation from the name to the formula is harder than for method (a). Method (a) may be more suitable for cursive text, and method (b) for compendia. If method (b) is used it should be used whenever more than one double bond is involved, but method (a) is to be used only under the special conditions detailed in the rule.

Examples:

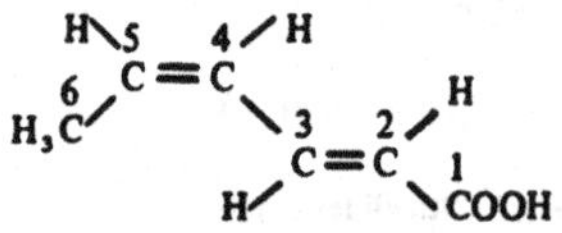

(a) (2*E*,4*Z*)-2,4-Hexadienoic acid
(b) (*E*,*Z*)-2,4-Hexadienoic acid

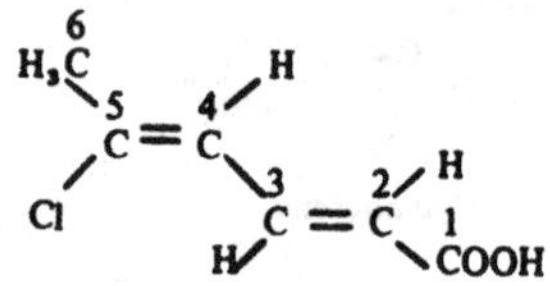

(a) (2*E*,4*Z*)-5-Chloro-2,4-hexadienoic acid
(b) (*Z*,*E*)5-Chloro-2,4-hexadienoic acid

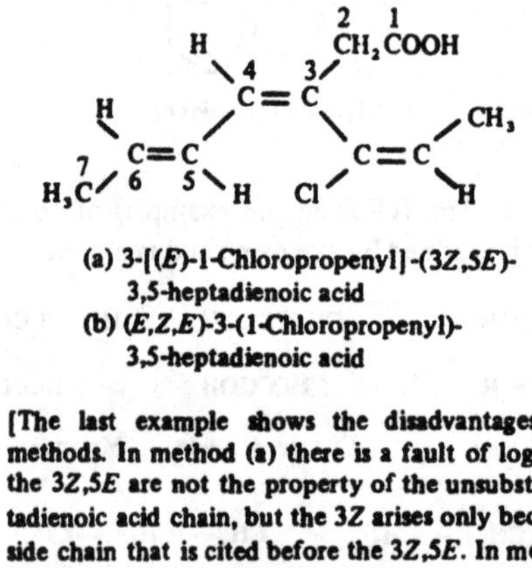

(a) 3-[(*E*)-1-Chloropropenyl]-(3*Z*,5*E*)-
3,5-heptadienoic acid
(b) (*E*,*Z*,*E*)-3-(1-Chloropropenyl)-
3,5-heptadienoic acid

[The last example shows the disadvantages of both methods. In method (a) there is a fault of logic, namely, the 3*Z*,5*E* are not the property of the unsubstituted heptadienoic acid chain, but the 3*Z* arises only because of the side chain that is cited before the 3*Z*,5*E*. In method (b) it is some trouble to assign the *E*,*Z*,*E* to the correct double bonds.]

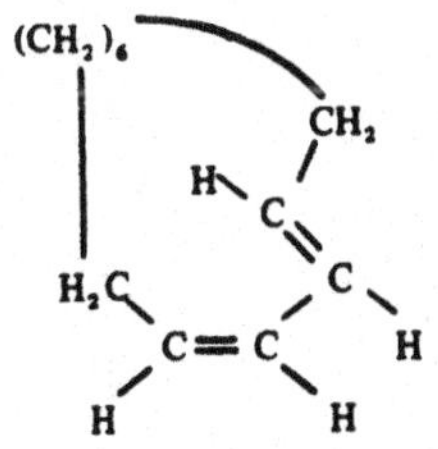

(a) (1Z,3E)-1,3-Cyclododecadiene
(b) (Z,E)-1,3-Cyclododecadiene

[The lower locant is assigned to the Z double bond.]

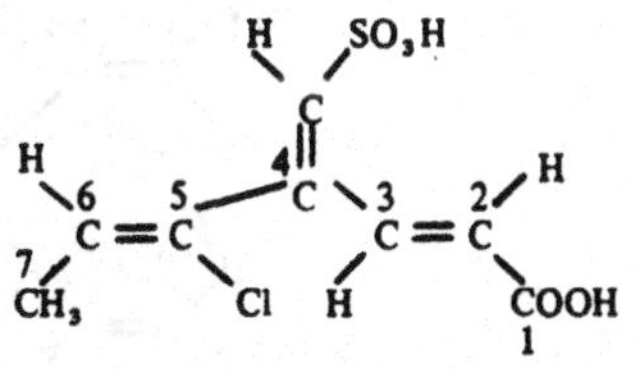

(a) 5-Chloro-4-(E-sulfomethylene)-
    (2E,5Z)-2,5-heptadienoic acid
(b) (Z,E,E)-5-Chloro-4-(sulfomethylene)-
    2,5-heptadienoic acid

[In application of the sequence rule, the relation of the SO_3H to CCl (rather than to C-3), and of the CH_3 to Cl, are decisive.]

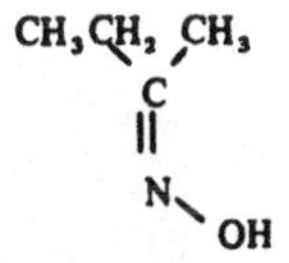

(a) Butanone (E)-oxime*
(b) (E)-Butanone oxime

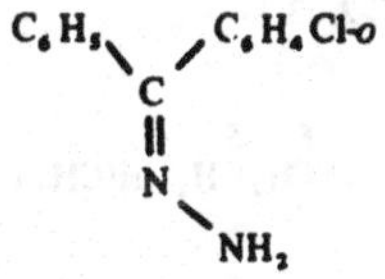

(a) 2-Chlorobenzophenone (Z)-hydrazone
(b) (Z)-2-Chlorobenzophenone hydrazone

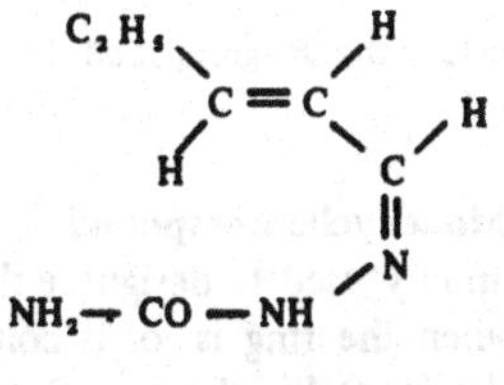

(a) (E)-2-Pentenal (Z)-semicarbazone
(b) (Z,E)-2-Pentenal semicarbazone

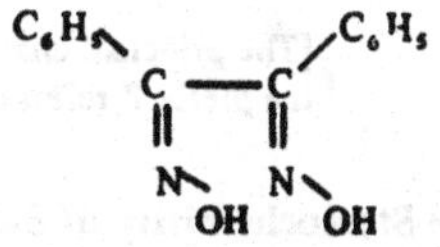

(a) Benzil (Z,E)-dioxime
(b) (Z,E)-Benzil dioxime

E-2.23. When Rule C-13.1 or E-2.22(b) permits alternatives, preference for lower locants and for inclusion in the principal chain is allotted as follows, in the order stated, so far as necessary: Z over E groups; *cis* over *trans* cyclic groups; R over S groups (also r over s, etc., as in the sequence rule); if the nature of these groups is not decisive, then the lower locant for such a preferred group at the first point of difference.

Examples:

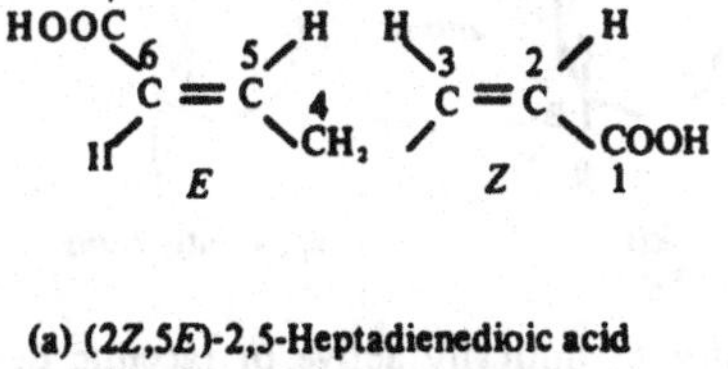

(a) (2Z,5E)-2,5-Heptadienedioic acid
(b) (E,Z)-2,5-Heptadienedioic acid

[The lower numbers are assigned to the Z double bond.]

*The terms *syn, anti,* and *amphi* are abandoned for such compounds.

$$\underset{Cl}{\overset{H}{\diagdown}}\overset{1}{C}=\overset{2}{C}\overset{H}{\diagup}$$

(a) 1-Chloro-3-[2-chloro-(*E*)-vinyl]-(1*Z*,3*Z*)-
1,3-pentadiene
(b) (*E,Z,Z*)-1-Chloro-3-(2-chlorovinyl)-
1,3-pentadiene

[According to Rule C-13.1 the principal chain must
include the C≡C–CH₃ group because this gives lower
numbers to the double bonds (1,3 rather than 1,4);
then the Cl-containing *Z* group is chosen for the remainder of the principal chain in accord with Rule
E-2.23.]

$$(R)\text{-}\underset{6}{CH_2}\underset{5}{CH_2}\underset{4}{CH(CH_3)}$$

(a,b) (*Z*)-(4*R*)-3-[(*S*)-*sec*-Butyl]-4-methyl-2-hexenoic acid

[The principal chain is chosen to include the (*R*)-group, and
the prefix *Z* refers to the (*R*)-group.]

E-3. Relative Stereochemistry of Substituents in Monocyclic Compounds[†]

Preamble. The prefixes *cis* and *trans* are commonly used to designate the positions of
substituents on rings relative to one another; when the ring is, or is considered to be,
rigidly planar or approximately so and is placed horizontally, these prefixes define which
groups are above and which below the (approximate) plane of the ring. This
differentiation is often important, so this classical terminology is retained in Subsection
E-3; since the difficulties inherent in end groups do not arise for cyclic compounds, it is
unnecessary to resort to the less immediately informative *E/Z* symbolism.

When the *cis–trans* designation of substituents is applied, rings are considered in their
most extended form; reentrant angles are not permitted; for example

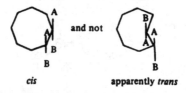

cis   apparently *trans*

The absolute stereochemistry of optically active or racemic derivatives of monocyclic
compounds is described by the sequence-rule procedure (see Rule E-5.9 and Appendix 2).
The relative stereochemistry may be described by a modification of sequence-rule
symbolism as set out in Rule E-5.10. If either of these procedures is adopted, it is then
superfluous to use also *cis* or *trans* in the names of individual compounds.

[†]Formulas in Examples to this Rule denote relative (not absolute) configurations.

E-3.1. When alternative numberings of the ring are permissible according to the Rules of Section C, that numbering is chosen which gives a *cis* attachment at the first point of difference; if that is not decisive, the criteria of Rule E-2.23 are applied. The prefixes *cis* and *trans* may be abbreviated to *c* and *t*, respectively, in names of compounds when more than one such designation is required.

Examples:

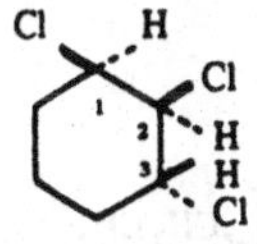

1,*c*-2,*t*-3-Trichlorocyclohexane 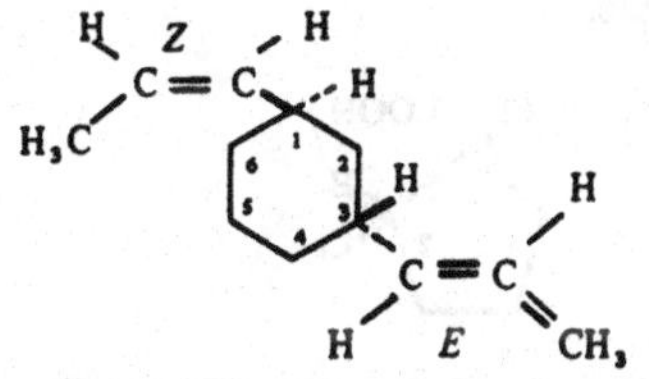 1-(*Z*)-Propenyl-*trans*-3-(*E*)-propenylcyclohexane

E-3.2. When one substituent and one hydrogen atom are attached at each of two positions of a monocycle, the steric relations of the two substituents are expressed as *cis* or *trans*, followed by a hyphen and placed before the name of the compound.

Examples:

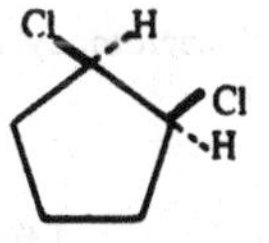

cis-1,2-Dichlorocyclopentane 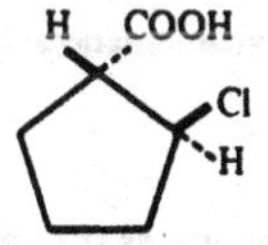 *trans*-2-Chloro-1-cyclopentanecarboxylic acid

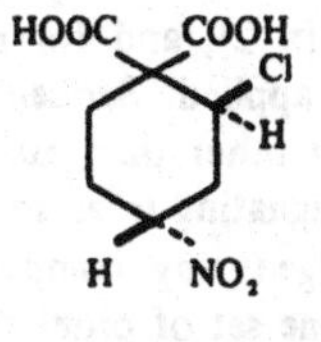

trans-2-Chloro-4-nitro-1,
1-cyclohexanedicarboxylic acid

E-3.3. When one substituent and one hydrogen atom are attached at each of more than two positions of a monocycle, the steric relations of the substituents are expressed by adding *r* (for *reference* substituent), followed by a hyphen, before the locant of the lowest numbered of these substituents and *c* or *t* (as appropriate), followed by a hyphen, before the locants of the other substituents to express their relation to the reference substituent.

Examples:

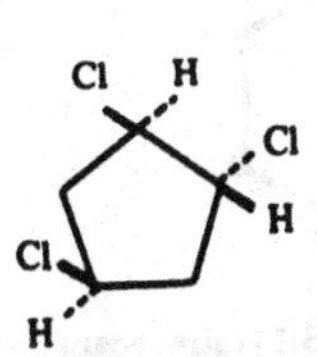

r-1,*t*-2,*c*-4-Trichlorocyclopentant *t*-5-Chloro-*r*-1, *c*-3-cyclohexanedicarboxylic acid
(not *r*-1, *t*-2, *t*-4, which would follow from the
alternative direction of numbering; see Rule
E-3.1)

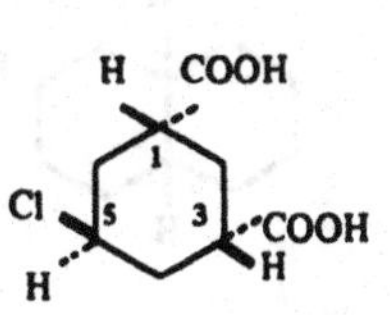

E-3.4. When two different substituents are attached at the same position of a monocycle, then the lowest numbered substituent named as suffix is selected for designation as reference group in accordance with Rule E-3.2 or E-3.3; or, if none of the substituents is named as suffix, then of the lowest numbered pair that one preferred by the sequence rule is selected as reference group; and the relation of the sequence-rule preferred group at each other position, relative to the reference group, is cited as *c* or *t* (as appropriate).

Examples:

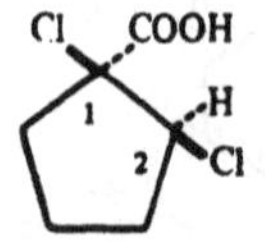

1,*t*-2-Dichloro-*r*-1-cyclopentanecarboxylic acid

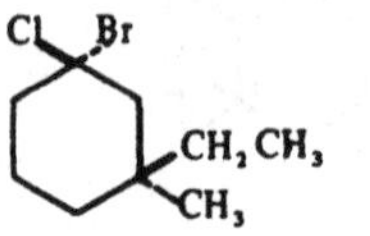

r-1-Bromo-1-chloro-*t*-3-ethyl-3-methylcyclohexane (alphabetical order of prefixes)

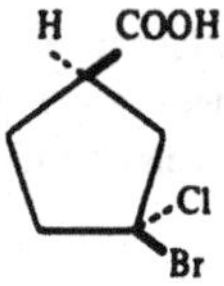

c-3-Bromo-3-chloro-*r*-1-cyclopentanecarboxylic acid

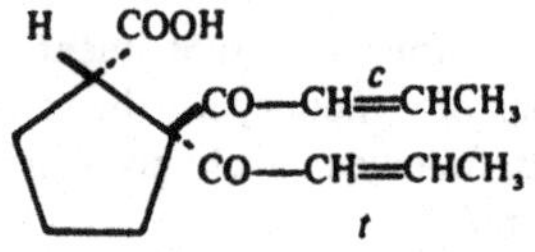

2-Crotonoyl-*t*-2-isocrotonoyl-*r*-1-cyclopentane-carboxylic acid

E-4. Fused Rings

Preamble. In simple cases the relative stereochemistry of substituted fused-ring systems can be designated by the methods used for monocycles. For the absolute stereochemistry of optically active and racemic compounds the sequence-rule procedure can be used in all cases (see Rule E-5.9 and Appendix 2), and for related relative stereochemistry the procedure of Rule E-5.10 can be applied. Sequence-rule methods are, however, not descriptive of geometrical shape for other than quite simple cases. There is as yet no generally acceptable system for designating in an immediately interpretable manner the stereochemistry of polycyclic bridged ring compounds (for instance, the *endo–exo* nomenclature, which should solve one set of problems, has been used in different ways). These and related problems (e.g., cyclophanes, catenanes) will be considered in a later document.

E-4.1. Steric relations at saturated bridgeheads common to two rings are denoted by *cis* or *trans*, followed by a hyphen and placed before the name of the ring system, according to the relative positions of the exocyclic atoms or groups attached to the bridgeheads. Such rings are said to be *cis* fused or *trans* fused.

Examples:

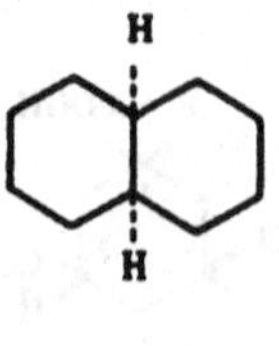

cis-Decalin

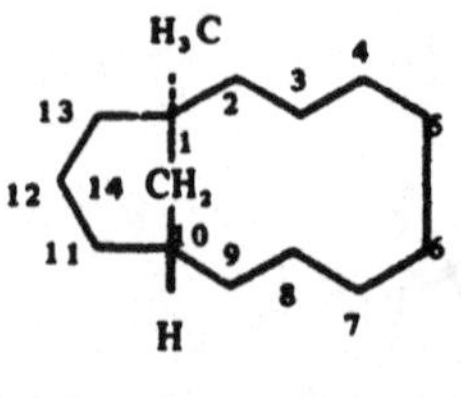

1-Methyl-*trans*-bicyclo[8.3.1]tetradecane

E-4.2. Steric relations at more than one pair of saturated bridgeheads in a polycyclic compound are denoted by *cis* or *trans*, each followed by a hyphen and, when necessary, the corresponding locant of the lower numbered bridgehead and a second hyphen, all placed before the name of the ring system. Steric relations between the nearest atoms* of *cis*- or *trans*-bridgehead pairs may be described by affixes *cisoid* or *transoid*, followed by a hyphen and, when necessary, the corresponding locants and a second hyphen, the whole placed between the designations of the *cis*- or *trans*-ring junctions concerned. When a choice remains among nearest atoms, the pair containing the lower numbered atom is selected; *cis* and *trans* are not abbreviated in such cases. In complex cases, however, designation may be more simply effected by the sequence-rule procedure (see Appendix 2).

Examples:

cis-cisoid-trans-Perhydrophenanthrene

cis-cisoid-4a, 10a-*trans*-Perhydroanthracene
or *rel*-(4aR, 8aS, 9aS, 10aS)-Perhydroanthracene[†]

trans-3a-*cisoid*-3a, 4a-*cis* -4a-Perhydrobenz[*f*] indene
or *rel*-(3aR, 4aS, 8aR, 9aR)-Perhydrobenz[*f*] indene

E-5. Chirality

E-5.1. The property of nonidentity of an object with its mirror image is termed chirality. An object, such as a molecule in a given configuration or conformation, is termed chiral when it is not identical with its mirror image; it is termed achiral when it is identical with its mirror image.

Notes: (1) Chirality is equivalent to handedness, the term being derived from the Greek Χειρ = hand.

(2) All chiral molecules are molecules of optically active compounds, and molecules of all optically active compounds are chiral. There is a 1:1 correspondence between chirality and optical activity.

(3) In organic chemistry the discussion of chirality usually concerns the individual molecule or, more strictly, a model of the individual molecule. The chirality of an assembly of molecules may differ from that of the component molecules, as in a chiral quartz crystal or in an achiral crystal containing equal numbers of dextrorotatory and levorotatory tartaric acid molecules.

(4) The chirality of a molecule can be discussed only if the configuration or conformation of the molecule is specifically defined or is considered as defined by

*The term "nearest atoms" denotes those linked together through the smallest number of atoms, irrespective of actual separation in space. For instance, in the second Example to this Rule, the atom 4a is "nearer" to 10a than to 8a.

†For the designation *rel*, see Rule E-5.10.

common usage. In such discussions structures are treated as if they were (at least temporarily) rigid. For instance, ethane is configurationally achiral although many of its conformations, such as (A), are chiral; in fact, a configuration of a mobile molecule is chiral only if all its possible conformations are chiral; and conformations of ethane such as (B) and (C) are achiral.

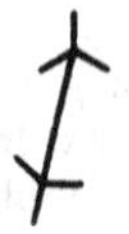

(A) 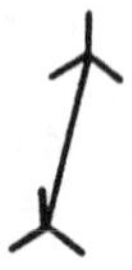   (B) 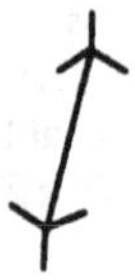   (C)

Examples:

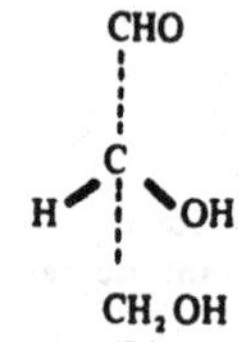

CHO   CHO   CH₂OH

H—C—OH   HO—C—H   H—C—OH

CH₂OH   CH₂OH   CH₂OH
(D) 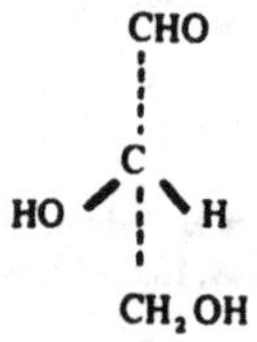   (E) 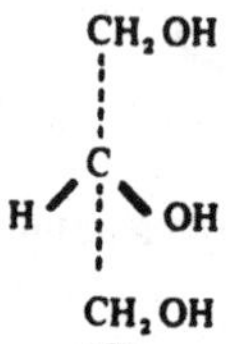   (F)

(D) and (E) are mirror images and are not identical, not being superposable. They represent chiral molecules. They represent (D) dextrorotatory and (E) levorotatory glyceraldehyde.

(F) is identical with its mirror image. It represents an achiral molecule, namely, a molecule of *1,2,3-*propanetriol (glycerol).

E-5.2. The term asymmetry denotes absence of any symmetry. An object, such as a molecule in a given configuration or conformation, is termed asymmetric if it has no element of symmetry.

Notes: (1) All asymmetric molecules are chiral, and all compounds composed of them are therefore optically active; however, not all chiral molecules are asymmetric since some molecules having axes of rotation are chiral.

(2) Notes (3) and (4) to Rule E-5.1 apply also in discussions of asymmetry.

Examples:

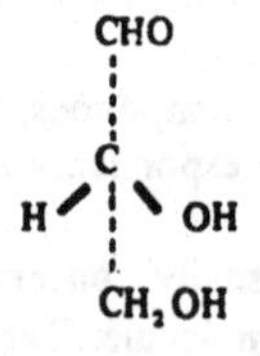

CHO

H—C—OH

CH₂OH

has no element of symmetry and represents a molecule of an optically active compound.

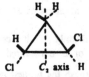

has a C_2 axis of rotation; it is chiral although not asymmetric, and is therefore a molecule of an optically active compound.

E-5.3. (a) An asymmetric atom is one that is tetrahedrally bonded to four different atoms or groups, none of the groups being the mirror image of any of the others.

(b) An asymmetric atom may be said to be at a chiral center since it lies at the center of a chiral tetrahedral structure. In a general sense, the term "chiral center" is not restricted to tetrahedral structures; the structure may, for instance, be based on an octahedron or tetragonal pyramid.

(c) When the atom by which a group is attached to the remainder of a molecule lies at a chiral center, the group may be termed a chiral group.

Notes: (1) The term "asymmetric," as applied to a carbon atom in rule E-5.3 (a), was chosen by van't Hoff because there is no plane of symmetry through a tetrahedron whose corners are occupied by four atoms or groups that differ in scalar properties. For differences of vector sense between the attached groups, see Rule E-5.8.

(2) In Subsection E-5 the word "group" is used to denote the series of atoms attached to one bond. For instance, in (i) the groups attached to C* are $-CH_3$, $-OH$, $-CH_2CH_3$, and $-COOH$; in (ii) they are $-CH_3$, $-OH$, $-COCH_2CH_2CH_2$, and $-CH_2CH_2CH_2CO$.

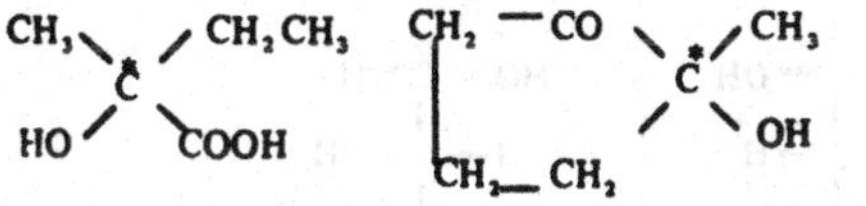

(i)   (ii)

(3) For the chiral axis and chiral plane (which are less common than the chiral center), see Appendix 2.

(4) There may be more than one chiral center in a molecule and these centers may be identical, or structurally different, or structurally identical but of opposite chirality; however, the presence of an equal number of structurally identical chiral groups of opposite chirality, and no other chiral group, leads to an achiral molecule. These statements apply also to chiral axes and chiral planes. Identification of the sites and natures of the various factors involved is essential if the overall chirality of a molecule is to be understood.

(5) Although the term "chiral group" is convenient for use in discussions it should be remembered that chirality attaches to molecules and not to groups or atoms. For instance, although the *sec*-butyl group may be termed chiral in dextrorotatory 2-*sec*-butyl-naphthalene, it is not chiral in the achiral compound $(CH_3CH_2)(CH_3)CH-CH_3$.

Examples:

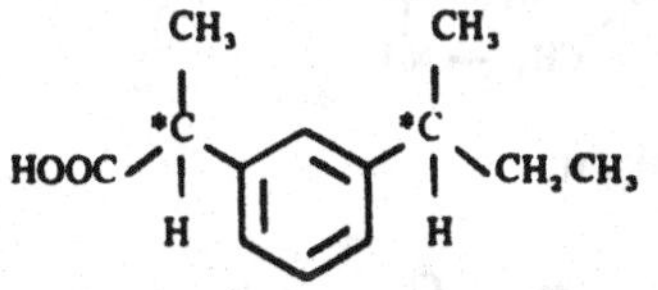

In this chiral compound there are two asymmetric carbon atoms, marked C*, each lying at a chiral center. These atoms form part of different chiral groups, namely, $-CH(CH_3)$ COOH and $-CH(CH_3)CH_2CH_3$

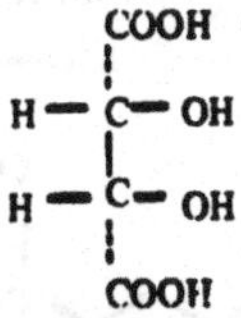

In this molecule (*meso*-tartaric acid) the two central carbon atoms are asymmetric atoms and each is part of a chiral group $-CH(OH)COOH$. These groups, however, although structurally identical, are of opposite chirality, so that the molecule is achiral.

E-5.4. Molecules that are mirror images of one another are termed enantiomers and may be said to be enantiomeric. Chiral groups that are mirror images of one another are termed enantiomeric groups.

Hence: enantiomerism (phenomenological)

Note: Although the adjective enantiomeric may be applied to groups, enantiomerism strictly applies only to molecules [see Note (5) to Rule E-5.3].

Examples: The following pairs of molecules are enantiomeric.

(i)

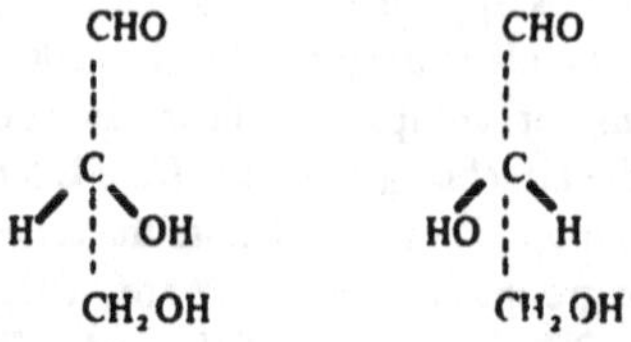

CHO
C
H   OH
CH₂OH

CHO
C
HO   H
CH₂OH

(ii)

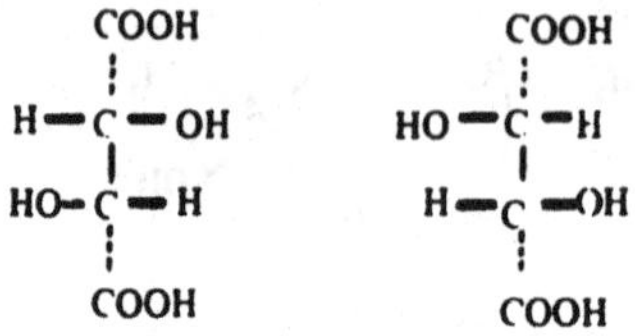

COOH
H—C—OH
HO—C—H
COOH

COOH
HO—C—H
H—C—OH
COOH

(iii)

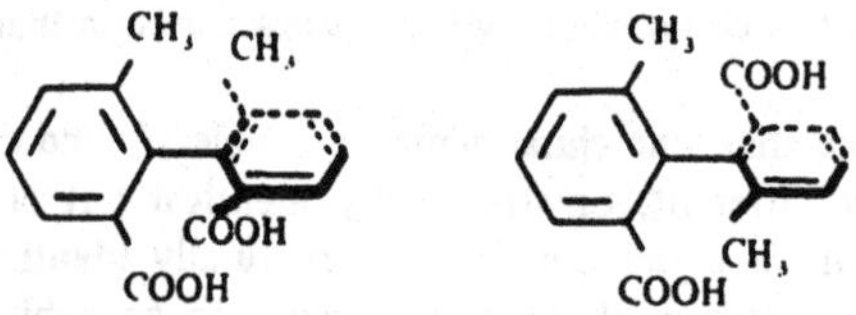

CH₃ CH₃
COOH
COOH

CH₃
COOH
CH₃
COOH

(iv)

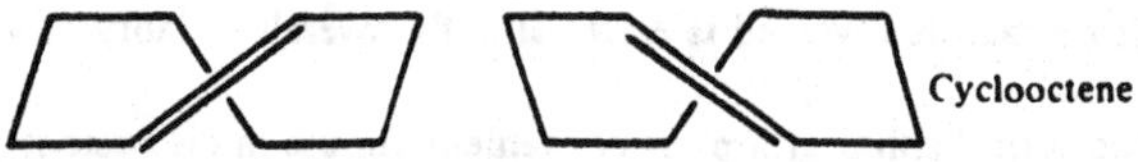

Cyclooctene

(v)

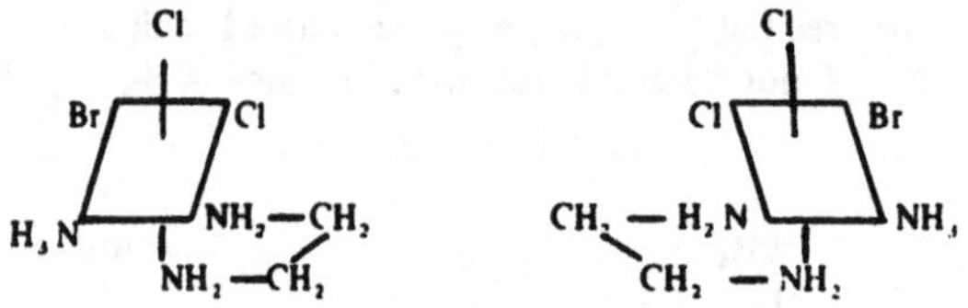

Cl
Br   Cl
H₂N   NH₂—CH₂
NH₂—CH₂

Cl
Cl   Br
CH₂—H₂N   NH₂
CH₂—NH₂

(vi)

CH₂CH₃
C
H
CH₃
Cl

CH₂CH₃
C
H
H₃C
Cl

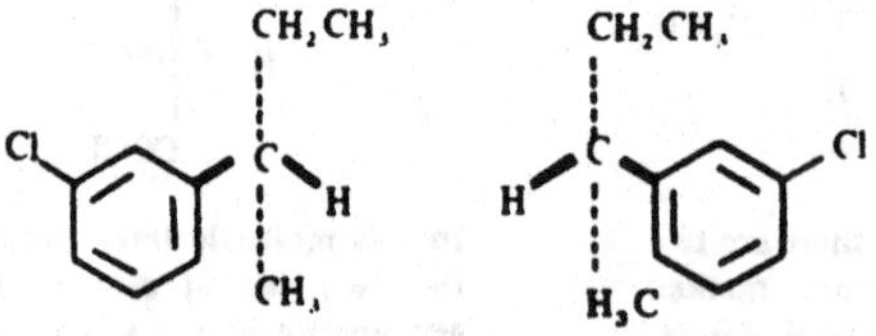

The *sec*-butyl groups in (vi) are enantiomeric.

E-5.5. When equal amounts of enantiomeric molecules are present together, the product is termed racemic, independently of whether it is crystalline, liquid, or gaseous. A homogeneous solid phase composed of equimolar amounts of enantiomeric molecules is termed a racemic compound. A mixture of equimolar amounts of enantiomeric molecules present as separate solid phases is termed a racemic mixture. Any homogeneous solid containing equimolar amounts of enantiomeric molecules is termed a racemate.

Examples: The mixture of two kinds of crystal (mirror-image forms) that separate below 28° from an aqueous solution containing equal amounts of dextrorotatory and levorotatory sodium ammonium tartrate is a racemic mixture.

The symmetrical crystals that separate from such a solution above 28°, each containing equal amounts of the two salts, provide a racemic compound.

E-5.6. Stereoisomers that are not enantiomeric are termed diastereoisomers.

Hence: diastereoisomeric (adjectival)
diastereoisomerism (phenomenological)

Note: Diastereoisomers may be chiral or achiral.
Examples:

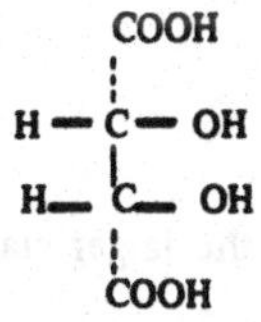

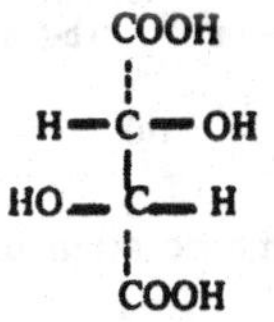

are diastereoisomers; the former is achiral, and the latter is chiral.

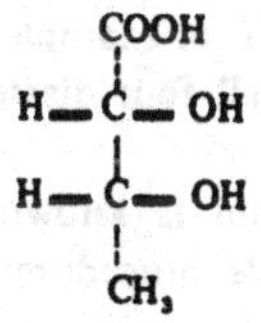

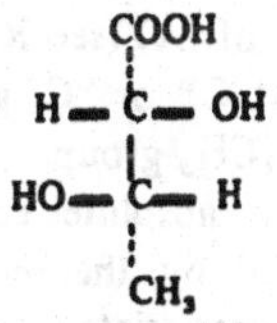

are diastereoisomers; both are chiral.

E-5.7. A compound whose individual molecules contain equal numbers of enantiomeric groups, identically linked, but no other chiral group, is termed a *meso* compound.
Example:

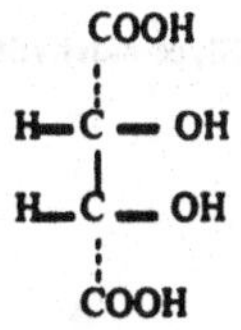

meso-Tartaric acid 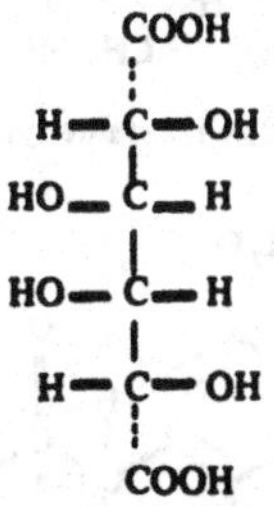   Galactaric acid

E-5.8. An atom is termed pseudoasymmetric when bonded tetrahedrally to one pair of enantiomeric groups (+)-a and (−)-a and also to two atoms or groups b and c that are different from group a, different from each other, and not enantiomeric with each other.
Examples:

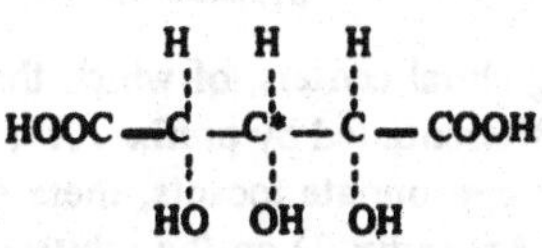

(A)   (B)

C* are pseudoasymmetric

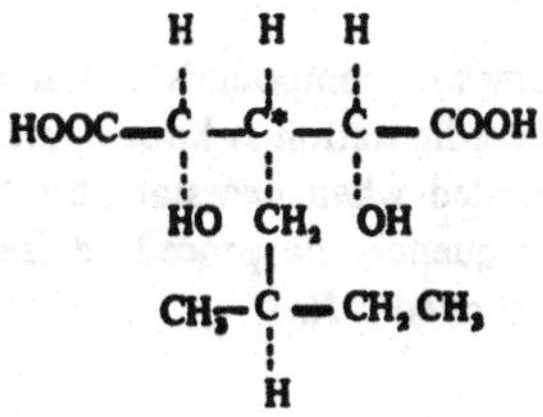

Notes: (1) The orientation, in space, of the atoms around a pseudoasymmetric atoms is not reversed on reflection; for a chiral atom (see Note to Rule E-5.3) this orientation is always reversed.

(2) Molecules containing pseudoasymmetric atoms may be achiral or chiral. If ligands b and c are both achiral, the molecule is achiral as in the first example to this Rule. If either or both of the nonenantiomeric ligands b and c are chiral, the molecule is chiral, as in the second example to this Rule, that is the molecule is not identical with its mirror image. A molecule (i) is also chiral if b and c are enantiomeric, that is, if the molecule can be symbolized as (ii), but then, by definition, it does not contain a pseudoasymmetric atom.

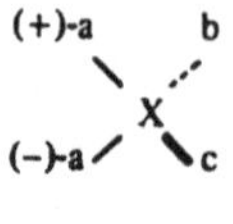

(i) 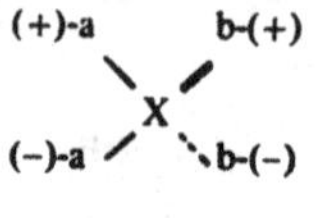   (ii)

(3) Compounds differing at a pseudoasymmetric atom belong to the larger class of diastereoisomers.

(4) In example (A), interchange of H and OH on C* gives a different achiral compound, which is an achiral diastereoisomer of (A) (see Rule E-5.6). In example (B), diastereoisomers are produced by inversion at C* or °C, giving in all four diastereo-isomers, all chiral because of the $-CH(CH_3)CH_2CH_3$ group.

E-5.9. Names of chiral compounds whose absolute configuration is known are differentiated by prefixes *R, S,* etc., assigned by the sequence-rule procedure (see Appendix 2), preceded when necessary by the appropriate locants.

Examples:

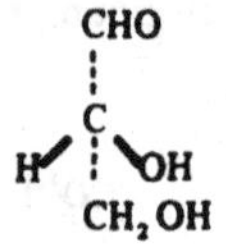

(*R*)-Glyceraldehyde 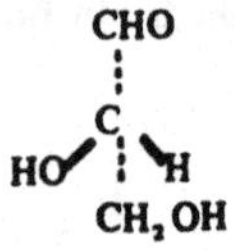   (*S*)-Glyceraldehyde

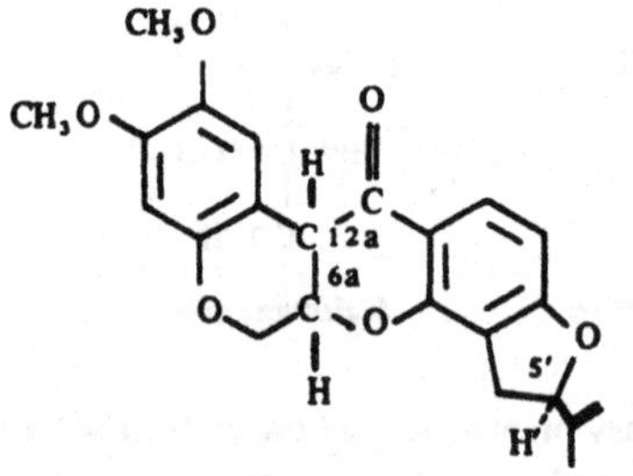

(6a*S*,12*S*,5'*R*)-Rotenone 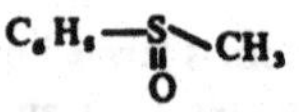   Methyl phenyl
                                     (*R*)-sulfoxide

E-5.10. (a) Names of compounds containing chiral centers, of which the relative but not the absolute configuration is known, are differentiated by prefixes *R*, S** (spoken R star, S star), preceded when necessary by the appropriate locants, these prefixes being assigned by the sequence-rule procedure (see Appendix 2) on the arbitrary assumption that the prefix first cited is *R*.

(b) In complex cases the stars may be omitted and, instead, the whole name is prefixed by *rel* (for *relative*).

(c) When only relative configuration is known, enantiomers are distinguished by a prefix (+) or (−), referring to the direction of rotation of plane-polarized light passing through them (wavelength, temperature, solvent, and/or concentration should also be specified, particularly when known to affect the sign).

(d) When a substituent of known absolute chirality is introduced into a compound of which only the relative configuration is known, then starred symbols R^*, S^* are used and not the prefix *rel.*

Note: This Rule does not form part of the procedure formulated in the sequence-rule papers by Cahn, Ingold, and Prelog (see Appendix 2).

Examples:

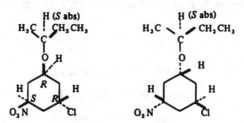

(1*R**, 3*S**,)-1-Bromo-3-chlorocyclohexane

rel-(1*R*,3*R*,5*R*)-1-Bromo-3-chloro-5-nitrocyclohexane

(1*R**,3*R**,5*S**)-[(1*S*)-*sec*-Butoxy]-3-chloro-5-nitrocyclohexane

E-5.11. When it is desired to express relative or absolute configuration with respect to a class of compounds, specialized local systems may be used. The sequence rule may, however, be used additionally for positions not amenable to treatment by the local system.

Examples:

gluco, arabino, etc., combined when necessary with D or L, for carbohydrates and their derivatives [see IUPAC-IUB Tentative Rules for Carbohydrate Nomenclature; see also *J. Org. Chem.*, 28, 281 (1963)].

D, L for amino acids and peptides [see Comptes rendus of the 16th IUPAC Conference, New York, N.Y., 1951., pp. 107–108; also published in *Chem. Eng. News*, 30, 4522 (1952)].

D, L, and a series of other prefixes and trivial names for cyclitols and their derivatives [see IUPAC-IUB Tentative Rules for the Nomenclature of Cyclitols, 1967, *IUPAC Inf. Bull.*, No. 32, 51 (1968); also published in *J. Biol. Chem.*, 243, 5809 (1968)].

α, β, and a series of trivial names for steroids and related compounds [see IUPAC-IUB Revised Tentative Rules for the Nomenclature of Steroids, 1967, *IUPAC Inf. Bull.*, No. 33, 23 (1968); also published in *J. Org. Chem.*, 34, 1517 (1969)].

The α, β system for steroids can be extended to other classes of compounds such as terpenes and alkaloids when their absolute configurations are known; it can also be combined with stars or the use of the prefix *rel* when only the relative configurations are known.

In spite of the Rules of Subsection E-2, *cis* and *trans* are used when the arrangement of the atoms constituting an unsaturated backbone is the most important factor, as, for instance, in polymer chemistry and for carotenoids. When a series of double bonds of the same stereochemistry occurs in a backbone, the prefix all-*cis* or all-*trans* may be used.

E-5.12. (a) An achiral object having at least one pair of features that can be distinguished only by reference to a chiral object or to a chiral reference frame is said to be prochiral, and the property of having such a pair of features is termed prochirality. A consequence is that, if one of the paired features of a prochiral object is considered to differ from the other, the resultant object is chiral.

(b) In a molecule an achiral center or atom is said to be prochiral if it would be held to be chiral when two attached atoms or groups, that taken in isolation are indistinguishable, are considered to differ.

Notes: (1) For a tetrahedrally bonded atom this requires a structure Xaabc (where none of the groups a, b, or c is the enantiomer of another).

(2) For a fuller exploration of this concept, which is of particular importance to biochemists and spectroscopists, and for its extension to axes, planes, and unsaturated compounds, see Hanson, K. R., *J. Am. Chem. Soc.*, 88, 2731 (1966).

Examples:

$$
\begin{array}{ccc}
& \text{CH}_3 & \text{CHO} \\
& | & | \\
& & \text{H} - \text{C} - \text{OH} \\
\text{H} - \text{C} - \text{H} & & \text{H} - \text{C} - \text{H} \\
& | & | \\
& \text{OH} & \text{OH} \\
& \text{(A)} & \text{(B)}
\end{array}
$$

In both examples (A) and (B), the methylene carbon atom is prochiral; in both cases it would be held to be at a chiral center if one of the methylene hydrogen atoms were considered to differ from the other. An actual replacement of one of these protium atoms by, say, deuterium would produce an actual chiral center at the methylene carbon atom; as a result, compound (A) would become chiral, and compound (B) would be converted into one of two diastereoisomers.

E-5.13. Of the identical pair of atoms or groups in a prochiral compound, that one which leads to an (*R*) compound when considered to be preferred to the other by the sequence rule (without change in priority with respect to other ligands) is termed *pro-R*, and the other is termed *pro-S*.

Example:

$$\begin{array}{c} CHO \\ | \\ H^1 \text{---} C \text{---} OH \\ | \\ H^2 \end{array}$$

H^1 is *pro-R*.
H^2 is *pro-S*.

E-6. Conformations

E-6.1. A molecule in a conformation into which its atoms return spontaneously after small displacements is termed a conformer.

Examples:

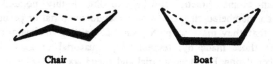

are different conformers.

E-6.2. (a) When, in a six-membered saturated ring compound, atoms in relative positions 1, 2, 4, and 5 lie in one plane, the molecule is described as in the chair or boat conformation according as the other two atoms lie, respectively, on opposite sides or on the same side of that plane.

Examples:

Chair   Boat

Note: These and similar representations are idealized, minor divergences being neglected.

(b) A molecule of a monounsaturated six-membered ring compound is described as being in the half-chair or half-boat conformation according as the atoms not directly bound to the doubly bonded atoms lie, respectively, on opposite sides or on the same side of the plane containing the other four (adjacent) atoms.

Examples:

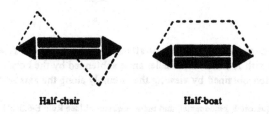

Half-chair   Half-boat

(c) A median conformation through which one boat form passes during conversion into the other boat form is termed a twist conformation. Similar twist conformations are involved in conversion of a chair into a boat form or vice versa.

Examples:

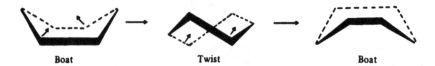

Boat   Twist   Boat

E-6.3. (a) Bonds to a tetrahedral atom in a six-membered ring are termed equatorial or axial according as they or their projections make a small or a large angle, respectively, with the plane containing a majority of the ring atoms.* Atoms or groups attached to such bonds are also said to be equatorial or axial, respectively.

Notes: (1) See, however, pseudoequatorial and pseudoaxial [Rule E-6.3(b)]. (2) The terms equatorial and axial may be abbreviated to e and a when attached to formulas; these abbreviations may also be used in names of compounds and are there placed in parentheses after the appropriate locants, for example, 1(e)-bromo-4(a)-chlorocyclohexane.

Examples:

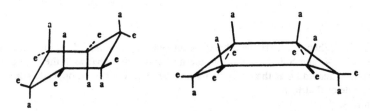

(b) Bonds from atoms directly attached to the doubly bonded atoms in a monounsaturated six-membered ring are termed pseudoequatorial or pseudoaxial according as the angles that they make with the plane containing the majority of the ring atoms approximate those made by, respectively, equatorial or axial bonds from a saturated six-membered ring. Pseudoequatorial and pseudoaxial may be abbreviated to e' and a', respectively, when attached to formulas; these abbreviations may also be used in names, then being placed in parentheses after the appropriate locants.

Example:

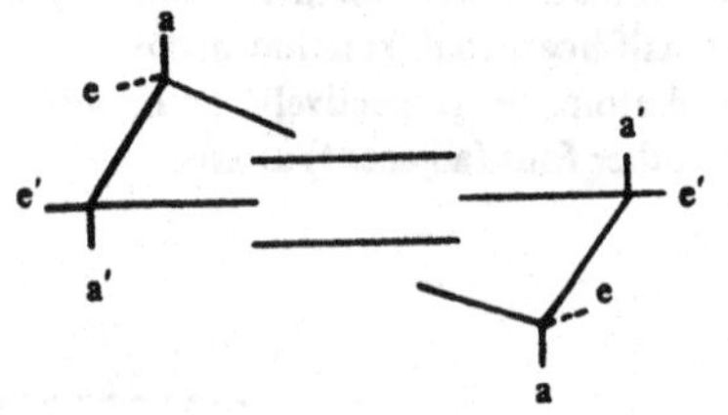

E-6.4. Torsion angle: In an assembly of attached atoms X—A—B—Y, where neither X nor Y is collinear with A and B, the smaller angle subtended by the bonds X—A and Y—B in a plane projection obtained by viewing the assembly along the axis A—B is termed the

*The terms axial, equatorial, pseudoaxial, and pseudoequatorial [see Rule E-6.3(b)] may be used also in connection with other than six-membered rings if, but only if, their interpretation is then still beyond dispute.

torsion angle (denoted by the Greek lower case letter theta θ or omega ω). The torsion angle is considered positive or negative according as the bond to the front atom X or Y requires rotation to the right or left, respectively, in order that its direction may coincide with that of the bond to the rear selected atom Y or X. The multiplicity of the bonding of the various atoms is irrelevant. A torsion angle also exists if the axis for rotation is formed by a collinear set of more than two atoms directly attached to each other.

Notes: (1) It is immaterial whether the projection be viewed from the front or the rear.

(2) For the use of torsion angles in describing molecules see Rule E-6.6.

Examples: (For construction of Newman projections, as here, see Rule E-7.2.)

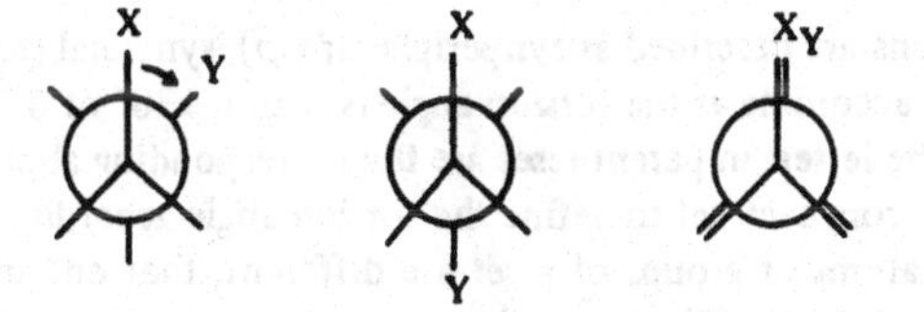

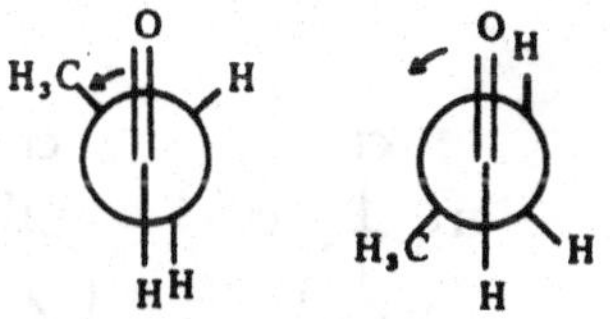

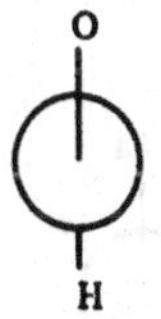

Newman projections of
propionaldehyde

Newman projection of
hydrogen peroxide
$\theta = \sim 180°$

E-6.5. If two atoms or groups attached at opposite ends of a bond appear one directly behind the other when the molecule is viewed along this bond, these atoms or groups are described as eclipsed, and that portion of the molecule is described as being in the eclipsed conformation. If not eclipsed, the atoms or groups and the conformation may be described as staggered.

Examples:

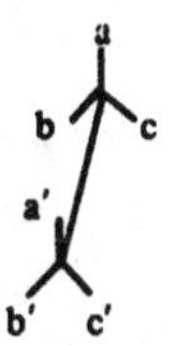

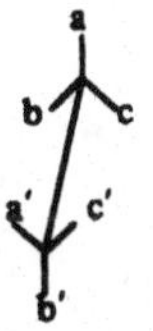

Eclipsed conformation.
The pairs a/a′, b/b′, and c/c′ are eclipsed.

Staggered conformation.
All the attached groups are staggered.

Projection of CH_3CH_2CHO.
The CH_3 and the H of the CHO are eclipsed.
The O and H's of CH_2 in CH_2CH_3 are
staggered.

E-6.6. Conformations are described as synperiplanar (*sp*), synclinal (*sc*), anticlinal (*ac*), or antiperiplanar (*ap*) according as the torsion angle is within ±30° of 0°, ±60°, ±120°, or ±180°, respectively; the letters in parentheses are the corresponding abbreviations. Atoms or groups are selected from each set to define the torsion angle according to the following criteria: (1) if all the atoms or groups of a set are different, that one of each set that is preferred by the sequence rule; (2) if one of a set is unique, that one; or (3) if all of a set are identical, that one which provides the smallest torsion angle.
Examples:

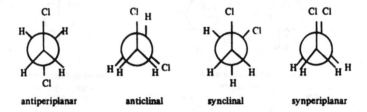

antiperiplanar   anticlinal   synclinal   synperiplanar

In the above conformations, all CH_2Cl-CH_2Cl, the two Cl atoms decide the torsion angle.

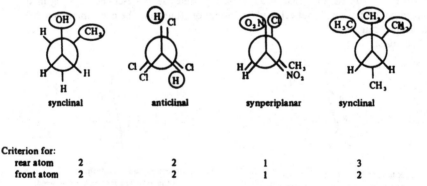

synclinal   anticlinal   synperiplanar   synclinal

Criterion for:				
rear atom	2	2	1	3
front atom	2	2	1	2

| | (CH₃)₂N–NH₂ synclinal* | CH₃CH₂–COCl anticlinal | (CH₃)₂CH–CONH₂ antiperiplanar |

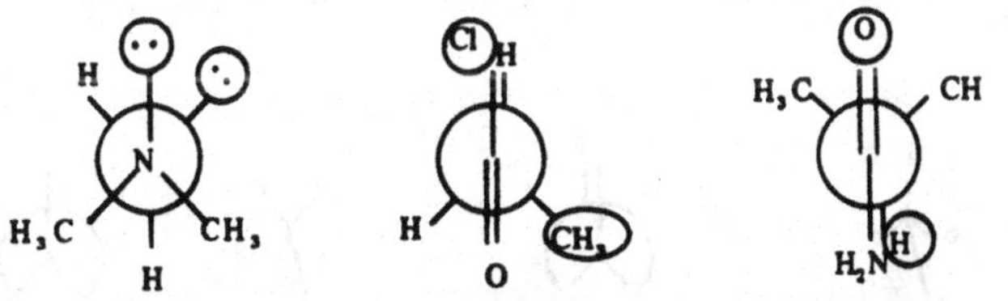

Criterion for:			
rear atom	2	2	2
front atom	2	1	1

E-7. Stereoformulas

E-7.1. In a Fischer projection the atoms or groups attached to a tetrahedral center are projected on to the plane of the paper from such an orientation that atoms or groups appearing above or below the central atom lie behind the plane of the paper and those appearing to left and right of the central atom lie in front of the plane of the paper, and that the principal chain appears vertical with the lowest numbered chain member at the top.

Examples:

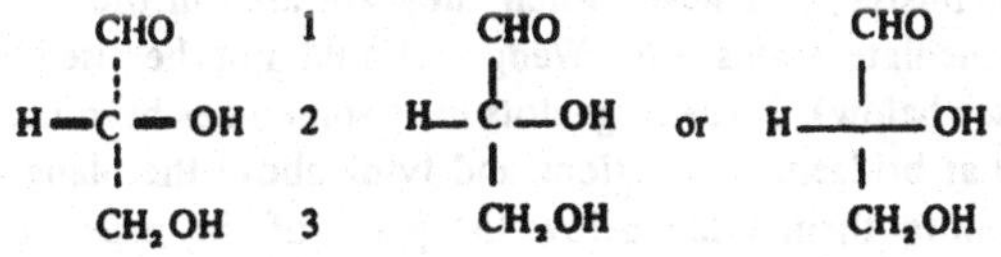

Orientation   Fischer projection

Notes: (1) The first of the two types of Fischer projection should be used whenever convenient.

(2) If a Fischer projection formula is rotated through 180° in the plane of the paper, the upward and downward bonds from the central atom still project behind the plane of the paper, and the sideways bonds project in front of that plane. If, however, the formula is rotated through 90° in the plane of the paper, the upward and downward bonds now project in front of the plane of the paper and the sideways bonds project behind that plane.

E-7.2. To prepare a Newman projection, a molecule is viewed along the bond between two atoms; a circle is used to represent these atoms with lines from outside the circle toward its center to represent bonds to other atoms; the lines that represent bonds to the nearer and the further atom end at, respectively, the center and the circumference of the circle. When two such bonds would be coincident in the projection, they are drawn at a small angle to each other.[†]

---

*The lone pair of electrons (represented by two dots) on the nitrogen atoms are the unique substituents that decide the description of the conformation (these are the "phantom atoms" of the sequence-rule symbolism).

[†]Cf. Newman, M. S., *Rec. Chem. Progr.*, 13, 111 (1952); *J. Chem. Educ.*, 33, 344 (1955); *Steric Effects in Organic Chemistry*, John Wiley & Sons, New York, 1956, 5.

Examples:

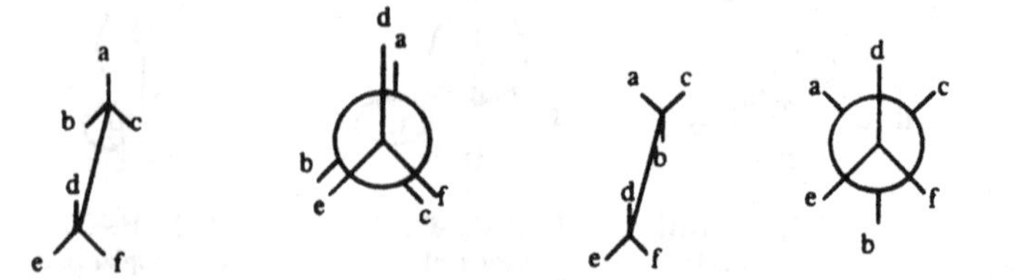

| Perspective | Newman projection | Perspective | Newman projection |

E-7.3. *General Note*; Formulas that display stereochemistry should be prepared with extra care so as to be unambiguous and, whenever possible, self-explanatory. It is inadvisable to try to lay down rules that will cover every case, but the following points should be borne in mind.

A thickened line (━) denotes a bond projecting from the plane of the paper toward an observer, a broken line (- - -) denotes a bond projecting away from an observer, and, when this convention is used, a full line of normal thickness (──) denotes a bond lying in the plane of the paper. A wavy line (∿) may be used to denote a bond whose direction cannot be specified or, if it is explained in the text, a bond whose direction it is not desired to specify in the formula. Dotted lines (· · · · · ·) should preferably not be used to denote stereochemistry, and never when they are used in the same paper to denote mesomerism, intermediate states, etc. Wedges should not be used as complement to broken lines (but see below). Single large dots have sometimes been used to denote atoms or groups attached at bridgehead positions and lying above the plane of the paper, with open circles to denote them lying below the plane of the paper, but this practice is strongly deprecated.

Hydrogen or other atoms or groups attached at sterically designated positions should never be omitted.

In chemical formulas, rings are usually drawn with lines of normal thickness, that is, as if they lay wholly in the plane of the paper even though this may be known not to be the case. In a formula such as (I) it is then clear that the H atoms attached at the A/B ring junction lie further from the observer than these bridgehead atoms, that the H atoms attached at the B/C ring junction lie nearer to the observer than those bridgehead atoms, and that X lies nearer to the observer than the neighboring atom of ring C.

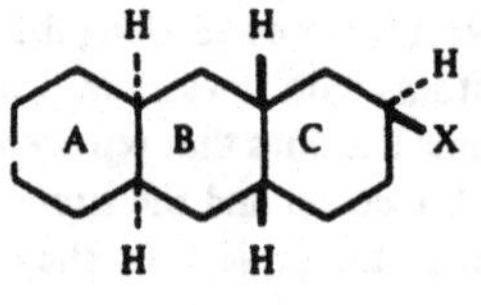

(I) 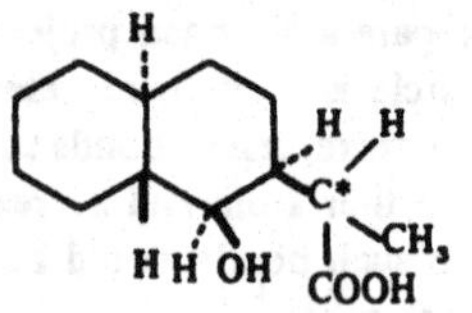   (II)

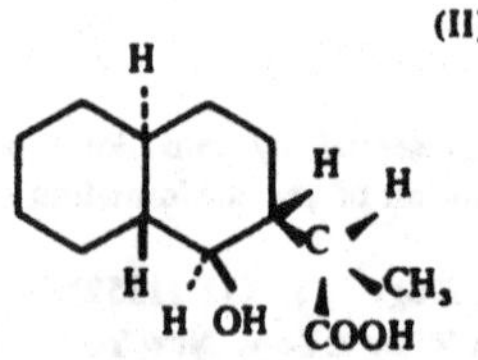

(III)

However, ambiguity can then sometimes arise, particularly when it is necessary to show stereochemistry within a group such as X attached to the rings that are drawn planar. For instance, in formula (II), the atoms O and C*, lying above the plane of the paper, are attached to ring B by thick bonds, but then, when showing the stereochemistry at C*, one finds that the bond *from* C* *to* ring B projects away from the observer and so should be a broken line. Such difficulties can be overcome by using wedges in place of lines, the broader end of the wedge being considered nearer to the observer, as in (III).

In some fields, notably for carbohydrates, rings are conveniently drawn as if they lay perpendicular to the plane of the paper, as represented in (IV); however, conventional formulas such as (V), with the lower bonds considered as the nearer to the observer, are so well established that is is rarely necessary to elaborate this to form (IV).

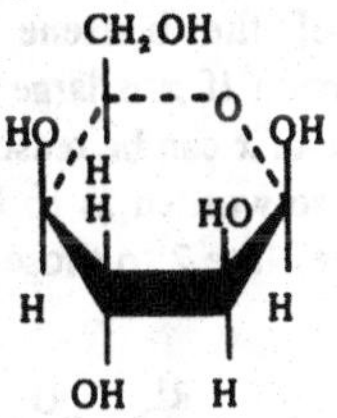

(IV) 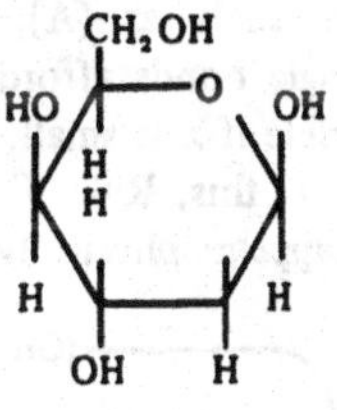   (V)

By a similar convention, in drawings such as (VI) and (VII), the lower sets of bonds are considered to be nearer than the upper to the observer. In (VII), note the gaps in the rear lines to indicate that the bonds crossing them pass in front (and thus obscure sections of the rear bonds). In some cases, when atoms have to be shown as lying in several planes, the various conventions may be combined, as in (VIII). In all cases the overriding aim should be clarity.

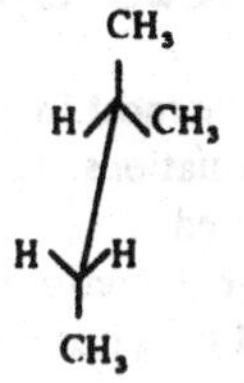

(VI) 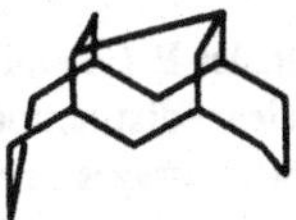   (VII) 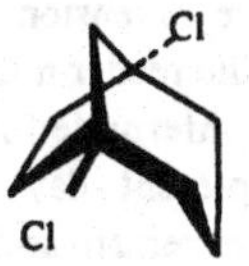   (VIII)

APPENDIX 1. CONFIGURATION AND CONFORMATION

See Rules E-1.4 and E-1.5.

Various definitions have been propounded to differentiate configurations from conformations.

The original usage was to consider as conformations those arrangements of the atoms of a molecule in space that can be interconverted by rotation(s) around a single bond, and as configurations those other arrangements whose interconversion by rotation requires bonds to be broken and then re-formed differently. Interconversion of different configurations will then be associated with substantial energies of activation, and the various species will be separable, but interconversion of different conformations will normally be associated with less activation energy, and the various species, if separable, will normally be more readily interconvertible. These differences in activation energy and stability are often large.

Nevertheless, rigid differentiation on such grounds meets formidable difficulties. Differentiation by energy criteria would require an arbitrary cut in a continuous series of values. Differentiation by stability of isolated species requires arbitrary assumptions about conditions and halflives. Differentiation on the basis of rotation around single bonds meets difficulties connected both with the concept of rotation and with the selection of single bonds as requisites, and these need more detailed discussion here.

Enantiomeric biaryls are nowadays usually considered to differ in conformation, any difficulty in rotation about the $1,1'$ bond due to steric hindrance between the neighboring groups being considered to be overcome by bond bending and/or bond stretching, even though the movements required must closely approach bond breaking if these substituents are very large. Similar doubts about the possibility of rotation occur with a molecule such as (A), where rotation of the benzene ring around the oxygen-to-ring single bonds affords easy interconversion if x is large but appears to be physically impossible if x is small; and no critical size of x can be reasonably established. For reasons such as this, Rules E-1.4 and E-1.5 are so worded as to be independent of whether rotation appears physically feasible or not (see Note 2 to those Rules).

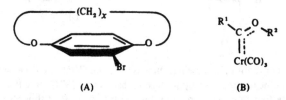

(A)   (B)

The second difficulty arises in the many cases where rotation is around a bond of fractional order between one and two, as in the helicenes, crowded aromatic molecules, metallocenes, amides, thioamides, and carbene-metal coordination compounds (such as B). The term conformation is customarily used in these cases and that appears a reasonable extension of the original conception, though it will be wise to specify the usage if the reader might be in doubt.

When interpreted in these ways, Rules E-1.4 and E-1.5 reflect the most frequent usage of the present day and provide clear distinctions in most situations. Nevertheless, difficulties remain and a number of other usages have been introduced.

It appears to some workers that once it is admitted that change of conformation may involve rotation about bonds of fractional order between one and two, it is then illogical to exclude rotation about classical double bonds because interconversion of open-chain *cis-trans* isomers depends on no fundamentally new principle and is often relatively easy, as for certain alkene derivatives such as stilbenes and for *azo* compounds, by irradiation. This extension is indeed not excluded by Rules E-1.4 and E-1.5, but if it is applied that fact should be explicitly stated.

A further interpretation is to regard a stereoisomer possessing some degree of stability (that is, one associated with an energy hollow, however shallow) as a configurational isomer, the other arrangements in space being termed conformational isomers; the term conformer (Rule E-6.1) is then superfluous. This definition, however, requires a knowledge of stability (energy relations) that is not always available.

In another view, a configurational isomer is any stereoisomer that can be isolated or (for some workers) whose existence can be established (for example, by physical methods); all other arrangements then represent conformational isomers; but it is then impossible to differentiate configuration from conformation without involving experimental efficiency or conditions of observation.

Yet another definition is to regard a conformation as a precise description of a configuration in terms of bond distances, bond angles, and dihedral angles.

In none of the above views except the last is attention paid to extension or contraction of the bond to an atom that is attached to only one other atom, such as –H or =O. Yet such changes in interatomic distance due to nonbonded interactions may be important, for instance, in hydrogen bonding, in differences due to crystal form, in association in solution, and in transition states. This area may repay further consideration.

Owing to the circumstances outlined above, the Rules E-1.4 and E-1.5 have been deliberately made imprecise, so as to permit some alternative interpretations, but they are not compatible with all the definitions mentioned above. The time does not seem ripe to legislate for other than the commoner usages or to choose finally between these. It is, however, encouraging that no definition in this field has (yet) involved atomic vibrations for which, in all cases, only time-average positions are considered.

Finally it should be noted that an important school of thought uses conformation with the connotation of "a particular geometry of the molecule, i.e., a description of atoms in space in terms of bond distances, bond angles, and dihedral angles," a definition much wider than any discussed above.

APPENDIX 2. OUTLINE OF THE SEQUENCE-RULE PROCEDURE

The sequence-rule procedure is a method of specifying the absolute molecular chirality (handedness) of a compound, that is, a method of specifying which of two enantiomeric forms each chiral element of a molecule exists. For each chiral element in the molecule it provides a symbol, usually R or S, which is independent of nomenclature and numbering. These symbols define the chirality of the specific compound considered; they may not be the same for a compound and some of its derivatives; and they are not necessarily constant for chemically similar situations within a chemical or a biogenetic class. The procedure is applied directly to a three-dimensional model of the structure, and not to any two-dimensional projection thereof.

The method has been developed to cover all compounds with ligancy up to four and with ligancy six,[*] and for all configurations and conformations of such compounds. The following is an outline confined to the most common situations; it is essential to study the original papers, especially the 1966 paper,[†] before using the sequence rule for other than fairly simple cases.

General Basis

The sequence rule itself is a method of arranging atoms or groups (including chains and rings) in an order of precedence, often referred to as an order of preference; for discussion this order can conveniently be generalized as a $>$ b $>$ c $>$ d, where $>$ denotes "is preferred to."

The first step, however, in considering a model is to identify the nature and position of each chiral element that it contains. There are three types of the chiral element, namely, the chiral center, the chiral axis, and the chiral plane. The chiral center, which is very much the most commonly met, is exemplified by an asymmetric carbon atom with the tetrahedral arrangement of ligands, as in (1). A chiral axis is present in, for instance, the chiral allenes such as (2) or the chiral biaryl derivatives. A chiral plane is exemplified by the plane containing the benzene ring and the bromine and oxygen atoms in the chiral compound (3), or by the underlined atoms in the cycloalkene (4). Clearly, more than one

---

[*]Ligancy refers to the number of bonds from an atom, independently of the nature of the bonds.
[†]Cahn, R. S., Ingold, C., and Prelog. V., *Angew. Chem. Int. Ed.*, 5, 385 (1966); errata, 5, 511 (1966); *Angew. Chem.*, 78, 413 (1966). Earlier papers: Cahn, R. S. and Ingold, C. K., *J. Chem. Soc.* (Lond.), 612 (1951); Cahn, R. S., Ingold, C., and Prelog, V., *Experientia*, 12, 81 (1956). For a partial, simplified account see Cahn, R. S., *J. Chem. Educ.*, 41, 116 (1964); errata, 41, 503 (1964).

type of chiral element may be present in one compound; for instance, group "a" in (2) migh be a *sec*-butyl group which contains a chiral center.

(1)   (2)

(3)   (4)

The Chiral Center

Let us consider first the simplest case, namely, a chiral center (such as carbon) with four ligands, a, b, c, and d, which are all different atoms tetrahedrally arranged as in CHFClBr. The four ligands are arranged in order of preference by means of the sequence rule; this contains five subrules, which are applied in succession so far as necessary to obtain a decision. The first subrule is all that is required in a great majority of actual cases; it states that ligands are arranged in order of decreasing atomic number, in the above case (a) Br > (b) Cl > (c) F > (d) H. There would be two (enantiomeric) forms of the compound and we can write these as (5) and (6). In the sequence-rule procedure the model is viewed from the side remote from the least-preferred ligand (d), as illustrated. Then, tracing a path from a to b to c in (5) gives a clockwise course, which is symbolized by (R) (Latin *rectus*, right; for right hand); in (6) it gives an anticlockwise course, symbolized as (S) (Latin *sinister*, left). Thus (5) would be named (R)-bromochlorofluoromethane, and (6) would be named (S)-bromochlorofluoromethane. Here already it may be noted that converting one enantiomer into another changes each R to S, and each S to R, always. It will be seen also that the chirality prefix is the same whether the alphabetical order is used, as above, for naming the substituents or whether this is done by the order of complexity (giving fluorochlorobromomethane).

(5), (R)   (6), (S)

Next, suppose we have $H_3C-CHClF$. We deal first with the atoms directly attached to the chiral center; so the four ligands to be considered are Cl > F > C (of CH_3) > H. Here the H's of the CH_3 are not concerned, because we do not need them in order to assign our symbol.

However, atoms directly attached to a center are often identical, as, for example, the underlined C's in $H_3\underline{C}-CHCl-\underline{C}H_2OH$. For such a compound we at once establish a preference (a) Cl > (b, c) $\underline{C},\underline{C}$ > (d) H. Then to decide between the two $\underline{C}$'s we work outward, to the atoms to which they in turn are directly attached and we then find which we can conveniently write as C(H,H,H) and C(O,H,H). We have to compare H,H,H with O,H,H, and since oxygen has a higher atomic number than hydrogen we have O > H and thence the complete order Cl > C (of CH_2OH) > C (of CH_3) > H, so that the chirality symbol can then be determined from the three-dimensional model.

$$-\underset{\underset{H}{\diagdown}}{\overset{\overset{H}{\diagup}}{C}}-H \quad \text{and} \quad -\underset{\underset{H}{\diagdown}}{\overset{\overset{O}{\diagup}}{C}}-H$$

We must next meet the first complication. Suppose that we have a molecule (7).

$$\text{(b) } H_3C-\underline{C}HCl-\underset{\underset{H \text{ (d)}}{|}}{\overset{\overset{Cl \text{ (a)}}{|}}{C}}-\underline{C}HF-OH \text{ (c)}$$

(7) (S)

To decide between the two C's we first arrange the atoms attached to them in *their* order of preference, which gives $\underline{C}$(Cl,C,H) on the left and $\underline{C}$(F,O,H) on the right. Then we compare the preferred atom of one set (namely, Cl) with the preferred atom (F) of the other set, and as Cl > F we arrive at the preferences a > b > c > d shown in (7) and chirality (S). If, however, we had a compound (8) we should have met $\underline{C}$(Cl,C,H) and $\underline{C}$(Cl,O,H) and, since the atoms of first preference are identical (Cl), we should have had to make the comparisons with the atoms of second preference, namely, O > C, which to the different chirality (R) as shown in (8).

$$\text{(c) } H_3C-\underline{C}HCl-\underset{\underset{H \text{ (d)}}{|}}{\overset{\overset{Cl \text{ (a)}}{|}}{C}}-\underline{C}HCl-OH \text{ (b)}$$

(8) (R)

Branched ligands are treated similarly. Setting them out in full gives a picture that at first sight looks complex but the treatment is in fact simple. For instance, in compound (9) a first quick glance again shows (a) Cl > (b, c) $\underline{C},\underline{C}$ > (d) H: When we expand the two $\underline{C}$'s we find they are both $\underline{C}$(C,C,H), so we continue exploration. Considering first the left-hand ligand we arrange the branches and their sets of atoms in order thus: C(Cl,H,H) > C(H,H,H). On the right-hand side we have C(O,$\underline{C}$,H) > C(O,$\underline{H}$,H) (because $\underline{C}$ > $\underline{H}$). We compare first the preferred of these branches from each side and we find C(Cl,H,H) > C(O,C,H) because Cl > O, and that gives the left-hand branch preference over the right-hand branch. That is all we need to do to establish chirality (S) for this highly branched compound (9). Note that it is immaterial here that, for the lower branches, the right-hand C(O,H,H) would have been preferred to the left-hand C(H,H,H); we did not need to reach that point in our comparisons and so we are not concerned with it; but we should have reached it if the two top (preferred) branches had both been the same CH_2Cl.

Rings, when we met during outward exploration, are treated in the same way as branched chains.

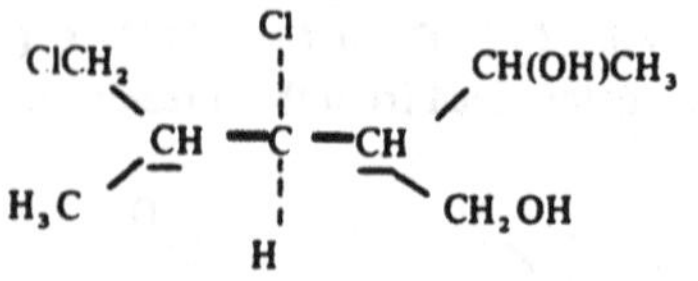

(9)

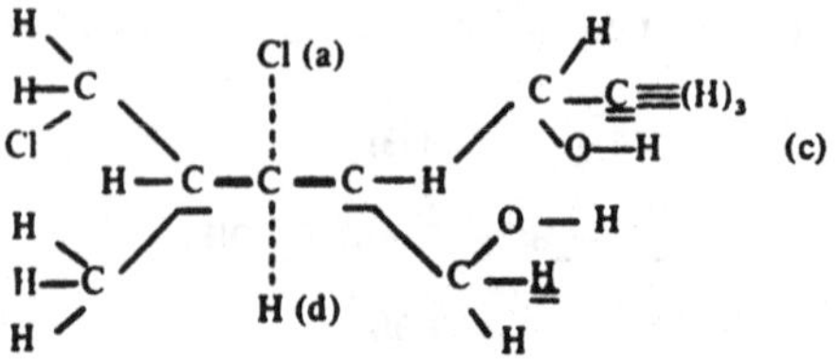

(9) (*S*)

With these simple procedures alone, quite complex structures can be handled; for instance, the analysis alongside Formula (10) for natural morphine explains why the specification is as shown. The reason for considering C-12 as C(C,C,C) is set out in the next paragraphs.

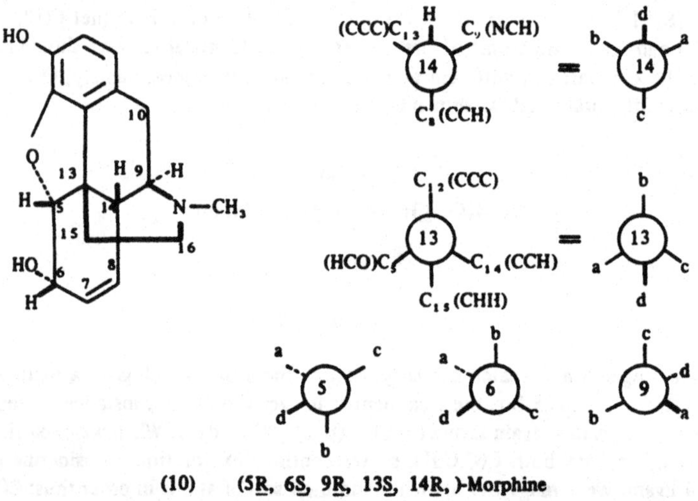

(10)   (5$\underline{R}$, 6$\underline{S}$, 9$\underline{R}$, 13$\underline{S}$, 14$\underline{R}$,)-Morphine

Now, using the sequence rule depends on exploring along bonds. To avoid theoretical arguments about the nature of bonds, simple classical forms are used. Double and triple bonds are split into two and three bonds, respectively. A $>$C=O group is treated as (i) (below) where the (O) and the (C) are duplicate representations of the atoms at the other end of the double bond. —C≡CH is treated as (ii) and —C≡N is treated as (iii).

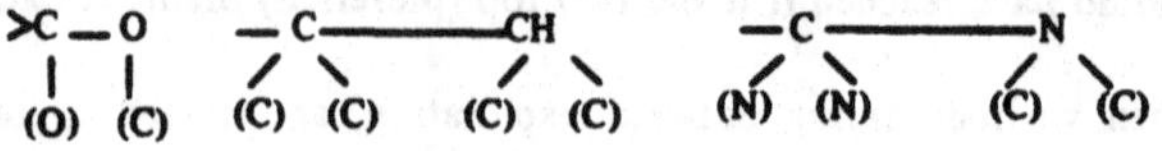

(i)   (ii)   (iii)

Thus in D-glyceraldehyde (11) the CHO group is treated as C(O,(O),H) and is thus preferred to the C(O,H,H) of the CH$_2$OH group, so that the chirality symbol is (R).

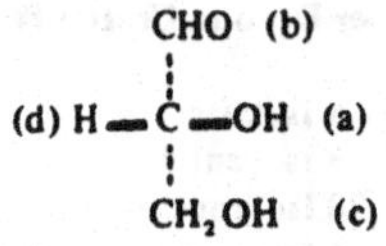

CHO (b)

(d) H —— C —— OH (a)

CH$_2$OH (c)

D-Glyceraldehyde
(11) (R)

Only the doubly bonded atoms themselves are duplicated, and not the atoms or groups attached to them; the duplicated atoms may thus be considered as carrying three phantom atoms (see below) of atomic number zero. This may be important in deciding preferences in certain complicated cases.

Aromatic rings are treated as Kekulé structures. For aromatic hydrocarbon rings it is immaterial which Kekulé structure is used because "splitting" the double bonds gives the same result in all cases; for instance, for phenyl the result can be represented as (12a) where "(6)" denotes the atomic number of the duplicate representations of carbon.

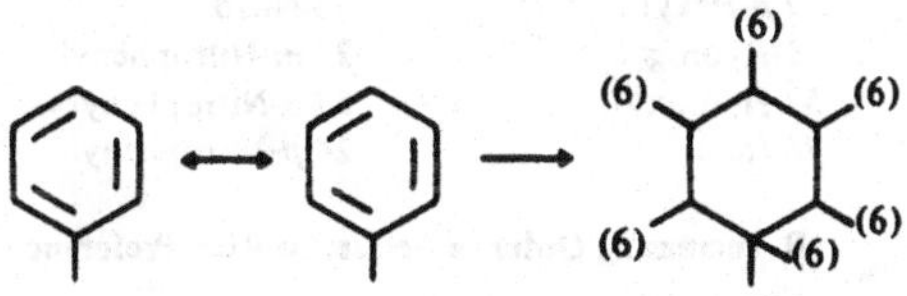

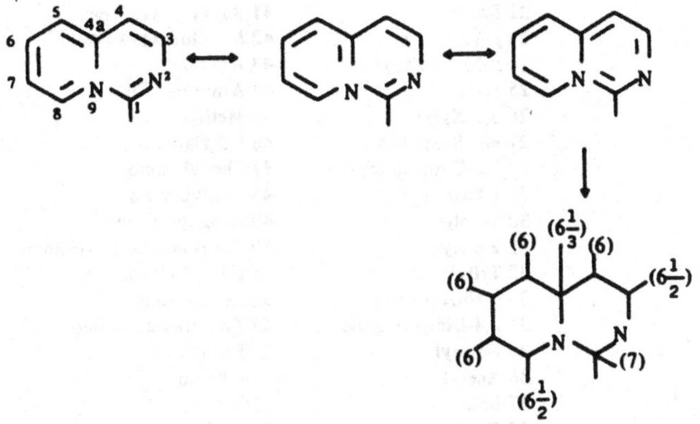

For aromatic hetero rings, each duplicate is given an atomic number that is the mean of what it would have if the double bond were located at each of the possible positions. A complex case is illustrated in (13). Here C-1 is doubly bonded to one or other of the nitrogen atoms (atomic number 7) and never to carbon, so its added duplicate has atomic number 7; C-3 is doubly bonded either to C-4 (atomic number 6) or to N-2 (atomic number 7), so its added duplicate has atomic number 6½; so has that of C-8; but C-4a may be doubly bonded to C-4, C-5, or N-9, so its added duplicate has atomic number 6.33.

One last point about the chiral center may be added here. Except for hydrogen, ligancy, if not already four, is made up to four by adding "phantom atoms" which have atomic number zero and are thus always last in order of preference. This has various uses but perhaps the most interesting is where nitrogen occurs in a rigid skeleton, as, for example, in α-isosparteine (14). Here the phantom atom can be placed where the nitrogen

SOME COMMON GROUPS IN ORDER OF SEQUENCE-RULE PREFERENCE[a]

A. Alphabetical Order (Higher Number Denotes Greater Preference)

64 Acetoxy	38 Carboxyl	9 Isobutyl	55 Nitroso
36 Acetyl	74 Chloro	8 Isopentyl	6 *n*-Pentyl
48 Acetylamino	17 Cyclohexyl	20 Isopropenyl	61 Phenoxy
21 Acetylenyl	52 Diethylamino	14 Isopropyl	22 Phenyl
10 Allyl	51 Dimethylamino	69 Mercapto	47 Phenylamino
43 Amino	34 2,4-Dinitrophenyl	58 Methoxy	54 Phenylazo
44 Ammonio $^+H_3N-$	28 3,5-Dinitrophenyl	39 Methoxycarbonyl	18 Propenyl
37 Benzoyl	59 Ethoxy	2 Methyl	4 *n*-Propyl
49 Benzoylamino	40 Ethoxycarbonyl	45 Methylamino	29 1-Propynyl
65 Benzoyloxy	3 Ethyl	71 Methylsulfinyl	12 2-Propynyl
50 Benzyloxycarbonylamino	46 Ethylamino	66 Methylsulfinyloxy	73 Sulfo
13 Benzyl	68 Fluoro	72 Methylsulfonyl	25 *m*-Tolyl
60 Benzyloxy	35 Formyl	67 Methylsulfonyloxy	30 *o*-Tolyl
41 Benzyloxycarbonyl	63 Formyloxy	70 Methylthio	23 *p*-Tolyl
75 Bromo	62 Glycosyloxy	11 Neopentyl	53 Trimethylammonio
42 *ter*-Butoxycarbonyl	7 *n*-Hexyl	56 Nitro	32 Trityl
5 *n*-Butyl	1 Hydrogen	27 *m*-Nitrophenyl	15 Vinyl
16 *sec*-Butyl	57 Hydroxy	33 *o*-Nitrophenyl	31 2,6-Xylyl
19 *tert*-Butyl	76 Iodo	24 *p*-Nitrophenyl	26 3,5-Xylyl

B. Increasing Order of Sequence Rule Preference

1 Hydrogen	20 Isopropenyl	39 Methoxycarbonyl[b]	58 Methoxy
2 Methyl	21 Acetylenyl	40 Ethoxycarbonyl[b]	59 Ethoxy
3 Ethyl	22 Phenyl	41 Benzyloxycarbonyl[b]	60 Benzyloxy
4 *n*-Propyl	23 *p*-Tolyl	42 *tert*-Butoxycarbonyl[b]	61 Phenoxy
5 *n*-Butyl	24 *p*-Nitrophenyl	43 Amino	62 Glycosyloxy
6 *n*-Pentyl	25 *m*-Tolyl	44 Ammonio $^+H_3N-$	63 Formyloxy
7 *n*-Hexyl	26 3,5-Xylyl	45 Methylamino	64 Acetoxy
8 Isopentyl	27 *m*-Nitrophenyl	46 Ethylamino	65 Benzoyloxy
9 Isobutyl	28 3,5-Dinitrophenyl	47 Phenylamino	66 Methylsulfinyloxy
10 Allyl	29 1-Propynyl	48 Acetylamino	67 Methylsulfonyloxy
11 Neopentyl	30 *o*-Tolyl	49 Benzoylamino	68 Fluoro
12 2-Propynyl	31 2,6-Xylyl	50 Benzyloxycarbonylamino	69 Mercapto HS-
13 Benzyl	32 Trityl	51 Dimethylamino	70 Methylthio CH_3S-
14 Isopropyl	33 *o*-Nitrophenyl	52 Diethylamino	71 Methylsulfinyl
15 Vinyl	34 2,4-Dinitrophenyl	53 Trimethylammonio	72 Methylsulfonyl
16 *sec*-Butyl	35 Formyl	54 Phenylazo	73 Sulfo HO_3S-
17 Cyclohexyl	36 Acetyl	55 Nitroso	74 Chloro
18 1-Propenyl	37 Benzoyl	56 Nitro	75 Bromo
19 *tert*-Butyl	38 Carboxyl	57 Hydroxy	76 Iodo

[a]ANY alteration to structure, or substitution, etc., may alter the order of preference.
[b]These groups are ROC(=O)–.

lone pair of electrons is; then N-1 appears as shown alongside the formula; and the chirality (*R*) is the consequence. The same applies to N-16. Phantom atoms are similarly used when assigning chirality symbols to chiral sulfoxides (see example to Rule E-5.9).

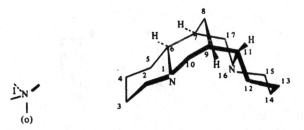

(14) (1R, 6R, 7S, 9S, 11R, 16R)-Sparteine

Symbolism

In names of compounds, the R and S symbols, together with their locants, are placed in parentheses, normally in front of the name, as shown for morphine (10) and sparteine (14), but this may be varied in indexes or in languages other than English. Positions within names are required, however, when more than a single series of numerals is used, as for esters and amines. When relative stereochemistry is more important than absolute stereochemistry, as for steroids or carbohydrates, a local system of stereochemical designation may be more useful and sequence-rule symbols need then be used only for any situations where the local system is insufficient.

Racemates containing a single center are labeled (RS). If there is more than one center the first is labeled (RS) and the others are (RS) or (SR) according to whether they are R or S when the first is R. For instance, the 2,4-pentanediols CH_3–CH(OH)–CH_2– CH(OH)–CH_3 are differentiated as

one chiral form (2R,4R)–
other chiral form (2S,4S)–
meso compound (2R,4S)–
racemic compound (2RS,4RS)–

Finally the principles by which some of the least rare of other situations are treated will be very briefly summarized.

Pseudoasymmetric Atoms

A subrule decrees that R groups have preference over S groups and this permits pseudoasymmetric atoms, as in abC(c-R)(c-S) to be treated in the same way as chiral centers, but as such a molecule is achiral (not optically active) it is given the lower case symbol r or s.

Chiral Axis

The structure is regarded as an elongated tetrahedron and viewed along the axis – it is immaterial from which end it is viewed; the nearer pair of ligands receives the first two positions in the order of preference, as shown in (15) and (16).

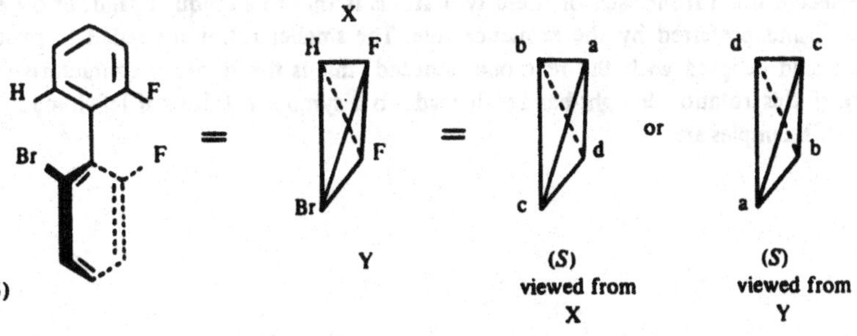

(15)

(S)
viewed from
X

(S)
viewed from
Y

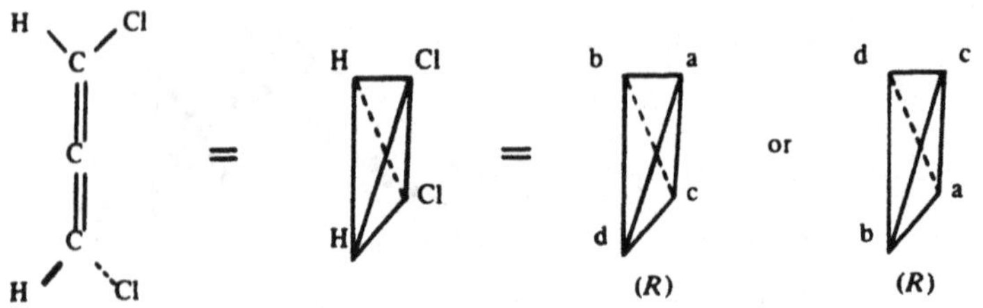

(16)

Chiral Plane

The sequence-rule-preferred atom directly attached to the plane is chosen as "pilot atom." In compound (3) this is the C of the left-hand CH₂ group. Now this is attached to the left-hand oxygen atom in the plane. The sequence-rule-preferred path from this oxygen atom is then explored in the plane until a rotation is traced which is clockwise (*R*) or anticlockwise (*S*) when viewed from the pilot atom. In (3) this path is O → C → C(Br) and it is clockwise (*R*).

Other Subrules

Other subrules cater for new chirality created by isotopic labeling (higher mass number preferred to lower) and for steric differences in the ligands. Isotopic labeling rarely changes symbols allotted to other centers.

Octahedral Structures

Extensions of the sequence rule enable ligands arranged octahedrally to be placed in an order of preference, including polydentate ligands, so that a chiral structure can then always be represented as one of the enantiomeric forms (17) and (18). The face 1–2–3 is observed from the side remote from the face 4–5–6 (as marked by arrows), and the path 1 → 2 → 3 is observed; in (17) this path is clockwise (R), and in (18) it is anticlockwise (S).

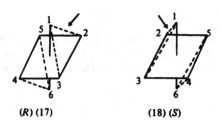

(R) (17)   (18) (S)

Conformations

The torsion angle between selected bonds from two singly bonded atoms is considered. The selected bond from each of these two atoms is that to a unique ligand, or otherwise to the ligand preferred by the sequence rule. The smaller rotation needed to make the front ligand eclipsed with the rear one is noted (this is the rotatory characteristic of a helix); if this rotation is right-handed it leads to a symbol *P* (plus); if left-handed to *M* (minus). Examples are

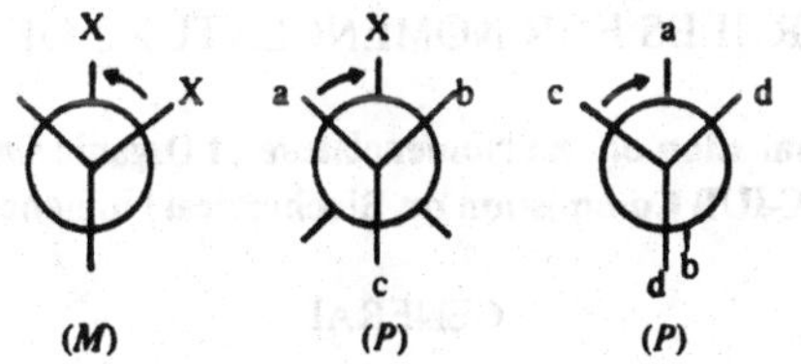

(M)   (P)   (P)

Details and Complications

For details and complicating factors the original papers should be consulted. They include treatment of compounds with high symmetry or containing repeating units (e.g., cyclitols), also π bonding (metallocenes, etc.), mesomeric compounds and mesomeric radicals, and helical and other secondary structures.

DEFINITIVE RULES FOR NOMENCLATURE OF STEROIDS*

IUPAC Commission on the Nomenclature of Organic Chemistry and
IUPAC-IUB Commission on Biochemical Nomenclature

GENERAL

Rule 2S–1 (Expanded from Rules S–1 and S–2)

1.1. Steroids are numbered and rings are lettered as in Formula (1). If one of the two methyl groups attached to C-25 is substituted it is assigned the lower

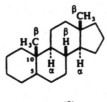

(1)

number (26); if both are substituted, that carrying the substituent cited first in the alphabetical order is assigned the lower number [cf. IUPAC Rule** C–15.11(e)]. For trimethyl steroids see Rule 2S–2.3, Note c.

1.2. If one or more of the carbon atoms shown in (1) is not present and a steroid name is used, the numbering of the remainder is undisturbed.

1.3. For a steroid the name, including stereochemical affixes, and its structural formula (see Rule 2S–1.4), denote the absolute configuration at each asymmetric center (see also Rule 2S–1.5). When the configuration at one or more centers is not known, this is indicated by Greek letter(s) ξ (xi) prefixed by the appropriate numeral(s).

(2)

1.4. When the rings of a steroid are denoted as projections on to the plane of the paper the formula is normally to be oriented as in (2). An atom or group attached to a ring depicted as in the orientation (2) is termed α(alpha) if it lies below the plane of the paper or β(beta) if it lies above the plane of the paper. In formulas, bonds to atoms or groups lying below the plane of the paper are shown as broken (—————) lines, and bonds to atoms or groups lying above the plane of the paper are shown as solid lines preferably thickened (————). Bonds to atoms or groups whose configuration is not known are denoted by wavy lines (∿∿∿).

---

*From IUPAC Commission on the Nomenclature of Organic Chemistry and IUPAC-IUB Commission on Biochemical Nomenclature, *Pure Appl. Chem.*, 31, 283–322 (1972). With permission.

**IUPAC Nomenclature of Organic Chemistry, Sections A, B, and C, Butterworths, London, 1971.

Notes: (1) Projections of steroid formulas should not be oriented as in Formula (3), (4), or (5) unless circumstances make it obligatory.

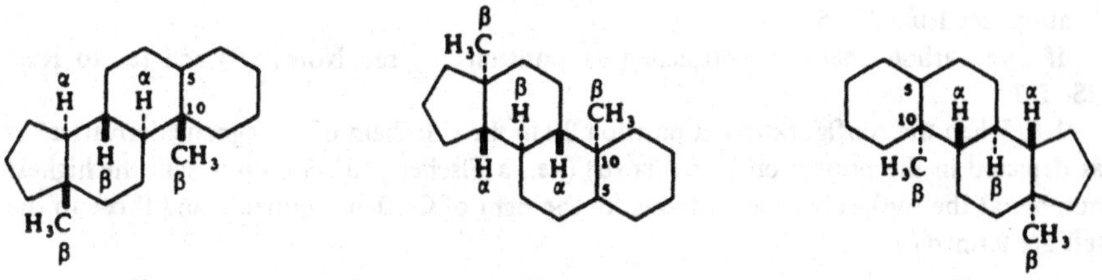

$$\beta$$
$$H_3C$$

(structures shown)

(3)   (4)   (5)

(2) With the preferred orientation (2), and with (3), α bonds appear as broken lines and β bonds as solid (thickened) lines. The reverse is true for (4) and (5). Wavy lines denote ξ bonds for all orientations of the formula.

(3) A perspective representation of the stereochemistry of Formula (2) as in (2a) or (2b) may also be used.

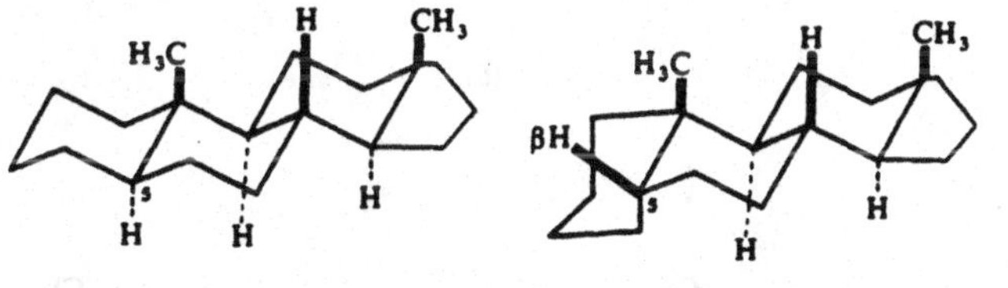

(2a)
A 5α-steroid

(2b)
A 5β-steroid

(For the significance of the prefixes 5 α- and 5 β- see Rule 2S-1.5.)

When steroid formulas are drawn in this way, bonds pointing upwards are, by convention, drawn bold and bonds pointing downwards are drawn broken; these representations correspond to the β and α bonds of projection formulas such as (2) and do not conform to the general practice that bold and broken lines denote bonds projecting, respectively, above and below the plane of the paper. Note, however, that the general practice is followed with chair and boat forms of spirostans (see Rule 2S-3.3).

(4) All hydrogen atoms and methyl groups attached at ring-junction positions must always be inserted as H and CH_3, respectively (Me may be used in place of CH_3 if editorial conventions require it). The practice, sometimes followed, of denoting methyl groups by bonds without lettering is liable to cause confusion and should be abandoned. This is essential in view of customs in other fields and applies also to other groups of compounds such as cyclic terpenes and alkaloids for which steroid conventions are commonly used.

1.5 Unless implied or stated to the contrary (see Rules 2S-3, 2S-4.3, 2S-5, and 2S-11), use of a steroid name implies that atoms or groups attached at the ring-junction positions 8, 9, 10, 13, and 14 are oriented as shown in Formula (2) (i.e., 8β, 9α, 10β, 13β, 14α), and a carbon chain attached at position 17 is assumed to be β-oriented (see Notes below). The configuration of hydrogen (or a substituent) at the ring-junction position 5 is always to be designated by adding α, β, or ξ after the numeral 5, this numeral and letter being placed immediately before the stem name. The configuration of substituents attached at other centers of asymmetry in the tetracyclic system A–D is stated by adding α, β, or ξ after the respective numerals denoting their position.

Notes: For the purpose of this Rule a carboxyl group at position 17 is not considered to constitute a carbon "chain" (for the nomenclature used see Rule 2S–4.3). For pentacyclic and hexacyclic derivatives see Rule 2S–3, and for stereochemical modifications see Rule 2S–5.

If two carbon chains are attached at position 17, see Notes (d) and (e) to Rule 2S–2.3.

1.6. When the configuration at position 20 in the sidechain of a pregnane derivative* is as depicted in the projection Formula (6) (i.e., a Fischer projection but with the highest number at the top), substituents shown to the right of C-20 are termed α and those to the left are termed β.

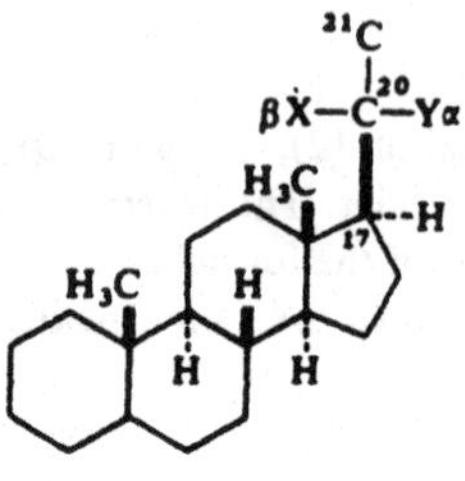

(6)

Examples:

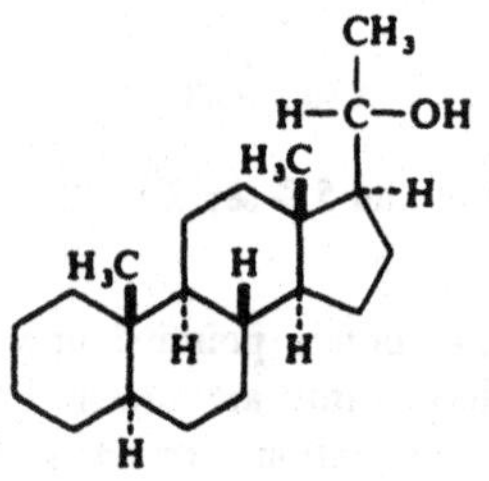

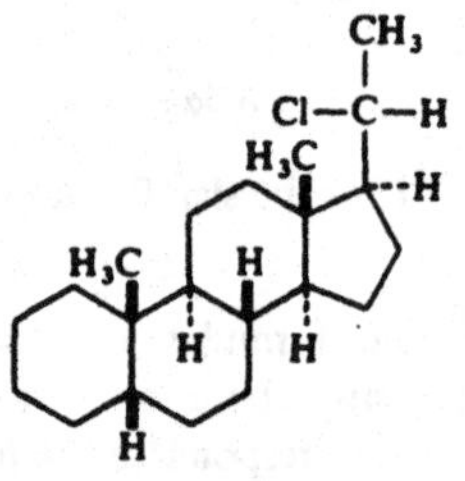

(7)
5α-Pregnan-20α-ol*

(8)
20β-Chloro-5β-pregnane*

Notes: (1) The 20α/20β-nomenclature is continued because of long tradition. When a longer sidechain is present at C-17 the sequence-rule procedure[†] is more generally convenient (see Rule 2S–1.7) and it may also be used to designate stereochemistry at C-20 in pregnanes, being particularly useful for 20-substituents that may cyclize with a substituent at another position [e.g., carboxylic acids as in Example (12)]. For 20-hydroxy-, 20-alkoxy-, 20-acyloxy-, 20-amino-, and 20-halogeno- derivatives of pregnane without a substituent on C-17 or C-21, 20α- is equivalent to (20S)-, and 20β- to (20R)-; however, these equivalences are sometimes reversed when additional substituents are present, e.g., on C-17 or C-21, and in such cases the references below[†] should be consulted.

*For the name "pregnane" see Rule 2S–2.3.
[†]Cahn, R. S., Ingold, C. K., and Prelog, V., *Angew. Chem. Int. Ed.*, 5, 385 (1966); *Angew. Chem.*, 78, 413 (1966); for a partial simplified account see Cahn, R. S., *J. Chem. Educ.*, 41, 116 (1964). See also IUPAC 1968 Tentative Rules for the Nomenclature of Organic Chemistry, Sections E, Fundamental Stereochemistry, *IUPAC Inf. Bull.*, No. 35, 71 (1969).

(2) When stereochemistry at C-20 is denoted by a Fischer-type projection, as in (6) to (11) or for cardenolides as (37) or bufanolides as (43), the 17,20-bond is preferably denoted by an ordinary line; the stereochemistry at C-17 is then

$$^{21}CH_3$$

$$H-^{20}C-OH \qquad but \qquad H-C-OH \qquad although \qquad H-C-OH$$

(9)	(10)	(11)
20α-ol (20S)	20α,21-diol (20R)	17,20α,21-triol (20S)

(12)	(13)
(20S)-16β-Hydroxypregnane-20-carboxylic acid lactone (≡ 20α)	(20S)-18,20-Epoxypregnane (≡ 20α)

adequately denoted by a thick or a broken bond to the H or to the other substituent (e.g., OH) at position 17. In such formulas, representing the 17,20-bond by a thick or a broken line cannot be correct for both C-17 and C-20; this has, however, frequently been done, then involving the additional convention that the way in which this bond is written is neglected when considering the stereochemistry at C-20.

1.7. The stereochemistry at C-20 and other positions in steroid sidechains longer than ethyl is described by the sequence-rule procedure.[†]

Examples:

(14)	(15)
(24R)-24-Methyl-5α-cholestan-3β-ol[*] (formerly 24α-methyl) (trivial name: campestanol)	(24S)-24-Methyl-5α-cholestan-3β-ol[**] (formerly 24β-methyl) (trivial name: ergostanol)

[†]Cahn, R. S., Ingold, C. K., and Prelog, V., Angew. Chem. Int., Ed., 5, 385(1966); Angew. Chem., 78, 413 (1966); for a partial simplified account see Cahn, R. S., J. Chem. Educ., 41, 116 (1964). See also IUPAC 1968 Tentative Rules for the Nomenclature of Organic Chemistry, Sections E, Fundamental Stereochemistry, IUPAC Inf. Bull., No. 35, 71, (1969).
[*]For the name "cholestane" see Rule 2S–2.3. These systematic names are preferred to the trivial names given below them.

Notes: (1) The sequence-rule procedure is also used when the sidechain is cyclized (see Rules 2S–3.3 and 2S–3.4).

(2) The backbone of a 17-side chain is best denoted as in the plane of the paper (lines of ordinary thickness), the 17,20-bond being similarly denoted. Except for pregnane derivatives, stereochemistry due to substituents on the chain is then indicated by the customary thick or broken lines denoting bonds that project, respectively, above and below the plane of the paper.

FUNDAMENTAL CARBOCYCLES

Rule 2S–2 (Expanded from Rules S–3.1 to S–3.5)

2.1. The parent tetracyclic hydrocarbon without methyl groups at C-10 and C-13 and without a sidechain at C-17 is named "gonane."

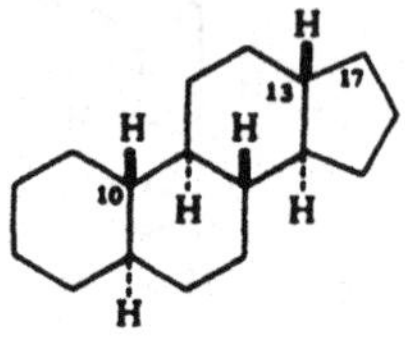

(16)	(17)
5α-Gonane	5β-Gonane

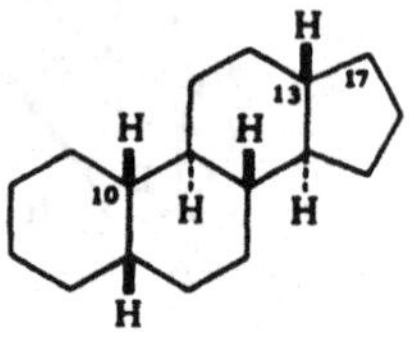

2.2. The hydrocarbon with a methyl group at C-13 but without a methyl group at C-10 and without a sidechain at C-17 is named "estrane."

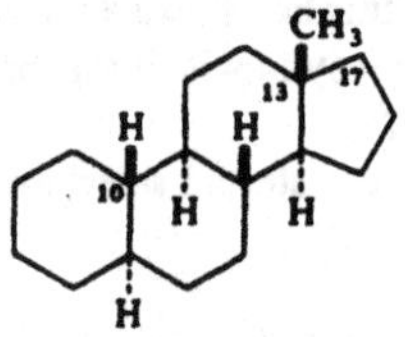

(18)	(19)
5α-Estrane	5β-Estrane

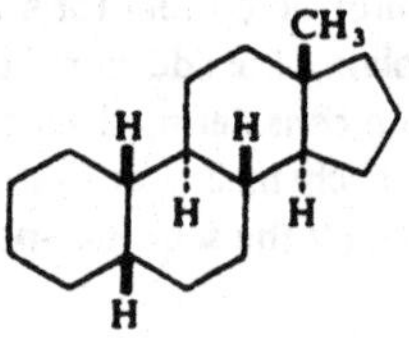

Note: Names of compounds having a methyl group attached to C-10 and a hydrogen atom attached to C-13 are to be based on 18-norandrostane (see Rules 2S–2.3 and 2S–6.1) and not on 10-methylgonane.

2.3. The following names are used for the hydrocarbons (20) and (21) with methyl groups at both C-10 and C-13.

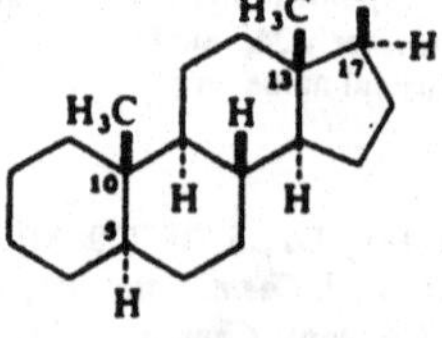

(20)	(21)

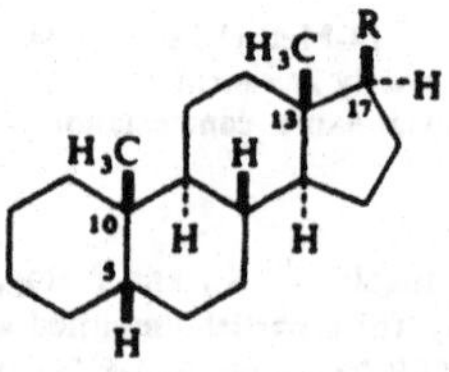

R	(20) 5α-Series	(21) 5β-Series
H	5α-Androstane	5β-Androstane (*not* testane)
C₂H₅	5α-Pregnane (*not* allopregnane)	5β-Pregnane
CH(CH₃)CH₂CH₂CH₃ *	5α-Cholane (*not* allocholane)	5β-Cholane
CH(CH₃)CH₂CH₂CH₂CH(CH₃)₂ *	5α-Cholestane	5β-Cholestane (*not* coprostane)
CH(CH₃)CH₂CH₂$\overset{24†}{CH}$(CH₃)CH(CH₃)₂ *	5α-Ergostane	5β-Ergostane
CH(CH₃)CH₂CH₂$\overset{24‡}{CH}$(C₂H₅)CH(CH₃)₂ *	5α-Stigmastane	5β-Stigmastane

*20R Configuration.
†24S Configuration.
‡24R Configuration.

Notes: (a) Unsaturation and substituents are denoted in the names of steroids by the usual methods of organic chemistry (cf. Rule 2S–4). Examples (22) to (25) illustrate some simple cases.

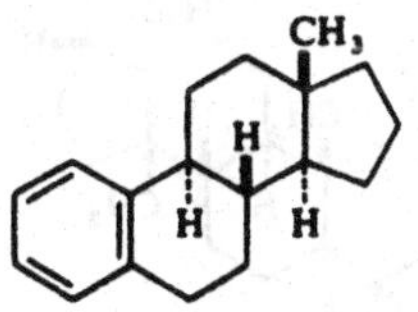

(22)

1,3,5(10)-Estratriene

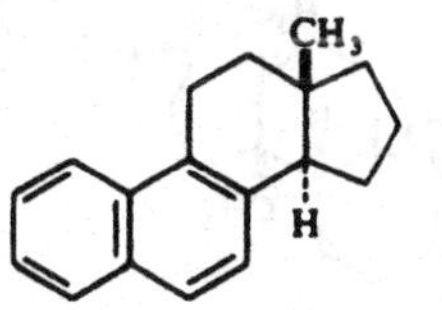

(23)

1,3,5(10),6,8-Estrapentaene

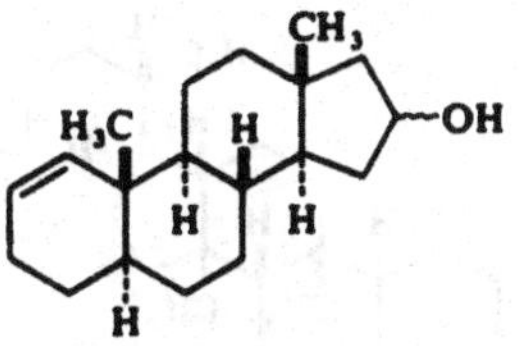

(24)

5α-Androst-1-en-16ξ-ol

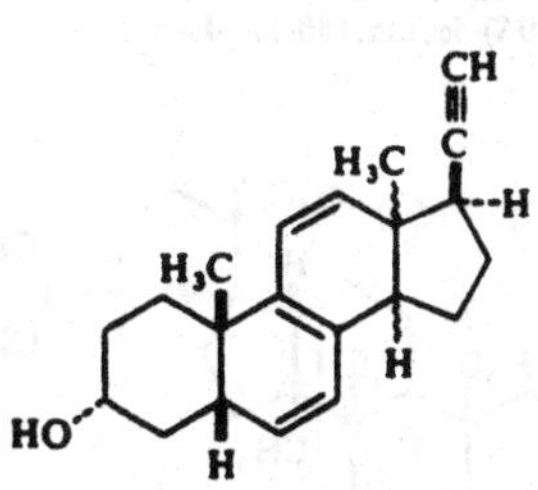

(25)

5β,13ξ,14ξ-Pregna-6,8,11-trien-20-yn-3α-ol

(b) The names "cholane," "cholestane," "ergostane," and "stigmastane" imply the configuration at C-20 shown in partial Formula (26); this is (20R) except for some derivatives containing additional substituents (cf. Notes to Rule 2S–1.6).

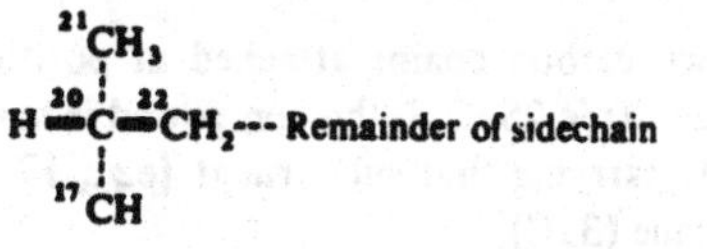

(26)

(c) Tetracyclic triterpenoids may be regarded as trimethyl steroids, the three additional methyl groups being numbered 30 (attached to C-4 with α configuration), 31 (attached to C-4 with β configuration), and 32 (attached to C-14); for example, 5α-lanostane (27) is 4,4,14α-trimethyl-5α-cholestane, the former name implying 14α, 20R configuration. Trivial names are common in this series of compounds, and some are illustrated in Examples (27) to (31A).

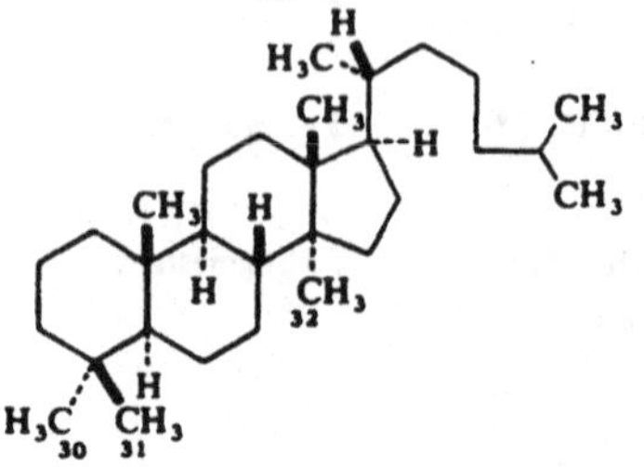

(27)

5α-Lanostane

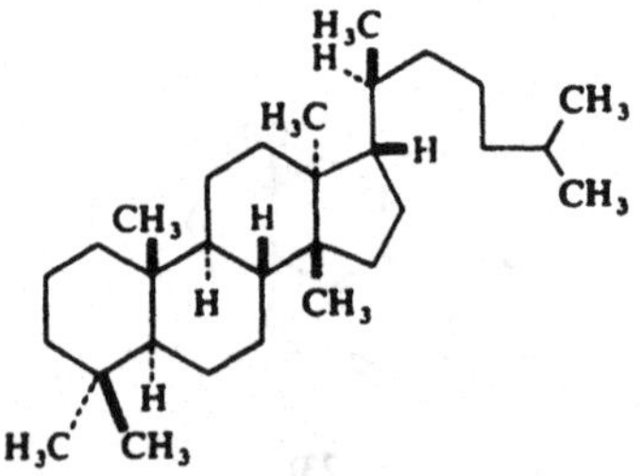

(28)

5α-Tirucallane
(20S)-5α,13α,14β,17α-Lanostane

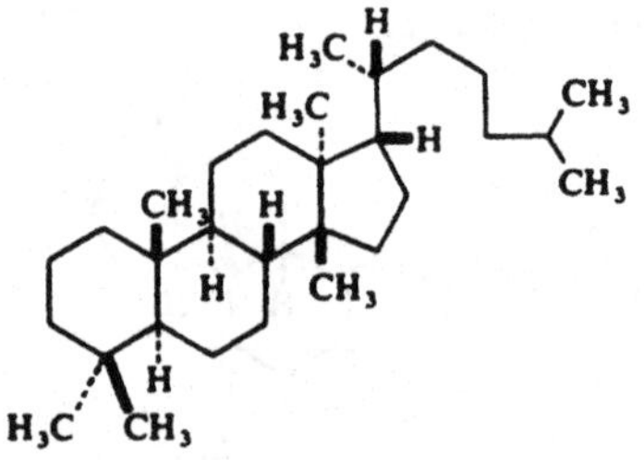

(29)

5α-Euphane
5α,13α,14β,17α-Lanostane
(20R implied in the name)

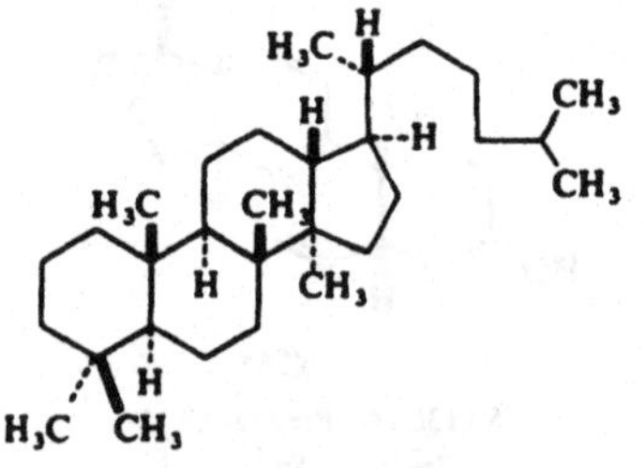

(30)

5α-Dammarane
8-Methyl-18-nor-5α-Lanostane (all configurations except ·5α are implied in the name)

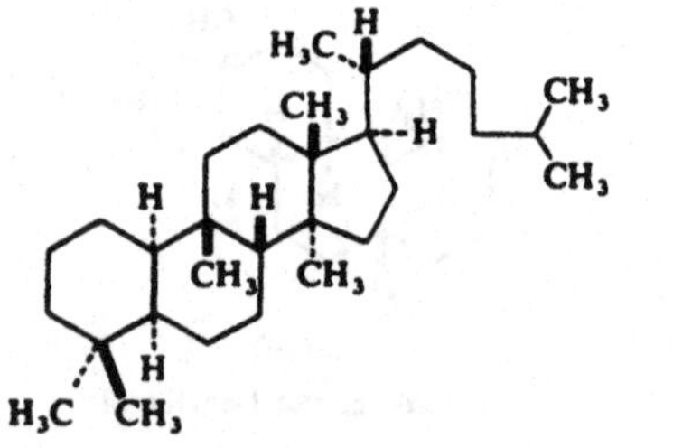

(31)

5α-Cucurbitane
19(10→9β)*abeo*-5α,10α-Lanostane (for the *abeo* nomenclature see Rule 2S–9)

(d) If a steroid has two carbon chains attached at position 17 and one of them is included in the table under Rule 2S–2.3, the compound is named as a 17-alkyl derivative of the steroid in the table carrying that substituent [e.g., 17-methyl-5α-pregnane (31B); 17-propyl-5α, 17α-cholestane (31C)].

(e) If a steroid has two carbon chains attached at position 17, neither of which is included in the table under Rule 2S–2.3, the compound is named as a 17,17-disubstituted androstane [e.g., 17,17-dimethyl-5α-androstane, (31D); 17α-methyl-17β-propyl-5α-androstane, (31E)].

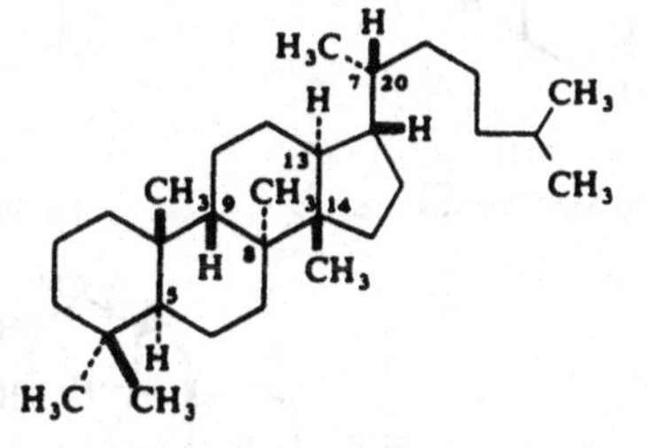

(31A)

5α-Protostane
(20*R*)-4,4,8,14-Tetramethyl-18-nor-5α,8α,9β,13α,14β,
17β(H)-cholestane. (This is an important
biogenetic precursor of tetracyclic
triterpenoids and steroids.)

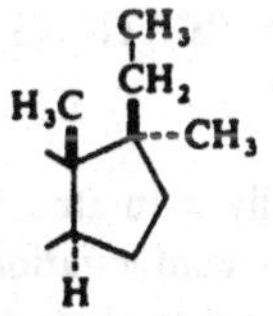

(31B)

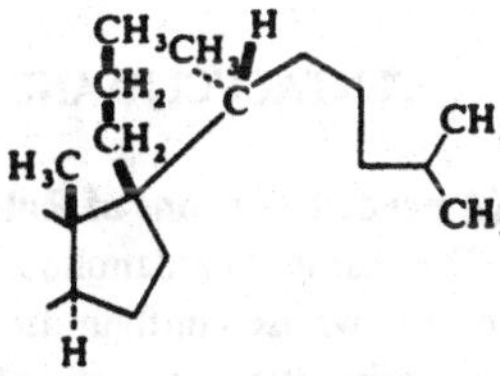

(31C)

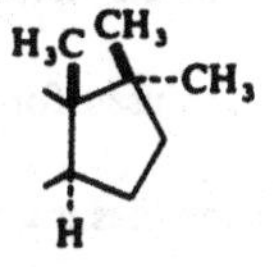

(31D)

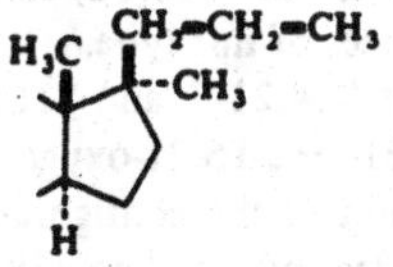

(31E)

2.4. When an additional ring is formed by means of a direct link between any two carbon atoms of the steroid ring system or the attached sidechain, the name of the steroid is prefixed by "cyclo," this prefix is preceded by the numbers of the positions joined by the new bond and the Greek letter (α, β, or ξ) denoting the configuration of the new bond, unless that designation is already implicit in the name.

Examples:

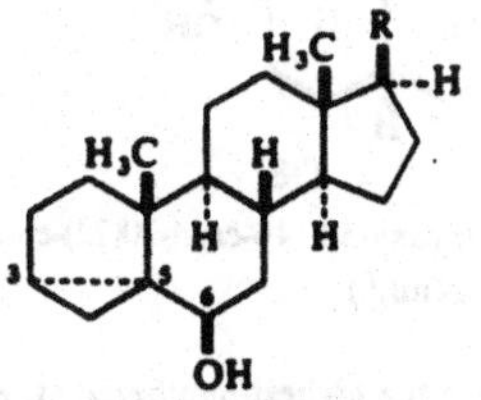

(32)

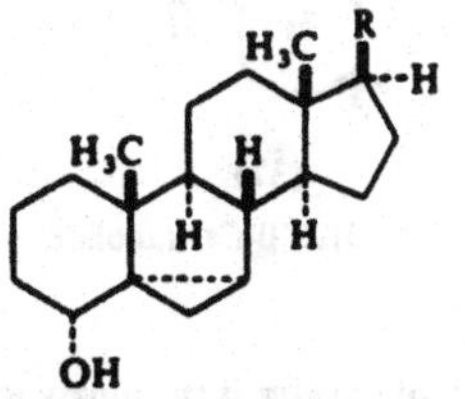

(33)

R = CH(CH₃)CH₂CH₂CH₂CH(CH₃)₂

3α,5-Cyclo-5α-cholestan-6β-ol   5,7α-Cyclo-5α-cholestan-4α-ol

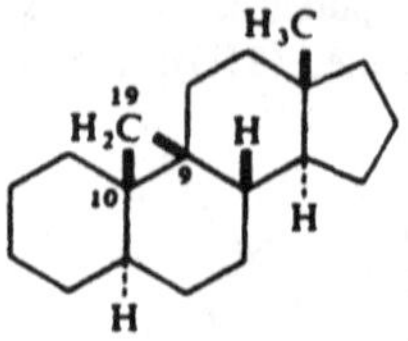

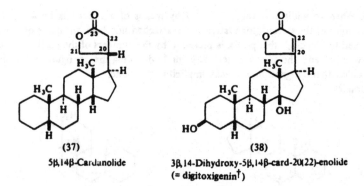

(34)
9,19-Cyclo-5α,9β-androstane

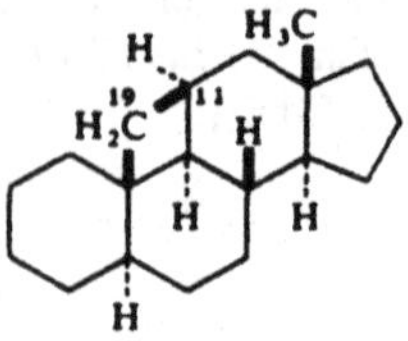

(35)
11β,19-Cyclo-5α-androstane

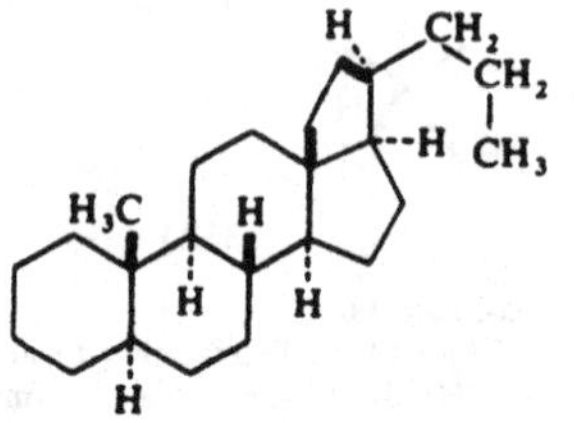

(36)
(20R)-18,21-Cyclo-5α-cholane

PENTACYCLIC AND HEXACYCLIC MODIFICATIONS

Rule 2S–3 (Amended Versions of Rules S–3.6 to S–3.9)

3.1. (a) The name "cardanolide" is used for the fully saturated system (37) of digitaloid lactones whose configuration is as illustrated (the configuration at position 20 is shown as a Fischer-type projection* and is the same as that in cholesterol, i.e., 20R). Notwithstanding Rule 2S–1.5, the configuration at position 14 must always be stated as an affix to the names of these compounds.

(b) Names such as "20(22)-cardenolide" are used for the naturally occurring unsaturated lactones of this type.

(c) The names "14,21-" and "16,21-epoxycardanolide" are used for the compounds containing a 14,21- or a 16,21-oxygen bridge, respectively.

Note: Statement of the configuration at C-14 for all cardanolides is a change from the earlier steroid Rules and is in line with current practice.

Examples:

(37)
5β,14β-Cardanolide

(38)
3β,14-Dihydroxy-5β,14β-card-20(22)-enolide
(= digitoxigenin[†])

---

*This method of drawing is customary for the steroids. Since the highest-numbered atom is at the top, the usual Fischer projection has been rotated in the plane of the paper through 180°.

[†] Denotes a trivial name; the systematic name is preferred.

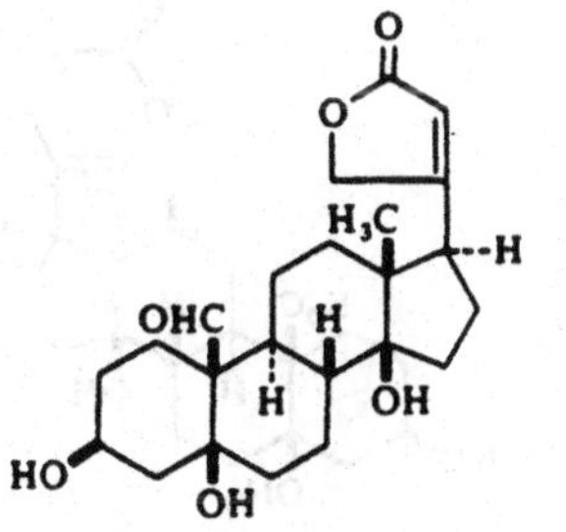

(39)

3β,5,14-Trihydroxy-19-oxo-5β,14β-card-
20(22)-enolide (= strophanthidin*)

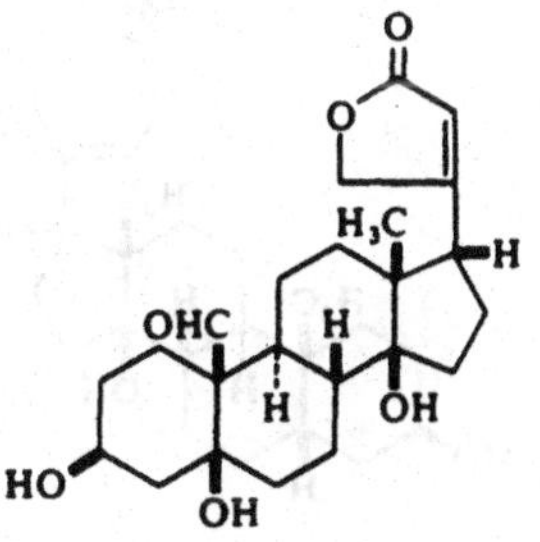

(40)

3β,5,14-Trihydroxy-19-oxo-5β,14β,17α-card-
20(22)-enolide (= 17α-strophanthidin*) (also
allostrophanthidin†)

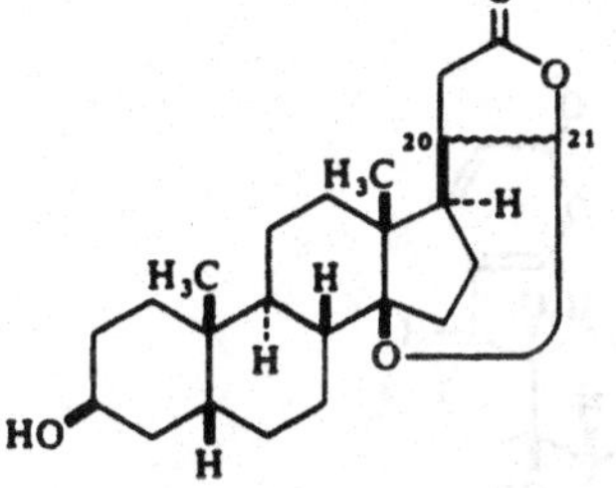

(41)

3β-Hydroxy-14,21ξ-epoxy-5β,14β,20ξ-
cardanolide (= isodigitoxigenin†)

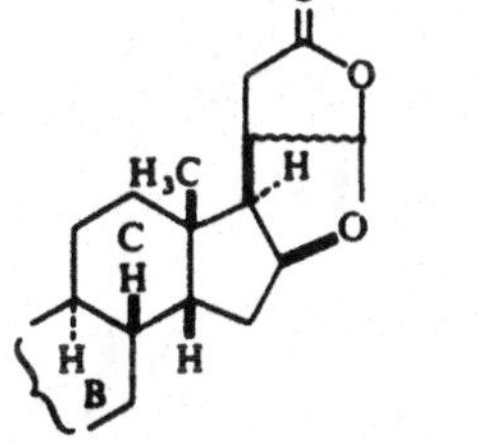

(42)

A 16β,21ξ-epoxy-14β,20ξ-cardanolide

3.2. The name "bufanolide" is used for the fully saturated system (43) of the squill-toad poison group of lactones, with the configuration at position 20 shown [this configuration is drawn as a Fischer-type projection (see Note to Rule 2S–3.1(a)) and is the same as in cholesterol, i.e., 20R]. Notwithstanding Rule 2S–1.5, the configuration at position 14 must always be stated as an affix to the names of these compounds. Unsaturated derivatives are named by replacing the suffix -anolide by -enolide, -adienolide etc.; thus, the name "20,22-bufadienolide" is used for the naturally occurring doubly unsaturated lactones.

Note: Statement of the configuration at C-14 for all bufanolides is a change from the earlier steroid Rules and is in line with current practice.

Examples:

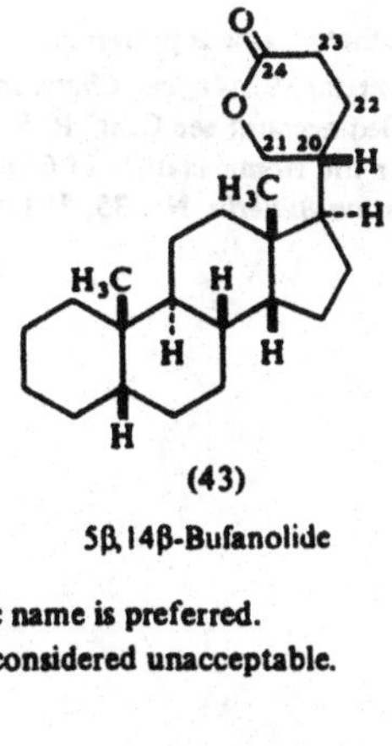

(43)

5β,14β-Bufanolide

* Denotes a trivial name; the systematic name is preferred.
† Denotes a previous trivial name now considered unacceptable.

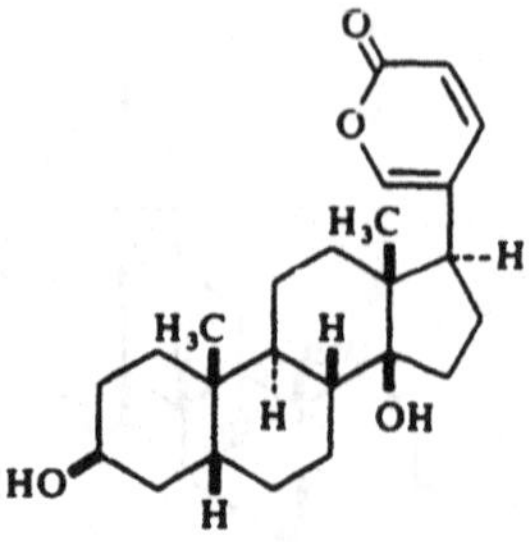

(44)

3β,14-Dihydroxy-5β,14β-bufa-20,22-dienolide
(= bufalin*)

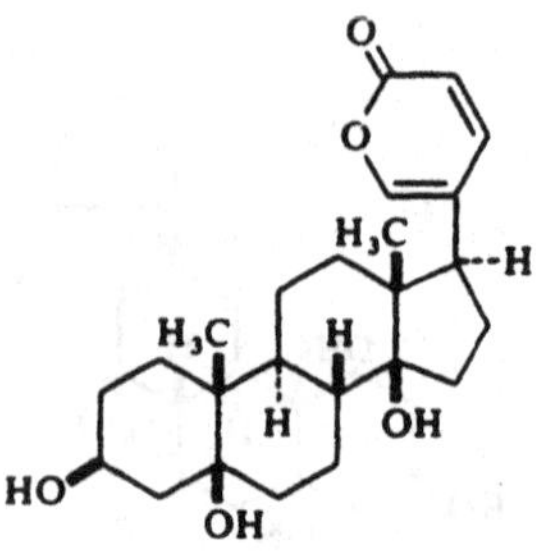

(45)

3β,5,14-Trihydroxy-5β,14β-bufa-20,22-
dienolide (= telecinobufagin*)

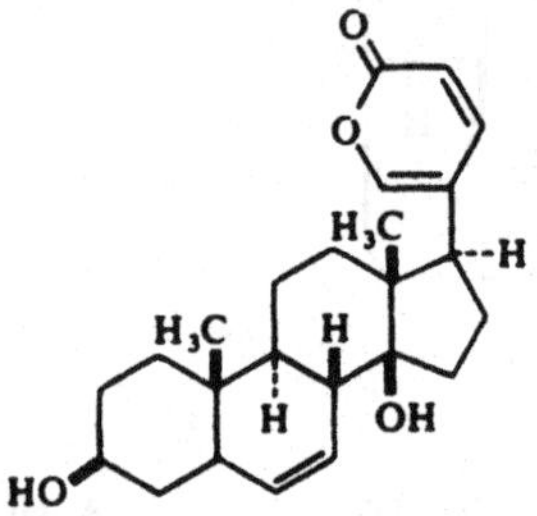

(46)

3β,14-Dihydroxy-14β-bufa-4,20,22-trienolide
(= scillarenin*)

3.3. The name "spirostan" is used for the compound of Structure (47) (this is a 16,22:22,26-diepoxycholestane); this name specifies the configurations shown for all the asymmetric centers except positions 5 and 25. A prefix 5α- or 5β- is added in the usual way (see Rule 2S–1.5). Configurations at C-16 and C-17, if different from those shown in Formula (47), are designated as 16β(H) and 17β(H). Configurations at C-20 and C-22, if different from those shown in Formula (47), are designated by the sequence-rule procedure[†] or, if unknown, by ξ. Steric relations of substituents at C-23, C-24, C-25, or C-26 are in all cases designated by the sequence-rule procedure[†] or, if unknown, by ξ.

*Denotes a trivial name; the systematic name is preferred.

[†]Cahn, R. S., Ingold, C. K., and Prelog, V., *Angew. Chem. Int. Ed.*, 5, 385 (1966); *Angew. Chem.*, 78, 413 (1966); for a partial simplified account see Cahn, R. S., *J. Chem. Educ.*, 41, 116 (1964). See also IUPAC 1968 Tentative Rules for the Nomenclature of Organic Chemistry, Sections E, Fundamental Stereochemistry, *IUPAC Information Bulletin*, No. 35, 71 (1969).

Examples:

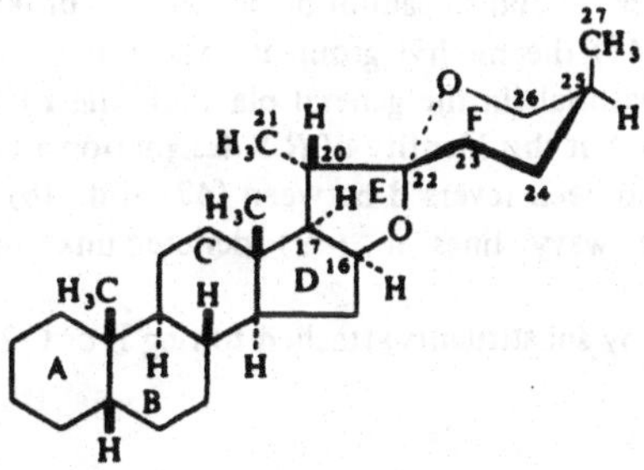

(47)

(25S)-5β-Spirostan

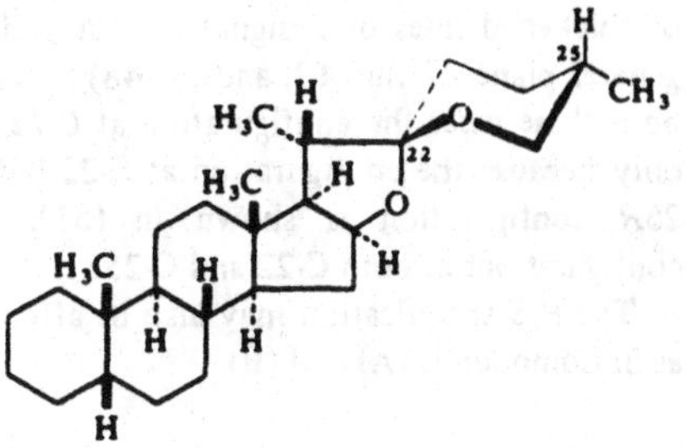

(48)

(22S,25S)-5β-Spirostan

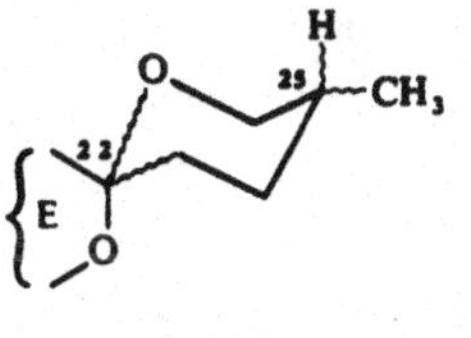

(49)

22ξ,25ξ-

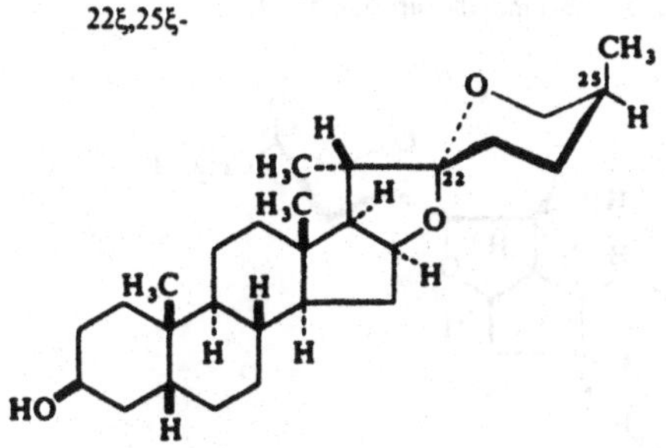

(50)

(25S)-5β-Spirostan-3β-ol
(= sarsasapogenin*)

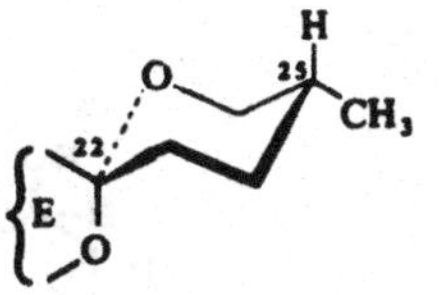

(51)

(25R)-

Notes: Several other methods have been used in the past for designating stereo-chemistry at C-22 and C-25 in the spirostans and related series; all involve serious difficulties (cf. The Basle Proposals, IUPAC *Information Bulletin*, No. 11; also Fieser, L. F. and Fieser, M., *The Steroids*, Reinhold, New York, 1959, chap. 21). The sequence-rule procedure is adopted in these Rules because it gives an unequivocal symbolism.

It is to be noted that, although ring E, like rings, A, B, C, and D, can conveniently be shown by projection on to the plane of the paper, yet ring F cannot be adequately represented in this way since the oxygen atom, C-26, C-24, and C-23 lie in one plane that is perpendicular to the plane of the paper. Ring F is conveniently drawn as in Formulas (47) to (51); in Formula (47), for instance, the broken line from C-22 to oxygen denotes that the oxygen atom and C-26 of ring F lie behind the plane of the paper and that consequently, C-23 and C-24 lie in front of the plane of the paper (configuration R at C-22). In partial Formula (48) the configuration at C-22 is reversed and must be stated in

*Denotes a trivial name; the systematic name is preferred.

the name (*S*). It is conventional to draw ring F as a chair, but this conformation is not implied in the name "spirostan," whatever the conformation of ring F, C-27 and the 25-hydrogen atom both lie in the plane of the paper and so cannot be denoted by broken or thickened lines or designated α or β. In (47) the methyl group is axial (above the general plane of ring F), and in (48) it is equatorial (in the general plane of ring F); in both these cases the configuration at C-25 is *S*, but this identity of *R,S* designation arises only because the configuration at C-22 has also been reversed between (47) and (48); a 25*R* configuration is shown in (51). The wavy lines in (49) denote unknown configurations at both C-22 and C-25.

The *R,S* specification may also be affected by substituents attached to ring F or C-27, as in Compounds (A) and (B).

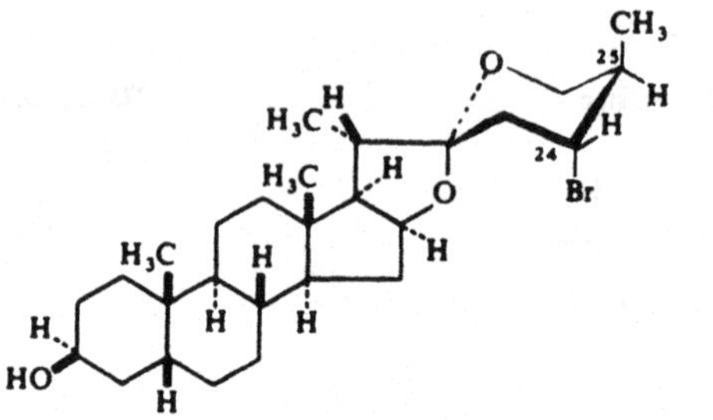

(A)

(24*R*,25*R*)-24-Bromo-5β-spirostan-3β-ol

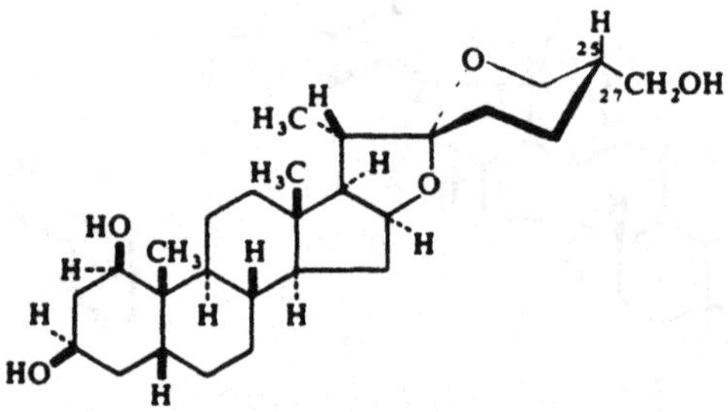

(B)

(25*S*)-5β-Spirostan-1β,3β,27-triol

3.4. The name "furostan" is used for the compound of Structure (52) (16β,22-epoxy-cholestane); this name specifies the configurations at all the asymmetric centers except positions 5, 22, and (if position 26 is substituted) also 25. Configuration at C-5 is designated by use of α or β in the usual way (see Rule 2S–1.5), and configurations at C-22 and, if necessary, C-25 by the sequence-rule procedure, or in all these cases by ξ if unknown.

Example:

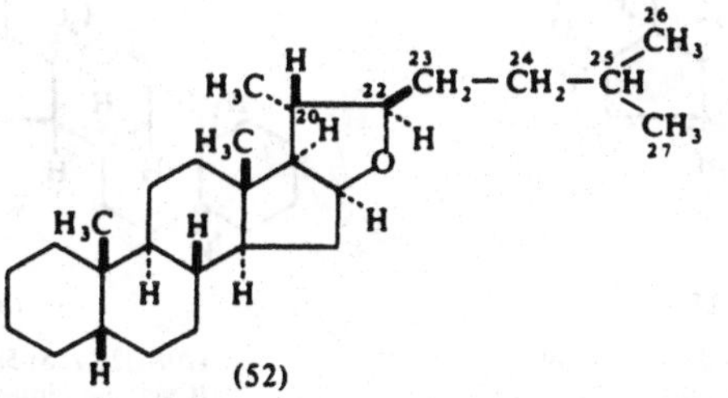

(52)

(22R)-5β-Furostan

Note: Representative examples of the new standard names and old names (standard names are preferred) for some common types of spirostan, furostan and derived structures are given in Table 1 and Formulas (53) to (59).

Table 1
SPIROSTANS AND FUROSTANS

Formula type	Standard name	Configurations implied in standard name	Old names (with trivial names for particular compounds in brackets)[a]
47	(25S)-Spirostan	20S,22R	Sapogenin (without prefix) Neogenin 25-L-Genin [Sarsasapogenin is (53)]
51	(25R)-Spirostan	20S,22R	Isogenin 25-D-Genin [Smilagenin is (25R)-5β-spirostan-3β-ol; Tigogenin is (25R)-5α-spirostan-3β-ol]
54	(20R,22S,25S)-Spirostan	–	Cyclopseudoneogenin
55	(20R,25R)-Spirostan	–	Cyclopseudoisogenin
56	(22R) (or S or ξ) (25R) (or S or ξ)-Furostan	20S	Dihydrogenin (26-ol) and dihydropseudogenin (26-ol) [Dihydrosarsasapogenin is 5β,22ξ,25S-furostan-3β,26-diol; dihydropseudotigogenin is (58); cf. (57).]
57	(25R) (or S or ξ)- Furost-20(22)-en	–	Pseudogenin [Pseudotigogenin is (57); pseudosarsasapogenin is (59); pseudosmilagenin is (25R)-5β-furost-20(22)-en-3β,26-diol].

[a]The standard name is preferred.

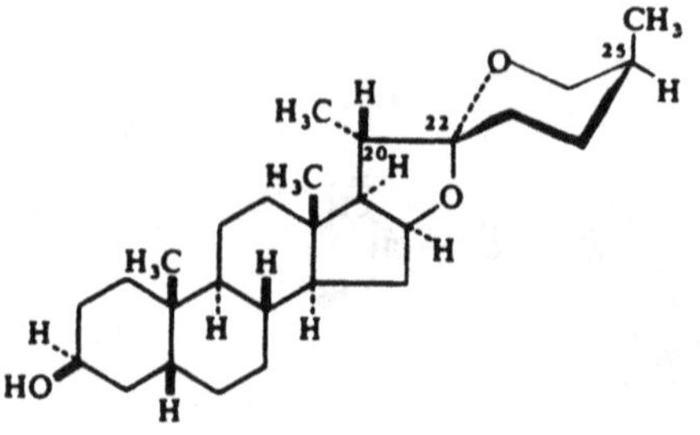

(53)
(25S)-5β-Spirostan-3β-ol
(Sarsasapogenin*)

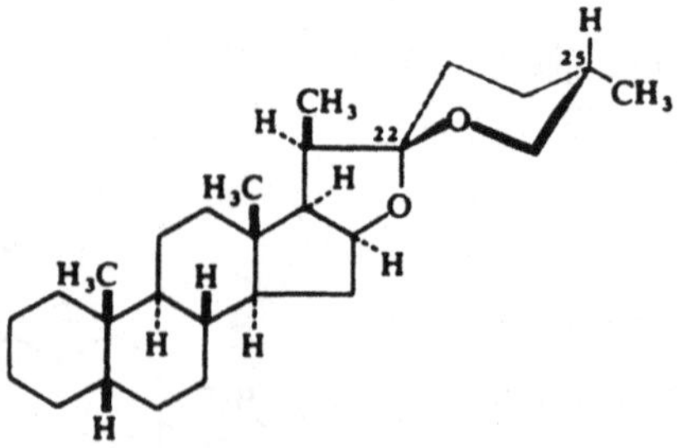

(54)
(20R,22S,25S)-5β-Spirostan
(Cyclopseudoneogenin*)

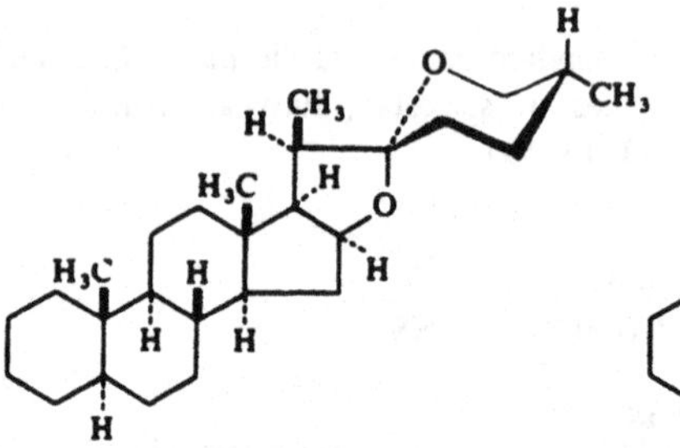

(55)
(20R,25R)-5α-Spirostan
(Cyclopseudoisogenin*)

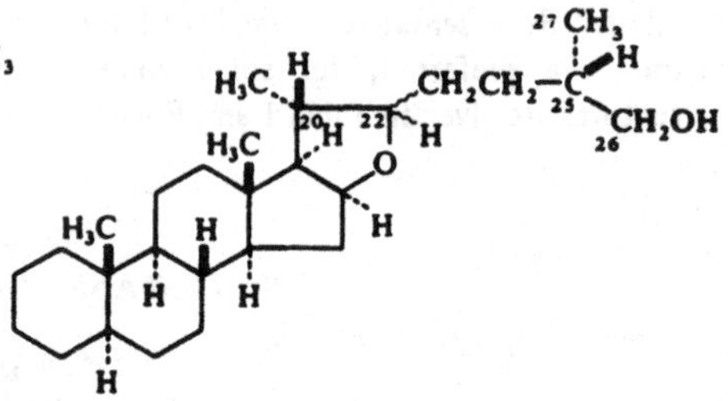

(56)
(20S,22ξ,25S)-5α-Furostan-26-ol
(Dihydrogenin*)

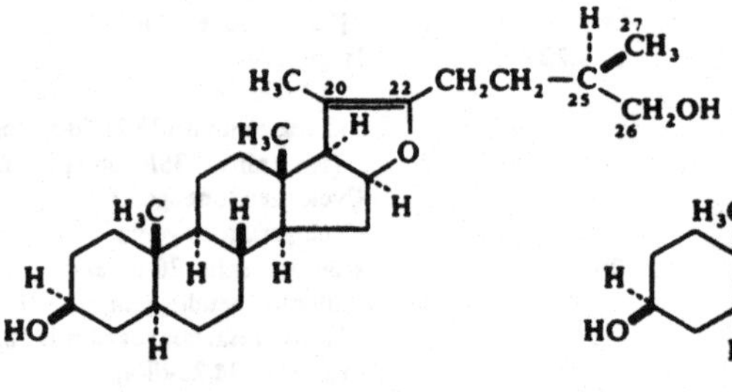

(57)
(25R)-5α-Furost-20(22)-en-3β,26-diol
(Pseudotigogenin*)

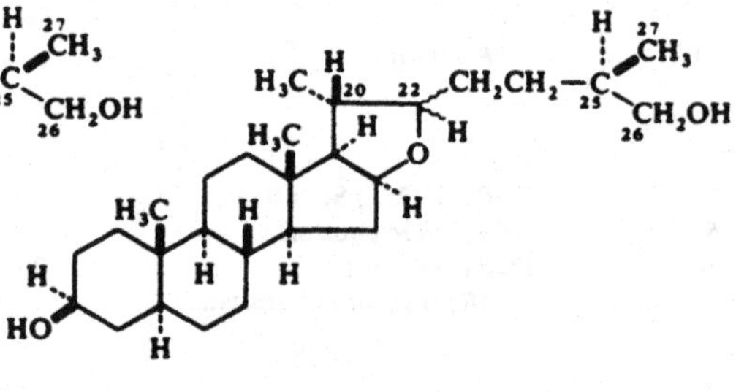

(58)
(20S,22ξ,25R)-5α-Furostan-3β,26-diol
(Dihydropseudotigogenin*)

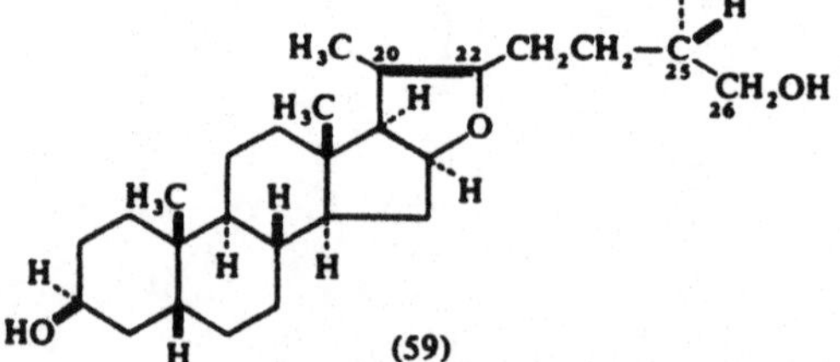

(59)
(25S)-5β-Furost-20(22)-en-3β,26-diol
(Pseudosarsasapogenin*)

*The standard name is preferred.

DERIVATIVES

Rule 2S–4 (Extended Version of Rule S–4)

4.1. Steroid derivatives that can be considered to be formed by modification of, or introduction of substituents into, a parent compound are named by the usual methods of organic chemistry (see *IUPAC Nomenclature of Organic Chemistry*, Sections A, B, and C, 1971).

Notes: For the benefit of the specialist, those rules of general substitutive nomenclature that apply most often to steroids are outlined here. For full details the IUPAC Rules cited above should be consulted.

I. Unsaturation is indicated by changing terminal "-ane" to "-ene," "-adiene," "-yne," etc. or "-an" to "-en," "-adien," "-yn," etc.; e.g., 5α-cholest-6-ene, 5β-cholesta-7,9(11)-diene, 5-spirosten; see also the names of Examples (22) to (25).[†]

II. Most substituents can be designated either as suffixes or as prefixes; a few can be named only as prefixes, the commonest of these being halogens, alkyl and nitro groups. When possible, one type of substituent must be designated as suffix. When more than one type is present that could be designated as suffix, one type only may be so expressed and the other types must be designated as prefixes. Choice for suffix is made according to an order of preference that is laid down in the Rules cited above; the most important part of this order, for steroids, is as follows, in decreasing preference: Onium salt, acid, lactone, ester, aldehyde, ketone, alcohol, amine, ether. Suffixes are added to the name of the saturated or unsaturated parent system, the terminal "e" of "-ane," "-ene," "-yne," "-adiene," etc. being elided before a vowel (presence or absence of numerals has no effect on such elisions). The following examples illustrate the use of these principles.

(a) *Acids.* Suffix for $-CH_3 \rightarrow -COOH$: -oic acid, suffix for $CH \rightarrow C-COOH$: -carboxylic acid.

Examples:

11-Oxo-5α-cholan-24-oic acid
(20S)-3α-Hydroxy-5-pregnene-20-carboxylic acid

(b) *Lactones, other than cardanolides and bufanolides.* The ending "-ic acid" or "-carboxylic acid" of the name of the hydroxy acid is changed to "-lactone" or "-carbolactone," respectively, preceded by the locant of the acid group and then the locant of the hydroxyl group: the prefix "hydroxy" is omitted for the lactonized hydroxyl group.

Examples:

3β-Hydroxy-5α-cholano-24,17α-lactone
(20R)-3β-Hydroxy-5-pregnene-20,18-carbolactone

(c) *Cardanolides and bufanolides.* The -olide ending of these names denotes the lactone grouping, and substituents must be named as prefixes.

(d) *Esters of steroid alcohols.* Special procedures are used. For esters of monohydric steroid alcohols, the steroid hydrocarbon radical name is followed by that of the acyloxy group in its anionic form. The steroid radical name is formed by replacing the terminal "e" of the hydrocarbon name by "yl" and inserting before this the locant and Greek letter, with hyphens, to designate the position and configuration.

[†]For uniformity with the IUPAC Rules cited above, the conventions of *Chemical Abstracts* are used also in the present Rules for the position of locants (positional numerals) and designation of unsaturation. In such matters, and in use of Δ to designate unsaturation (which is not recommended by IUPAC), authors should respect the house customs of the journals to which their papers are submitted.

Example:

5α-Cholestan-3β-yl acetate

For esters of polyols the name of the polyol [cf. (g) below] is followed by that of the acyloxy group(s) in its anionic form, with locants when necessary.
Examples:

5β-Cholestane-3α,12α-diol diacetate
5β-Cholestane-3α,12α-diol 3-acetate 12-benzoate
Estradiol-17β 17-monoacetate

When an acid, lactone or spirostan group is also present, the ester group is designated by an acyloxy prefix.
Example:

(25S)-3β-Acetoxy-5β-spirostan

(e) *Aldehydes.* Suffixes: -al (denotes change of $-CH_3$ to $-CHO$, i.e., without change in the number of carbon atoms); -aldehyde (denotes change of $-COOH$ to $-CHO$, i.e., without change in the number of carbon atoms; name derived from that of the acid). Prefix: oxo- (denotes change of $> CH_2$ to $> CO$, thus also of $-CH_3$ to $-CHO$, with no change in the number of carbon atoms).
Examples:

5α-Androstan-19-al
5α-Cholan-24-aldehyde
19-Oxo-5α, 17α(H)-etianic acid

Other methods are used for introduction of additional carbon atoms as $-CHO$ groups.
(f) *Ketones.* Suffix: -one; prefix: oxo-.
Examples:

5β-Androstan-3-one
5-Pregnene-3,20-dione
11-Oxo-5α-cholan-24-oic acid

(g) *Alcohols.* Suffix: -ol; prefix: hydroxy-.
Examples:

5β-Cholestane-3α, 11β-diol
3α-Hydroxy-5α-androstan-17-one

Notes: (1) Composite suffixes -olone and -onol, to denote simultaneous presence of hydroxyl and ketonic groups, are not permitted by IUPAC Rules and should not be used.
(2) A few trivial names exist for hydroxy ketones, such as testosterone for 17β-hydroxy-4-androsten-3-one (see Rule 2S-4.2).
(h) *Amines.* Suffix: -amine; prefix: amino-.
The suffix may be attached to the name of the parent compound or of its radical.
Examples:

5-Androsten-3β-amine or 5-Androsten-3β-ylamine
3β-(Dimethylamino)-5α-pregnan-20α-ol

(i) *Ethers.* Ethers are named as alkoxy derivatives when another group is present that has priority for citation as suffix.

Examples:

3β-Ethoxy-5α-cholan-24-oic acid
17β-Methoxy-4-androsten-3-one

When no such other group is present, ethers of steroid monoalcohols may be named by stating the name of the steroid hydrocarbon radical, followed by the name of the alkyl (or aryl, etc.) radical, and lastly by "ether;" in English these three parts of the name are printed as separate words, for example, 5α-androstan-3β-yl methyl ether. For ethers of steroid polyols the same system may be used but with the name of the steroid hydrocarbon radical replaced by the name of the polyol; for partially etherified polyols, locant(s) precede the names of the alkyl (or aryl, etc.) group(s); for example, 5α-pregnene-3β,17,20α-triol trimethyl ether, 5α-pregnene-3β,17,20α-triol 3,17-dimethyl ether, cortisol 21-methyl ether.

4.2. The following are examples of trivial names retained for important steroid derivatives, these being mostly natural compounds of significant biological activity.

Aldosterone	18,11-Hemiacetal of 11β,21-dihydroxy-3,20-dioxo-4-pregnene-18-al
Androsterone	3α-Hydroxy-5α-androstan-17-one
Cholecalciferol*	9,10-Seco-5,7,10(19)-cholestatrien-3β-ol (for seco see Rule 2S–8)
Cholesterol	5-Cholesten-3β-ol
Cholic acid	3α,7α,12α-Trihydroxy-5β-cholan-24-oic acid
Corticosterone	11β,21-Dihydroxy-4-pregnene-3,20-dione
Cortisol	11β,17,21-Trihydroxy-4-pregnene-3,20-dione
Cortisol acetate	Cortisol 21-acetate
Cortisone	17,21-Dihydroxy-4-pregnene-3,11,20-trione
Cortisone acetate	Cortisone 21-acetate
Deoxycorticosterone	21-Hydroxy-4-pregnene-3,20-dione (i.e., the 11-deoxy derivative of corticosterone)
Ergocalciferol*	9,10-Seco-5,7,10(19),22-ergostatetraen-3β-ol (for seco see Rule 2S–8)
Ergosterol	5,7,22-Ergostatrien-3β-ol
Estradiol-17α	1,3,5(10)-Estratriene-3,17α-diol
Estradiol-17β	1,3,5(10)-Estratriene-3,17β-diol
Estriol	1,3,5(10)-Estratriene-3,16α,17β-triol
Estrone	3-Hydroxy-1,3,5(10)-estratrien-17-one
Lanosterol	8,24-Lanostadien-3β-ol
Lithocholic acid	3α-Hydroxy-5β-cholan-24-oic acid
Progesterone	4-Pregnene-3,20-dione
Testosterone	17β-Hydroxy-4-androsten-3-one

*Included in the List of Trivial Names for Miscellaneous Compounds of Biochemical Importance published by the IUPAC-IUB Commission of Biochemical Nomenclature: see, for example, *IUPAC Inf. Bull.*, No. 25, 19 (1966), *J. Biol. Chem.*, 241, 2987 (1966), or *Biochim. Biophys. Acta*, 107, 1 (1965).

Note: If these trivial names are used as a basis for naming derivatives or stereoisomers, the derived trivial name must make the nature of the modification completely clear and is preferably accompanied at first mention by the full systematic name. For example, in steroid papers "epi" is often used with trivial names to denote inversion at one center; the name "11-epicortisol" defines the compound fully since cortisol is already defined as the 11β-alcohol; but the name "epicortisol" does not define the compound and is inadequate.

4.3. Androstane-17-carboxylic acids may be called "etianic acids," although the former (systematic) name is preferred. The orientation of the hydrogen atoms at positions 5 and 17 must in all cases be indicated as 5α or 5β, and 17α(H) or 17β(H), respectively.

Examples:

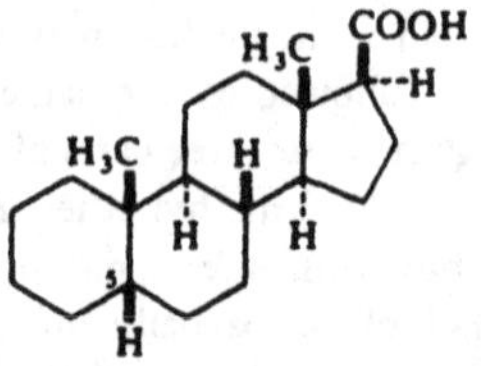

(60)

5β-Androstane-17β-carboxylic acid (systematic) or 5β,17α(H)-etianic acid (trivial)

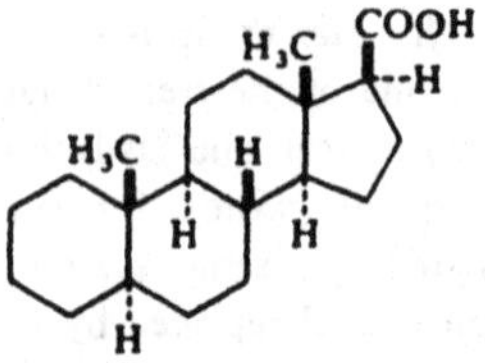

(61)

5α-Androstane-17β-carboxylic acid (systematic) or 5α,17α(H)-etianic acid (trivial)

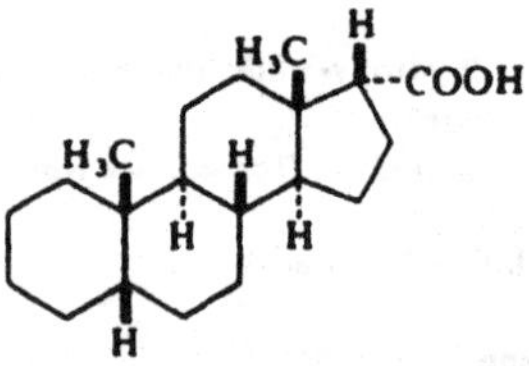

(62)

5β-Androstane-17α-carboxylic acid (systematic) or 5β,17β(H)-etianic acid (trivial)

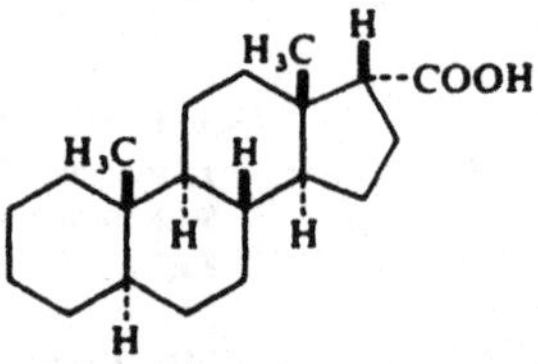

(63)

5α-Androstane-17α-carboxylic acid (systematic) or 5α,17β(H)-etianic acid (trivial)

STEREOCHEMICAL MODIFICATIONS

Rule 2S–5 (Extended Version of Rule S–5)

5.1. If, as for instance in a synthetic compound, there is stereochemical inversion at all the asymmetric centers whose configurations do not require to be specified in a name, the italicized prefix *ent-* (a contracted form of *enantio-*) is placed in front of the complete name of the compound. This prefix denotes inversion at all asymmetric centers (including those due to named substituents) whether these are cited separately or are implied in the name.

Examples:

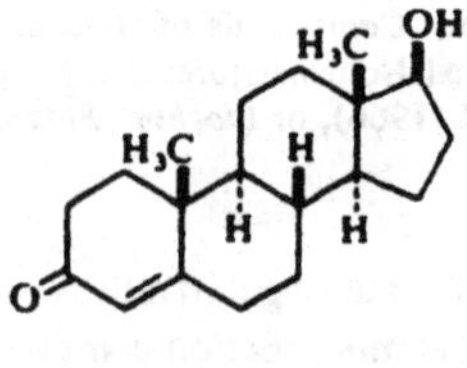

(64)

17β-Hydroxy-4-androsten-3-one
(Testosterone)

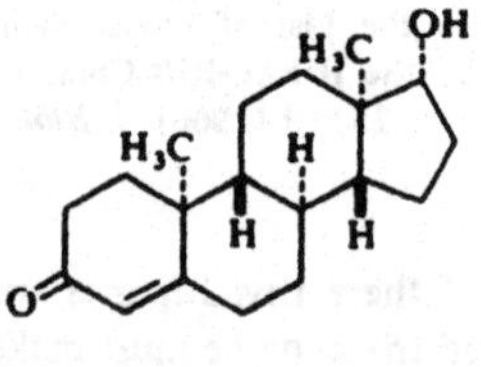

(65)

ent-17β-Hydroxy-4-androsten-3-one
(*ent*-Testosterone)

Note: When Roman or Arabic numerals are used to enumerate formulae, the prefix *ent-* may be used to indicate the enantiomer. Thus, e.g., (65) above may be designated (*ent-64*).

5.2. If there is stereochemical inversion at a minority of the asymmetric centers whose configurations do not require to be specified in a name, the configuration of the hydrogen atoms or substituents at the affected bridgeheads, or the carbon chain (if any) at position 17, are stated by means of a prefix or prefixes α or β, each with its appropriate positional numeral, placed before the stem name laid down in the preceding Rules.

Examples:

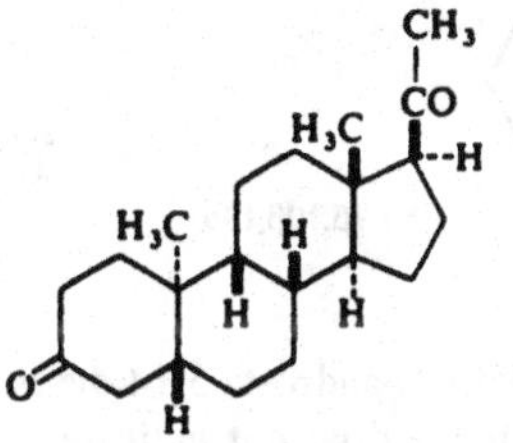

(66)
5β,9β,10α-Pregnane-3,20-dione

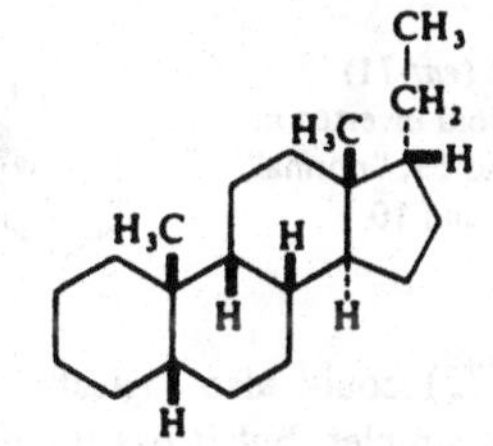

(67)
5β,9β,17α-Pregnane

Note: The prefix *retro*, indicating 9β,10α-configuration, is not recommended for systematic nomenclature.

5.3. The enantiomer of a compound designated as in Rule 2S–5.2 is given the same name preceded by *ent-*.

Note: This Rule covers the compounds in which there is inversion at a majority, but not all, of the asymmetric centers that do not require to be specified in the name.

Examples:

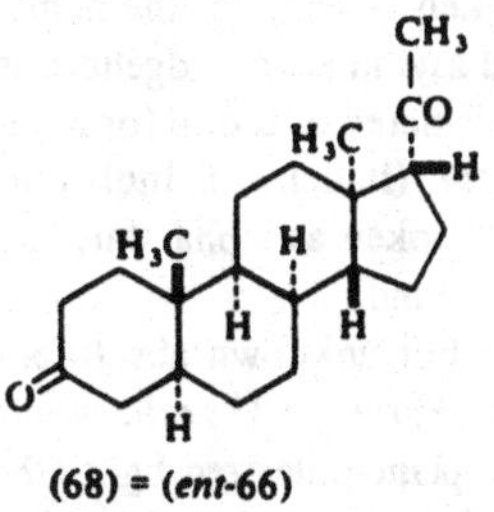

(68) = (*ent*-66)
ent-5β,9β,10α-Pregnane-3,20-dione
(not 5α,8α,13α,14β,17α-pregnane-3,20-dione)

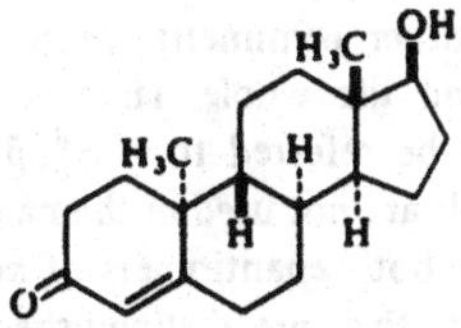

(69)
ent-17α-Hydroxy-13α,14β-androst-4-en-3-one
(not 17β-hydroxy-8α,9β,10α-androst-4-en-3-one)

5.4. If there is stereochemical inversion at half of the asymmetric centers whose configurations are implied in the stem name of a "normal" steroid [e.g., (70)], the prefixes to be specified in the name of the stereoisomer are that set that includes the number occurring first in the series 8, 9, 10, 13, 14, 17, without or with the prefix *ent-* as appropriate.

	Configuration at asymmetric centers	Name
(70) "Normal" steroid	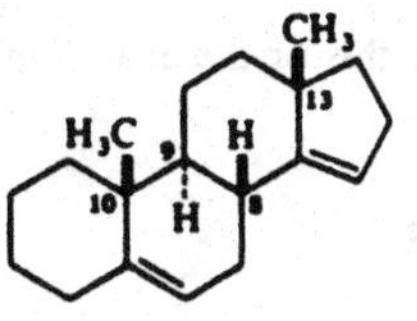 8β,9α,10β,13β	5,14-An-drostadiene

(71)
Steroid inverted at
8 and 10; "normal"
at 9 and 13

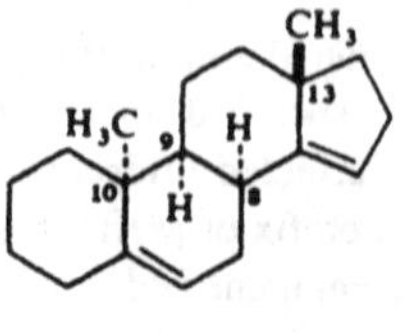

8α,9α,10α,13β

8α,10α-
Androsta-
5,14-diene

(72) (*ent*-71)
Steroid inverted at
9 and 13; "normal"
at 8 and 10

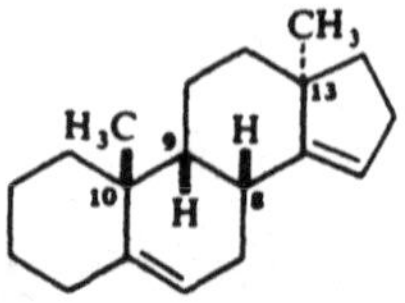

8β,9β,10β,13α

ent-8α,10α-
Androsta-
5,14-diene

Note: (72) could also logically be named "9β,13α-androsta-5,14-diene;" this name might seem simpler, but it has the disadvantage that it does not indicate that (72) is the enantiomer of (71).

5.5. Racemates, as for instance obtained by synthesis, are named by use of an italicized prefix *rac*- (an abbreviation of *racemo*-), placed before the complete name of the compound, the enantiomer chosen for naming being that required by Rules 2S–5.1 to 2S–5.4.

Example: A racemate composed of (64) and (65) (=*ent*-64) is named:

rac-17β-Hydroxy-4-androsten-3-one or *rac*-testosterone

5.6. (a) When the relative, but not the absolute, configuration of two or more asymmetric centers in a steroid derivative is known, as for instance for a compound obtained by synthesis, the 10β configuration is taken as basis for the name; or, if C-10 is not asymmetric or is absent, the lowest-numbered asymmetric bridgehead is designated α (or *R*); the other asymmetric centers are then considered as α or β (or *R* or *S*) relative to that one; and the whole name is prefixed by *rel*- (italicized). Individual asymmetric centers may be referred to as α*, β*, *R**, or *S** (spoken as alpha star, R star, etc.) but these symbols are not used in the name of the compound.

(b) When both enantiomers of known relative, but unknown absolute, configuration are prepared, they are distinguished by a prefix (+)-*rel*- or (-)-*rel*-, where the *plus* or *minus* sign refers to the direction of rotation of plane-polarized light (the wavelength, solvent, temperature, and/or concentration must be added when known to affect this sign).

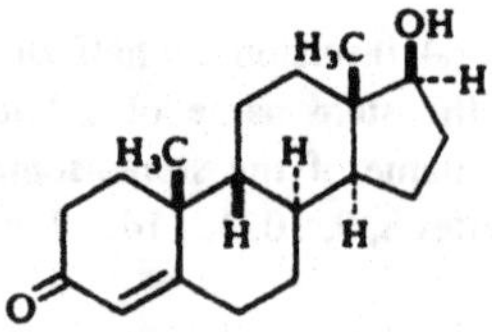

(73)

The dextrorotatory form having either this or the enantiomeric configuration would be named:

(+)-*rel*-17β-Hydroxy-8α,9β-androst-4-en-3-one

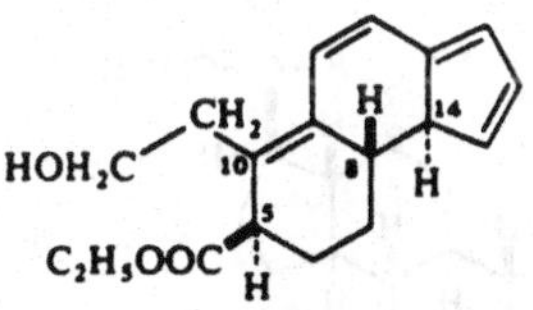

(74A)   equal to   (74B)

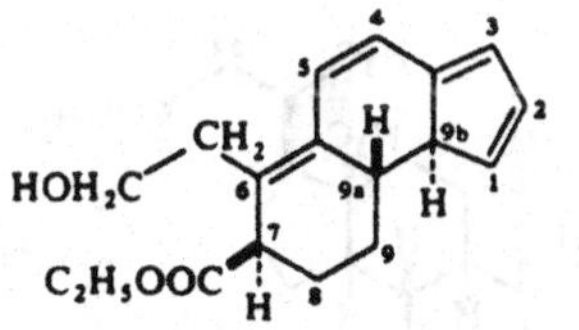

(74A) *rel*-(Ethyl-2-hydroxy-*A*-nor-2,3-seco-5α-gona-9,11,13(17),15-tetraen-3-oate)

(for seco see Rule 2S–8 and for nor see Rule 2S–7)

(or (74B) *rel*-[(7*R*.9a*S*,9b*S*)-Ethyl 8,9,9a,9b-tetrahydro-6-(2-hydroxyethyl)-7*H*-

cyclopenta[*a*]-naphthalene-7-carboxylate]

Note: At some stage in synthetic work on steroids, names of intermediates have to be changed from a system used in general organic chemistry to the steroid system. The names (74A) and (74B) illustrate such a change and it should be noted (i) that not merely the name but also the numbering are usually changed and (ii) that the steroid name usually avoids the need to specify the configuration at each asymmetric center. The latter factor will often indicate at what point in a synthesis the change of nomenclature is desirable.

SHORTENING OF SIDECHAINS AND ELIMINATION OF METHYL GROUPS

Rule 2S–6 (Expanded from Rule S–6)

6.1. Elimination of a methylene group from a steroid sidechain (including a methyl group) is indicated by the prefix "nor-," which in all cases is preceded by the number of the carbon atom that disappears. When alternatives are possible, the number attached to nor is the highest permissible. Elimination of two methylene groups is indicated by the prefix "dinor-."

Examples:

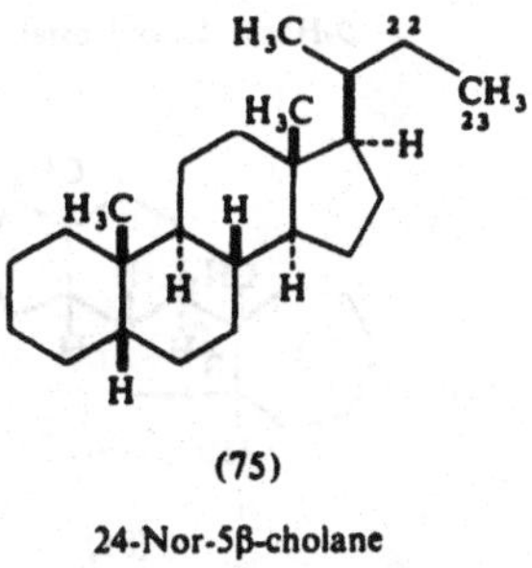

(75)   (76)

24-Nor-5β-cholane   18-Nor-4-pregnene-3,20-dione

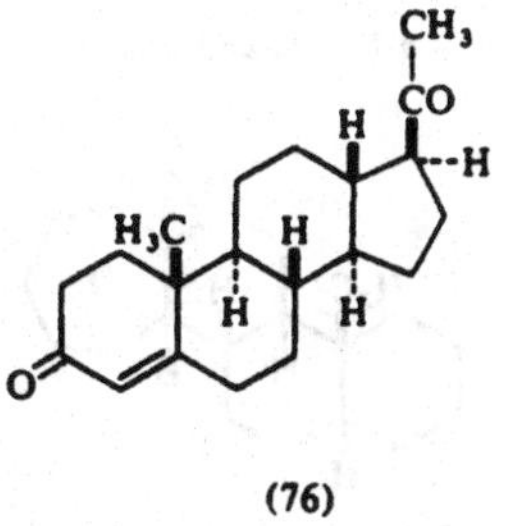

Exceptions: By Rules 2S–2.1 and 2S–2.2 the names gonane (for 18,19-dinorandrostane) and estrane (for 19-norandrostane) constitute exceptions to the above Rule 2S–6.1. The names gonane and estrane are used also as parent names for their derivatives.

However, 18-nor- and 19-nor- are used with other trivial names, as in 19-norpregnane, 18,19-dinorspirostan, 18-norestrone.

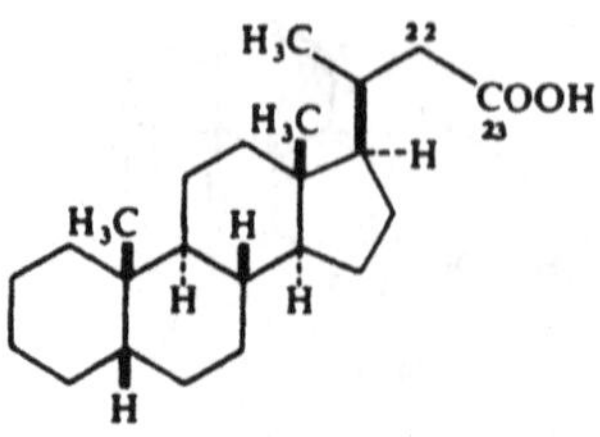

(77)

24-Nor-5β-cholan-23-oic acid   18,19-Dinor-5α-pregnane-20α-carboxylic acid

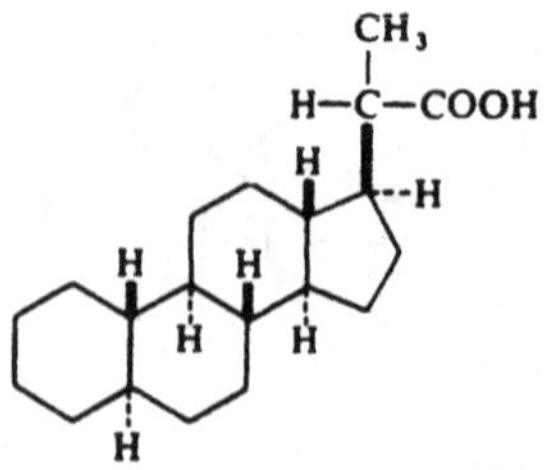

The compound produced by shortening the 17-sidechain of pregnane is named 17-methylandrostane rather than 21-norpregnane, (see also Note to Rule 2S–2.2).

RING CONTRACTION OR EXPANSION

Rule 2S–7 (Amended Version of Rule S–7)

7.1. Ring contraction and ring expansion (other than insertion of atoms between directly linked bridgeheads or, when a steroid sidechain is present, between C-13 and C-17) are indicated by prefixes "nor" and "homo," respectively, preceded by an italic capital letter indicating the ring affected. For loss or insertion of two methylene groups, "dinor" and "dihomo" are used. "Homo" and "nor," when occurring in the same name, are cited in alphabetical order.*

Examples:

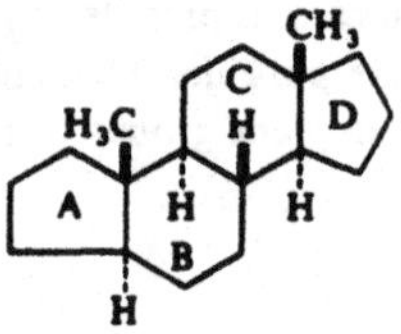

(78)   (79)

A-Nor-5α-androstane   *D*-Homo-5α-androstane

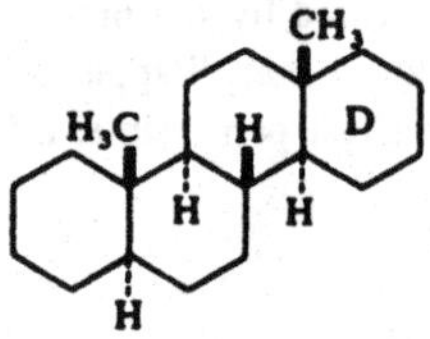

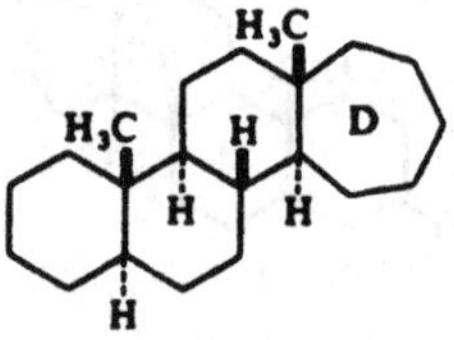

(80)   (81)

D-Dihomo-5α-androstane   *A*-Homo-*B*-nor-5α-androstane

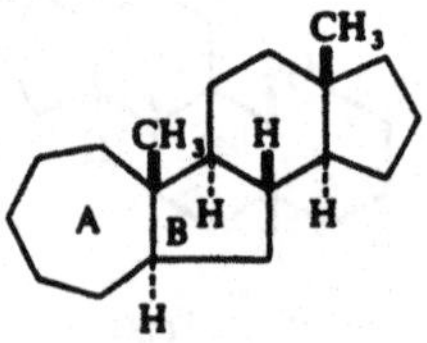

Notes: (a) By too extended use, this nomenclature can be applied to compounds whose steroid character is excessively modified. It is recommended that it be confined to steroids containing at least one angular methyl group, or a steroid 17-sidechain, or a

---

*Alphabetical order is used for any combination of the prefixes cyclo, homo, nor, and seco; they are placed after any prefixes denoting substituents and before any stereochemical prefixes required by Rule 2S–1.5, or, if there are none of the latter, then immediately before the stem name.

steroidal group on ring *D* (e.g., a spirostan); also that no more than two of the steroid rings may be altered by any combination of the operations denoted by "nor" and "homo." When these conditions are not met, general systematic nomenclature should be used.

(b) Names incorporating "homo" and "nor" are normally preferred to alternatives incorporating "cyclo" and "seco" [cf. Example (86)].

7.2. On ring contraction the original steroid numbering is retained, and only the highest number(s) of the contracted ring, exclusive of ring junctions, is deleted.

Example:

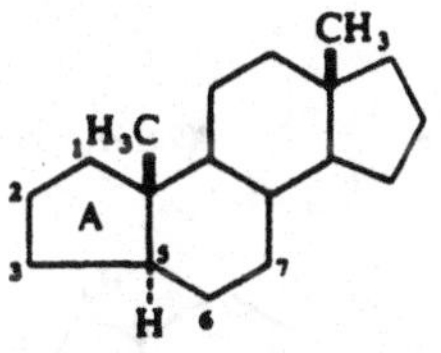

(82)

A-Nor-5α-androstan (number 4 is omitted)

7.3. On ring expansion (other than insertion of atoms between directly linked bridgeheads or, when a 17-sidechain is present, between C-13 and C-17), the letter a (and b etc. as necessary) is added to the highest number in the ring enlarged exclusive of ring junctions, and this letter and number are assigned to the last peripheral carbon atom in the order of numbering of the ring affected.

Examples:

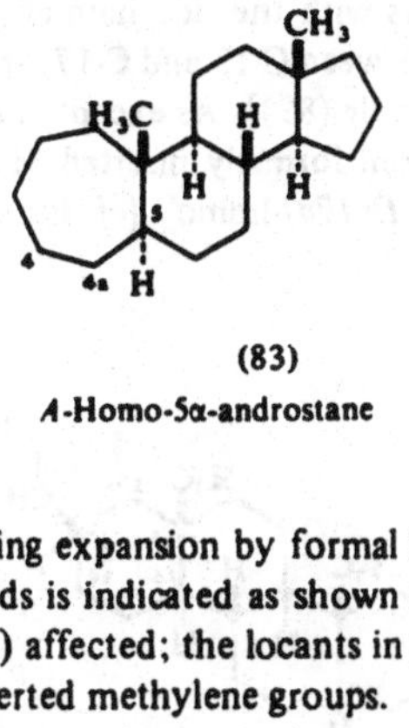

(83)	(84)
A-Homo-5α-androstane	3-Hydroxy-*D*-dihomo-1,3,5(10)-estratrien-17b-one

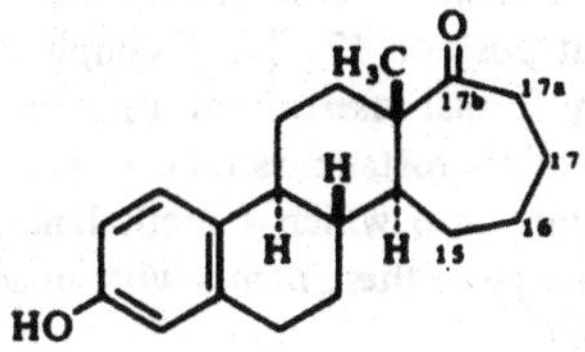

7.4. Ring expansion by formal insertion of a methylene group between directly linked bridgeheads is indicated as shown in the following table. The italic capital letters denote the ring(s) affected; the locants in parentheses (which are included in the name) are those of the inserted methylene groups.

CH₂ added between	Prefix used
C-5 and C-10	*AB(10a)*-Homo
C-8 and C-9	*BC(8a)*-Homo
C-8 and C-14	*C(14a)*-Homo
C-9 and C-10	*B(9a)*-Homo
C-13 and C-14	*CD(13a)*-Homo

Examples:

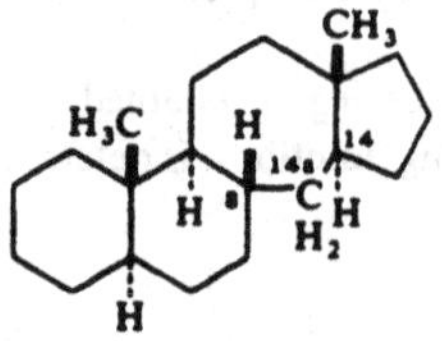

(85)

C(14a)-Homo-5α-androstane

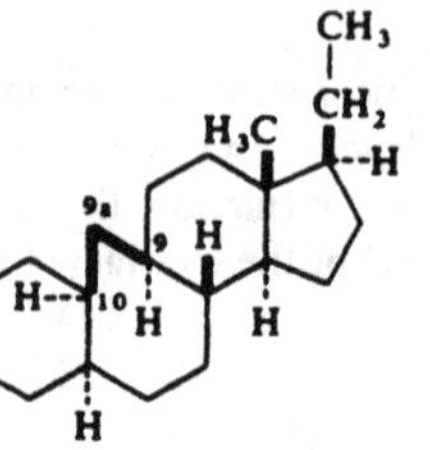

(86)

B(9a)-Homo-19-nor-5α,10α(H)-pregnane*

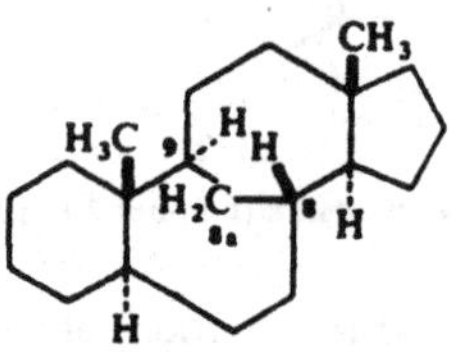

(87)

BC(8a)-Homo-5α-androstane

7.5. Expansion of ring *D* by insertion of atoms between C-13 and C-17: The names "*D*-homopregnane," "*D*-homocholane," etc. are used only for the isomer with the sidechain at position 17a [cf. Example (88)]. Isomers with the sidechain at position 17 (formed by formal insertion of a methylene group between C-13 and C-17) are named as derivatives of androstane, estrane, or gonane [cf. Example (89)]. As exceptions, furostans and spirostans into which a methylene group has been formally inserted between C-13 and C-17 are given these names with an added prefix "*D(17a)*-homo" [cf. Example (90)].
Examples:

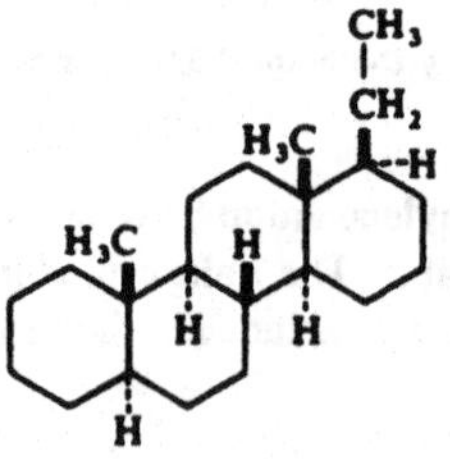

(88)

D-Homo-5α-pregnane

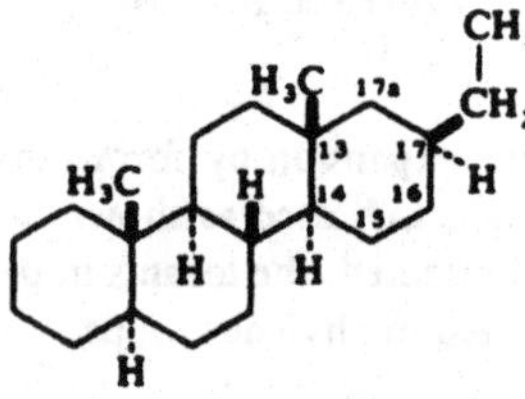

(89)

17β-Ethyl-*D*-homo-5α-androstane

*This name is preferred to 9β,19-cyclo-9,10-seco-5α,10α(H)-pregnane [see Note (b) to Rule 2S–7.1]. This skeleton is contained in some *Buxus* alkaloids.

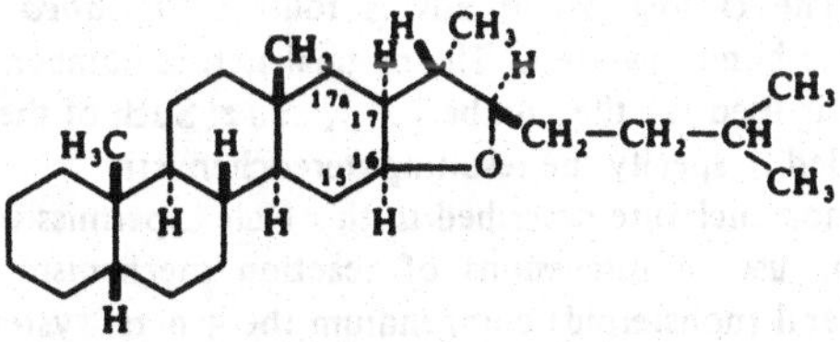

(90)

(22R)-D(17a)-Homo-5β-furostan

RING FISSION

Rule 2S–8 (Unchanged from Rule S–7.4)

8.1. Fission of a ring, with addition of a hydrogen atom at each terminal group thus created, is indicated by the prefix "seco-," the original steroid numbering being retained.*

Examples:

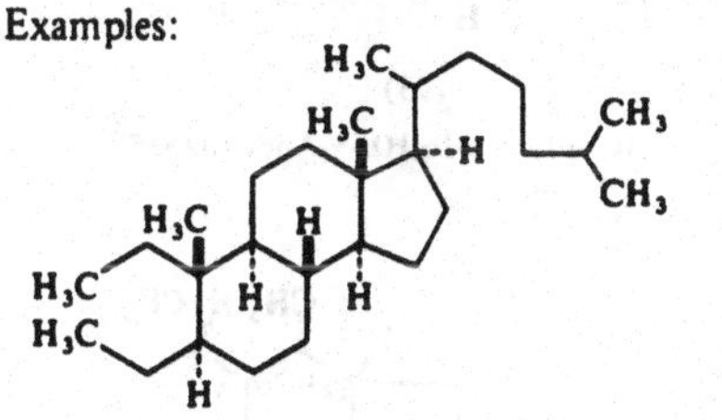

(91)

2,3-Seco-5α-cholestane

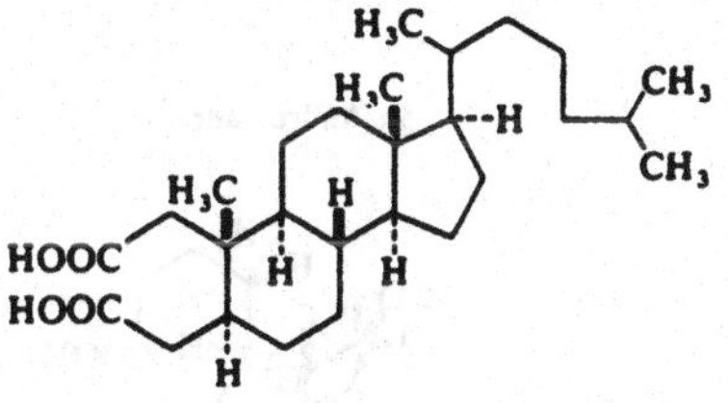

(92)

2,3-Seco-5α-cholestane-2,3-dioic acid

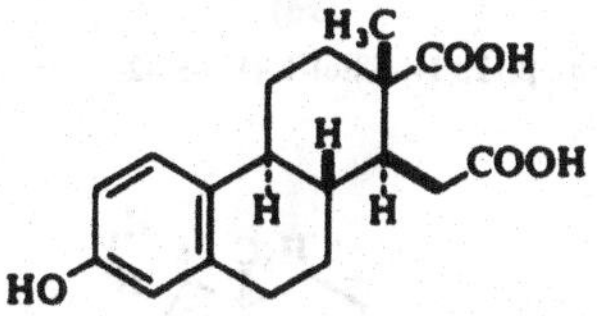

(93)

3-Hydroxy-16,17-seco-1,3,5(10)-estratriene-16,17-dioic acid

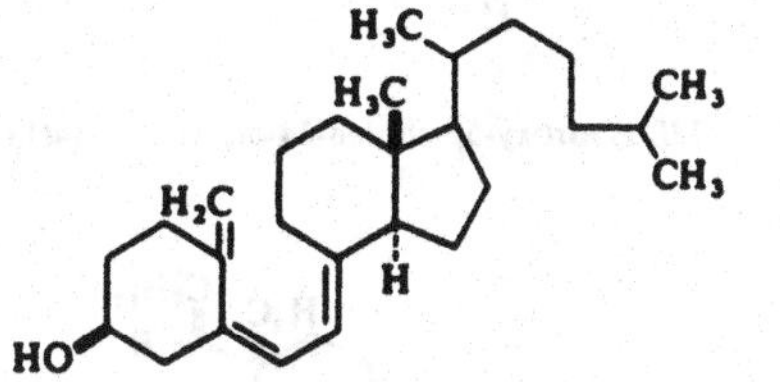

(94)

9,10-Seco-5,7,10(19)-cholestatrien-3β-ol
(trivial name: cholecalciferol†)

MODIFICATION BY BOND MIGRATION (*abeo* SYSTEM)

Rule 2S–9

9.1. A compound that does not possess a steroid skeleton but may be considered formally to arise from a steroid by bond migration may be given the name laid down in the preceding Rules for the steroid in question, to which is attached a prefix of the form $x(y \to z)abeo$-. This prefix is compiled as follows: A numeral denoting the stationary (unchanged) end of the migrating bond (x) is followed by parentheses enclosing (i) the number denoting the original position (y) from which the other end of this bond has migrated, (ii) an arrow, and (iii) the number (z) denoting the new position to which the

---

*If more than one ring is opened, general systematic nomenclature may be preferable. The principles of Note (a) to Rule 2S–7.1 apply also to seco-steroids.
†This trivial name is retained (see Rule 2S–4.2).

bond has moved. The closing parenthesis is followed by *abeo-* (Latin, I go away) (italicized) to indicate bond migration. The original steroid numbering is retained for the new compound and is used for the numbers x, y, and z. Such of the customary letters as are necessary are added to specify the resulting stereochemistry.

Note: The *abeo* nomenclature described in this Rule is permissive, not compulsory. It is most suitable for use in discussions of reaction mechanism and biogenesis. For registration in a general (nonsteroid) compendium the general systematic names may be preferable, particularly when names of steroid type can be conveniently assigned by the homo-nor method. Differences in numbering between *abeo* names and other systematic names should be particularly noted [cf. Example (96)].

Examples:

5α-Androstane   (95)   5(10 → 1)*abeo*-1α(H),5α-Androstane **

12β-Hydroxy-5β-cholan-24-oic acid   (96)   14(13 → 12)*abeo*-5β,12β(H)-Chol-13(17)-en-24-oic acid‡

5α-Cholestane   (97)   14(8 → 9)*abeo*-5α,9ξ-Cholestane*†

**Name according to Rule 2S–7.4 ("homo-nor" system): 9aβ-Methyl-*B(9a)*-homo-*A*-nor-5α,10α-estrane.
‡The name of this compound according to Rule 2S–7.4 ("homo-nor" system) is as follows: (4R)-4-(17α-Methyl-*D*-homo-*C*-nor-18-nor-5β-androst-17-en-17-yl)pentanoic acid, or 17-(1R)-3-Carboxy-1-methylpropyl]-17a-methyl-*D*-homo-*C*-nor-18-nor-5β-androst-17-ene.
*The configuration at C-9, if known, is assigned by the sequence-rule procedure. (97) cannot conveniently be named by the "homo-nor" system.
†The "homo-nor" system is not appropriate.

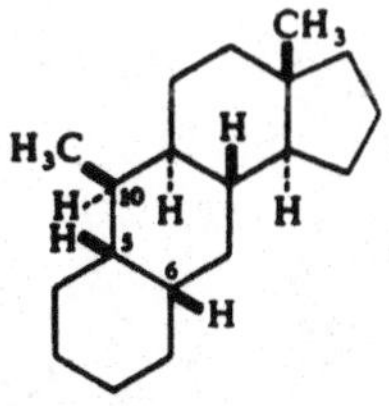

(98)

1(10→6)*abeo*-5β.6β(H)-Androstane (an anthrasteroid)†

HETEROCYCLIC MODIFICATIONS

Rule 2S–10 (Unchanged from Rule S–7.5)

10.1. If hetero atoms occur in the ring system of a steroid the replacement ("oxa-aza") system of nomenclature is used with steroid names and numbering (cf. IUPAC Rule B–4; also Introduction to IUPAC Rules C–0.6).**

Example:

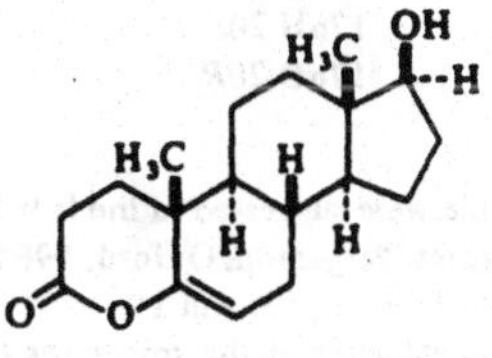

(99)

17β-Hydroxy-4-oxa-5-androsten-3-one

STEROID ALKALOIDS

Rule 2S–11

11.1 When readily possible, systematic names for steroid alkaloids are derived from pregnane or some other steroid parent name. Trivial names for other steroid alkaloids are chosen so that the name for the saturated system ends in "-anine." In names for unsaturated compounds this ending is changed to "-enine," "-adienine," etc., as appropriate. When asymmetry exists at positions 8, 9, 10, 13, 14, 16, 17, 20 or 23, it is implied in the name, as set out in Table 2 and the following formulas, and divergences are designated as laid down in Rule 2S–5. Configurations at positions 5, 22, and 25 must be specified with the name. Sequence-rule symbols are used for positions numbered 20 or higher.

Examples: Typical examples of parent names for groups of alkaloids are given in the table below and the corresponding formulas. It must be noted that substitution or unsaturation may alter the R,S designations for derivatives.

†The "homo-nor" system is not appropriate.

**IUPAC, *Nomenclature of Organic Chemistry, Sections A, B, and C,* Butterworths, London, 1971.

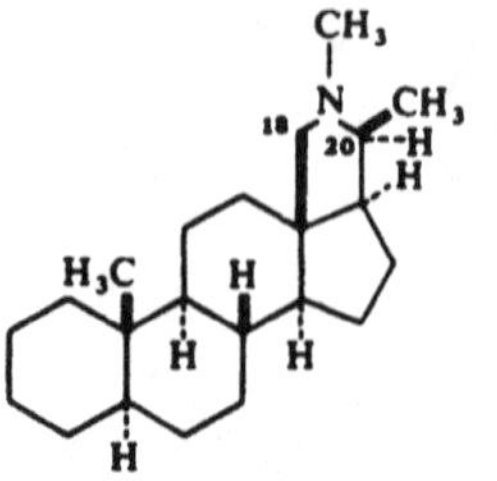

(100)

5α-Conanine*

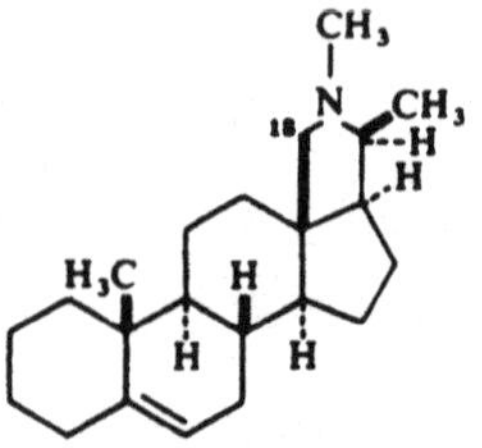

(101)

5-Conenine*

Table 2
PARENT NAMES FOR GROUPS OF STEROID ALKALOIDS[a]

Formula	Name of parent	Stereochemistry[b] implied in the name, as shown in the formula	Stereochemistry to be indicated by sequence-rule prefixes (or ξ)
100	Conanine	17αH,20S	–
102	Tomatanine[c]	16αH,17αH,20S	22, 25
103	Solanidanine[d]	16αH,17αH,20S	22, 25
104	Cevanine[e]	13βH,17αH,20R	22, 25
105	Veratranine[e,f]	17αH.20S	22, 25
106	Jervanine[e,f]	17αO,20R	22, 23, 25

[a]Some of the names in this table were suggested in the Introduction to *Optical Rotatory Power, Ia Steroids,* Tables des Constantes. Pergamon, Oxford, 1965, pp. 2a and 2f.

[b]Additional to that at positions 8, 9, 10, 13, and 14.

[c]The compounds are oxa-aza-analogues of the spirostans (which are dioxa spiro compounds). Formulae are conveniently drawn analogously to those of the spirostans.

[d]This group includes rubijervine and isorubijervane.

[e]These structures contain a D-homo-C-nor skeleton, with the stereochemistry shown. However, they are commonly considered as 14(13→12)*abeo* structures and are numbered as such.

[f]Jervanine, as defined here, is the same as veratranine except for addition of an epoxy bridge, but it is convenient to have two separate names: the veratranine skeleton [see (105)] is present in the alkaloid veratramine. It should be noted that the name 5α-jervane has been used for the rearranged hydrocarbon skeleton (107) [Fried, J. and Klingsberg, A., *J. Am. Chem. Soc.,* 75, 4934 (1953)], for which the *abeo*-type numbering given in (107) is here recommended.

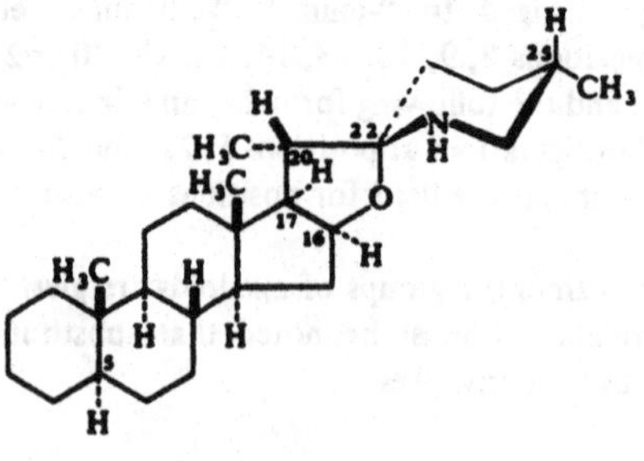

(102)

(22S,25S)-5α-Tomatanine

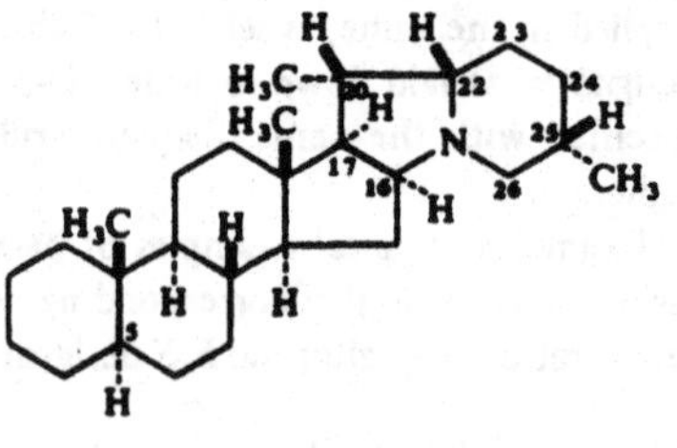

(103)

(22S,25S)-5α-Solanidanine

*Cf. Haworth, R. D. and Michael, M., *J. Chem. Soc.,* p. 4973 (1957).

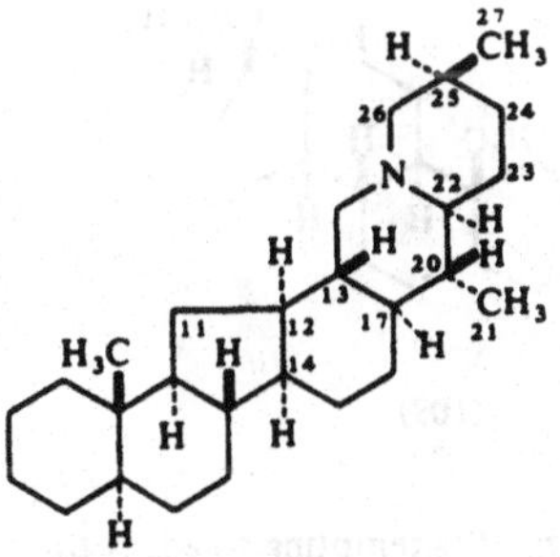

(104)

(22S,25S)-5α-Cevanine

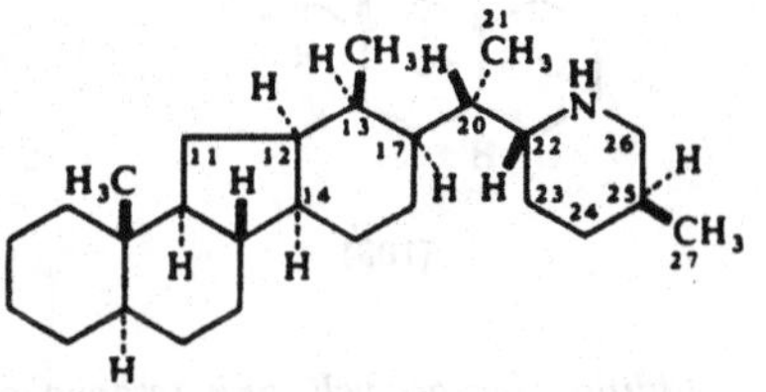

(105)

(22R,25S)-5α-Veratranine

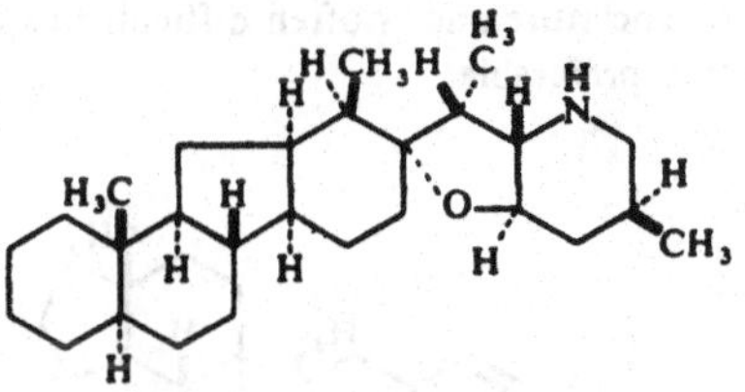

(106)

(22S,23R,25S)-5α-Jervanine

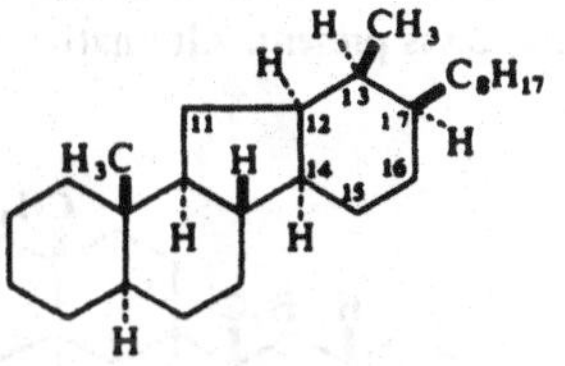

(107)

5α-Jervane*

APPENDIX

Guidelines for Steroids Containing Additional Rings

1. *General.* When additional rings are formed within, or on, a steroid nucleus, situations often arise where either the resemblance to a normal steroid is obscured or the steroid-type name becomes so complex that recourse to general systematic nomenclature is preferable. On the other hand, the general rules, with one exception, are based on that form of each component that contains the maximum number of conjugated double bonds, the whole fused system is then renumbered, and the stereochemistry must be defined separately for each chiral position; the final name resulting is then cumbrous and in a form that is often barely recognizable by a steroid specialist chemist and even less so by a biochemist or biologist. The paragraphs below give suggestions as to how general nomenclature may be modified to incorporate steroid names, but without an attempt to legislate rigidly or to cover every case. The decision whether any one compound shall receive such a modified steroid name or a general systematic name is left to authors and editors in the particular circumstances of each case. Nor are the requirements of journals and compendia or abstracts necessarily identical.

2. *Rings derived from functional groups.* Bivalent functional groups such as –O– and –O–O– linked to two different positions, thus forming additional rings, are named by the ordinary methods of organic chemistry; for example, (108) is 3α,9-epidioxy-5α-androstan-17-one. Similarly, methylendioxy derivatives are best named as such, e.g., (109) 2α,3α-methylenedioxy-5-pregnene. In the same way, lactones and acetals formed by linkage between two different positions of a steroid skeleton are best named as such instead of by framing the name on the newly modified ring system.

*Cf. Fried, J. and Klingsberg, A., *J. Am. Chem. Soc.*, 75, 4934 (1953).

(108)   (109)

3. *Additional carbocyclic or heterocyclic fused rings.* It is tempting to adapt the simple substitutive procedure for fusion of steroid nuclei with simple carbocyclic rings, particularly if the latter are saturated. Thus (110) might be named 2α,3β-tetramethylene-5α-androstane.* However, formation of additional rings by alkylene ($-[CH_2]_x-$) prefixes is not in accord with IUPAC nomenclature and is often difficult to apply when unsaturation is present. Alternatives are thus preferable.

(110)   (111)

The exceptional case (Rule A–23.5) referred to above enables 2,3-benz-5α-androst-2-ene to be a name for (111), and a slight extension of the rule would allow (110) to be called 2β,3α-cyclohexano-5α-androstane. Such methods might be used in simple cases but these too become difficult when complex ring systems are fused and often when unsaturation is present in the additional component.

For a general procedure it is better to modify systematic IUPAC general practice to permit the steroid component to be cited in a reduced state, the reason why modification is necessary at all being of course the wish to keep the description of the stereochemistry as simple as possible. The suggestions below are closely similar to present practices of *Chemical Abstracts.*

An additional carbocyclic component is cited in its most unsaturated form by its fusion name (usually ending in -o), placed in front of the name of the steroid component, and the position of fusion is indicated by·numerals in square brackets; for instance, benz[2,3]-5α-androst-2-ene for (111). Here note that the unsaturation of the benzo ring causes unsaturation also in the steroid component and this must be cited (-2-ene). Similarly, (112) is naphth[2′,3′:2,3]-5α-androst-2-ene; the steroid *A* ring is still considered partially unsaturated even though it may be preferable to write the naphthalene double bonds as in the formula shown; note also that the locants for the nonsteroid component receive primes, and that, when choice is possible, its locants for ring fusion are as low as possible and in the same direction as in the steroid component (i.e., not 6′,7′:2,3 or 3′,2′:2,3).

---

*For simplicity, nomenclature in this Appendix is mostly described in terms of androstane, and partial formulas are to be understood accordingly. The principles, however, are general.

(112)   (113)   (114)

The reduced compound (110) is then 2β,3α,3',4',5',6'-hexahydrobenz[2,3]-5α-andro-stane. Note the citation of the configuration at the new ring junction positions and that the steroid component is now cited in its saturated state.

Two further points can be illustrated with (113). Consider first the hydrocarbon where X = H. The additional ring is cited as cyclopropa- denoting an unsaturated three-membered ring as in (114). In (114) the position of the "extra" (indicated) hydrogen must be cited as 3'H. Reduction of (114) to (113; X = H) adds 2α,3α-dihydro to the name, which thus becomes 2α, 3α-dihydro-3'H-cycloprop[2,3]-5α-androstane. If X were not hydrogen but, say, OH, the hydro prefixes would still be needed to show the state of hydrogenation and the OH group would be named additionally; in such cases it is preferable to state the configuration for the OH group that is present rather than that of the H atom that has been replaced; the name then becomes 2α,3-dihydro-3'H-cyclo-prop[2,3]-5β-androstan-3α-ol.

The same fundamental principle can be used for heterocyclic components, but conveniently modified to accord with general nomenclature as follows: (a) the heterocyclic component is cited after the steroid component (to permit modification of the ending for salt formation, etc.), and (b) the position of fusion of the heterocyclic component is cited by letters as in the standard IUPAC and *Ring Index* method. Thus, (115) is 2'-methyl-2'H-5α-androst-2-eno[3,2-c]pyrazole; note the numbering of the pyrazole ring so that numbers for ring fusion are as low as possible; if the methyl group in (115) were replaced by hydrogen, the double bonds would be placed in the mesomeric pyrazole ring just as in (115) so as to retain this low numbering for ring fusion. In the isomer (116) the steroid component is no longer unsaturated and is therefore cited as androstano-; the full name for (116) is 1'-methyl-1'H-5α-androstano[3,2-c]pyrazole.

(115)   (116)

Further problems arise when ring fusion involves a quaternary carbon atom. The name for (117), for instance, could be built up as follows: To 5α-pregnane is fused an isoxazole skeleton, giving (118); into this, only one double bond can be introduced, so that one hydrogen atom must be added as indicated hydrogen, which gives a 4'βH- prefix and a skeleton (119). The last step, inserting the double bond, gives the full name 4'βH-5α-pregnano[16.17-d]isoxazole, even though it appears in (117) as if the hetero-cyclic ring should be named as the partly hydrogenated system isoxazoline.

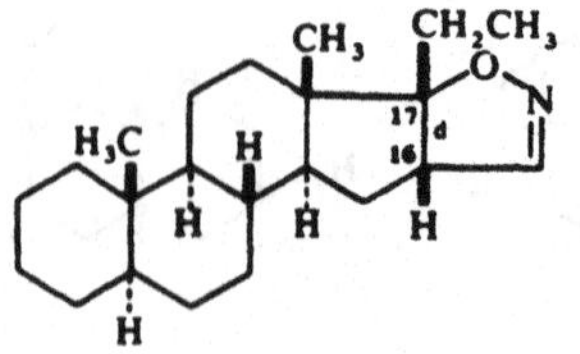

(117) 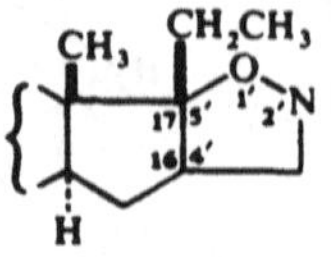   (118) 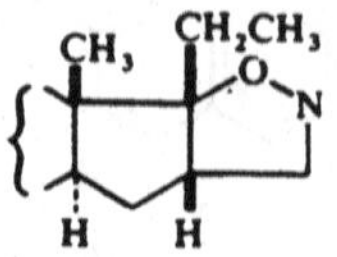   (119)

Not all such fusions cause all these complications. For instance, for (120) one fuses androstane to azirine, obtaining a skeleton into which one inserts a double bond as in the hypothetical compound (121); then, clearly, (120) is 1′,3′-dihydro-1′-methyl-5α-andro-stano[5,6-*b*]azirine.

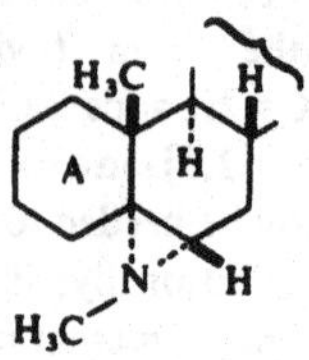

(120) 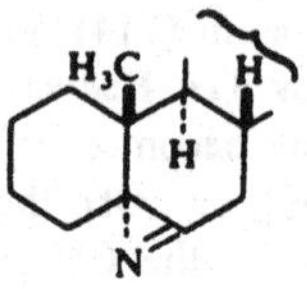   (121)

4. *Stereochemistry.* Stereochemistry in additional rings that lie in the approximate plane of rings *A–D* is cited as α or β, but in other cases by means of sequence-rule symbols.

5. *Spiro derivatives.* Spiro derivatives of steroids are named in accordance with the principles laid down in IUPAC Rules A–41, A–42, B–10, and B–11. Additional stereochemistry due to the spiro junction and substituents in the nonsteroid ring is designated by the sequence-rule procedure. Alternative names permitted by IUPAC Rules are illustrated for (122) and (123).

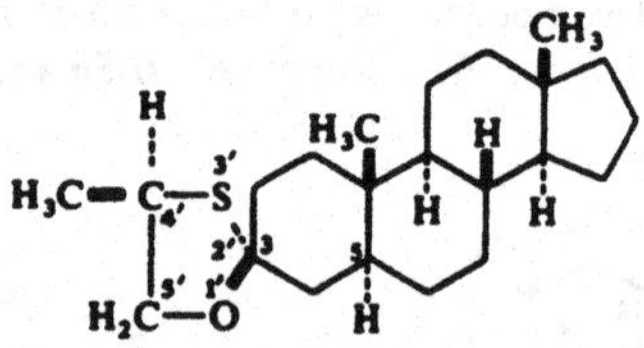

(122)

4′*R*-Methyl-(*R*)-spiro[5α-androstane-3,2′-(1′,3′-oxathiolane)]
or 5α-androstane-3(*R*)-spiro-2′-(4′*R*-methyl-1′,3′-oxathiolane)

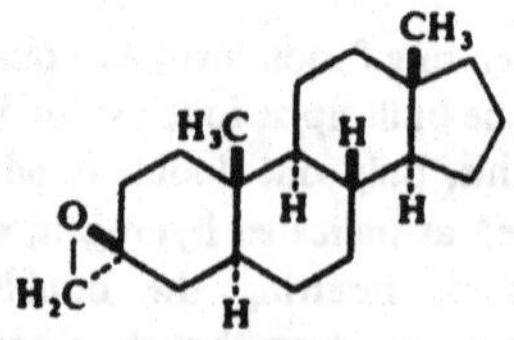

(123)

(3*S*)-Spiro[5α-androstane-3,2′-oxirane]
or (3*S*)-5α-androstane-3-spiro-2′-oxirane

NOMENCLATURE OF CYCLITOLS RECOMMENDATIONS (1973)*

IUPAC Commission on the Nomenclature of Organic Chemistry
and IUPAC-IUB Commission on Biochemical Nomenclature

EVOLUTION OF CYCLITOL NOMENCLATURE

The typical stereochemical feature of cyclitols is exemplified by Formula A, usually drawn more simply as B or C, in which the ring is considered as being planar and nearly perpendicular to the plane of the paper with hydrogen atoms and hydroxyl groups above or below the plane of the ring.

A   B   C

In 1900, Maquenne[3] devised a fractional notation whereby numerals in the numerator denote hydroxyl or other groups (not hydrogen) above the plane of the ring while numerals in the denominator denote hydroxyl or other groups (not hydrogen) below that plane. Thus the above compound received a stereochemical prefix 1,2,4,5 -, which may be more conveniently printed as 1,2,4,5/3,6-.

Maquenne did not, however, specify exactly how the numerals were to be assigned to the individual positions, and as the chemistry of cyclitols developed, these assignments were made in different ways. Several systems of nomenclature were proposed.[4,5] Most notably, a logical and self-consistent system was developed (but not assembled as a set of rules) by Posternak,[6] and his system was widely used, though with occasional variants by others. The variety of names that resulted is illustrated in Table 1, which gives also the names derived by application of the Recommendations below.

It is an advantage of the Posternak system that the resulting fractional prefix describes not only the relative positions of the substituents but also the absolute configuration of a compound; no additional prefix such as D or L, or R or S, is needed to differentiate enantiomers since pairs of enantiomers receive different fractional prefixes. This very feature, however, entails serious disadvantages. The fractional prefix gives no indication whether a compound so specified is chiral or achiral, and for a pair of enantiomers gives no indication that they have the same relative configuration, i.e., that they are enantiomers. This is contrary to the practice in the rest of chemical literature, whereby enantiomers receive identical names except for a specific prefix denoting the chirality. Also, specification of racemates becomes somewhat cumbrous by this system.

An alternative method of assigning numerals, based in part on previous practice[4,5] and on proposals made by McCasland,[7] was recommended by a majority of the Joint Cyclitol Nomenclature Subcommittee, and was adopted by the parent IUPAC and IUPAC-IUB

*From IUPAC Commission on the Nomenclature of Organic Chemistry and IUPAC-IUB Commission on Biochemical Nomenclature, *Pure Appl. Chem.*, 37, 283–297 (1974). With permission.

Table 1
EXAMPLES OF CYCLITOLS NAMED BY DIFFERENT SYSTEMS[a]

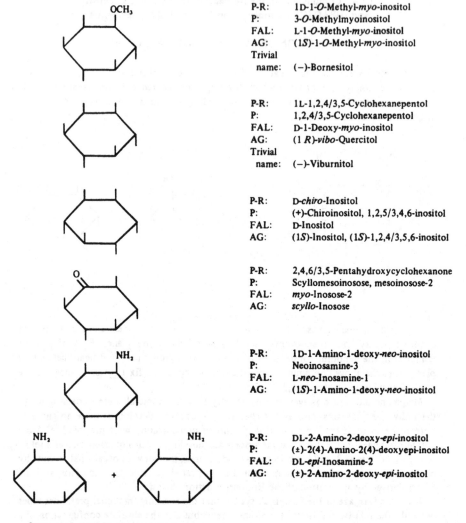

P-R:	1D-1-*O*-Methyl-*myo*-inositol
P:	3-*O*-Methylmyoinositol
FAL:	L-1-*O*-Methyl-*myo*-inositol
AG:	(1*S*)-1-*O*-Methyl-*myo*-inositol
Trivial name:	(−)-Bornesitol

P-R:	1L-1,2,4/3,5-Cyclohexanepentol
P:	1,2,4/3,5-Cyclohexanepentol
FAL:	D-1-Deoxy-*myo*-inositol
AG:	(1 *R*)-*vibo*-Quercitol
Trivial name:	(−)-Viburnitol

P-R:	D-*chiro*-Inositol
P:	(+)-Chiroinositol, 1,2,5/3,4,6-inositol
FAL:	D-Inositol
AG:	(1*S*)-Inositol, (1*S*)-1,2,4/3,5,6-inositol

P-R:	2,4,6/3,5-Pentahydroxycyclohexanone
P:	Scyllomesoinosose, mesoinosose-2
FAL:	*myo*-Inosose-2
AG:	*scyllo*-Inosose

P-R:	1D-1-Amino-1-deoxy-*neo*-inositol
P:	Neoinosamine-3
FAL:	L-*neo*-Inosamine-1
AG:	(1*S*)-1-Amino-1-deoxy-*neo*-inositol

P-R:	DL-2-Amino-2-deoxy-*epi*-inositol
P:	(±)-2(4)-Amino-2(4)-deoxyepi-inositol
FAL:	DL-*epi*-Inosamine-2
AG:	(±)-2-Amino-2-deoxy-*epi*-inositol

[a]P-R = Present Recommendations
P = = Posternak[6]
FAL = Fletcher, Anderson, and Lardy[4]
AG = Angyal and Gilham[5]

Nomenclature Commissions in 1967.[1] By this method, enantiomers receive identical fractional prefixes that specify relative configuration, but they also receive an additional prefix D or L, which specifies the chirality.

When the Tentative Rules were published in 1968,[1] it seemed advisable to set out detailed Rules for Posternak's system because it had been widely used in the literature up to that date. These nonpreferred Rules were, therefore, given in Part C of the Tentative Rules. However, this system has not been widely used during the past few years, and the "nonpreferred" Rules are therefore omitted from these Recommendations.

The present Recommendations are essentially identical with the Tentative Rules, but they have been extensively rearranged in format for the convenience of their users.

RECOMMENDATIONS

A. Cyclitols with only Hydroxyl or Substituted Hydroxyl Groups
1. Inositols
Rule I-1.* Configuration Prefixes

I-1.1. 1,2,3,4,5,6-Cyclohexanehexols are termed generically "inositols." Individual inositols are differentiated by use of an italicized prefix and hyphen, as follows, the locants (positional numbers) being assigned according to criteria ii. and vi. of Rule I-4.

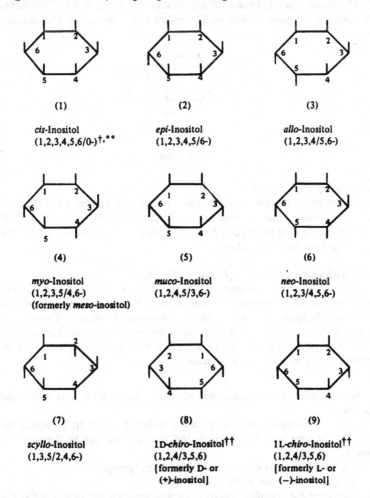

(1)	(2)	(3)
cis-Inositol	epi-Inositol	allo-Inositol
(1,2,3,4,5,6/0-)†,**	(1,2,3,4,5/6-)	(1,2,3,4/5,6-)
(4)	(5)	(6)
myo-Inositol	muco-Inositol	neo-Inositol
(1,2,3,5/4,6-)	(1,2,4,5/3,6-)	(1,2,3/4,5,6-)
(formerly meso-inositol)		
(7)	(8)	(9)
scyllo-Inositol	1D-chiro-Inositol††	1L-chiro-Inositol††
(1,3,5/2,4,6-)	(1,2,4/3,5,6)	(1,2,4/3,5,6)
	[formerly D- or	[formerly L- or
	(+)-inositol]	(−)-inositol]

*I- (for Inositol) is attached to the Rule members as a general identifying prefix.
†Preferred to "all-cis-" in this and similar cases. The zero is inserted for clarity.
**Throughout the examples, a simple vertical stroke standing alone signifies a bond to a hydroxyl group.

††For absolute configurational prefixes, see Rule I-10.

I-1.2. The numberings of Formulas (1) to (9) are retained for derivatives of the inositols. Within this framework, criteria iv. and v. of Rule I-4 are used to decide between alternatives. These arise because (a) in several of the parent inositols [(1), (5), (6), (7), (8), and (9)] there are two or more fully equivalent starting points for numbering that may not be equivalent in the derivatives, and (b) criterion vi. of Rule I-4 does not apply to chiral derivatives of the *meso*-inositols [(1) to (7)]. The application of criteria iv. and v. to a pair of enantiomers gives each pair of mirror-related positions the same number. Typically one enantiomer will be numbered clockwise, the other counterclockwise.

2. Other Cyclitols
Rule I-2. Trivial Names
I-2. The trivial name (+)-quercitol is permitted for 1L-1,3,4/2,5-cyclohexanepentol (for derivation of this name see below). The generic name "quercitols" is abandoned.

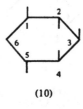

(10)

(+)-Quercitol

Rule I-3. Description of Structure
I-3. The structure of cyclitols other than the inositols are described by use of the IUPAC 1971 Rules for the Nomenclature of Organic Chemistry, Section C,[8] with the proviso that cyclitols are named as substituted cycloalkanepolyols even when some or all of the hydroxyl groups are substituted.

Rule I-4. Assignment of Locants (Positional Numbers)
I-4. Locants (positional numbers) are assigned to the carbon atoms of the ring, and thus the direction of numbering is described, with reference to the steric relations and nature of the substituents attached to the ring. The substituents lying above the plane of the ring constitute a set, and those lying below the plane another set. Lowest locants are related to one set of the substituents according to the following criteria, which are applied successively until a decision is reached:

i. to the substituents considered as a numerical series, without regard to configuration;

ii. if one set of substituents is more numerous than the other, to the more numerous;

iii. if the sets are equally numerous and one of them can be denoted by lower numbers, to that set;

iv. to substituents other than unmodified hydroxyl groups;

v. to the substituent first in alphabetical order;[9]

vi. − for *meso*-compounds only−to those positions that lead to an L rather than a D designation when Rule I-10 is applied to the lowest-numbered asymmetric carbon atom.

Notes: (1) "Lowest numbers" are those that, when considered as a single ascending series, contain the lower number at the first point of difference, e.g., 1,2,3,6 is lower than 1,2,4,5.

(2) Criterion vi. is needed only for compounds with *meso*-configuration, being

required only for problems involving prochirality.[10] It can be simply applied by noting that it causes numbering to be clockwise when the formula is oriented so that the substituent on the lowest-numbered asymmetric carbon atom of the ring projects upwards.

(3) When two or more positions are fully equivalent it is immaterial which is chosen as the starting point.

Rule I-5. Relative Configuration

I-5.1. The relative configurations at ring positions of a cyclitol, other than an inositol or a derivative thereof, are described by means of a fraction. The numerator of the fraction consists of the locants (assigned as described above) of the set of substituents that lies above or below the plane of the ring, these numbers being arranged in ascending order and separated by commas. The denominator contains the locants of the other set. Conventionally, the set of locants containing the lowest numbers is cited as numerator.

I-5.2. When only hydroxyl or substituted hydroxyl groups are involved, the fraction also serves as a list of locants. Its position in the name is that usually assigned to the list of locants (see examples).

Note: (1) The fraction may be written with a horizontal or a sloping division line, e.g.,

$\frac{1,2,4}{3,5,6}$ or 1,2,4/3,5,6,·.

Examples* (showing also which criteria of Rule I-4 were applied):

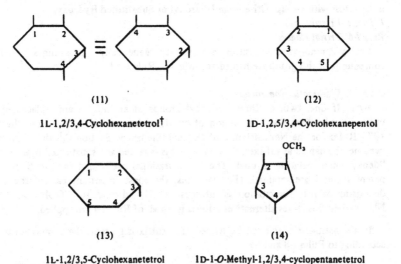

(11)

1L-1,2/3,4-Cyclohexanetetrol[†]

(12)

1D-1,2,5/3,4-Cyclohexanepentol

(13)

1L-1,2/3,5-Cyclohexanetetrol

(14)

1D-1-O-Methyl-1,2/3,4-cyclopentanetetrol

*As exceptions to general nomenclature, but in accord with carbohydrate nomenclature, ethers and esters of cyclitols may be named either by using prefixes such as 1-O-methyl, 1-O-acetyl, etc., or by adding 1-methyl ether, 1-acetate, etc., after the name of the polyol. For simplicity, only the former alternative is used in these examples.

†For allocation of D and L to these and other enantiomers in the examples, see Rule I-10.

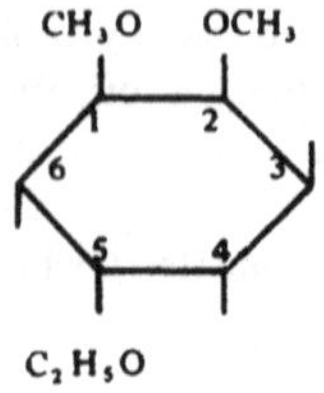

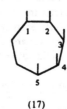

(15)

1L-5-*O*-Ethyl-1,2-di-*O*-methyl-*neo*-inositol
Note: numbers 1,2,5 for substituents are
lower than 2,3,5 or 2,4,5 or 2,5,6)

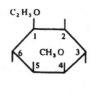

(16)

1L-1-*O*-Ethyl-4-*O*-methyl-*muco*-inositol

(17)

1,2,3,4,5/0-Cycloheptanepentol

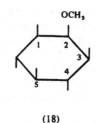

(18)

2-*O*-Methyl-*myo*-inositol

B. Cyclitols with Groups Other than Hydroxyl or Substituted Hydroxyl

1. Inositol Derivatives

Rule I-6. Trivial Names

I-6. χ-Amino-χ-deoxyinositols are termed generically "inosamines," individual compounds of this group are named according to Rule I-7.1.

Rule I-7. Systematic Nomenclature

I-7.1. If one, two, or three hydroxyl groups of an inositol are replaced by other univalent substituents with retention of configuration, and if, according to the IUPAC 1971 Rules for the Nomenclature of Organic Chemistry, Section C,[8] these substituents need not be named as suffixes; the compound is regarded as a substituted inositol and the "deoxy" nomenclature is used. The configurational prefix and the numbering of the parent inositol are retained. (For cyclitols, the most important part of the order of decreasing priority for citation as suffix is COOH and modified COOH, $=0$, OH, SH, NH_2.) When this leaves alternatives criteria iv. to vi. of Rule I-4 are applied.

If a substituent that must be named as a suffix is present, the compound is named according to Rules I-8 and I-9.

I-7.2. Inositol derivatives in which one carbon atom carries a substituent additional to a hydroxyl are named as substituted inositols, provided that the substituent does not rank above hydroxyl for citation as suffix. (If it does, Rule I-9.2 applies.) For the disubstituted position in such compounds the configurational prefix refers to the hydroxyl group.

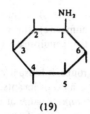

(19)

1D-1-Amino-1-deoxy-*myo*-inositol

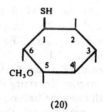

(20)

1L-1-Deoxy-1-mercapto-6-*O*-methyl-*chiro*-inositol*

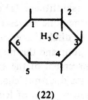

(21)

1,3,5-Triamino-1,3,5-trideoxy-*scyllo*-inositol

(22)

2-*C*-Methyl-*myo*-inositol†

2. Other Cyclitols
Rule I-8. Trivial Names

I-8. 2,3,4,5,6-Pentahydroxycyclohexanones are termed generically "inososes;" the individual compounds are named according to Rule I-9. The trivial name (−)-quinic or L-quinic acid is preferred for the following compound (see the last example to Rule I-9):

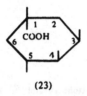

(23)

(−)-Quinic acid; L-Quinic acid;
1L-1(OH),3,4/5-Tetrahydroxy-
cyclohexanecarboxylic acid

Rule I-9. Systematic Nomenclature

I-9.1. Cyclitols containing substituents other than hydroxyl or modified hydroxyl (excepting inositols covered by Rule I-7) are named and numbered according to the above-mentioned IUPAC Rules, with the proviso that *O*-substituents are named as such (see Rule I-3). Substituted hydroxyl groups are not named as alkoxy, aryloxy, or acyloxy groups. When these rules leave alternatives available, the criteria ii. to vi. of Rule I-4 are applied. Relative configuration is indicated as prescribed in Rule I-5.1. Except when it is serving as a locant set, the fraction describing the configuration is placed in parentheses, and it becomes the first element in the name, except for the configurational prefix (Rule I-10).

---

*IUPAC Rule C-502 is compatible with a name 1L-6-*O*-methyl-1-thio-*chiro*-inositol but that name does not accord with the instruction in Rule I-7.1 to use the "deoxy" nomenclature.
†The prefix *C*- is added to denote substitution on carbon in accordance with carbohydrate nomenclature.[11]

Notes: (1) The IUPAC Rule C-10[8] provides that one type of group be chosen as suffix, named as suffix, and given the lowest possible number(s), the remaining types being named as prefixes. For choice of suffix, see the penultimate (parenthetical) sentence in Rule I-7.1.

(2) When there are substituents other than hydroxyl groups, it is usually impracticable to use the fraction describing the relative configuration as a list of locants. In stipulating that, in such cases, the fraction be placed in front of the *complete* name of the compound (including *O*-substituents), the present Recommendations differ from the Tentative Rules.

I-9.2. Cyclitol derivatives in which one carbon atom carries a substituent additional to hydroxyl are named (a) as substituted cycloalkanepolyols or (b) as hydroxy derivatives, according as a substituent (a) does not or (b) does rank above hydroxyl for citation as suffix. When the Rule leaves alternatives available, the criteria ii. to vi. of Rule I-4 are applied. For the disubstituted positions in such compounds, the fractional prefix refers to the hydroxyl group and this may be specified for clarity where necessary.

Note: Replacement of the hydrogen of amino, mercapto, or hydroxyl groups by other atoms or groups does not change the numbering of cyclitol derivatives except when it affects criterion iv. or v. of Rule I-4. However, the IUPAC Rules[8] require that the ring carbon atom carrying as a substituent a trisubstituted ammonio (R_3N^+), acid, oxo, cyano, or acyl group, or a derivative thereof, receive the locant 1; such cases will be relatively rare in cyclitol chemistry. A convenient alternative for "onium" salts is to use the terminology exemplified by methiodide, hydrochloride, sulfate, etc.

Examples:

(24)

(1,4/2,3,5,6)-2,3,5,6-Tetraamino-1,4-cyclohexanediol

(25)

(1,4,5/2,3)-5-Amino-1,2,3,4-cyclopentanetetrol

(26)

1L-(1/2,3,4,5)-5-Amino-1,2,3,4-cyclohexanetetrol

(27)

1D-(1,2/4,5)-4-Amino-5-mercapto-1-*O*-methyl-1,2-cyclohexanediol

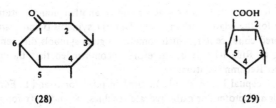

(28)   (29)

2L-2,3,5/4,6-Pentahydroxycyclohexanone   1L-(1,5/2,3,4)-2,3,4,5-Tetrahydroxycyclopentane-
                                                carboxylic acid

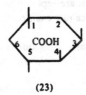

(23)

1L-1(OH),3,4/5-Tetrahydroxycyclohexanecarboxylic
acid (L-quinic acid) (This numbering is opposite to
former usage.)

C. Absolute Configuration
Rule I-10. Absolute Configuration

I-10. The absolute configuration of a cyclitol is specified by making a vertical Fischer-Tollens type of projection of the structure, with C-1 at the top and with C-2 and C-3 on the front edge of the ring. The configuration is then designated as D if the hydroxyl group at the lowest-numbered chiral center (or other substituent if no hydroxyl group is present there) projects to the right, and as L if it projects to the left (of Figure 1). The prefix D or L, followed by a hyphen, is written before the name of the compound and may be preceded by the locant of the defining center. Racemic compounds are designated by the prefix DL.

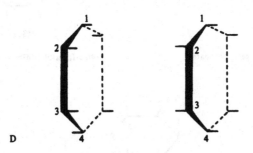

D   L

FIGURE 1.

Notes: (1) The mere absence of a prefix D, L, or DL indicates that the compound has a *meso*-configuration; thus, the prefix D, L, or DL should not be omitted.

(2) A simple way of applying this Rule is as follows: When the formula is drawn in such a way that the substituent on the *lowest*-numbered asymmetric carbon atom is above the plane of the ring, and the numbering is clockwise, the compound is L; if anti-clockwise, it is D [see Examples (8) and (9)].

(3) In a great majority of cases the lowest-numbered chiral center is position 1, so that it would be reasonable that D or L should be preceded by the locant of the defining

center only when it is not 1. However, according to another nomenclature system for cyclitols[4] and also for the related carbohydrate field, the symbols D and L are assigned to the *highest*-numbered chiral center, which sometimes gives symbols different from those assigned according to Rule I-10. It is, therefore, recommended that the numeral 1 be included (as in these Recommendations).

(4) Small Roman capital letters should be used in print for D and L. For compounds containing cyclitols and protein or carbohydrate residues, D_c and L_c (c for cyclitol) may be used alongside D_s, L_s, D_g, and L_g.[12] Cyclitol nomenclature may also be combined with the use of the sequence rule[2] or the stereospecific numbering (*sn*) system,[13] where necessary.

(5) When many hydroxyl groups are replaced by other substituents, it may be simpler to use the sequence rule.[2] Sequence-rule examples are given in Table 1, also in Reference 2.

Examples: Many examples of chiral compounds are named in the preceding examples [e.g., (11) to (16) and (26) to (29)]. The following are additional.

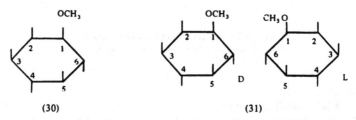

(30)

1D-1-*O*-Methyl-*myo*-inositol
[D-(−)-Bornesitol]

(31)

DL-1-*O*-Methyl-*myo*-inositol

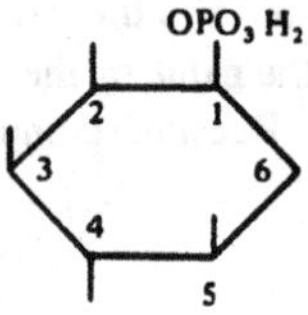

(32)

1D-*myo*-Inositol 1-(dihydrogen phosphate)

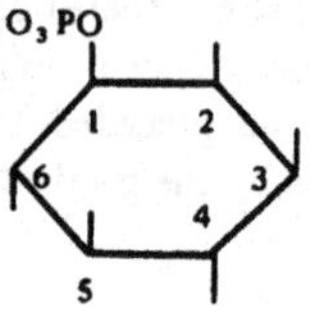

(33)

1L-*myo*-Inositol 1-(dihydrogen phosphate)

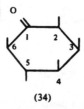

(34)

1   2L-2,3,4,6/5-Pentahydroxycyclohexanone

REFERENCES

1. IUPAC-IUB, IUPAC Information Bulletin No. 32, 51 (1968); *Eur. J. Biochem.*, 5, 1 (1968); *Arch. Biochem. Biophys.*, 128, 269 (1968); *J. Biol. Chem.*, 243, 5809 (1968); *Biochem. J.*, 112, 17 (1969); *Biochim. Biophys. Acta*, 165, 1 (1968); *Hoppe-Seyler's Z. Physiol. Chem.*, 350, 523 (1969) (German language version); *Bull. Soc. Chim. Biol.*, 51, 3 (1969) (French language version).
2. Cahn, R. S., Ingold, C., and Prelog, V., *Angew. Chem.*, 78, 413 (1966); *Angew. Chem. Int. Ed.*, 5, 385 (1966); IUPAC 1968 Tentative Rules, Section E, *J. Org. Chem.*, 35, 2849 (1970).
3. Maquenne, L., *Les Sucres et leur Principaux Dérivés*, Gauthiers-Villars, Paris, 1900; also Georges Carré et C. Naud, Paris, 1900.
4. Fletcher, H. G., Jr., Anderson, L., and Lardy, H. A., *J. Org. Chem.*, 16, 1238 (1951).
5. Angyal, S. J. and Gilham, P. T., *J. Chem. Soc.*, 3691 (1957).
6. Posternak, T., *The Cyclitols*, Hermann, Paris, 1965.
7. McCasland, G. E., *Adv. Carbohydr. Chem.*, 20, 11 (1965).
8. IUPAC Definitive Rules for *Nomenclature of Organic Chemistry*, Section C, 2nd ed., Butterworths, London, 1971.
9. IUPAC Definitive Rules for *Nomenclature of Organic Chemistry*, Section C, 2nd ed., Butterworths, London, 1971, Rule C-16.3.
10. Hanson, K. R., *J. Am. Chem. Soc.*, 88, 2731 (1966).
11. IUPAC-IUB, IUPAC Information Bulletin No. 7, Carbohydrate Nomenclature-1, IUPAC, Oxford, 1970; *J. Biol. Chem.*, 247, 613 (1972).
12. IUPAC, *J. Am. Chem. Soc.*, 82, 5575, (1960).
13. IUPAC-IUB, *Eur. J. Biochem.*, 2, 127 (1967); *Biochem. J.*, 105, 897 (1967).

TENTATIVE RULES FOR CARBOHYDRATE NOMENCLATURE
PART 1 (1969)*

IUPAC Commission on the Nomenclature of Organic Chemistry (CNOG)
and IUPAC-IUB Commission on Biochemical Nomenclature (CBN)

PREAMBLE

Scope of the Rules

These Rules deal with the acyclic and cylic forms of monosaccharides and their simple derivatives; oligasaccharides are also dealt with briefly.

Carbohydrate chemistry continues to provide a very fruitful field of research, such that it will be necessary, in the near future, to promulgate further Rules to cover the needs of developing areas, e.g., branched-chain and unsaturated monosaccharides, other carbohydrate acyclic and heterocyclic derivatives, conformational problems, and poly-saccharides.

Use of the Rules

These Rules are additional to the Definitive Rules for the Nomenclature of Organic Chemistry[1] and are intended to govern those aspects of the nomenclature of carbohydrates not covered by those rules.

1. The Structure Named

These Rules are designed to name first a parent monosaccharide represented in the Fischer projection of the acyclic form and then its cyclic forms and derivatives.

The numbering system used in monosaccharides is based on the location of the (potential) carbonyl group. Modification of that group or introduction of further similar groups can therefore often destroy the uniqueness of the numbering system and permit a derivative to be named from more than one parent. In order to determine the unique systematic name of a derivative it is important to follow the procedure of establishing the Fischer projection of the appropriate parent monosaccharide, naming that according to the Rules, and thereafter deriving the name of any derivative.

2. Conventional Representations

a. The Fischer projection – In this representation of a monosaccharide, the carbon chain is written vertically with carbon atom number 1 at the top. The groups projecting to left and right of the carbon chain are considered as being in front of the plane of the paper. The optical antipode with the hydroxyl group at the highest-numbered asymmetric carbon atom on the right is then regarded as belonging to the D-series. It is now known that this convention represents the absolute configuration.

b. The Haworth representation – The Haworth representation of the cyclic forms of monosaccharides can be derived from the Fischer projection, as follows. The monosaccharide is depicted with the carbon-chain horizontal and in the plane of the paper, the potential carbonyl group being to the right. The oxygen bridge is then depicted as being formed behind the plane of the paper.

The heterocyclic ring is therefore located in a plane approximately perpendicular to the plane of the paper and the groups attached to the carbon atoms of that ring are above and below the ring. The carbon atoms of the ring are not shown.

*From IUPAC Commission on the Nomenclature of Organic Chemistry and IUPAC-IUB Commission on Biochemical Nomenclature, *IUPAC Inf. Bull. Append. Tentative Nomencl. Sym. Units Stand.*, No. 32, August 1973. With permission.

Groups that appear to the right of the vertical chain in the Fischer projection (A and D below) then appear below the plane of the ring in the Haworth representation (B, C, and E below). However, at the asymmetric carbon atom (C-5 in A; C-4 in D) involved via oxygen in ring formation with the carbon atom of the carbonyl group, a formal double inversion must be envisaged to obtain the correct Haworth representation.

In the pyranose forms of D-aldohexoses C-6 will always be above the plane. In the furanose forms of D-aldohexoses the position of C-6 will depend on the configuration at C-4; it will, for example, be above the plane in D-glucofuranoses (e.g., C) but below the plane in D-galactofuranoses (e.g., E):

Examples:

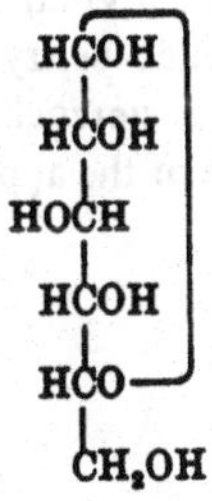

(A) 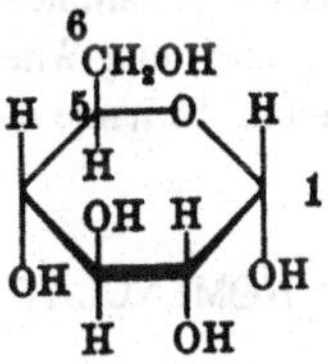   (B) 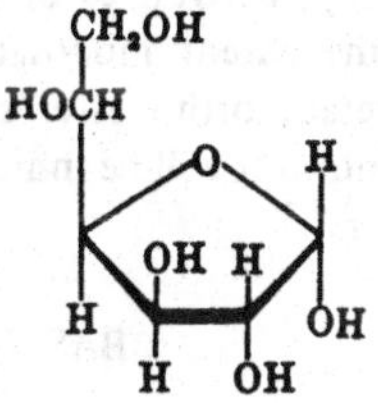   (C)

α-D-Glucopyranose   α-D-Glucofuranose
(Fischer)   (Haworth)   (Haworth)

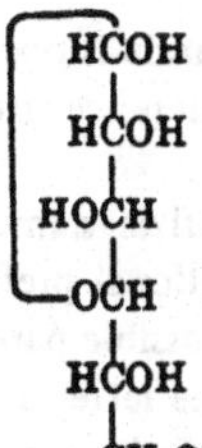

(D) 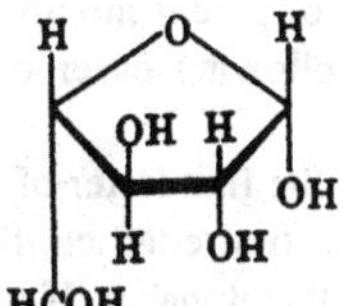   (E) 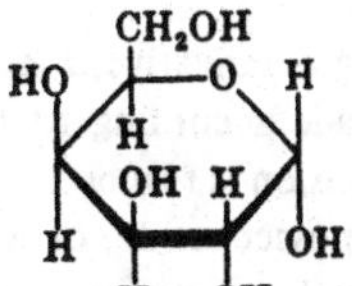   (F)

α-D-Galactofuranose   α-D-Galactopyranose
(Fischer)   (Haworth)   (Haworth)

3. The Reference Carbon Atom and the Anomeric Prefix

a. The reference carbon atom - This is defined as the highest-numbered asymmetric carbon atom in the monosaccharide chain.

b. The anomeric prefix – In a definitive name, the anomeric prefix (α or β) relates the configuration at the anomeric (or glycosidic) center to that of the reference carbon atom.

The anomer having the same orientation, in the Fischer projection, at the anomeric carbon atom and at the reference carbon atom is designated α: the anomer having opposite orientations, in the Fischer projection, is designated β.

The anomeric prefix (α or β) can only be used in conjunction with, and having the above-defined relation to, the configurational prefix (D or L) denoting the configuration at the reference carbon atom. Further, it may be used only when the locant of the anomeric center is smaller than that of the reference carbon atom.

4. Numbering of Monosaccharides

The basic principle for the numbering of monosaccharides gives the (potential) carbonyl group the lower of the possible numbers (cf. Rule Carb-4). This numbering system is usually retained even when a modification introduces a group which, on the basis of general   ·ganic chemical nomenclature, would have priority over the (potential) carbonyl group   .g., in uronic acids the (potential) carbonyl group retains locant one, despite the norm∴ priority of the carboxyl group].

In ketoaldonic acids, the carboxyl group that replaces the original (formal) aldehyde group retains the locant one.

5. New Asymmetric Centers

Not infrequently, derivatives of monosaccharides contain asymmetric carbon atoms not present in the parent monosaccharide. Examples include benzylidene derivatives, certain other acetals, ortho ester structures, etc. When the stereochemistry at such a carbon atom is known it will be indicated in the name by use of the appropriate Sequence Rule symbol, R or S.[2]

BASIS OF NOMENCLATURE

Rule Carb-1

The basis for the naming and numbering of a monosaccharide or monosaccharide derivative is the structure of the parent monosaccharide ($C_nH_{2n}O_n$), represented in the Fischer projection of the acyclic form.

Choice of Parent Structure
Rule Carb-2

If, in naming a derivative, a choice of parent monosaccharide is possible, the selection of parent is made according to the following order of preference, treated in the order given until a decision is reached.

(a) The monosaccharide, of which the first letter of the trivial name (Rule Carb-5), or of the configurational prefix, or of the first cited configurational prefix of a systematic name (Rule Carb-8), occurs earliest in the alphabet. If two possible parents have the same initial letter, then the choice will be made according to the letter at the first point of difference in the trivial name, the configurational prefix of the systematic name, etc. Examples: Allose before glucose, glucose before gulose, *allo-* before *gluco-*, *gluco-* before *gulo-*.

(b) The configurational symbol D- before L-.

(c) The monosaccharide which gives the point(s) of modification of the $>$ CH(OH) chain the lowest locant(s).*

(d) The monosaccharide which gives the lowest locants* to the substituents, present in the derivative.

(e) The monosaccharide which, when the substituents have been placed in alphabetical order, results in the first-cited substituent having the lowest locant.*

Trivial and Systematic Names
Rule Carb-3

In naming monosaccharides or monosaccharide derivatives, either trivial or systematic names can be used for the parent monosaccharide.

---

*Lowest locants are defined as follows: When a series of locants containing the same number of terms are compared term by term, that series is "lowest" which contains the lowest number on the occasion of the first difference (see IUPAC, *Nomenclature of Organic Chemistry, Section C,* 1965, p. 23, footnote).

Trivial names are defined in Rule Carb-5.

Systematic names are formed by adding one or more configurational prefixes (Rule Carb-8) to the appropriate stem name (Rule Carb-6).

Rule Carb-4

The names "aldose" and "ketose" are used in a generic sense to denote monosaccharides in which the (potential) carbonyl group is terminal (aldehydic) or nonterminal (ketonic), respectively. In an aldose, the carbon atom of the (potential) carbonyl group is atom number one; in a ketose it has the lower number possible.

Rule Carb-5

The trivial names of the acyclic aldoses with three, four, five, or six carbon atoms are retained, and are used in preference to their systematic names for the aldoses and for the formation of names of their derivatives. The trivial names of these aldoses are

Triose:	Glyceraldehyde (glycerose is not recommended)
Tetroses:	Erythrose, threose
Pentoses:	Arabinose, lyxose, ribose, xylose
Hexoses:	Allose, altrose, galactose, glucose, gulose, idose, mannose, talose

Rule Carb-6

The "stem names" of the acyclic aldoses having three, four, five, six, seven, eight, nine, ten, etc., carbon atoms in the chain are triose, tetrose, pentose, hexose, heptose, octose, nonose, decose, etc.

The "stem names" of the acyclic ketoses having four, five, six, seven, eight, nine, ten, etc., carbon atoms in the chain are tetrulose, pentulose, hexulose, hepulose, actulose, nonulose, deculose, etc.

Configurational Symbols and Prefixes

Rule Carb-7

Configurational relationships are denoted by the symbols D and L which in print will be small capital roman letters and which are not abbreviations for "dextro" and "laevo." Racemic forms may be indicated by DL. Such symbols are affixed by a hyphen immediately before the monosaccharide trivial name (Rule Carb-5) or before each configurational prefix (Rule Carb-8) of a systematic name, and are employed only with compounds that have been related definitely to the reference standard glyceraldehyde (see Rule Carb-8). The configurational symbol should not be omitted, if known.

If the sign of the optical rotation under specified conditions is to be indicated, this is done by adding (+) or (-). Racemic forms may be indicated by (±). With compounds optically compensated intramolecularly the prefix "*meso*" is used where appropriate.

Examples: D-Glucose or D(+)-glucose, D-fructose or D(-)-fructose, DL-glucose or (±)-glucose.

Rule Carb-8

The configuration of a $>$CHOH group or a set of two, three, or four contiguous $>$CHOH groups (or wholly or partly derivative groups, such as $>$CHOCH$_3$, $>$CHOCOCH$_3$, or $>$CHNH$_2$) is designated by the appropriate one of the following configurational prefixes, which are (except for *glycero-*) derived from the trivial names of the aldoses mentioned in Rule Carb-5. When used in systematic names these prefixes are to be uncapitalized and are italicized in print. They are affixed by a hyphen to the stem name defined in Rule Carb-6. There may be more than one configurational prefix in a name.

Each prefix is D or L according to whether the configuration at the reference carbon atom in the Fischer projection is the same as, or the opposite of, that in D(+)-glyceraldehyde.

Only the Fischer projections of the D-prefixes are given below; X is the group with the lowest-numbered carbon atom(s).

One >CHOH group:

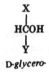

D-*glycero-*

Two >CHOH groups:

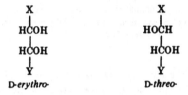

D-*erythro-*   D-*threo-*

Three >CHOH groups:

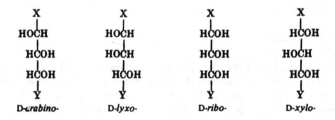

D-*arabino-*   D-*lyxo-*   D-*ribo-*   D-*xylo-*

Four >CHOH groups:

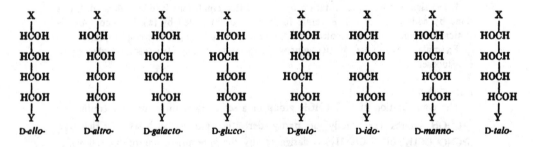

D-*allo-*   D-*altro-*   D-*galacto-*   D-*gluco-*   D-*gulo-*   D-*ido-*   D-*manno-*   D-*talo-*

The systematic name for a monosaccharide is then formed by using the configurational symbols and prefixes with the appropriate stem name (Rule Carb-6).

For sets of more than four contiguous $>$CHOH groups see Rule Carb-9.

The trivial names, which are preferred, of the acyclic aldoses with four to six carbon atoms (Rule Carb-5) thus corresponds to the following systematic names.

Trivial	Systematic
D-Erythrose	D-*erythro*-Tetrose
D-Threose	D-*threo*-Tetrose
D-Arabinose	D-*arabino*-Pentose
D-Lyxose	D-*lyxo*-Pentose
D-Ribose	D-*ribo*-Pentose
D-Xylose	D-*xylo*-Pentose
D-Allose	D-*allo*-Hexose
D-Altrose	D-*altro*-Hexose
D-Galactose	D-*galacto*-Hexose
D-Glucose	D-*gluco*-Hexose
D-Gulose	D-*gulo*-Hexose
D-Idose	D-*ido*-Hexose
D-Mannose	D-*manno*-hexose
D-Talose	D-*talo*-hexose

Note: (Anglo-American Usage). Since 1952, usage in the United States and the United Kingdom has been based on a different significance for configurational prefixes in that they have been related to a sequence of *consecutive but not necessarily contiguous asymmetric groups*.

Examples:

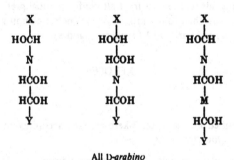

All D-*arabino*

N and M are each a single nonasymmetric carbon center or a sequence of nonasymmetric carbon centers.

Ketoses and Deoxysaccharides. Prefixes with this significance were used when N is the methylene group of a deoxy compound or the keto group of a ketose containing not more than four asymmetric carbon centers, but not the keto group of higher-sugar ketose.

Examples: Names according to this usage are given in notes to the subsequent Rules.

Multiple Configurational Prefixes
Rule Carb-9

An acyclic monosaccharide containing more than four contiguous asymmetric carbon atoms is named by adding two or more prefixes, together indicating the configurations at all the asymmetric carbon atoms, to the stem name defined in Rule Carb-6.

The configurational prefixes employed are given in Rule Carb-8. The sequence of $(4n + m$; where n is 1 or more and m is 0, 1, 2, or 3) asymmetric carbon atoms is divided, beginning at the asymmetric carbon atom next to the functional group, into (n) sets of four asymmetric carbon atoms, and a final set (m) of less than four. The order of citation of these prefixes commences at the end farthest from carbon number one.

The locants corresponding to the configurational prefixes may be inserted in the name, if desired. In such cases, all locants are given and immediately precede the appropriate configurational prefixes.

Examples:

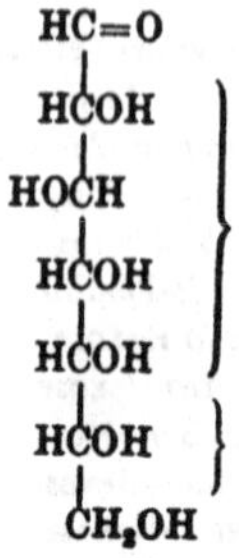

HC=O

HCOH

HOCH

HCOH

HCOH

HCOH

CH₂OH

HC=O

HOCH

HOCH

HCOH

HCOH

HOCH

HOCH

CH₂OH

D-*glycero*-D-*gluco*-
Heptose or 6-D-
glycero-2,3,4,5-
D-*gluco*-heptose

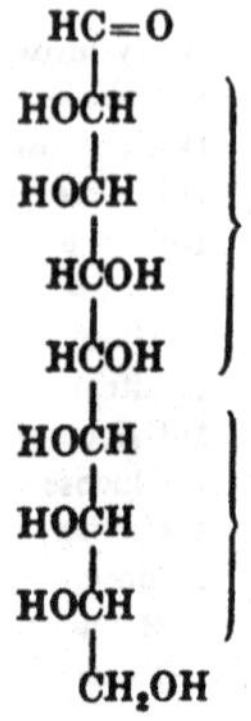

L-*ribo*-D-*manno*-
Nonose, or 6,7,8-
L-*ribo*-2,3,4,5-D-
manno-nonose

Comment. Compounds that require multiple configurational prefixes but which do not necessarily contain more than four contiguous asymmetric carbon atoms are covered by Rule Carb-10 (ketoses) and Carbon-14 (deoxysaccharides).

KETOSES

Rule Carb-10

Ketoses are classified as 2-ketoses, 3-ketoses, etc., according to the position of the (potential) carbonyl group (see Rule Carb-4).

The systematic name of an individual ketose is obtained by affixing, before the stem name (Rule Carb-6) and by means of a hyphen, the locant of the (potential) carbonyl group. The locant is preceded by the configurational prefix or prefixes (Rule Carb-8) for the groups of asymmetric centers present.

If more than one configurational prefix is needed, the order of their citation commences at the end farthest from carbon atom number one.

The locant two may be omitted from the name of a 2-ketose when no ambiguity can arise.*

When the carbonyl group is at the middle carbon atom of a ketose containing an uneven number of carbon atoms in the chain two names are possible. That name will be selected as accords with the order of precedence given in Rule Carb-2.

*In this text, the locant is always retained for the sake of clarity.

Examples:

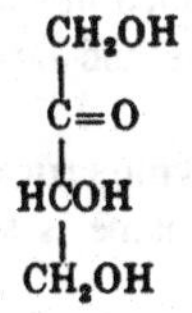

D-*glycero*-2-Tetrulose

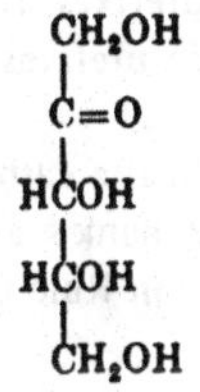

D-*erythro*-2-Pentulose

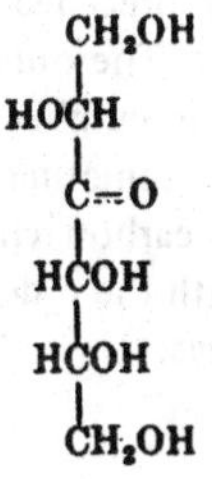

D-*erythro*-L-*glycero*-3-Hexulose†

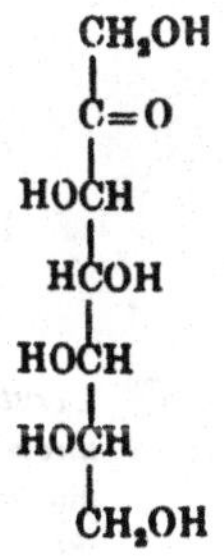

L-*gluco*-2-Heptulose

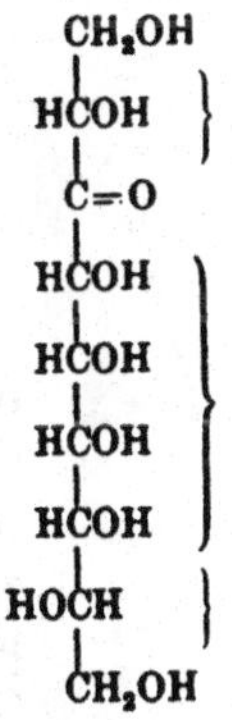

L-*glycero*-D-*allo*-D-*glycero*-3-Nonulose

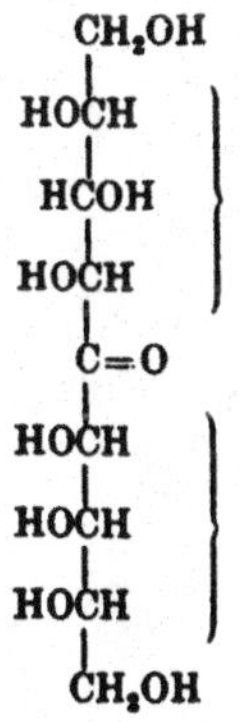

L-*ribo*-L-*xylo*-5-Nonulose (not D-*xylo*-D-*ribo*-5-nonulose) [see Rule Carb-2(a)]

The following are examples of nonsystematic names of ketoses that are established by usage and may be retained.

D-Ribulose for	D-*erythro*-2-Pentulose
D-Xylulose for	D-*threo*-2-Pentulose
Sedoheptulose for	D-*altro*-2-Heptulose
D-Fructose for	D-*arabino*-2-Hexulose
D-Psicose for	D-*ribo*-2-Hexulose
D-Sorbose for	D-*xylo*-2-Hexulose
D-Tagatose for	D-*lyxo*-2-Hexulose

DIKETOSES

Rule Carb-11

Monosaccharide derivatives containing two (potential) ketonic carbonyl groups have the general name diketose.

The systematic name of an individual diketose is derived by the use of the termination "odiulose" in place of the termination "ulose" characteristic of the monoketose (Rule

†Name according to Anglo-American usage: D-*arabino*-3-Hexulose.

Carb-6). The locants of the (potential) carbonyl groups are the lowest possible numbers (see Rule Carb-4) and are inserted together with a hyphen before the stem name. They are in turn preceded by configurational prefixes, the latter as prescribed in Rules Carb-8 and Carb-9. The order of citation of these prefixes commences at the end farthest from carbon atom number one.

Note. It sometimes happens that, when the carbonyl groups are symmetrically placed along the carbon chain, two systematic names are possible; that name is selected as accords with the order of precedence given in Rule Carb-2.

Examples:

CH_2OH	CH_2OH	CH_2OH	CH_2OH
$C=O$	$C=O$	$C=O$	$HCOH$
$C=O$	$HCOH$	$HOCH$	$HOCH$
$HCOH$	$HOCH$	$C=O$	$C=O$
CH_2OH	$C=O$	$HCOH$	$C=O$
	CH_2OH	CH_2OH	$HOCH$
			$HOCH$
			CH_2OH
D-*glycero*-2,3-Pentodiulose	L-*threo*-2,5-Hexodiulose	D-*glycero*-L-*glycero*-2,4-Hexodiulos* (not D-*glycero*-L-*glycero*-3,5-hexodiulose) [See Rule Carb-2(b)]	L-*erythro*-L-*threo*-4,5-Octodiulose† (not L-*threo*-D-*erythro*-4,5-octodiulose) [See Rule Carb-2 (a)]

ALDOKETOSES

Rule Carb-12

Monosaccharide derivatives containing a (potential) aldehyde carbonyl group and a (potential) ketonic carbonyl group have the general name aldoketose.

Names of individual aldoketoses are formed in the same way as those of diketoses, but by the use of the termination "osulose" in place of the termination "ose" of the corresponding aldose (Rule Carb-6). The carbon atom of the (potential) aldehydic carbonyl group is numbered one, and this locant is not cited in the name. The locant of the (potential) ketonic carbonyl group is given unless it is two; it may then be omitted.**

Examples:

$HC=O$	$HC=O$
$C=O$	$HOCH$
$HCOH$	$C=O$
$HCOH$	$HCOH$
CH_2OH	$HCOH$
	CH_2OH
D-*erythro*-2-Pentosulose	D-*erythro*-L-*glycero*-3-Hexosulose††

*Name according to Anglo-American usage: D-*threo*-2,4-Hexodiulose.
†Name according to Anglo-American usage: L-*altro*-4,5-Octodiulose.
**In this text, the locant is always retained for the sake of clarity.
††Name according to Anglo-American usage: D-*arabino*-3-Hexulose.

```
        HC=O
         |
         C=O
         |
        HOCH
         |
        HCOH
         |
        HOCH
         |
        HOCH
         |
        CH₂OH
```

1-*gluco*-2-Hep-
tosulose

Comment: 2-Aldoketoses have also been named as "osones" but this practice is not recommended.

DIALDOSES

Rule Carb-13

Monosaccharide derivatives containing two (potential) aldehydic carbonyl groups have the general name "dialdose." Names of individual dialdoses are formed in the same way as those of diketoses, but by the use of the termination "odialdose" in place of the termination "odiulose." Locants are not needed.

Examples:

```
   HC=O            HC=O            HC=O
    |               |               |
   HCOH            HCOH            HCOH
    |               |               |
   HOCH            HOCH            HOCH
    |               |               |
   HC=O            HOCH            HCOH
                    |               |
                   HCOH            HCOH
                    |               |
                   HC=O            HC=O
```

L-*threo*-Tetro-   *meso-galacto*-   D-*gluco*-Hexo-
dialdose   Hexodialdose[†]   dialdose (not L-
                                              gulo-hexodial-
                                              dose

DEOXY-MONOSACCHARIDES AND AMINO-MONOSACCHARIDES

Rule Carb-14

(a) The replacement of an alcoholic hydroxyl group of a monosaccharide, or monosaccharide derivative, by a hydrogen atom is expressed by using the prefix "deoxy," preceded by the appropriate locant and followed by a hyphen together with a systematic or trivial name (Rule Carb-3). The systematic name consists of a stem name with such configurational prefixes as express the configurations at the asymmetric centers present in the deoxy-compound. The order of citation of the configurational prefixes commences at the end farthest from carbon atom number one.

A trivial name may be used only if the transformation of the saccharide into the deoxy-compound does not alter the configuration at any asymmetric center.

---

†The prefix *meso*- may precede the name of such symmetrical compounds for the sake of the clarity.

Examples:

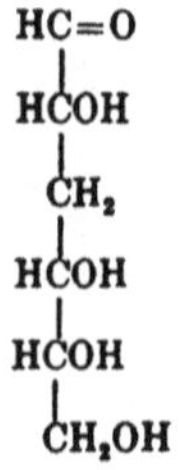

$$
\begin{array}{cccc}
\text{HC=O} & \text{CH}_2\text{OH} & \text{HC=O} & \text{HC=O} \\
| & | & | & | \\
\text{HCOH} & \text{C=O} & \text{CH}_2 & \text{HCOH} \\
| & | & | & | \\
\text{CH}_2 & \text{HCOH} & \text{HOCH} & \text{HCOH} \\
| & | & | & | \\
\text{HCOH} & \text{CH}_2 & \text{HCOH} & \text{HOCH} \\
| & | & | & | \\
\text{HCOH} & \text{CH}_2\text{OH} & \text{HOCH} & \text{HCOH} \\
| & & | & | \\
\text{CH}_2\text{OH} & & \text{CH}_2\text{OH} & \text{CH}_3
\end{array}
$$

3-Deoxy-D-
erythro-D-*glycero*-
hexose*

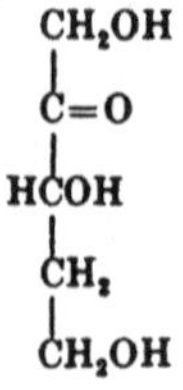

4-Deoxy-D-
glycero-2-pen-
tulose

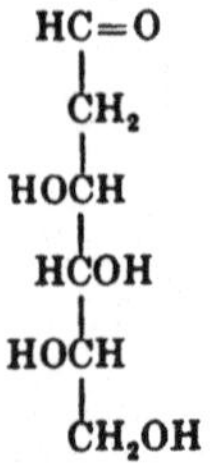

2-Deoxy-L-*xylo*-
hexose

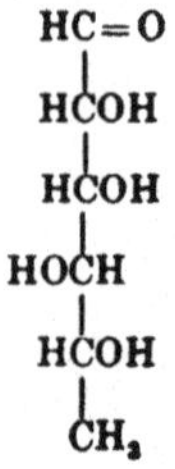

6-Deoxy-D-gulose

Trivial names of 6-deoxy-hexoses established by usage may be retained and used for the formation of names of derivatives.

Examples:

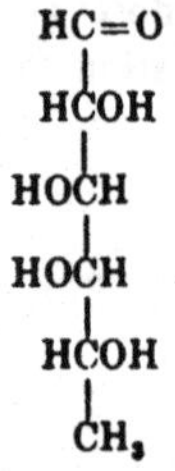

$$
\begin{array}{cc}
\text{HC=O} & \text{HC=O} \\
| & | \\
\text{HCOH} & \text{HCOH} \\
| & | \\
\text{HOCH} & \text{HCOH} \\
| & | \\
\text{HOCH} & \text{HOCH} \\
| & | \\
\text{HCOH} & \text{HOCH} \\
| & | \\
\text{CH}_3 & \text{CH}_3
\end{array}
$$

D-Fucose (6-
Deoxy-D-galac-
tose)

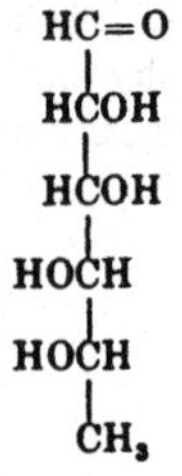

L-Rhamnose (6-
Deoxy-L-man-
nose)

The following is established as a trivial name for biochemical use: Deoxyribose for 2-deoxy-D-*erythro*-pentose.

(b) The replacement of an alcoholic hydroxyl group of a monosaccharide, or monosaccharide derivative, by an amino group is envisaged as substitution of the appropriate hydrogen atom of the corresponding deoxy-monosaccharide by the amino group.

Substition in the amino group is indicated by use of the prefix *N* (Rule Carb-15) unless the substituted amino group has a trivial name (for example: CH_3CONH-, acetamido).

The stereochemistry at the carbon atom carrying the amino group is expressed according to Rule Carb-8.

*Name according to Anglo-American usage: 3-Deoxy-D-*ribo*-hexose.

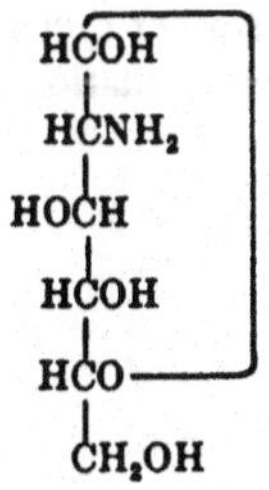

HCOH
HCNH$_2$
HOCH
HCOH
HCO
CH$_2$OH

2-Amino-2-deoxy-
α-D-glucopyranose

HCOH
HCNH—COCH$_3$
HOCH
HCOH
HCO
CH$_2$OH

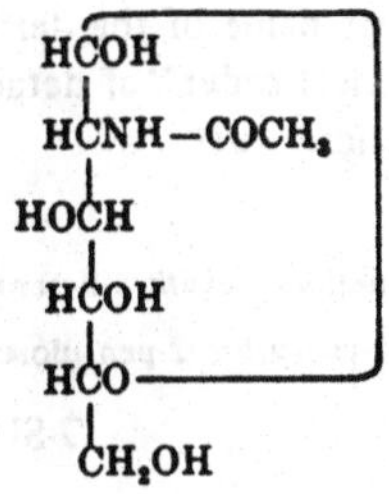

2-Acetamido-2-
deoxy-α-D-gluco-
pyranose

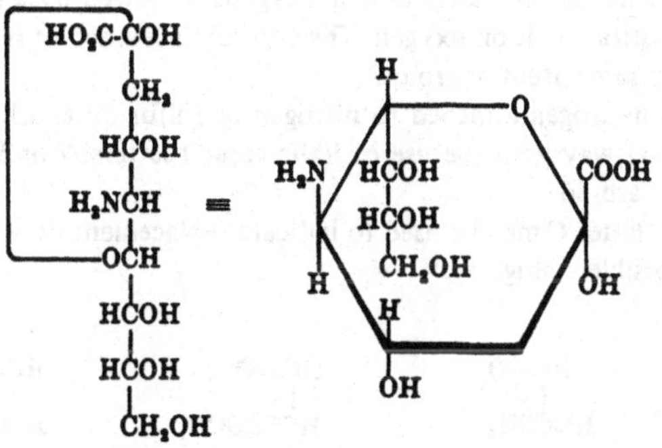

HO$_2$C-COH
CH$_2$
HCOH
H$_2$NCH
OCH
HCOH
HCOH
CH$_2$OH

(A)

≡

H
O
H$_2$N HCOH
HCOH
CH$_2$OH
H
H
COOH
OH
OH

(A) 5-Amino-3,5-dideoxy-α-D-*glycero*-D-*galacto*-2-nonulo-
pyranosonic acid

CHO
HCNH$_2$
OCH
HCOH
HCOH
CH$_2$OH

HC—COOH
CH$_3$

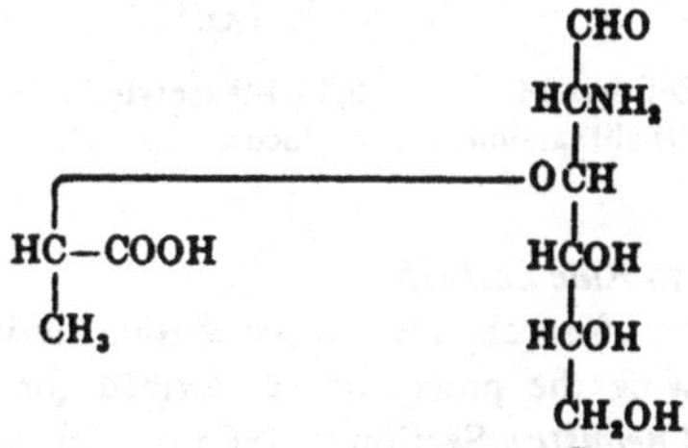

(B)

(B) 2-Amino-3-O-[1-(S)-carboxyethyl]-2-deoxy-
aldehydo-D-glucose

Trivial names accepted for biochemical usage:

D-Galactosamine for   2-Amino-2-deoxy-D-galactopyranose
                                             (the name chondrosamine is not recommended)
D-Glucosamine for   2-Amino-2-deoxy-D-glucopyranose
D-Mannosame for   2-Amino-2-deoxy-D-mannopyranose
Neuraminic acid for   5-Amino-3,5-dideoxy-α-D-*glycero*-
                                       D-*galacto*-2-nonulopyranosonic acid
Muramic acid for   2-Amino-3-O-[1-(S)-carboxyethyl]-
                                       2-deoxy-aldehydo-D-glucose

When the complete name of the derivative includes other prefixes, "deoxy" takes its place in the alphabetical order* of detachable prefixes; in citation the alphabetical order is preferred to numerical order.

Examples:

4-Amino-4-deoxy-3-*O*-methyl-D-*erythro*-2-pentulose

4-Deoxy-4-(ethylamino)-D-*erythro*-2-pentulose

O-SUBSTITUTION

Rule Carb-15

Replacement of the hydrogen atom of an alcoholic hydroxyl group of a saccharide or saccharide derivative by another atom or group is denoted by placing the name of this atom or group before the name of the parent compound. The name of the atom or group is preceded by an italic capital letter *O* (for oxygen), followed by a hyphen in order to make clear that substitution is on oxygen. The *O* prefix need not be repeated for multiple replacements by the same atom or group.

Replacement of hydrogen attached to nitrogen or sulfur by another atom or group is indicated in a similar way with the use of italic capital letters *N* or *S* (for examples see Rules Carb-24 and Carb-36).

The italic capital letter *C* may be used to indicate replacement of hydrogen attached to carbon, to avoid possible ambiguity.*

Examples:

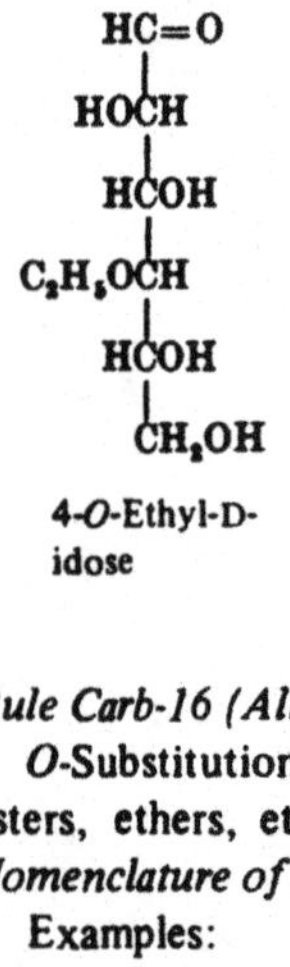

$HC=O$	$HC=O$	$HC=O$	$HC=O$
$HOCH$	$HOCCH_3$	$HCOCOCH_3$	$HCOH$
$HCOH$	$HCOC_2H_5$	$HOCH$	$HCOH$
C_2H_5OCH	$HCOH$	$HCOCOCH_3$	$HOCH$
$HCOH$	CH_2OH	$HCOH$	$HOCH$
CH_2OH		CH_2OH	$CH_2OSO_2C_6H_4CH_3\text{-}p$
4-*O*-Ethyl-D-idose	3-*O*-Ethyl-2-*C*-methyl-D-arabinose	2,4-Di-*O*-acetyl-D-glucose	6-*O*-Tosyl-L-mannose

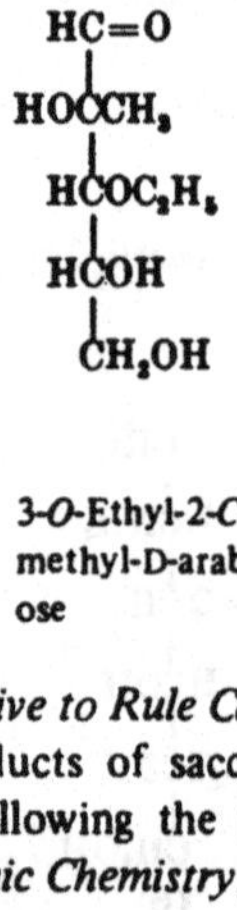

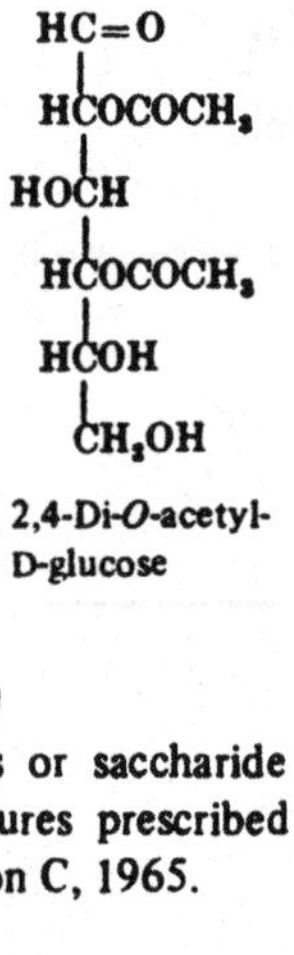

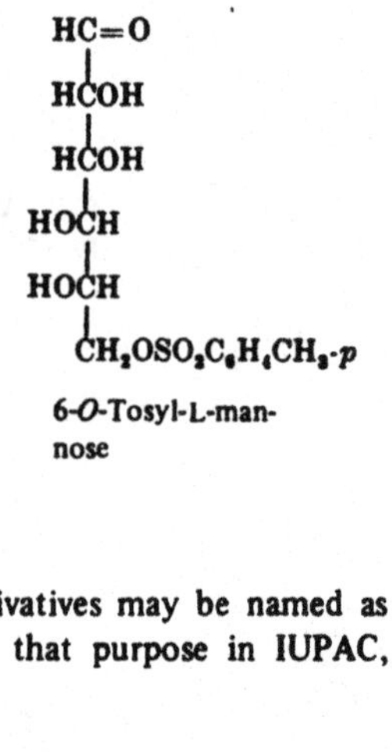

Rule Carb-16 (Alternative to Rule Carb-15)

O-Substitution products of saccharides or saccharide derivatives may be named as esters, ethers, etc., following the procedures prescribed for that purpose in IUPAC, *Nomenclature of Organic Chemistry*, Section C, 1965.

Examples:

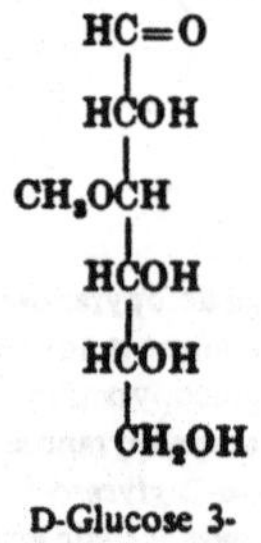

$HC=O$	$HC=O$	$HC=O$
$HCOH$	$HCOH$	$HCOCOC_6H_5$
CH_3OCH	CH_3COOCH	$HCOH$
$HCOH$	$HCOH$	$HOCH$
$HCOH$	$HCOH$	$HCOH$
CH_2OH	CH_2OH	CH_3
D-Glucose 3-methyl ether	D-Glucose 3-acetate	6-Deoxy-D-gulose 2-benzoate

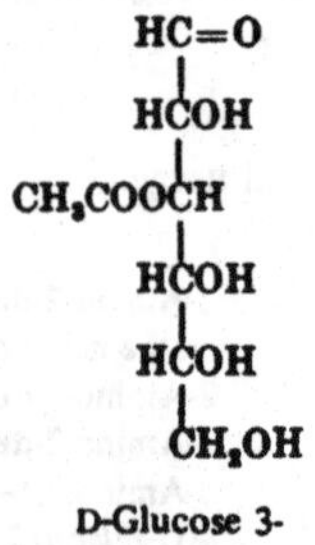

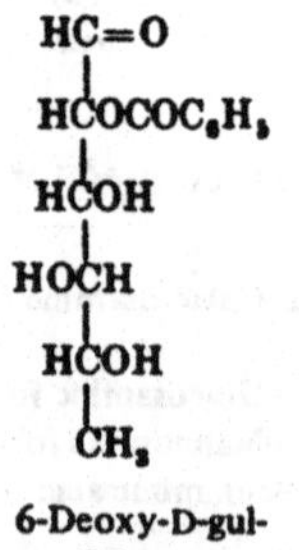

*See IUPAC, *Nomenclature of Organic Chemistry, Section C,* 1965, Rules C-16.1 and C-16.4.

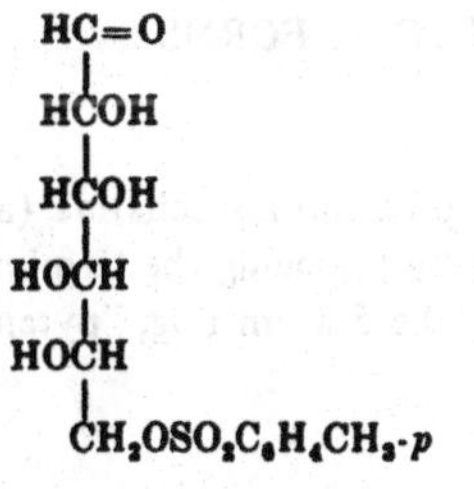

```
        HC=O                          HC=O
        HCOH                          HCOH
        HCOH                          HOCH
        HOCH                          HCOH
        HOCH                          HCOH
  CH₂OSO₂C₆H₄CH₃-p              CH₂OPO₃K₂
```

L-Mannose 6-*p*-toluenesul-
fonate (not ó-tosylate); (see
Rule C-641.5, Examples)

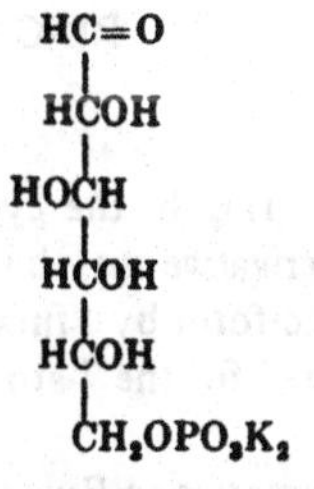

D-Glucose 6-(di-
potassium phos-
phate) (Permitted
biochemical
usage: Glucose
6-phosphate)

ACYCLIC FORMS

Rule Carb-17

The acyclic nature of a monosaccharide or monosaccharide derivative containing an uncyclized carbonyl group may be stressed by inserting the italicized prefix "*aldehydo*" or "*keto*," respectively, immediately before the configurational prefix(es) or before the trivial name. These prefixes may be abbreviated to "*al*" and "*ke*."

Examples:

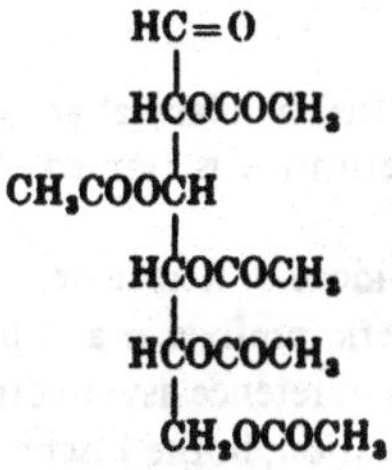

```
        HC=O                         CH₂OCOCH₃
      HCOCOCH₃                          CO
    CH₃COOCH                        CH₃COOCH
      HCOCOCH₃                       HCOCOCH₃
      HCOCOCH₃                       HCOCOCH₃
     CH₂OCOCH₃                      CH₂OCOCH₃
```

2,3,4,5,6-Penta-
O-acetyl-*alde-
hydo*-D-glucose
aldehydo-D-
Glucose 2,3,4,5,
6-pentaacetate

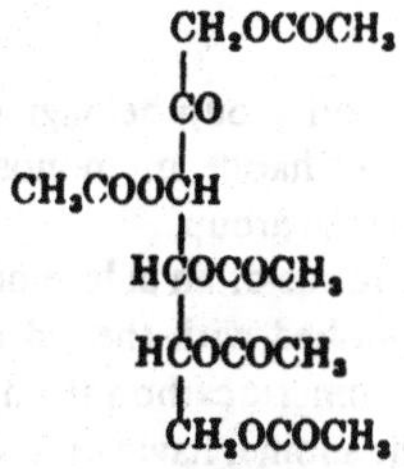

1,3,4,5,6-Penta-
O-acetyl-*keto*-D-
fructose *keto*-
D-Fructose
1,3,4,5,6-pent-
aacetate

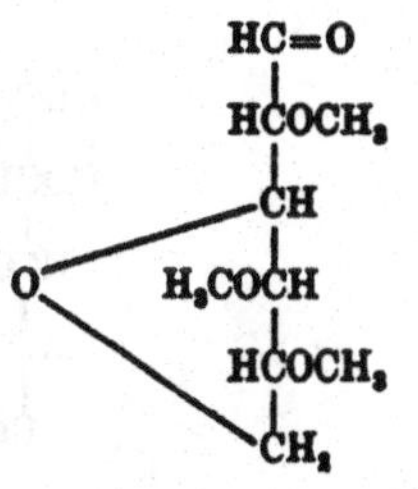

```
        HC=O                          CH₂OH
      HCOCH₃                        H₃COCH
        CH                             C=O
  O   H₃COCH                        HCOCH₃
      HCOCH₃                        HCOCH₃
        CH₂                        CH₂OCH₃
```

3,6-Anhydro-
2,4,5-tri-*O*-
methyl-*aldehydo*-
D-galactose

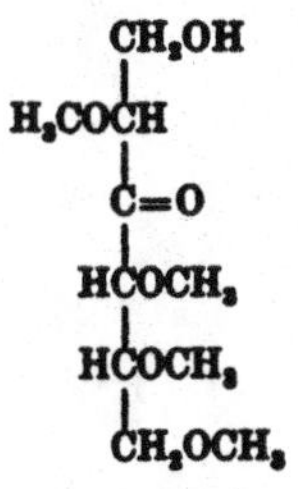

2,4,5,6-Tetra-*O*-
methyl-*keto*-D-
erythro-L-*glycero*-
3-hexulose*

*Name according to Anglo-American usage: 2,4,5,6-Tetra-*O*-methyl-*keto*-D-*arabino*-3-hexulose.

RING SIZE IN CYCLIC FORMS

Rule Carb-18

The size of the ring in the cyclic form of a monosaccharide (aldose or ketose) or monosaccharide derivative may be indicated by replacing the terminal letters "se" of the name of the acyclic form by "furanose" for the 5-atom ring, "pyranose" for the 6-atom ring, and "septanose" for the 7-atom ring.

Rule Carb-19 (Alternative to Rule Carb-18)

The size of the ring in the cyclic form of a monosaccharide (aldose or ketose) or monosaccharide derivative may be indicated by two numerals, placed in parentheses, and joined to the end of the name of the acyclic compound by a hyphen. These numerals denote the two carbon atoms to which the ring oxygen atom is attached, the carbon atom of the potential carbonyl group being cited first.

Rule Carb-20

For cyclic forms of ketoses, diketoses, dialdoses, and aldoketoses, the names constructed according to Rule Carb-18 may, when necessary, be followed by a pair of numerals, these numerals having the same significance as in Rule Carb-19.

Comment. Examples of the application of Rules Carb-18 to Carb-20 are given in Rules Carb-21 to Carb-23. The system of Rule Carb-18 is preferred, but that of Rule Carb-19 is advantageous in special cases.

ANOMERS

Rule Carb-21

The free hydroxyl group belonging to the internal hemiacetal grouping of the cyclic form of a monosaccharide or monosaccharide derivative is termed the "anomeric" or "glycosidic" hydroxyl group.

The two cyclic forms of an aldose or ketose, or aldose or ketose derivative (termed anomers), are distinguished with the aid of the anomeric prefixes α and β, relating the configuration at the anomeric carbon atom to that at the reference asymmetric carbon atom of the compound; the anomer having the same configuration, in the Fischer projection, at the anomeric and the reference carbon atom is designated α.

The anomeric prefix, α or β, followed by a hyphen, is placed immediately in front of the configurational symbol, D or L, of the trivial name or of the configurational prefix denoting the group of asymmetric carbon atoms that includes the reference carbon atom (see Preamble, paragraph 3).

Examples:

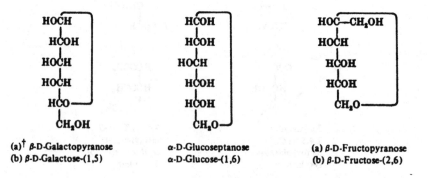

(a)† β-D-Galactopyranose   α-D-Glucoseptanose   (a) β-D-Fructopyranose
(b) β-D-Galactose-(1,5)   α-D-Glucose-(1,6)   (b) β-D-Fructose-(2,6)

†(a), (b), and (c), here and subsequently, refer to names coined in terms of Rules Carb-18, Carb-19, and Carb-20, respectively.

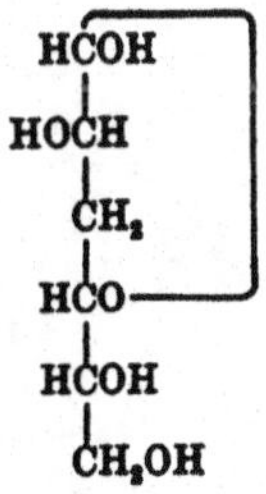

```
 HCOH ┐           ┌─HCOH
 HOCH │           │  HCOH
  CH₂ │           │  HOCH
 HCO──┘           │  HCOH
 HCOH             └──OCH
 CH₂OH              HCOH
                    CH₂OH
```

(a) 3-Deoxy-α-D-
erytho-L-*glycero*-
hexofuranose*
(b) 3-Deoxy-α-D-
erythro-L-*glycero*-
hexose-(1,4)

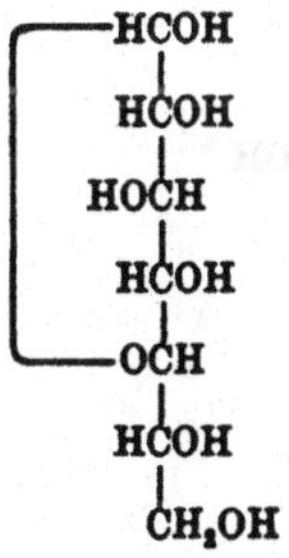

(a) α-D-*glycero*-L-
ido-Heptopyranose
(b) α-D-*glycero*-L-
ido-Heptose-(1,5)

Rule Carb-22

With ketones that have the (potential) carbonyl group located between two >CHOH groups, each separated from the carbonyl group by two, three, or four carbon atoms of the chain, ring-closure may take place towards either end of that chain. Likewise, with dialdoses, diketoses and aldoketoses ring-closure may take place from either (potential) carbonyl group towards the center of the chain.

In each case both cyclic forms have the same monosaccharide parent that dictates the basis of the name and numbering of each form (cf. Rule Carb-2). In one form the locant of the anomeric or glycosidic hydroxyl group is lower than that of the reference carbon atom; that cyclic form is named according to Rules Carb-18 and Carb-21. In the other the locant of the anomeric or glycosidic hydroxyl group must be higher than that of the reference carbon atom. This precludes (see Preamble, paragraph 3) the use of α and β to define the two anomers (Rule Carb-21), and the appropriate Sequence Rule symbol, *R* or *S* (see Preamble, paragraph 5), must be used, in place of α or β, to indicate the configuration at the anomeric carbon atom.

*Name, according to Anglo-American usage: 3-Deoxy-α-D-*arabino*-hexofuranose.

Examples:

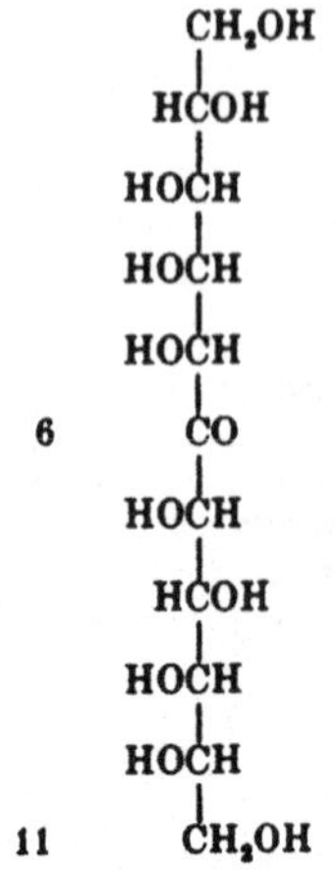

CH₂OH
HCOH
HOCH
HOCH
HOCH
6   CO
HOCH
HCOH
HOCH
HOCH
11   CH₂OH

CH₂OH
HCOH
—OCH
HOCH
HOCH
6   —COH
HOCH
HCOH
HOCH
HOCH
11   CH₂OH

=

11

L-*gluco*-L-*altro*-6-
Undeculose (not L-
talo-D-*gulo*-6-Unde-
culose) (*cf.* Rule
Carb-2)

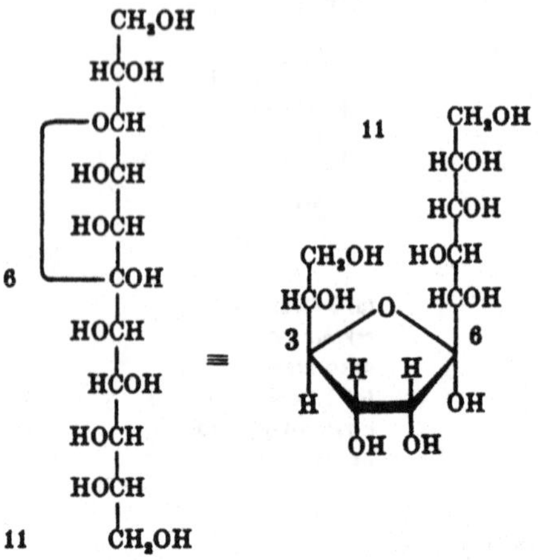

(b) (6S)-L-*gluco*-L-*altro*-6-Undeculose-(6,3)
(c) (6S)-L-*gluco*-L-*altro*-6-(Undeculofuranose-(6,3)

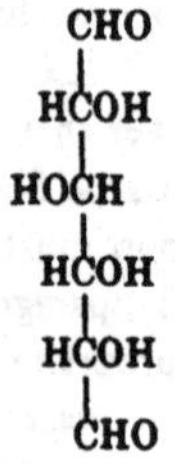

CHO
HCOH
HOCH
HCOH
HCOH
CHO

CHO
HCO—
HOCH
HCOH
HCOH
HCOH

D-*gluco*-Hexo-
dialdose (not L-
gulo-hexodial-
dose) (*cf.* Rules
Carb-2 and Carb-
11)

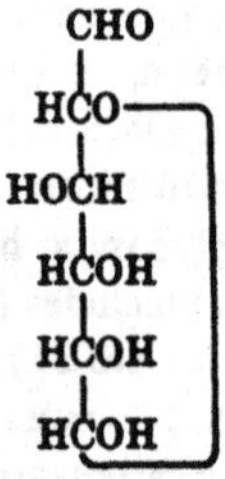

(c) (6R)-D-*gluco*-
Hexodialdopyra-
nose-(6,2)
(b) (6R)-D-*gluco*-
Hexodialdose-(6,2)

GLYCOSIDES

Rule Carb-23

Mixed acetals, resulting from the replacement of the hydrogen atom of the anomeric or glycosidic hydroxyl group by a group X, derived from an alcohol or phenol (XOH), are named "glycosides." The term "glycoside" is used in a generic sense only, and may not be applied to specific compounds. Glycosides are named by replacing the terminal "e" of the name of the corresponding cyclic form of the saccharide or saccharide derivative by "ide" and placing before the word thus obtained, as a separate word, the name of the group X.

Examples:

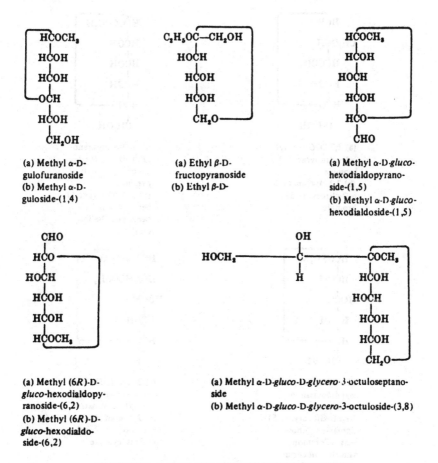

(a) Methyl α-D-gulofuranoside
(b) Methyl α-D-guloside-(1,4)

(a) Ethyl β-D-fructopyranoside
(b) Ethyl β-D-

(a) Methyl α-D-*gluco*-hexodialdopyranoside-(1,5)
(b) Methyl α-D-*gluco*-hexodialdoside-(1,5)

(a) Methyl (6*R*)-D-*gluco*-hexodialdopyranoside-(6,2)
(b) Methyl (6*R*)-D-*gluco*-hexodialdoside-(6,2)

(a) Methyl α-D-*gluco*-D-*glycero*-3-octuloseptanoside
(b) Methyl α-D-*gluco*-D-*glycero*-3-octuloside-(3,8)

GLYCOSYL RADICALS AND GLYCOSYLAMINES

Rule Carb-24

(a) The radical formed by detaching the anomeric or glycosidic hydroxyl group from the cyclic form of a monosaccharide or monosaccharide derivative is named by replacing the terminal 'e' of the name of the monosaccharide or monosaccharide derivative by "yl." The general name of these radicals if "glycosyl" (glycofuranosyl, glycopyranosyl, glycoseptanosyl) radical.

Examples:

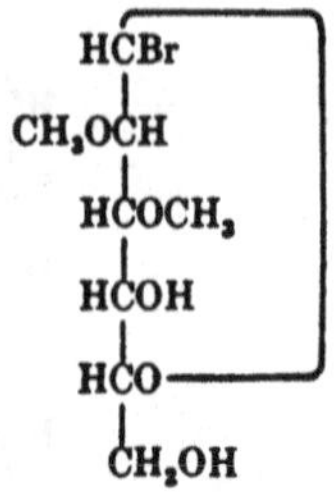

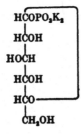

HCBr
|
CH₂OCH
|
HCOCH₃
|
HCOH
|
HCO
|
CH₂OH

(a) 2,3-Di-*O*-methyl-
α-D-altropyranosyl
bromide
(b) 2,3-Di-*O*-methyl-
α-D-altrosyl-(1,5)
bromide

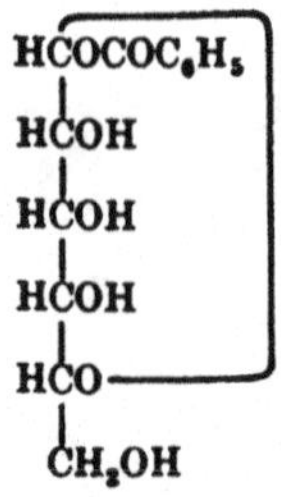

HCOCOC₆H₅
|
HCOH
|
HCOH
|
HCOH
|
HCO
|
CH₂OH

(a) α-D-Allopyrano-
syl benzoate (or 1-
O-benzoyl-α-D-allo-
pyranose)
(b) α-D-Allosyl-(1,5)
benzoate [or 1-*O*-
benzoyl-α-D-allose-
(1,5)]

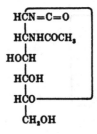

HCOPO₃K₂
|
HCOH
|
HOCH
|
HCOH
|
HCO
|
CH₂OH

(a) α-D-Glucopyran-
osyl dipotassium
phosphate
(b) α-D-Glucosyl-(1,5)
dipotassium phos-
phate (Common
name for biochem-
ical usage: α-Glucose
1-phosphate

HCN=C=O
|
HCNHCOCH₃
|
HOCH
|
HCOH
|
HCO
|
CH₂OH

(a) 2-Acetamido-2-
deoxy-α-D-glucopy-
ranosyl isocyanate
(b) 2-Acetamido-2-
deoxy-α-D-glucosyl-
(1,5) isocyanate

(b) The replacement of the glycosidic hydroxyl group of a cyclic form of a monosaccharide derivative by an amino group is indicated by adding the suffix "amine" to the name of the glycosyl radical.

Example:

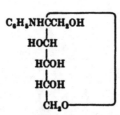

C₆H₅NHCCH₂OH
|
HOCH
|
HCOH
|
HCOH
|
CH₂O

(a) *N*-Phenyl-β-D-fructopy-
ranosylamine
(b) *N*-Phenyl-β-D-fructosyl-
(2,6)-amine

GLYCOSYLOXY RADICALS

Rule Carb-25

The radical formed by removal of the hydrogen atom from the anomeric or glycosidic hydroxyl group of the cyclic form of a monosaccharide or monosaccharide derivative is named by replacing the terminal "e" of the name of the saccharide by "yloxy."

Examples:

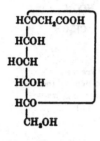

HCOCH$_2$COOH

HCOH

HOCH

HCOH

HCO——

CH$_2$OH

(a) α-D-Glucopyrano-
syloxyacetic acid
(b) α-D-Glucosyloxy-(1,5)-
acetic acid

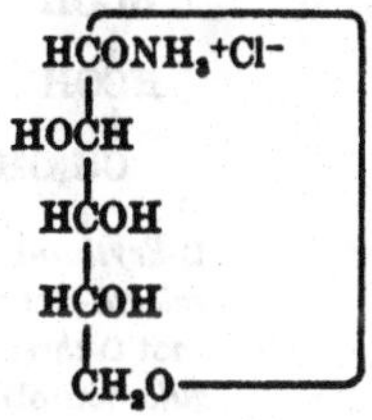

HCONH$_3$+Cl⁻

HOCH

HCOH

HCOH

CH$_2$O——

(a) α-D-Arabinopyra-
nosyloxyammonium
chloride
(b) α-D-Arabinosyloxy-
(1,5)-ammonium
chloride

ALDITOLS

Rule Carb-26

(a) Names for the polyhydric alcohols (alditols) of the saccharide series are derived from the names of the corresponding acyclic aldoses by changing the suffix "ose" to "itol."

If the same alditol can be derived from two different aldoses preference is given to that name which accords with the order of precedence given in Rule Carb-2.

Examples:

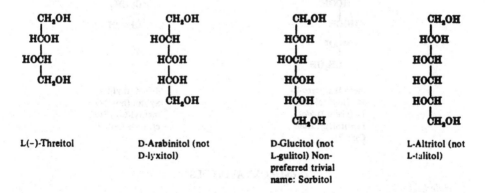

CH$_2$OH

HCOH

HOCH

CH$_2$OH

L(-)-Threitol

CH$_2$OH

HOCH

HCOH

HCOH

CH$_2$OH

D-Arabinitol (not
D-lyxitol)

CH$_2$OH

HCOH

HOCH

HCOH

HCOH

CH$_2$OH

D-Glucitol (not
L-gulitol) Non-
preferred trivial
name: Sorbitol

CH$_2$OH

HCOH

HOCH

HOCH

HOCH

CH$_2$OH

L-Altritol (not
L-talitol)

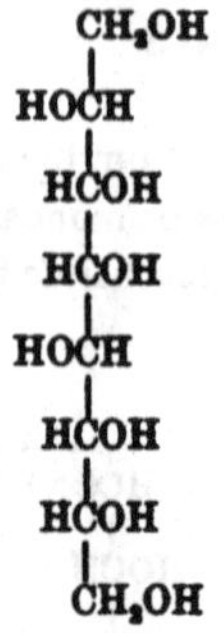

CH$_2$OH
HOCH
HCOH
HCOH
HOCH
HCOH
HCOH
CH$_2$OH

D-*Erythro*-L-
galacto-Octitol
(not D-*threo*-L-
gulo-octitol)

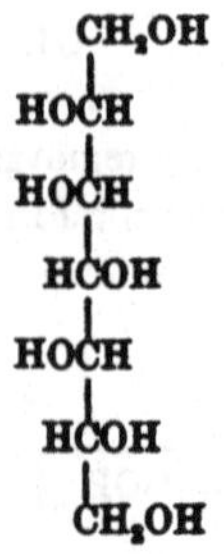

CH$_2$OH
HOCH
HOCH
HCOH
HOCH
HCOH
CH$_2$OH

D-*glycero*-L-
gulo-Heptitol (not
D-*glycero*-D-*ido*-
heptitol)

Note. Names such as "mannite" for mannitol are deprecated.

(b) To the trivial names of alditols optically compensated intramolecularly, which have no D- or L-prefix, the prefix *meso-* may be added for the sake of clarity.

Examples: *meso*-erythritol, *meso*-ribitol, *meso*-xylitol, *meso*-allitol, *meso*-galactitol.

The prefixes D and L must however be used (i) in the names of *meso*-alditols containing more than four contiguous asymmetric carbon atoms in order to define the steric relation of the configurational prefixes cited and (ii) in naming derivatives of *meso*-alditols that have become asymmetric by substitution.

Examples:

(i)
CH$_2$OH 1
HCOH
HOCH
HCOH
HOCH
HCOH
CH$_2$OH 7

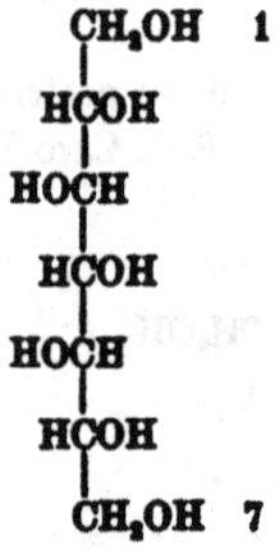

meso-D-*glycero*-L-
ido-Heptitol (not
L-*glycero*-D-*ido*-
heptitol; *cf.* Rule
Carb-2)

(ii)
CH$_2$OH 1
HCOH
HOCH
HCOCH$_3$
CH$_2$OH 5

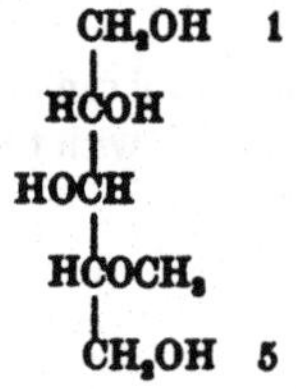

4-*O*-Methyl-D-
xylitol (not 2-*O*-
methyl-L-xylitol;
cf. Rule Carb-2)

ω-DEOXYALDITOLS

Rule Carb-27

The name of an aldose derivative having a terminal CH$_3$ and CH$_2$OH group is derived from that of the appropriate alditol (Rule Carb-2) by use of the prefix "deoxy."

Examples:

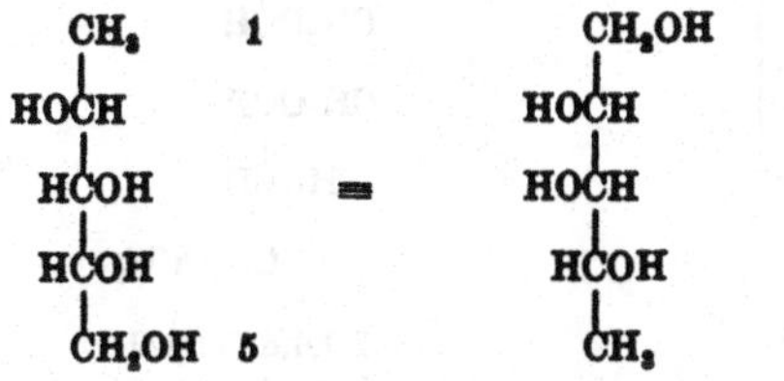

$$
\begin{array}{ccc}
\text{CH}_3 \quad 1 & \qquad & \text{CH}_2\text{OH} \\
\text{HOCH} & & \text{HOCH} \\
\text{HCOH} \quad = & & \text{HOCH} \\
\text{HCOH} & & \text{HCOH} \\
\text{CH}_2\text{OH} \quad 5 & & \text{CH}_3 \\
\end{array}
$$

1-Deoxy-D-arabinitol (not 5-deoxy-D-lyxitol)

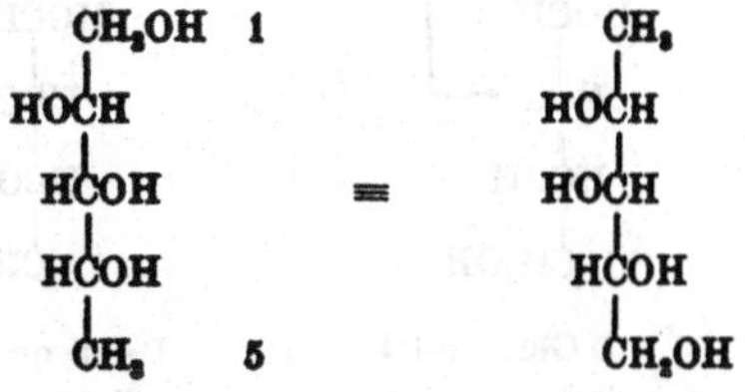

$$
\begin{array}{ccc}
\text{CH}_2\text{OH} \quad 1 & \qquad & \text{CH}_3 \\
\text{HOCH} & & \text{HOCH} \\
\text{HCOH} \quad = & & \text{HOCH} \\
\text{HCOH} & & \text{HCOH} \\
\text{CH}_3 \quad 5 & & \text{CH}_2\text{OH} \\
\end{array}
$$

5-Deoxy-D-arabinitol (not 1-deoxy-D-lyxitol)

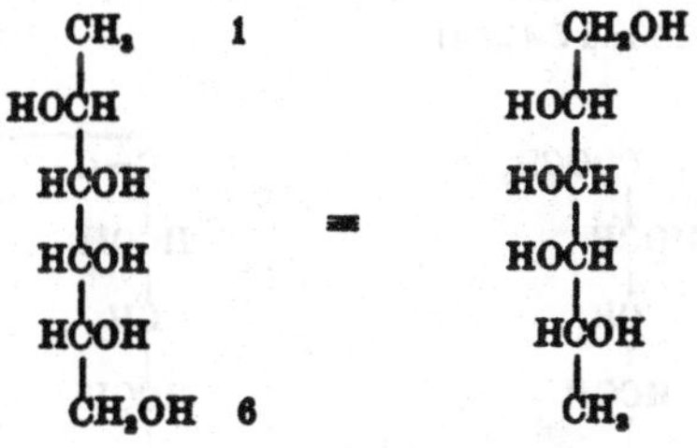

$$
\begin{array}{ccc}
\text{CH}_3 \quad 1 & \qquad & \text{CH}_2\text{OH} \\
\text{HOCH} & & \text{HOCH} \\
\text{HCOH} & & \text{HOCH} \\
\text{HCOH} \quad = & & \text{HOCH} \\
\text{HCOH} & & \text{HCOH} \\
\text{CH}_2\text{OH} \quad 6 & & \text{CH}_3 \\
\end{array}
$$

1-Deoxy-D-altritol (not 6-deoxy-D-talitol)

ALDONIC ACIDS

Rule Carb-28

Monocarboxylic acids formally derived from aldoses, having three or more carbon atoms in the chain, by oxidation of the aldehydic group, are named aldonic acids, and are divided into aldotrionic acid, aldotetronic acids, aldopentonic acids, aldohexonic acids, etc., according to the number of carbon atoms in the chain. The names of individual compounds of this type are formed by replacing the ending "oso" of the systematic or trivial name of the aldose by "onic acid."

Derivatives of these acids formed by change in the carboxyl group (salts, esters, lactones, acyl halides, amides, nitriles, etc.,) are named according to the IUPAC Nomenclature of Organic Chemistry, Section C, 1965, Rule C-4.

Examples:

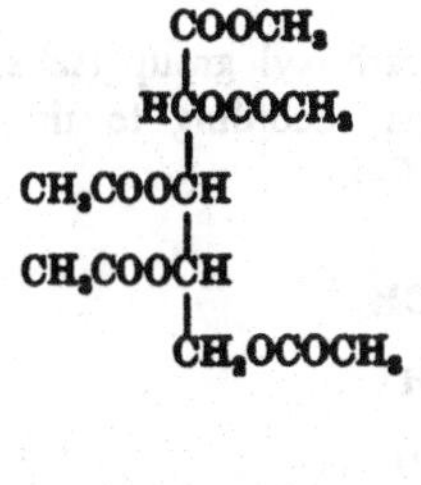

$$
\begin{array}{ccc}
\text{COOCH}_3 & \text{COONa} & \text{COOH} \\
\text{HCOCOCH}_3 & \text{HCOH} & \text{HCNH}_2 \\
\text{CH}_3\text{COOCH} & \text{HOCH} & \text{HOCH} \\
\text{CH}_3\text{COOCH} & \text{HCOH} & \text{HCOH} \\
\text{CH}_2\text{OCOCH}_3 & \text{HCOH} & \text{HCOH} \\
 & \text{CH}_2\text{OH} & \text{CH}_2\text{OH} \\
\end{array}
$$

Methyl tetra-*O*-acetyl-L-arabinonate or methyl L-arabinonate tetraacetate (*cf*. Rule C-463)

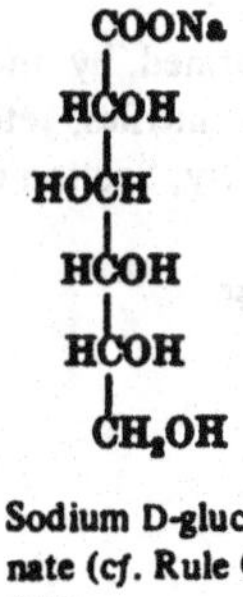

Sodium D-gluconate (*cf*. Rule C-461)

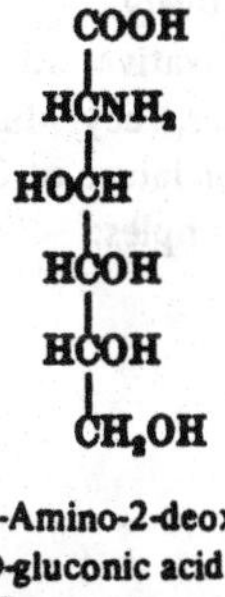

2-Amino-2-deoxy-D-gluconic acid (Common name for biochemical usage: D-Glucosaminic acid)

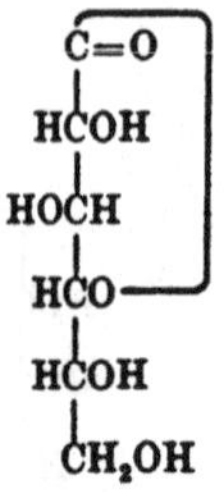

$$
\begin{array}{c}
\overset{|}{C}=O \\
H\overset{|}{C}OH \\
HO\overset{|}{C}H \\
H\overset{|}{C}O\!-\! \\
H\overset{|}{C}OH \\
\overset{|}{C}H_2OH
\end{array}
$$

D-Glucono-1,4-
lactone or, less
preferred, D-
glucono-γ-lac-
tone

$$
\begin{array}{c}
\overset{|}{C}=O \\
H\overset{|}{C}OH \\
HO\overset{|}{C}H \\
H\overset{|}{C}OH \\
H\overset{|}{C}O\!-\! \\
\overset{|}{C}H_2OH
\end{array}
$$

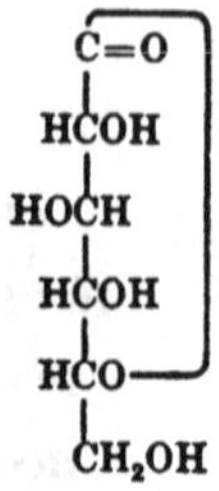

D-Glucono-1,5-
lactone or, less
preferred, D-
glucono-δ-lac-
tone

$$
\begin{array}{c}
CN \\
H\overset{|}{C}OCH_3 \\
CH_3O\overset{|}{C}H \\
CH_3O\overset{|}{C}H \\
HO\overset{|}{C}H \\
\overset{|}{C}H_2OCH_3
\end{array}
$$

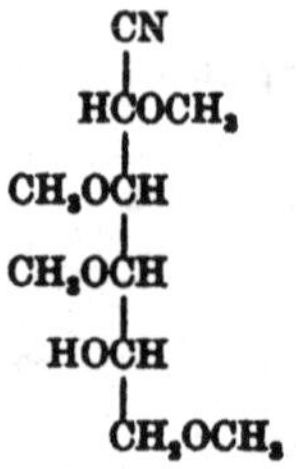

2,3,4,6-Tetra-*O*-
methyl-L-altron-
onitrile

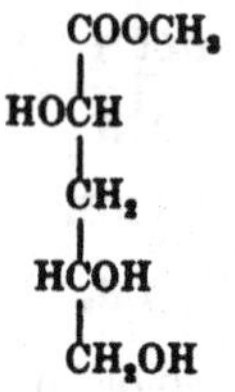

(*cf.* Rules c-472.1 and C-472.4)

$$
\begin{array}{c}
COOCH_3 \\
HO\overset{|}{C}H \\
\overset{|}{C}H_2 \\
H\overset{|}{C}OH \\
\overset{|}{C}H_2OH
\end{array}
$$

Methyl 3-deoxy-
D-*glycero*-L-
glycero-penton-
ate*

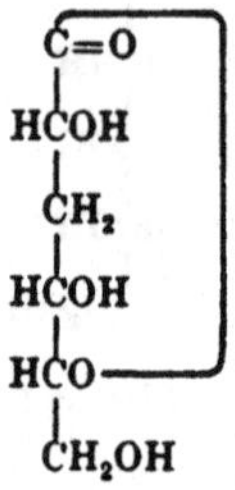

$$
\begin{array}{c}
\overset{|}{C}=O \\
H\overset{|}{C}OH \\
\overset{|}{C}H_2 \\
H\overset{|}{C}OH \\
H\overset{|}{C}O\!-\! \\
\overset{|}{C}H_2OH
\end{array}
$$

3-Deoxy-D-*erythro*-
D-*glycero*-hexono-
1,5-lactone†

KETOALDONIC ACIDS

Rule Carb-29

Keto-carboxylic acids formally derived by oxidation of a secondary alcoholic hydroxyl
group of an aldonic acid have the general name ketoaldonic acids.

The carbon atom of the carboxyl group is numbered one.

Names of individual ketoaldonic acids, or of the glycosides derived from such
compounds, are formed by replacing the ending "ose" or "oside" of the appropriate
ketose, or of the glycoside derived there from, by "osonic acid" or "osidonic acid,"
respectively.

Derivatives of these acids formed by modifying the carboxyl group (salts, esters,
lactones, acyl halides, amides, nitriles, etc.,) are named according to the IUPAC
Nomenclature of Organic Chemistry, Section C, 1965, Rule C-4.

Examples:

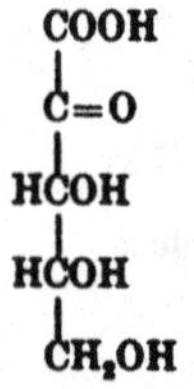

$$
\begin{array}{c}
COOH \\
\overset{|}{C}=O \\
H\overset{|}{C}OH \\
H\overset{|}{C}OH \\
\overset{|}{C}H_2OH
\end{array}
$$

D-*erythro*-2-
Pentulosonic
acid

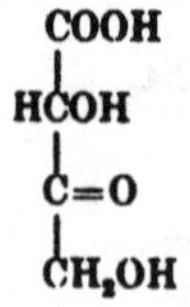

$$
\begin{array}{c}
COOH \\
H\overset{|}{C}OH \\
\overset{|}{C}=O \\
\overset{|}{C}H_2OH
\end{array}
$$

D-*glycero*-3-Tetru-
losonic acid

*Name according to Anglo-American usage: Methyl 3-deoxy-D-*threo*-pentonate.
†Name according to Anglo-American usage: 3-Deoxy-D-*ribo*-hexono-1,5-lactone.

```
      COOH          HOOC—COH┐        HOC—C═O┐
      |             |        |       |       |
    HOCH          HOCH       |     HOCH       |
      |             |        |       |       |
     C═O          HCOH       |     HCOH       |
      |             |        |       |       |
    HCOH          HCOH       |     HCO────────┘
      |             |        |       |
    HCOH          CH₂O───────┘    OCH₂
      |
    CH₂OH
```

D-erythro-L- | α-D-arabino-2-Hexu- | β-D-arabino-2-Hexu-
glycero-3-Hexu- | lopyranosonic acid | lopyranosono-1,5-
losonic acid* | (Common name for | lactone
 | biochemical usage: 2- |
 | Keto-D-gluconic acid) |

```
  HOOC—COCH₃┐        H₂COCCONH₂┐
  |          |        |         |
 HOCH        |      HOCH        |
  |          |        |         |
 HCOH        |      HCOH        |
  |          |        |         |
 HCOH        |      HCOH        |
  |          |        |         |
 CH₂O────────┘     OCH₂─────────┘
```

Methyl α-D-arabino- | Methyl β-D-arabino-
2-hexulopyranosido- | 2-hexulopyranosido-
nic acid | namide

Comment. Parentheses are suitably inserted where it is necessary to distinguish between an ester alkyl group and the hemiacetal alkyl group of a glycoside of a ketoaldonic acid.

```
 C₂H₅OOC—COCH₃┐        NaOOC—COC₂H₅┐
 |             |        |           |
 HOCH          |      HOCH          |
 |             |        |           |
 HCOH          |      HCOH          |
 |             |        |           |
 HCOH          |      HCOH          |
 |             |        |           |
 CH₂O──────────┘     CH₂O───────────┘
```

Ethyl (methyl α-D-arabino- | Sodium (ethyl α-D-arabino-2-
2-hexulopyranosid)onate | hexulopyranosid)onate

URONIC ACIDS

Rule Carb-30

The monocarboxylic acids formally derived by oxidation of the terminal CH₂OH group of aldoses having four or more carbon atoms in the chain, or of glycosides derived from these aldoses, to a carboxyl group are named "uronic acids." The names of the individual compounds of this type are formed by replacing (a) the "ose" of the systematic or trivial name of the aldose by "uronic" acid or (b) the "oside" of the name of the glycoside by "osiduronic acid."

*Name according to Anglo-American usage: D-arabino-3-Hexulosonic acid.

The carbon atom of the (potential) aldehydic carbonyl group (not that of the carboxyl group) is numbered one.

Derivatives of these acids formed by change in the carboxyl group (salts. esters, lactones, acyl halides, amides, nitriles, etc.,) are named according to IUPAC, *Nomenclature of Organic Chemistry*, Section C, 1965, Rule C-4.

Examples:

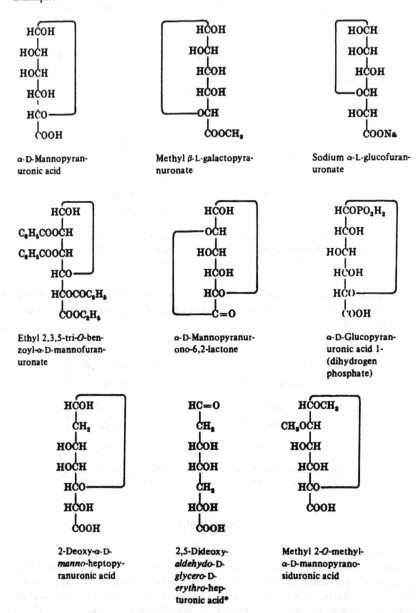

α-D-Mannopyranuronic acid

Methyl β-L-galactopyranuronate

Sodium α-L-glucofuranuronate

Ethyl 2,3,5-tri-*O*-benzoyl-α-D-mannofuranuronate

α-D-Mannopyranurono-6,2-lactone

α-D-Glucopyranuronic acid 1-(dihydrogen phosphate)

2-Deoxy-α-D-*manno*-heptopyranuronic acid

2,5-Dideoxy-*aldehydo*-D-*glycero*-D-*erythro*-hepturonic acid*

Methyl 2-*O*-methyl-α-D-mannopyranosiduronic acid

---

*Name according to Anglo-American usage: 2,5-Dideoxy-*aldehydo*-D-*ribo*-hepturonic acid.

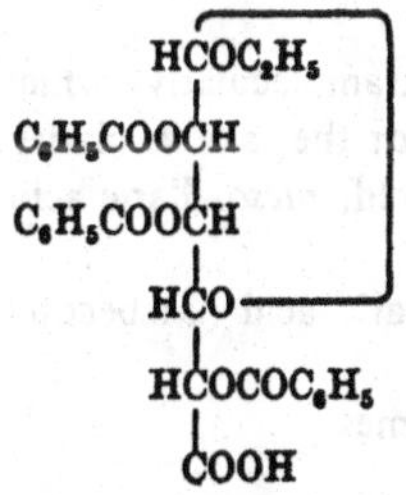

HCOC₂H₅ ... Ethyl structures

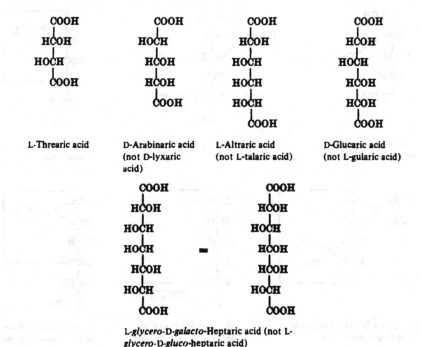

$$HCOC_2H_5$$
$$C_6H_5COOCH$$
$$C_6H_5COOCH$$
$$HCO$$
$$HCOCOC_6H_5$$
$$COOH$$

Ethyl 2,3,5-tri-*O*-benzoyl-
α-D-mannofuranosidu-
ronic acid

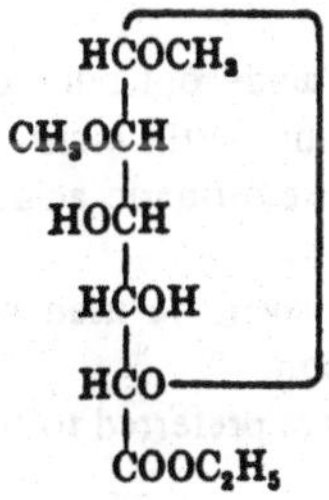

$$HCOCH_3$$
$$CH_3OCH$$
$$HOCH$$
$$HCOH$$
$$HCO$$
$$COOC_2H_5$$

Ethyl (methyl 2-*O*-
methyl-α-D-mannopyra-
nosid)uronate

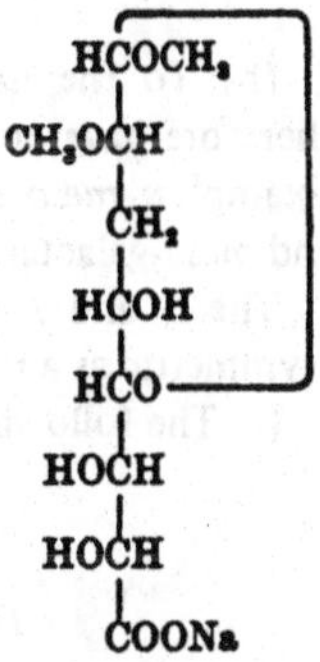

$$HCOCH_3$$
$$CH_3OCH$$
$$CH_2$$
$$HCOH$$
$$HCO$$
$$HOCH$$
$$HOCH$$
$$COONa$$

Sodium (methyl 3-
deoxy-2-*O*-methyl-β-
L-*manno*-L-*glycero*-
octopyranosid)uron-
ate†

ALDARIC ACIDS

Rule Carb-31

The dicarboxylic acids formed by oxidation of both terminal groups of an aldose to carboxyl groups are called "aldaric acids." Names of individual compounds of this type are formed by replacing the ending "oso" of the systematic or trivial name of the corresponding aldose by "aric acid." Choice between the several possible names is based on the order of precedence given in Rule Carb-2.

Examples:

(a) Names requiring D or L:

$$COOH$$
$$HCOH$$
$$HOCH$$
$$COOH$$

L-Threaric acid

$$COOH$$
$$HOCH$$
$$HCOH$$
$$HCOH$$
$$COOH$$

D-Arabinaric acid
(not D-lyxaric
acid)

$$COOH$$
$$HCOH$$
$$HOCH$$
$$HOCH$$
$$HOCH$$
$$COOH$$

L-Altraric acid
(not L-talaric acid)

$$COOH$$
$$HCOH$$
$$HOCH$$
$$HCOH$$
$$HCOH$$
$$COOH$$

D-Glucaric acid
(not L-gularic acid)

$$COOH$$
$$HCOH$$
$$HOCH$$
$$HOCH$$
$$HCOH$$
$$HOCH$$
$$COOH$$

═

$$COOH$$
$$HCOH$$
$$HOCH$$
$$HCOH$$
$$HCOH$$
$$HOCH$$
$$COOH$$

L-*glycero*-D-*galacto*-Heptaric acid (not L-
glycero-D-*gluco*-heptaric acid)

†Name according to Anglo-American usage: Sodium (methyl 3-deoxy-2-*O*-methyl-L-*glycero*-β-L-*galacto*-octopyranosid) uronate.

(b) To the names of aldaric acids optically compensated intramolecularly, which therefore have no D or L prefix, the prefix *meso-* may be added for the sake of clarity. Examples: *meso*-erythraric acid, *meso*-ribaric acid, *meso*-xylaric acid, *meso*-allaric acid, and *meso*-galactaric acid.

The D and L prefix must, however, be used when a *meso*-aldaric acid has become asymmetric as a result of substitution.

(c) The following trivial names are preferred to the systematic names.

COOH	COOH	COOH
HCOH	HOCH	HCOH
HOCH	HCOH	HCOH
COOH	COOH	COOH
(+)-Tartaric acid	(−)-Tartaric acid	*meso*-Tartaric
(L-threaric acid)	(D-threaric acid)	acid (erythraric
(*RR*-Tartaric acid)	(*SS*-Tartaric acid)	acid) (*RS*-Tartaric acid)

CYCLIC ACETALS

Rule Carb-32

Cyclic acetals formed by the reaction of saccharides or saccharide derivatives with aldehydes or ketones are named in accordance with Rule Carb-15, bivalent radical names being used as prefixes, the names of such radicals following the rules of general organic chemical nomenclature. In indicating more than one cyclic acetal grouping of the same kind, the appropriate pairs of locants are separated typographically when the exact placement of the acetal groups is known.

Examples:

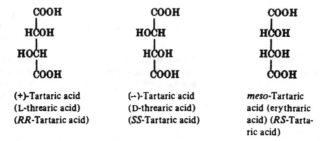

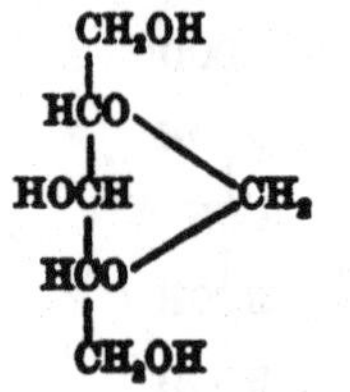

2,4-*O*-Methylenexylitol

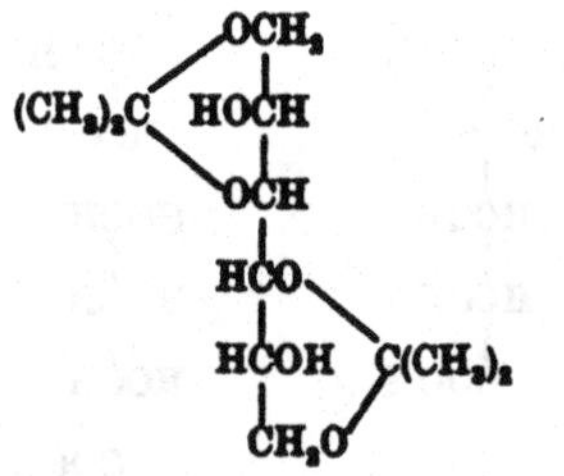

1,3:4,6-Di-*O*-isopropylidene-D-mannitol

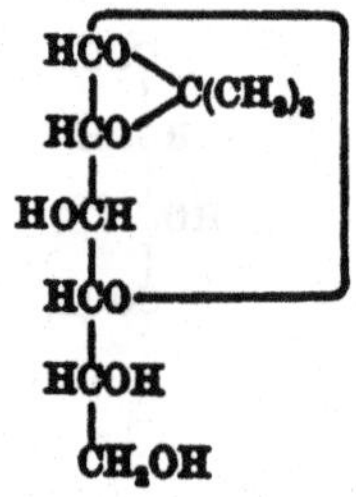

1,2-*O*-Isopropylidene-α-glucofuranose

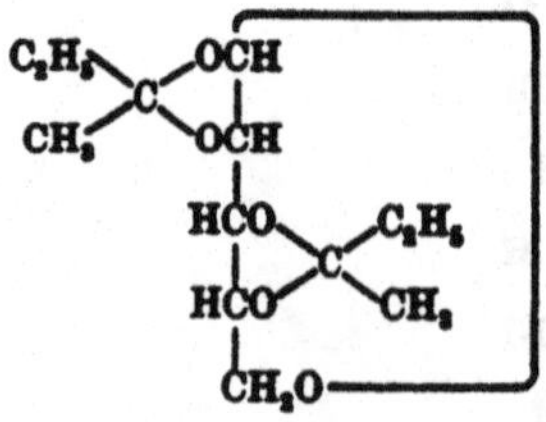

1,2:3,4-Di-*O*-*sec*-butylidene-β-D-arabinopyranose

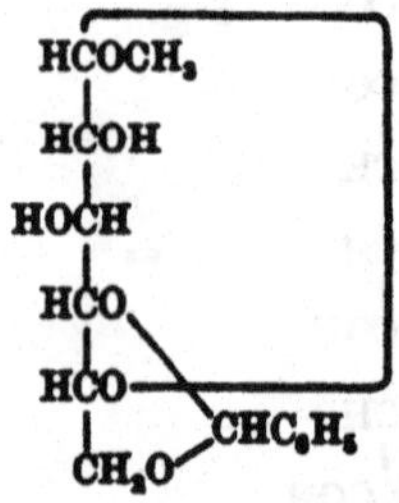

Methyl 4,6-*O*-benzylidene-α-D-glucopyranoside

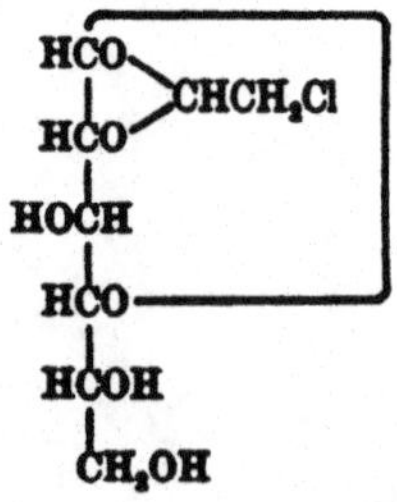

1,2-*O*-(2-Chloroethylidene)-α-D-glucofuranose

Note. It is to be noted that in the last three examples new asymmetric centers have been introduced at the carbonyl carbon atom of the aldehyde or ketone that has reacted with the saccharide.

When known, the stereochemistry at such a new center is indicated by use of the appropriate *R* or *S* symbol (see the Preamble, section 5), placed in parentheses, immediately before the name of the bivalent radical corresponding to the original aldehyde or ketone.

Example:

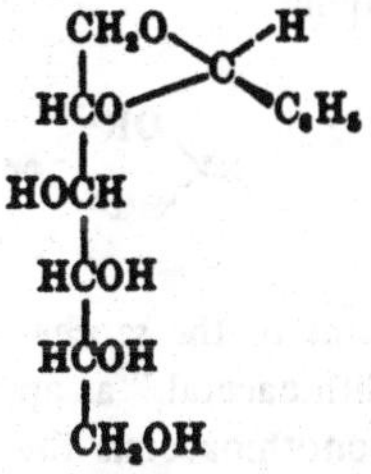

1,2-*O*-(*R*)-Benzylidene-
D-glucitol

ORTHO ESTERS

Rule Carb-33

The "glycosides of ortho ester structure" are named (a) as cyclic acetals, according to Rule Carb-32, or (b) as ortho esters, according to Rule C-464.1,* with the name of the saccharide as the first term of the name.

Examples:

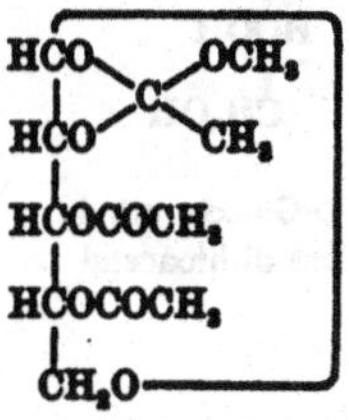

(a) 3,4-Di-*O*-acetyl-
1,2-*O*-(1-methoxy-
ethylidene)-α-D-
ribopyranose
(b) α-D-Ribopyra-
nose 3,4-diacetate
1,2-(methyl ortho-
acetate)

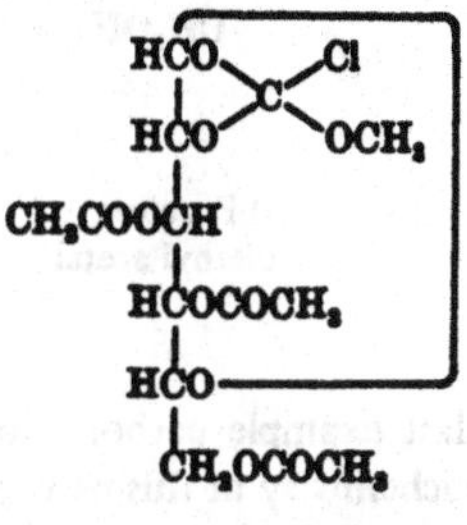

(a) 3,4,6-Tri-*O*-acetyl-1,2-*O*-(1-
chloro-1methoxy-methylene)-
α-D-glucopyranose
(b) α-D-Glucopyranose 3,4,6-
triacetate 1,2-(methyl chloroorthoformate)

Note. In each example a new asymmetric center has been introduced at the carbon atom of the hypothetical ortho acid.

When known, the stereochemistry at such a new center are indicated by use of the appropriate *RS* symbol (see the Preamble, section 5), placed in parentheses, immediately before that part of the name that includes the new asymmetric center.

*IUPAC, *Nomenclature of Organic Chemistry, Section C;* see Reference 1.

Examples:

(a) 3,4,6-Tri-*O*-acetyl-1,2-*O*-(R)-(1-chloro-1-methoxymethylene-α-D-glucopyranose
(b) α-D-Glucopyranose 3,4,6-triacetate 1,2-(R)-methyl chloroorthoformate)

ACETALS AND THIOACETALS

Rule Carb-34

The compounds obtained by transforming the carbonyl group of a saccharide or saccharide derivative into the grouping

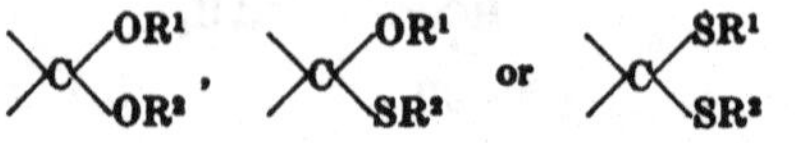

$$\underset{OR^2}{\overset{OR^1}{>C<}} \, , \quad \underset{SR^2}{\overset{OR^1}{>C<}} \quad or \quad \underset{SR^2}{\overset{SR^1}{>C<}}$$

are named by placing after the name of the saccharide or saccharide derivative the term "acetal," monothioacetal," or "dithioacetal," as appropriate, preceded by the names of the radicals R^1 and R^2. With monothioacetals the mode of bonding of two different radical R^1 and R^2 is indicated by the use of the prefixes *O* and *S*.

Examples:

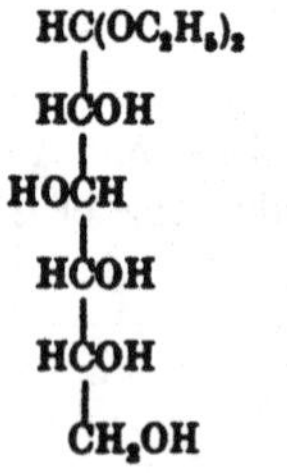

```
HC(OC₂H₅)₂        CH₂OH           S—CH₂         SC₂H₅
   |                 |          HC<               |
 HCOH            C(OC₂H₅)₂         S—CH₂      HCOCH₃
   |                 |                |           |
 HOCH             HOCH            HOCH         HCOH
   |                 |                |           |
 HCOH             HCOH            HCOH         HOCH
   |                 |                |           |
 HCOH             HCOH            HCOH         HCOH
   |                 |                |           |
 CH₂OH            CH₂OH           HCOH         HCOH
                                    |           |
                                  CH₂OH       CH₂OH
```

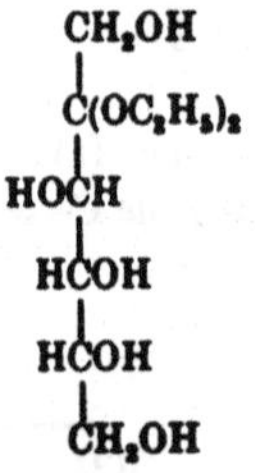

D-Glucose diethyl   D-Fructose   D-Glucose ethyl-   D-Glucose *S*-ethyl
acetal   diethyl acetal   ene dithioacetal   *O*-methyl mono-
                                                               thioacetal

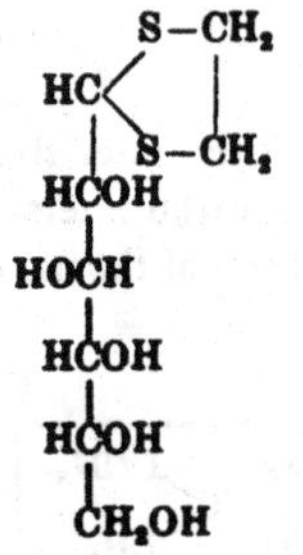

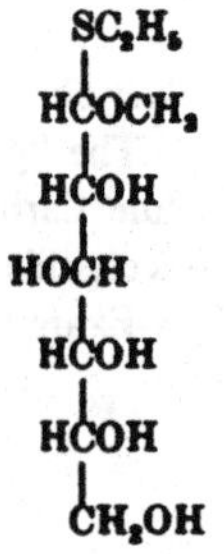

Note. In the last example carbon atom number one has become asymmetric. When known, the stereochemistry at this new asymmetric center will be indicated by use of the Sequence Rule Symbol, *R* or *S* (see the Preamble, section 5), preceded by the locant of the new asymmetric center and both placed in parentheses, at the beginning of the name.

Example:

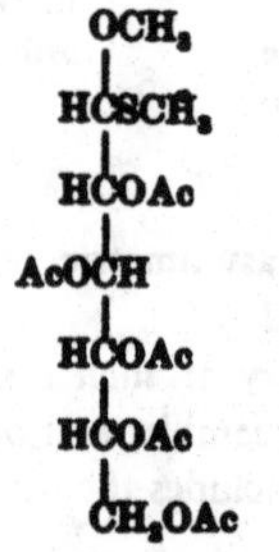

```
     OCH₃
      |
  HCSCH₃
      |
  HCOAc
      |
 AcOCH
      |
  HCOAc
      |
  HCOAc
      |
  CH₂OAc
```

(1*R*)-2,3,4,5,6-
Penta-*O*-acetyl-D-
glucose dimethyl
monothioacetal

HEMIACETALS

Rule Carb-35

The compounds obtained by transforming the carbonyl group of the acyclic form of a saccharide, or saccharide derivative, into the grouping

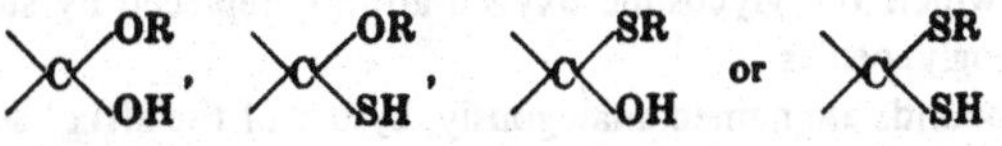

are named as indicated in Rule Carb-34, by using the endings "hemiacetal," "monothio-hemiacetal," or "dithiohemiacetal," as appropriate. The two isomers of a monothiohemi-acetal are differentiated by use of *O* and *S* prefixes.

Examples:

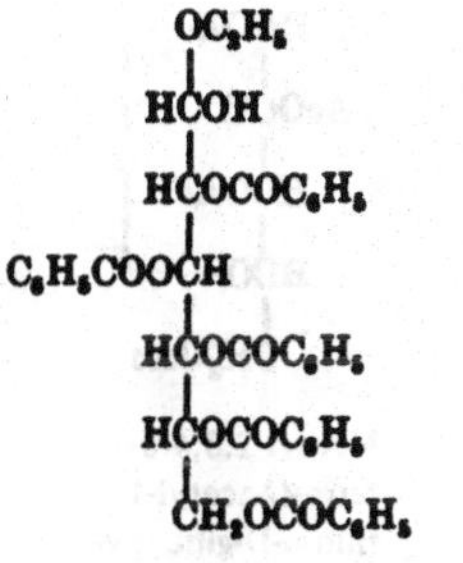

OC_2H_5	SC_2H_5
HCOH	HCSH
HCOCOC$_6$H$_5$	HCOCOC$_6$H$_5$
C$_6$H$_5$COOCH	C$_6$H$_5$COOCH
HCOCOC$_6$H$_5$	HCOCOC$_6$H$_5$
HCOCOC$_6$H$_5$	HCOCOC$_6$H$_5$
CH$_2$OCOC$_6$H$_5$	CH$_2$OCOC$_6$H$_5$
2,3,4,5,6-Penta-*O*-benzoyl-D-glucose ethyl hem-iacetal	2,3,4,5,6-Penta-*O*-benzoyl-D-glucose ethyl di-thiohemiacetal

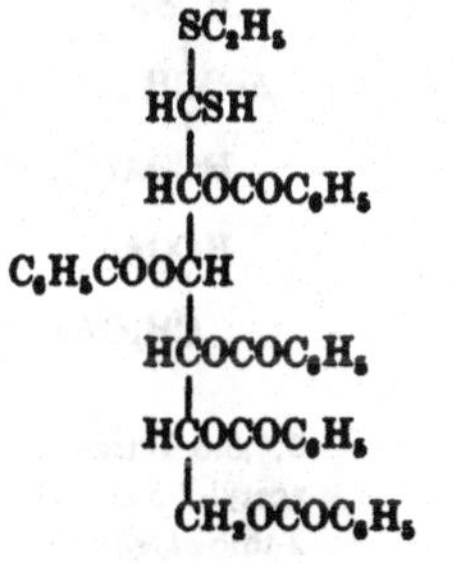

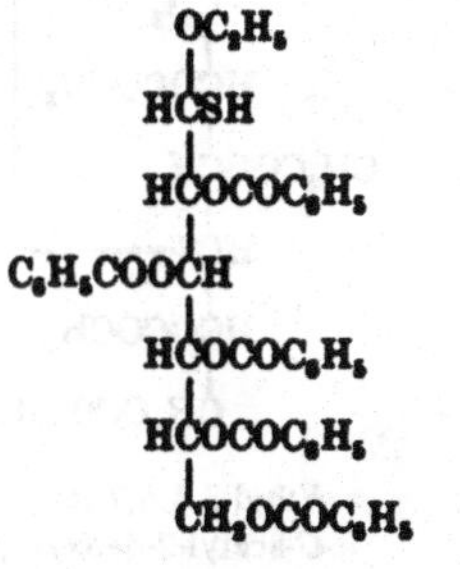

OC_2H_5	SC_2H_5
HCSH	HCOH
HCOCOC$_6$H$_5$	HCOCOC$_6$H$_5$
C$_6$H$_5$COOCH	C$_6$H$_5$COOCH
HCOCOC$_6$H$_5$	HCOCOC$_6$H$_5$
HCOCOC$_6$H$_5$	HCOCOC$_6$H$_5$
CH$_2$OCOC$_6$H$_5$	CH$_2$OCOC$_6$H$_5$
2,3,4,5,6-Penta-*O*-benzoyl-D-glucose *O*-ethyl monothiohemiacetal	2,3,4,5,6-Penta-*O*-benzoyl-D-glucose *S*-ethyl monothiohemiace-tal

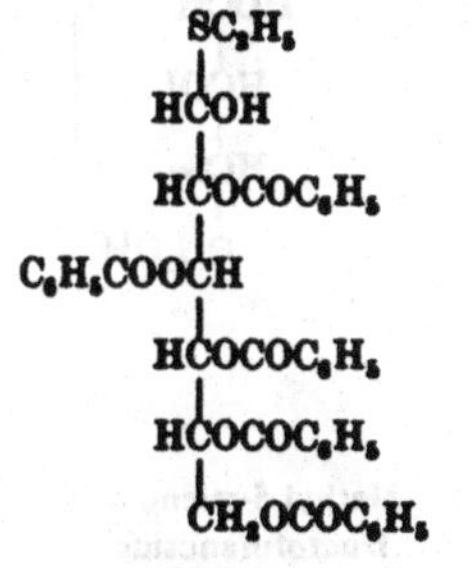

Note. In these compounds carbon atom number one has become asymmetric. When known, the stereochemistry at this new asymmetric center is indicated as described in the Note to Rule Carb-34.

OTHER SULFUR MONOSACCHARIDES

Rule Carb-36

Replacement of a hydroxyl oxygen atom of an aldose or ketose, or of the oxygen atom of the carbonyl group of the acyclic form of an aldose or ketose, by sulfur is indicated by placing the (nondetachable) affix "thio," preceded by the appropriate locant, before the systematic or trivial name of the aldose or ketose.

Replacement of the ring oxygen atom of the cyclic form of an aldose or ketose by sulfur is indicated in the same way, the number of the highest numbered carbon atom of the ring being used as locant.

Glycosides in which the glycosidic oxygen atom is replaced by sulfur are designated generically as "thioglycosides."

Selenium compounds are named analogously, by use of the affix "seleno."

Note. It should be noted that the appropriate affix is thio, not thia; the latter is used in systematic organic chemical nomenclature to indicate replacement of CH_2 by S.

Examples:

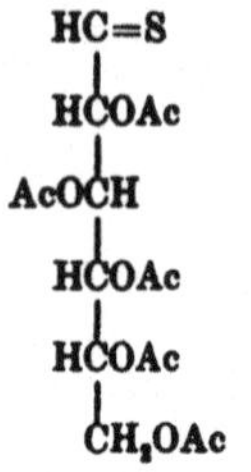

2,3,4,5,6-Penta-
O-acetyl-1-thio-
aldehydo-D-
glucose

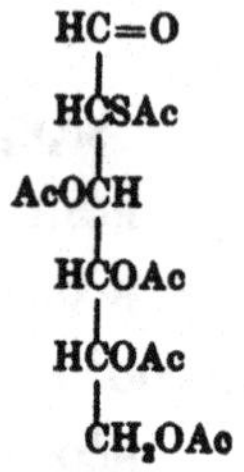

3,4,5,6-Tetra-*O*-
acetyl-2-*S*-acetyl-
2-thio-*aldehydo*-
D-glucose

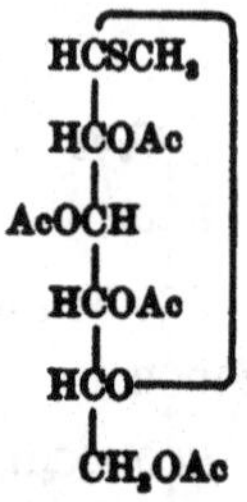

Methyl 2,3,4.6-
tetra-*O*-acetyl-1-
thio-α-D-glucopy-
ranoside

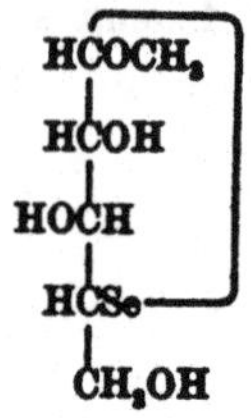

Methyl 4-seleno-
α-D-xylofurano-
side

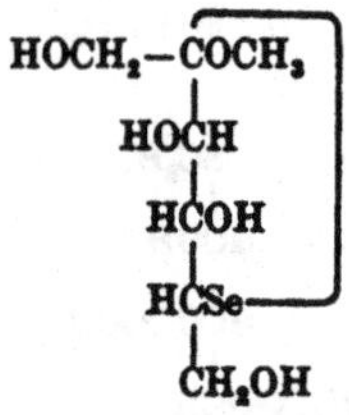

Methyl 5-seleno-α-D-
fructofuranoside

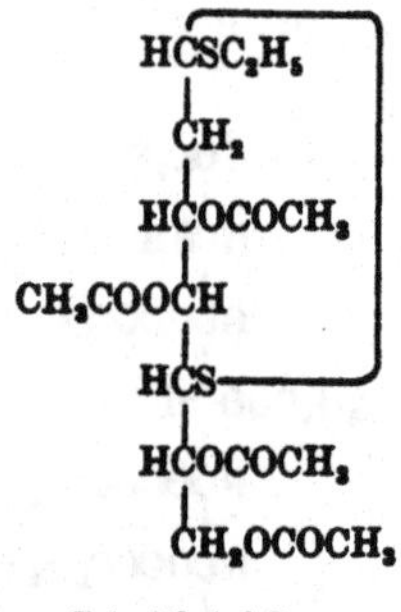

Ethyl 3,4,6,7-tetra-
O-acetyl-2-deoxy-1,5-
dithio-α-D-*gluco*-hep-
topyranoside

INTRAMOLECULAR ANHYDRIDES

Rule Carb-37

An intramolecular ether (commonly called an intramolecular anhydride), formed by elimination of water from two alcoholic hydroxyl groups of a single molecule of a monosaccharide (aldose or ketose) or monosaccharide derivative, is named by attaching the (detachable) prefix "anhydro" by a hyphen before the monosaccharide name; this prefix, in turn, is preceded by a pair of locants identifying the two hydroxyl groups involved.

Examples:

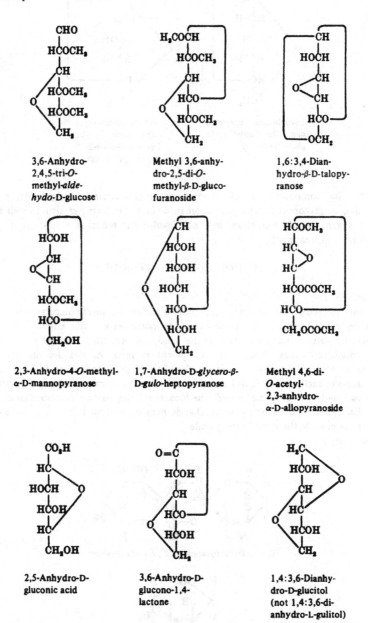

3,6-Anhydro-
2,4,5-tri-*O*-
methyl-*alde-
hydo*-D-glucose

Methyl 3,6-anhy-
dro-2,5-di-*O*-
methyl-β-D-gluco-
furanoside

1,6:3,4-Dian-
hydro-β-D-talopy-
ranose

2,3-Anhydro-4-*O*-methyl-
α-D-mannopyranose

1,7-Anhydro-D-*glycero*-β-
D-*gulo*-heptopyranose

Methyl 4,6-di-
O-acetyl-
2,3-anhydro-
α-D-allopyranoside

2,5-Anhydro-D-
gluconic acid

3,6-Anhydro-D-
glucono-1,4-
lactone

1,4:3,6-Dianhy-
dro-D-glucitol
(not 1,4:3,6-di-
anhydro-L-gulitol)

Trivial names for anhydro-monosaccharides established by usage but not recommended (because of possible confusion with polysaccharide names based on the use of the
termination -an) are

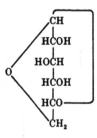

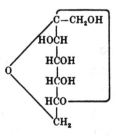

Levoglucosan (preferred
name: 1,6-Annydro-β-D-
glucopyranose)

Sedoheptulosan (pre-
ferred name: 2,7-An-
hydro-β-1)-*altro*-2-
heptulopyranose)

Note. The compounds usually known as monosaccharide anhydrides, glycose anhydrides, or glycosans (whose formation involves the reducing group). as well as the anhydro sugars (whose formation does not involve the reducing group) are not here differentiated in treatment.

INTERMOLECULAR ANHYDRIDES

Rule Carb-38

An intermolecular cyclic acetal (commonly called an intermolecular anhydride), formed by condensation of two monosaccharide molecules with the elimination of two molecules of water, is named by placing the word "dianhydride" after the names of two parent monosaccharides. When the two parent monosaccharides are different, the sequence of their citation is according to the order of preference given in Rule Carb-2. The position of each anhydride link is indicated by a pair of locants showing the positions of the two hydroxyl groups involved; the locants relating to one monosaccharide (in a mixed dianhydride, the second monosaccharide named) is primed. Both pairs of locants immediately precede the word "dianhydride."

Examples:

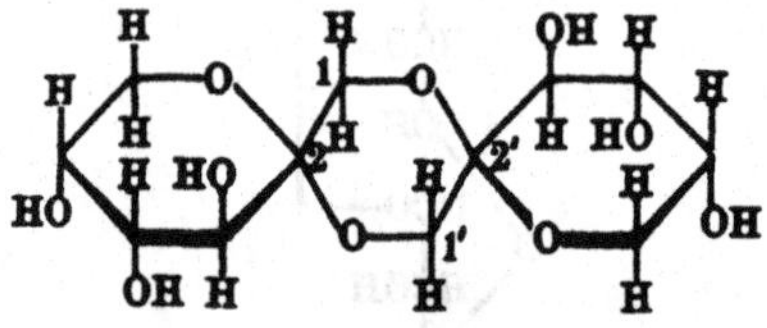

Di-α-D-fructopyranose 1,2'; 2,1'-dianhydride

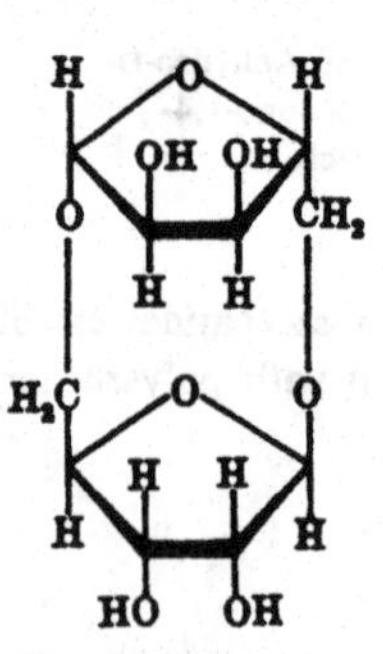

Di-β-D-ribofuranose
1,5'; 5,1'-dianhydride

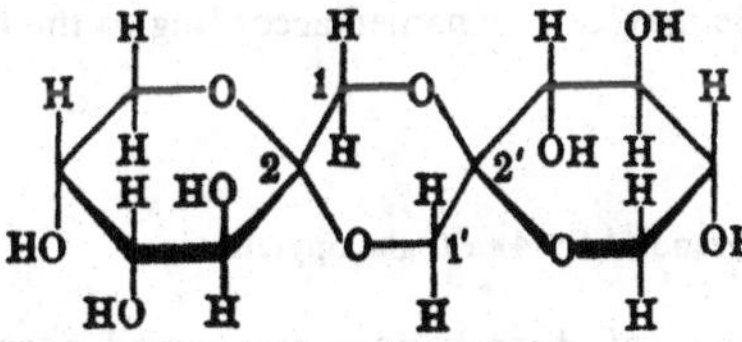

α-D-Fructopyranose α-D-sorbopyranose 1,2'; 2,1'-
dianhydride

OLIGOSACCHARIDES

An oligosaccharide is a compound which, on complete hydrolysis, gives monosaccharide units only, in relatively small number per molecule (in contrast to the
high-polymeric polysaccharides).

Comment. Most of the naturally occurring oligosaccharides have well established and
useful common names (for example, cellobiose, lactose, maltose, melizitose, raffinose,
stachyose, and sucrose) which were assigned before their complete structures were
known. Rational names may be assigned as described in the following Rules.

Disaccharides
Rule Carb-39

(a) *Nonreducing*. A nonreducing disaccharide is named, from its component
monosaccharide parts, as a glycosyl glycoside.

Example:

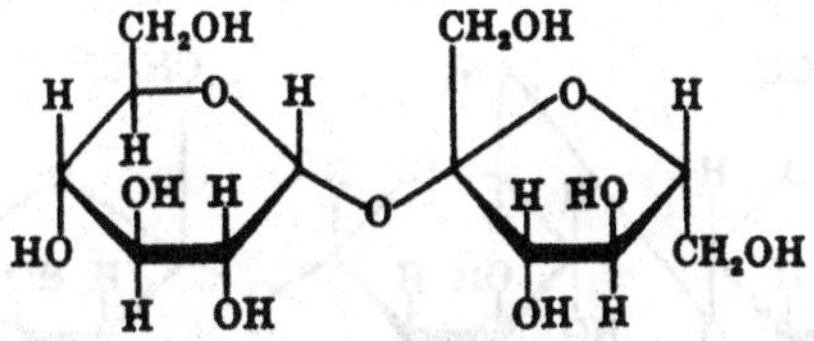

Sucrose: β-D-Fructofuranosyl α-D-glucopyranoside
(not α-D-glucopyranosyl β-D-fructofuranoside; alphabetical order of monosaccharide units, see Rule
Carb-2)

(b) *Reducing*. A reducing disaccharide is named, from its component monosaccharide
parts, as a glycosylglycose.

Example:

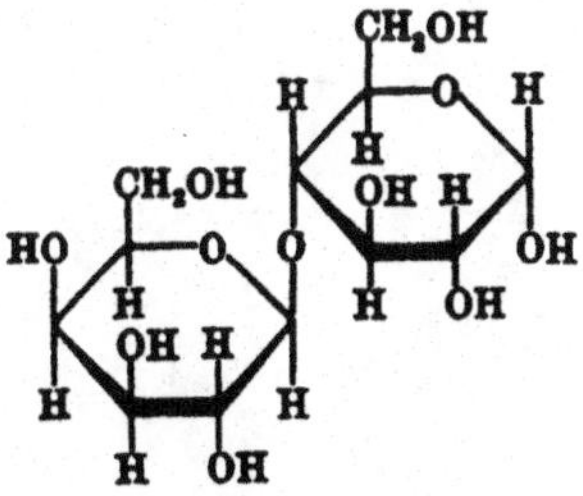

α-Lactose: 4-*O*-β-D-Galactopyranosyl-
α-D-glucopyranose

A reducing disaccharide may also be named according to the method described in Rule Carb-40.

Example:

α-Lactose: *O*-β-D-Galactopyranosyl-(1→4)-α-D-glucopyranose

(c)*Derivatives*. Derivatives of disaccharides are named according to the rules for monosaccharides.

Examples:

Methyl α-lactoside: Methyl 4-*O*-β-D-galactopyranosyl-α-D-glucopyranoside, or methyl *O*-β-D-galacto-pyranosyl-(1→4)-α-D-glucopyranoside

2-Amino-2-deoxy-4-*O*-(β-D-galactopyranosyl)-α-D-glucopyranose, or *O*-*j*-D-galactopyranosyl-(1→4)-2-amino-2-deoxy-α-D-glucopyranose

Trisaccharides and Higher Oligosaccharides
Rule Carb-40

(a) *Nonreducing*. A nonreducing trisaccharide is named as a glycosylglycosyl glycoside, from its component monosaccharide parts. Higher nonreducing oligosaccharides are named similarly.

Between the name of one glycosyl radical and the next are placed two locants which indicate the respective positions involved in this glycosidic union; these locants are separated by an arrow (pointing from the locant corresponding to the glycosyl carbon atom to the locant corresponding to the hydroxylic carbon atom involved) and are enclosed in parentheses.

Example:

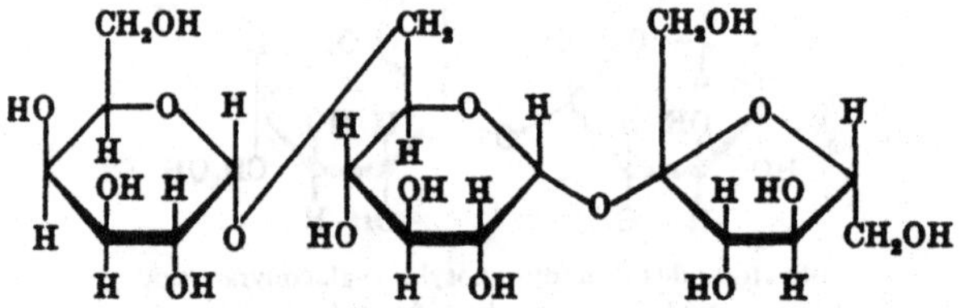

Raffinose: *O*-α-D-galactopyranosyl-(1→6) α-D-glucopyranosyl β-D-fructofuranoside

(b) *Reducing*. A reducing trisaccharide is named as a glycosylglycosylglycose, from its component monosaccharide parts. Higher reducing oligosaccharides are named similarly.

Examples:

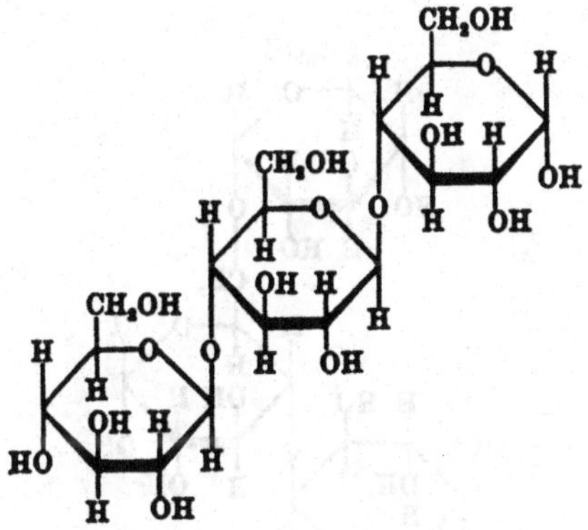

α-Cellotriose: *O*-β-D-Glucopyranosyl-(1→4)-*O*-β-D-glucopyranosyl-(1→4)-α-D-glucopyranose

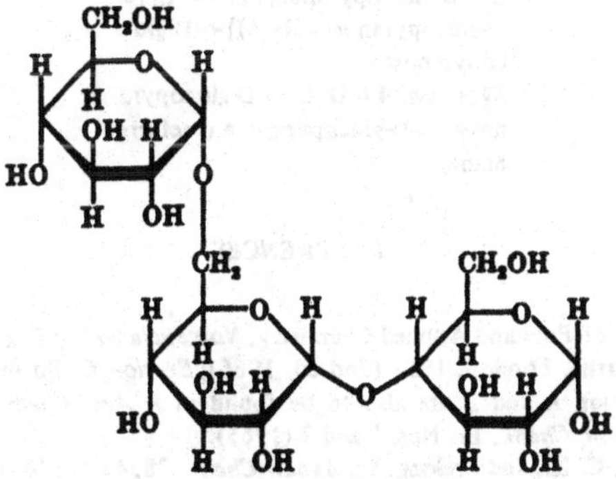

Panose: *O*-α-D-Glucopyranosyl-(1→6)-*O*-α-D-glucopyranosyl-(1→4)-α-D-glucopyranose

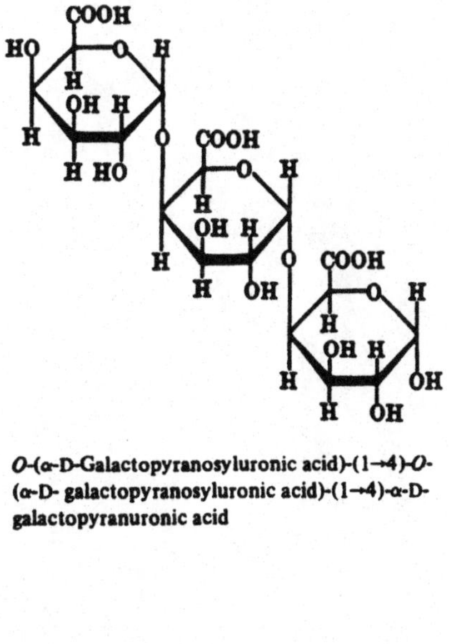

O-(α-D-Galactopyranosyluronic acid)-(1→4)-*O*-(α-D- galactopyranosyluronic acid)-(1→4)-α-D-galactopyranuronic acid

(c) *Reducing, branched.* By inserting one glycosyl substituent in brackets, it is distinguished from the second glycosyl substituent.

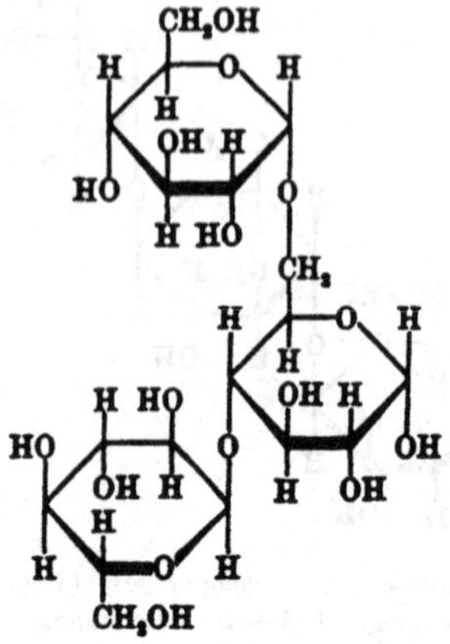

O-α-D-Glucopyranosyl-(1→4)-*O*-[α-D-glucopyranosyl-(1→6)]-α-D-glucopyranose
Synonym:4,6-Di-*O*-(α-D-glucopyranosyl)-α-D-glucopyranose (preferred name)

REFERENCES

1. International Union of Pure and Applied Chemistry, *Nomenclature of Organic Chemistry, Sections A and B*, Butterworths, London, 1957 (2nd ed. 1966); *Section C*, Butterworths, London, 1965. Editorial note: Section A and B are also to be found in *J. Am. Chem. Soc.*, 82, 5545 (1960); Section C in *Pure Appl. Chem.*, 11, Nos. 1 and 2 (1965).
2. Chan, R. S., Ingold, C. K., and Prelong, V., *Agnew Chem.*, 78, 413 (1966); *Agnew Chem. Int. Ed.*, 5, 385 (1966); IUPAC Tentative Rules for the Nomenclature of Organic Chemistry, *IUPAC Inf. Bull.*, 35, 71 (1969); [see also *Eur. J. Biochem.*, 18, 151 (1971)].

Carbohydrates

Table 1
NATURAL ALDITOLS, INOSITOLS, INOSOSES, AND AMINO ALDITOLS AND INOSAMINES

Substance[a] (synonym) derivative	Chemical formula	Melting point °C	Specific rotation[b] $[\alpha]_D$	Reference[c]	Chromatography, R value, and reference[d]			
					ELC	GLC	PPC	TLC
(A)	(B)	(C)	(D)	(E)	(F)	(G)	(H)	(I)
Alditols								
Glycerol (glycerine)	$C_3H_8O_3$	20	None (meso)	1	24rib (2)	4.69 (3)	32f (4)	62f (5)
Triacetate	$C_9H_{14}O_6$	4	None	1		3.60 (6)		
Trimethyl ether	$C_6H_{14}O_3$	Oil, bp 148	None	1		8xyll (7)		
Trimethylsilyl ether						5.94 (8)		
Tris-(o-nitrobenzoate)	$C_{24}H_{17}N_3O_{12}$	190–192	None	9egp				67f (35t)
1-Deoxyglycerol[e] (1,2-propanediol, propylene glycol)	$C_3H_8O_2$	Oil, bp 188–189	Racemic	1,10	5rib (2)	3.00 (11)	35f (12)	80f (5)
Bis-(p-nitrobenzoate)	$C_{17}H_{14}N_2O_8$	125–126		9egp				
Erythritol	$C_4H_{10}O_4$	118–120	None (meso)	13	53rib (2)	14.1 (3)	23f (4)	51f (5)
Tetraacetate	$C_{12}H_{18}O_8$	85	None	13		13.2 (6)		
Tetramethyl ether	$C_8H_{18}O_4$		None			26xyll (7)		
Trimethylsilyl ether						28.5 (14)		
Tetrakis-(p-nitrobenzoate)	$C_{32}H_{22}N_4O_{16}$	251–252	None	9egp				
1,4-Dideoxy-erythritol (2,3-butylenglycol)	$C_4H_{10}O_2$	25,34	None (meso)	15	6rib (2)		55f (12)	

[a] In order of increasing carbon chain length in the parent compounds grouped in the classes — alditols, inositols, inososes, amino alditols, and inosamines.

[b] $[\alpha]_D$ for 1–5 g solute; c, per 100 ml aqueous solution at 20–25°C unless otherwise given.

[c] References for melting point and specific rotation data. Letter indicates the reference also has chromatographic data according to: c = column, e = electrophoresis, g = gas, p = paper, and t = thin-layer.

[d] R value times 100, given relative to that of the compound indicated by abbreviation: f = solvent front, gal = galactose, glc = glucose, glcl = glucitol, glcn = glucosamine, myol = myo-inositol, perl = perseitol, pinl = pinitol, rib = ribose, sorl = sorbitol, suc = sucrose, xyll = xylitol, (as the pentaacetate or the pentamethyl ether, as pertains), and aral = arabinitol (as the pentaacetate). Under gas chromatography (Column GLC or G) numbers without code indication signify retention time in minutes. The conditions of the chromatography are correlated with the reference given in parentheses and are found in Table 5.

[e] Said to exist as a phosphate ester also.[18]

[f] Data given are for the enantiomorphic isomer.

[g] The author names as 3-dehydroquinic acid, but it is actually 5-dehydroquinic.

[h] The early given name, l-quercitol, of this compound does not make it the enantiomorph of d-quercitol; other isomeric relations are involved.

[i] This compound is isomeric with the previous one in regard to the N-methyl group position.

Table 1 (continued)
NATURAL ALDITOLS, INOSITOLS, INOSOSES, AND AMINO ALDITOLS AND INOSAMINES

Substance[a] (synonym) derivative (A)	Chemical formula (B)	Melting point °C (C)	Specific rotation[b] $[\alpha]_D$ (D)	Reference[c] (E)	Chromatography, R value, and reference[d]			
					ELC (F)	GLC (G)	PPC (H)	TLC (I)
Alditols (continued)								
Dibenzoate	$C_{18}H_{18}O_4$	77	-13	16				
1,4-Dideoxy-D-threitol	$C_4H_{10}O_2$	19	+1.4	15				
Diacetate	$C_8H_{14}O_4$	Oil, bp 192–194 (745 mm)		17				
Bis-(p-nitrobenzoate)	$C_{18}H_{16}N_2O_8$	142–144	-52.7 ± 0.5 (c 4, CHCl₃)	18				
L-Threitol	$C_4H_{10}O_4$	88–89	-4.5	19,22p	96rib (2)		144glc[f] (20)	
Tetraacetate	$C_{12}H_{18}O_{10}$	Oil, bp 145	-32 (C₂H₅OH)		45xyll[f] (21)			
Trimethylsilyl ether						27.5[f] (14)		
Di-O-benzylidene ether	$C_{18}H_{18}O_4$	(0.05 mm) 218–220	+87.2 (c 0.4, acetone)	22p				
Tetra-(p-nitrobenzoate)	$C_{32}H_{22}N_4O_{16}$	219–221[f]		23				
1,4-Dideoxy-L-threitol	$C_4H_{10}O_2$	Oil, bp ca 170	+12.4	18				
Bis-(p-nitrobenzoate)	$C_{18}H_{16}N_2O_8$	141–143	+52 (CHCl₃)	18				
1,4-Dideoxy-DL-threitol	$C_4H_{10}O_2$	7.6	Racemic	24				
Diacetate	$C_8H_{14}O_4$	41–41.5	Racemic	24				
D-Arabinitol (D-arabitol)	$C_5H_{12}O_5$	103	+7.8 (c 8, borax solution)	25	124rib (2)	38.1 (3)	14f (4)	32f (26)
Pentaacetate	$C_{15}H_{22}O_{10}$	76	+37.2 (CHCl₃)	27				
L-Arabinitol	$C_5H_{12}O_5$	101–102	-7.2 (c 9. borax solution) -32 (c 0.4, 5% molybdate)	28p, 30cp 29		38.1 (3)		70f (31)
Pentaacetate	$C_{15}H_{22}O_{10}$	72–73		30		44.4 (6) 105xyll (7) 40glcl (32)		
Pentamethyl ether	$C_{10}H_{22}O_5$							
Trimethylsilyl ether								
Ribitol (adonitol)	$C_5H_{12}O_5$	102	None (meso)	33	76rib (2)	39.9 (3)	14f (4)	37f (26)
Pentaacetate	$C_{15}H_{22}O_{10}$	51	None	34		40.0 (6)		

Table 1 (continued)

NATURAL ALDITOLS, INOSITOLS, INOSOSES, AND AMINO ALDITOLS AND INOSAMINES

Substance[a] (synonym) derivative (A)	Chemical formula (B)	Melting point °C (C)	Specific rotation[b] $[\alpha]_D$ (D)	Reference[c] (E)	Chromatography, R value, and reference[d]			
					ELC (F)	GLC (G)	PPC (H)	TLC (I)
			Alditols (continued)					
Pentamethyl ether	$C_{10}H_{22}O_5$		None			60xylI (7)		
Trimethylsilyl ether			None			32.8, 38.5 (35g)		92f (35t)
Xylitol	$C_5H_{12}O_5$	61,92.5–93.5	None (meso)	28,36	155rib (2)	30.3 (3)	14f (4)	26f (26)
Pentacetate	$C_{15}H_{22}O_{10}$	62.5–63	None	36		52.8 (6)		
Pentamethyl ether	$C_{10}H_{22}O_5$		None			100xylI (7)		
Trimethylsilyl ether			None			46myol (84)		
Galactitol (dulcitol)	$C_6H_{14}O_6$	186–187	None (meso)	37e	145rib (2)		7f (4)	24f (5)
Hexaacetate	$C_{18}H_{26}O_{12}$	167.5–168.5	None	37g		144.4 (6)		
Hexamethyl ether	$C_{12}H_{26}O_6$	78	None			388xylI (7)		
Trimethylsilyl ether	$C_{24}H_{62}O_6Si_6$			84		12.47 (38)		
D-Glucitol (sorbitol)	$C_6H_{14}O_6$	112	–1.8 (15°)	39	161rib (2)		8f (4)	22f (5)
Hexaacetate	$C_{18}H_{26}O_{12}$	99	+12.5 (c 0.8, $CHCl_3$)	40,41		144.4 (6)		
Hexamethyl ether								
Trimethylsilyl ether						246xylI (7)		
1,5-Anhydro-D-glucitol (polygalitol)	$C_6H_{12}O_5$	140–141	+42.4	42		27 (32)		
Tetraacetate	$C_{14}H_{20}O_9$	73–74	+38.9 ($CHCl_2$)	43				
L-Iditol	$C_6H_{14}O_6$	73.5	–3.5 (c 10)	43,45	173rib (2)		92sorl (44)	
Hexaacetate	$C_{18}H_{26}O_{12}$	121.5	–25.7 ($CHCl_3$)	46		153xylIf (21)		
D-Mannitol	$C_6H_{14}O_6$	166	–0.21	29	130rib (2)	38.1 (3)	8f (4)	27f (5)
Hexaacetate	$C_{18}H_{26}O_{12}$	126	+16 (5% molybdate)	47,48		127.2 (6)		83f (50a)
Hexamethyl ether	$C_{12}H_{26}O_6$		+18.8 (acetic acid)			284xylI (7)		
Trimethylsilyl ether						9.46 (8)		
1,5-Anhydro-D-mannitol (styrachitol)	$C_6H_{12}O_5$	157	–49.9	49				
Tetraacetate	$C_{14}H_{20}O_9$	66–67	–20.9 (C_2H_5OH)	51				
D-Mannitol 1-acetate	$C_6H_{14}O_7$	124–125	+4	52cp				
D-glycero-D-galacto-	$C_6H_{16}O_7$	183–185,188	–1.1	53,54	140rib (2)		100perl (55a)	

Table 1 (continued)

NATURAL ALDITOLS, INOSITOLS, INOSOSES, AND AMINO ALDITOLS AND INOSAMINES

Substance[a] (synonym) derivative (A)	Chemical formula (B)	Melting point °C (C)	Specific rotation[b] $[\alpha]_D$ (D)	Reference[c] (E)	Chromatography, R value, and reference[d]			
					ELC (F)	GLC (G)	PPC (H)	TLC (I)
Alditols (continued)								
Heptitol (L-*glycero*-D-*manno*-heptitol, perseitol)			+24.5 (5% molybdate)	29				
Heptaacetate	C₂₁H₃₀O₁₄	119–120.5	–14 (CHCl₃)	53				
D-*glycero*-D-*gluco*-Heptitol (L-*glycero*-D-*talo*-heptitol, β-sedoheptitol)	C₇H₁₆O₇	131–132	+46 (5% molybdate)	55c	171rib (2)		>120suc (55b)	
Tri-*O*-methylene-β-sedoheptitol	C₁₀H₁₆O₇	Sublimes 130, 276–278d	–23.3 (c 0.4, CHCl₃)	56				
D-*glycero*-D-*ido*-Heptitol	C₇H₁₆O₇		0.0	57c	168rib (2)	621aral (57b)	78–82 gal (57a)	
Heptaacetate	C₂₁H₃₀O₁₄	180–181	+24 (CHCl₃)	57				
Heptabenzoate	C₂₈H₄₄O₁₄	111–112	None (meso)	57c				
L-*glycero*-D-*ido*-Heptitol	C₇H₁₆O₇	175–176	None	57		719aral (57b)	74gal (57a)	
Heptaacetate D-*glycero*-	C₂₁H₃₀O₁₄	153	+2.6	58				
D-*glycero*-D-*manno*-Heptitol (D-*glycero*-D-*talo*-heptitol, volemitol)	C₇H₁₆O₇		+55 (5% molybdate)	29	140rib (2)			
Heptaacetate	C₂₁H₃₀O₁₄	62	+36.1 (CHCl₃)	58,59				
D-*erythro*-D-*erythro*-D-*galacto*-Octitol	C₈H₁₈O₈ · H₂O	169–170	–11 (5% molybdate)	55c			83perl (55a)	
Octaacetate	C₂₄H₃₂O₁₆	99–100	+2 (CHCl₃)	55				
Inositols								
Asteritol (an inositol monomethyl ether)	C₇H₁₄O₆	Sublimes, melts 164	+157 (c 0.01)	60			32f (60)	
Betitol (a dideoxyinositol)	C₆H₁₂O₄	224		61				

Table 1 (continued)
NATURAL ALDITOLS, INOSITOLS, INOSOSES, AND AMINO ALDITOLS AND INOSAMINES

Substance[a] (synonym) derivative (A)	Chemical formula (B)	Melting point °C (C)	Specific rotation $[\alpha]_D$ (D)	Reference[c] (E)	Chromatography, R value, and reference[d]			
					ELC (F)	GLC (G)	PPC (H)	TLC (I)
Inositols (continued)								
D-Bornesitol (D-*myo*-inositol monomethyl ether)	$C_7H_{14}O_6$	201–202	+31.4	62	20rib (2)			
Pentaacetate	$C_{17}H_{24}O_{11}$	138–139	+11.8 (c 0.8, acetone)	62				
Trimethylsilyl ether						86myol (84)		
L-Bornesitol (1-*O*-methyl L-*myo*-inositol)	$C_7H_{14}O_6$	205–206	−32.1	63,65cp	15glc (82)		19glc (66)	
Pentaacetate	$C_{17}H_{24}O_{11}$	142–143,157	−11.2 (CHCl₃)	64		8.27 (93)		
Conduritol (a 2,3-dehydro-2,3-dideoxy-inositol)	$C_6H_{10}O_4$	142–143	None (meso)	67				
Dihydroconduritol	$C_6H_{12}O_4$	204	None	68				
Tetraacetate	$C_{14}H_{18}O_8$	bp 165 (0.6 mm)	None	68				
Dambonitol (1,3-di-*O*-methyl-*myo*-inositol)	$C_8H_{16}O_6$	206,210	None (meso)	69,70	0glc (82)		20f (70)	
Tetraacetate	$C_{16}H_{24}O_{10}$	202	None	71c				
D-Inositol [*d*-inositol, *chiro*- (+)-inositol, (+)-inositol, D-*chiro*-inositol]	$C_6H_{12}O_6$	246–247d	+60,+65	72c, 73	83glc (82)		17f 12f (72, 74)	
		230–235	+68	74				
Hexaacetate	$C_{18}H_{24}O_{12}$	215–220	+64.5	74,75				
Hexabenzoate	$C_{48}H_{36}O_{12}$	252–253	−64.1					
L-Inositol [*l*-inositol, *levo*-inositol, *chiro*-(−)-inositol]	$C_6H_{12}O_6$	247		1,76p	23rib (2)		49pinl (132)	
Hexaacetate		96		1				
Trimethylsilyl ether						82myol (84)		
D,L-Inositol	$C_6H_{12}O_6$	253	Racemic	77				
Hexaacetate	$C_{18}H_{24}O_{12}$	111	None	77				
Hexabenzoate	$C_{48}H_{36}O_{12}$	213	None	78cp		9.62 (93)		

Table 1 (continued)
NATURAL ALDITOLS, INOSITOLS, INOSOSES, AND AMINO ALDITOLS AND INOSAMINES

Substance[a] (synonym) derivative (A)	Chemical formula (B)	Melting point °C (C)	Specific rotation[b] $[\alpha]_D$ (D)	Reference[c] (E)	Chromatography, R value, and reference[d]			
					ELC (F)	GLC (G)	PPC (H)	TLC (I)
Inositols (continued)								
Trimethylsilyl ether 1-*O*-Methyl-(+)-inositol	$C_7H_{14}O_6$	207–208	+60.7	75		13.3 (79)		
Pentaacetate	$C_{17}H_{24}O_{11}$	110.5–111.5	+29.1 (CHCl$_3$)	75	32glc[f] (82)			
1-*O*-Methyl-*muco*-inositol	$C_7H_{14}O_6$	Gum		80cp,81	30glc (80)		109pinl (81)	
Pentaacetate	$C_7H_{14}O_6$	bp ca 200 (vac)		80				
Pentabenzoate	$C_{42}H_{34}O_{11}$	Amorphous 95–100		80				
myo-Inositol (*meso*-inositol)	$C_6H_{12}O_6$	225–227	None (meso)	72p	16rib (2)		2f (4)	27f (50b)
Hexaacetate	$C_{18}H_{24}O_{12}$	206–208 221–213	None	83cp 85		13.42 (93)		79f (50a)
Trimethylsilyl ether	$C_{24}H_{60}O_6Si_6$	118–119		84g		10.3, 24.3 (8, 79)		
neo-Inositol	$C_6H_{12}O_6$	314		85,86	43rib (2)	9.17 (93)		
Hexaacetate	$C_{18}H_{24}O_{12}$	251–253		86cpt				
Laminitol (6-*C*-methyl-*myo* inositol)	$C_7H_{14}O_6$	226–269	–3	87c, 88cp	83glc (87a)		10f (87b)	
Hexaacetate	$C_{18}H_{20}O_{12}$	153	–19.6 ± 1 (CHCl$_3$)	88			27f (87c)	
Leucanthemitol (a dehydro dideoxy inositol)	$C_8H_{10}O_4$	131–132	+101.5	89,90			85–80f (89)	
Dihydroleucanthemitol	$C_6H_{12}O_4$	161	–40	90				
Liniodendritol (1,4-di-*O*-methyl-*myo*-inositol)	$C_8H_{16}O_6$	224	–25	66,91			52glc (66)	
Tetraacetate	$C_{14}H_{24}O_{10}$	139	–24	91				
Mytilitol (a *C*-methyl-*scyllo*-inositol)	$C_7H_{14}O_6$	259	None (meso)	92	<10sorl (94)			
Hexaacetate	$C_9H_{18}O_{12}$	180–181	None	92				
d-Ononitol [(+)-ononitol, 4-*O*-methyl-L-*myo*-inositol]	$C_7H_{14}O_6$	172	+6.6	64	60glc (82)		32f (66)	

Table 1 (continued)
NATURAL ALDITOLS, INOSITOLS, INOSOSES, AND AMINO ALDITOLS AND INOSAMINES

Substance[a] (synonym) derivative (A)	Chemical formula (B)	Melting point °C (C)	Specific rotation [α]_D (D)	Reference[c] (E)	Chromatography, R value, and reference[d]			
					ELC (F)	GLC (G)	PPC (H)	TLC (I)
Inositols (continued)								
Pentaacetate	$C_{17}H_{24}O_{11}$	121	-11.1 (c 0.8, CHCl₃)	65cp				
Trimethylsilyl ether								
d-Pinitol [(+)-pinitol, 3-O-methyl-(+)-inositol]	$C_7H_{14}O_6$	185–186	+65.5	95,96	35rib (2)	80myol (84)	9f (4)	
Pentaacetate	$C_{17}H_{24}O_{11}$	98	+8.6 (C₂H₅OH)	97		7.07 (93)		
l-Pinitol [(-)-pinitol, 3-O-methyl-(-)-inositol]	$C_7H_{14}O_6$	186	-65	98,99	27rib (2)			
Trimethylsilyl ether						64myol (84)	7f (4)	
l-Quebrachitol (1L-2-O-methyl-chiro-inositol)	$C_7H_{14}O_6$	190–191	-80.2 (28°)	100–102p				
Pentaacetate	$C_{17}H_{24}O_{11}$	96–98	-25.1 (29° CHCl₃)	100,101		6.90 (93)		
Trimethylsilyl ether								
allo-Quercitol (5-deoxy-allo-inositol)	$C_6H_{12}O_5$	262–263		103egt		58 (84)	140glc (103)	
Pentaacetate	$C_{16}H_{22}O_{10}$							
d-Quercitol [(+)-proto-quercitol, 4-deoxy-(+)-inositol]	$C_6H_{12}O_5$	235	+24.2	104,105	31glc (82)	11.9 (128)		
Pentaacetate	$C_{16}H_{22}O_{10}$	155	+61	106		8.4 (128)		
Pentabenzoate	$C_{41}H_{32}O_{10}$	238–239	-26	105,107				
l-Quercitol [(-)-proto-quercitol]	$C_6H_{12}O_5$	154–155	-62.8 (ethyl acetate)	105				
Pentabenzoate	$C_{41}H_{32}O_{10}$							
d-Quinic acid (a dideoxy carboxy-dextro-inositol)	$C_7H_{12}O_6$	164	+44 (c 10)	61				
l-Quinic acid	$C_7H_{12}O_6$	162	-42.1	108			45f (109c)	
Tetraacetate								
Trimethylsilyl ether	$C_{13}H_{30}O_{10}$	130–136	-22.5 (C₂H₅OH)	110				

Table 1 (continued)
NATURAL ALDITOLS, INOSITOLS, INOSOSES, AND AMINO ALDITOLS AND INOSAMINES

Substance[a] (synonym) derivative (A)	Chemical formula (B)	Melting point °C (C)	Specific rotation[b] $[\alpha]_D$ (D)	Reference[c] (E)	Chromatography, R value, and reference[d]			
					ELC (F)	GLC (G)	PPC (H)	TLC (I)
			Inositols (continued)					
5-Dehydroquinic acid	$C_7H_{10}O_6$	134–136,140–142	−82.4 (28°, C_2H_5OH)	111,112cp		8.47,2.1 (8,113)	30f^g (109)	
Protocatechuic Trimethylsilyl ether	$C_7H_6O_3$	201–202		111				
Scyllitol (*scyllo*-inositol, cocositol)	$C_6H_{12}O_6$	352–353	None (meso)	114,115	7rib (2)	4.6 (113)	0f (4)	
Hexaacetate	$C_{18}H_{24}O_{12}$	299–300	None	114,115		22.25 (93) 93myol (84)		
Trimethylsilyl ether	$C_{24}H_{60}O_6Si_6$	179–180	None	84		9.8, 18.4 (8,79)		
O-Methyl-*scyllo*-inositol	$C_7H_{14}O_6$	243	None (meso)	116cp			65pinl (132)	
Pentaacetate	$C_{17}H_{24}O_{11}$	192–193	None	116t				
Sequoyitol (5-*O*-methyl *myo*-inositol)	$C_7H_{14}O_6$	234–235	None (meso)	117	25rib (2)		27f (72)	
Pentaacetate	$C_7H_{24}O_{11}$	198	None	117				
Shikimic acid (3,4-anhydroquinic acid)	$C_7H_{10}O_5$	183–184	−200 (16°)	118,119		9.76 (93)	60f (109)	
Methyl shikimate		190–191	−161 (c 0.6)	120				
Triacetate	$C_9H_{12}O_8$	115	−136 (CH_3OH)	121				
Trimethylsilyl ether	$C_{13}H_{16}O_8$	Syrup	−60	120				
5-Dehydroshikimic acid	$C_7H_8O_5$	150–152	−57.5 (28°, C_2H_5OH)	122		8.94,2.7 (8,113)	50f^g (109)	
Methyl ester	$C_8H_{10}O_5$	124–126	−47.1±3 (c 0.2, C_2H_5OH)	122				
Trimethylsilyl ether Validitol [1S-(3,4,6/5)-3-hydroxymethyl-4,5,6-trihydroxy-cyclohexane]	$C_7H_{14}O_4$	119–121	−39	123		6.9 (113)		
Deoxyvaliditol [1S-(4,6/5)-3-methyl-4,5,6-trihydroxy-cyclohexane]	$C_7H_{14}O_3$		−19.4	123				

Table 1 (continued)

NATURAL ALDITOLS, INOSITOLS, INOSOSES, AND AMINO ALDITOLS AND INOSAMINES

Substance[a] (synonym) derivative (A)	Chemical formula (B)	Melting point °C (C)	Specific rotation[b] $[\alpha]_D$ (D)	Reference[c] (E)	Chromatography, R value, and reference[d]			
					ELC (F)	GLC (G)	PPC (H)	TLC (I)
Inositols (continued)								
Viburnitol [l-quercitol,[h] a deoxy *levo*-inositol, (−)-*vibo*-quercitol, 1-deoxy-D-*myo*-inositol]	$C_6H_{12}O_5$	174; 179–180; 158–159	−73.9; −49.5±1	124; 125,126; 127	31glc (82); <10sorl (94)		65pinl (132)	
Pentaacetate	$C_{16}H_{22}O_{10}$	112–113; 122–126		127; 124–126		9.5 (128)		
Bioinose (*myo*-inosose-2, *scyllo*-inosose, a dehydro or keto inositol)	$C_6H_{10}O_6$	196–197	None (meso)	129			43pinl (132c)	
Pentaacetate	$C_{16}H_{20}O_{11}$	121–213	None	129				
Phenylhydrazone	$C_{12}H_{16}N_2O_6$	220–222	None	130				
Trimethylsilyl ether	$C_{21}H_{40}O_6Si_5$	98		84		75myol (84)		
myo-Inosose-1 (*vibo*-inosose, *d*-inosose, L-*myo*-inosose-1)	$C_6H_{10}O_6$	138–139	+19.6	131			27pinl (132c)	
Phenylhydrazone	$C_{12}H_{16}N_2O_5$	196–197	−55.3 (C_5H_5N-C_2H_5OH)	131				
Trimethylsilyl ether						9.53 (8)		
2,3-Didehydro-D-inositol	$C_6H_8O_6$	No constants known		133				
Bis-(phenylhydrazone)	$C_{18}H_{20}N_4O_4$	217d	−250→−222 (24 hr, c 0.5, C_5H_5N-C_2H_5OH 1:1)	133				
2,3-Didehydro-L-inositol	$C_6H_8O_6$	No constants known		133				
Bis-(phenylhydrazone)	$C_{18}H_{20}N_4O_4$	217d	+240→+214 (24 hr c 0.8, C_5H_5N-C_2H_5OH 1:1)	133				
2,3-Didehydro-4-deoxy-*epi*-inositol	$C_6H_8O_6$	No constants known		134				
Bis-(phenylhydrazone)	$C_{18}H_{20}N_4O_3$	198–199	+54.8 (C_5H_5N-C_2H_5OH 1:1)	134			15f (134)	

Table 1 (continued)

NATURAL ALDITOLS, INOSITOLS, INOSOSES, AND AMINO ALDITOLS AND INOSAMINES

Substance[a] (synonym) derivative (A)	Chemical formula (B)	Melting point °C (C)	Specific rotation[b] $[\alpha]_D$	Reference[c] (E)	Chromatography, R value, and reference[d] ELC (F)	GLC (G)	PPC (H)	TLC (I)
Amino Alditols and Inosamines								
2-Aminoethanol (ethanolamine)	C_2H_7NO	Oil, bp 171	None	1				
Hydrochloride	$C_2H_7NO \cdot HCl$	100	None	1				
Picrate	$C_8H_{10}N_4O_8$	158	None	1				
Trimethylsilyl ether		No constants known	None			3.14 (8)		
A 2-amino-2,4-dideoxy-1-O-methyl-tetritol	$C_5H_{13}NO_2$			135				
N-acetyl acetate	$C_9H_{17}NO_4$	Oil, bp 91 (0.1 μ)		135				
Actinamine (1,3-dideoxy-1,3-N,N'-dimethyl-myo-inositol)	$C_8H_{18}N_2O_4$	135–136		136,137c				
Dihydrochloride	$C_8H_{18}N_2O_4 \cdot HCl$	>300		136				
N,N'-Diacetyl tetraacetate	$C_{20}H_{30}N_2O_{10}$	205–206		136				
Bluensidine (3-O-carbamoyl-1-deoxy-1-guanidino-scyllo-inositol)	$C_8H_{16}N_4O_8$	No constants known		138				
Hydrochloride	$C_8H_{16}N_4O_4 \cdot HCl$	190–194d	+1±0.5	138				
N,N'-Diacetyl tetraacetate	$C_{20}H_{32}N_4O_{12}$	250–251d	+5 (c 0.9, CHCl₃)	138				
neo-Inosamine-2 (2-amino-2-deoxy-neo-inositol)	$C_6H_{13}NO_5$	239–241d	None (meso)	139,140				
Hydrochloride	$C_6H_{15}NO_5 \cdot HCl$	217–221d	None	139,140				
N-Acetyl	$C_{18}H_{25}NO_{11}$	277–278	None	139,140				
scyllo-Inosamine	$C_6H_{13}NO_5 \cdot HCl$	No constants known	141	141		47glcn (149)		
N-Acetyl pentaacetate	$C_{18}H_{25}NO_{11}$	209–301	None (meso)	142				
Streptamine (1,3-diamino-1,3-dideoxy-scyllo-inositol)	$C_6H_{14}N_2O_4$	>290 (205s)	None (meso)	143				

Table 1 (continued)
NATURAL ALDITOLS, INOSITOLS, INOSOSES, AND AMINO ALDITOLS AND INOSAMINES

Substance[a] (synonym) derivative (A)	Chemical formula (B)	Melting point °C (C)	Specific rotation[b] $[\alpha]_D$ (D)	Reference[c] (E)	Chromatography, R value, and reference[d]			
					ELC (F)	GLC (G)	PPC (H)	TLC (I)
Amino Alditols and Inosamines (continued)								
Dihydroiodide	$C_6H_{13}N_2O_4 \cdot 2HI$	>280d	None	143				
N,N'-Diacetyl tetraacetate	$C_{16}H_{26}N_2O_{10}$	342–345d	None	143				
2-Deoxystreptamine	$C_6H_{14}N_2O_3$	221–223	None (meso)	144				
Dihydrobromide	$C_6H_{14}N_2O_3 \cdot 2HBr$	283–286d	None	145				
N,N'-Diacetyl triacetate	$C_{16}H_{24}N_2O_8$	340–350	None	144				
Deoxy-N-methyl-streptamine (hyosamine)	$C_7H_{16}N_2O_3$	183–186	+39.8	146				
		160–162	−31.1	146				
	$C_7H_{16}N_2O_3 \cdot H_2O$	130–133d	−17.8	147[i]				
N,N'-Diacetyl triacetate	$C_{17}H_{26}N_2O_8$	204	Racemic	144				
Diplcrate		238–240d	None (meso)	147				
Streptidine (1,3-dideoxy-1,3-diguanidino-scyllo-inositol)	$C_9H_{16}N_6O_4$			143				
N,N'-Diacetyl tetraacetate	$C_{20}H_{30}N_6O_{10}$	342–345	None	143				
Diplcrate	$C_{20}H_{24}N_{12}O_{18}$	284–285d	None	148				
Validamine (1S-(1,2,4/3,5)-5-hydroxy-methyl-2,3,4-trihydroxy-cyclohexylamine)	$C_7H_{13}NO_4$	No constants known	+60.6	150				
Hydrochloride	$C_7H_{15}NO_4 \cdot HCl$	229–232d	+57.4 (N HCl)	123				
Hydroxyvalidamine	$C_7H_{15}NO_5$	164–165	+80.7	123				
epi-Validamine	$C_7H_{15}NO_4$	210	+5.8	150				
Validenamine (1,6-dehydro-validamine)	$C_7H_{13}NO_4$	No constants known		150				
Hydrochloride	$C_7H_{15}NO_4 \cdot HCl$		+68.6 (N HCl)	150				
N-Acetyl tetraacetate	$C_{17}H_{23}NO_9$	95	+30.2 (CHCl_3)	150				

Compiled by George G. Maher.

Table 1 (continued)
NATURAL ALDITOLS, INOSITOLS, INOSOSES, AND AMINO ALDITOLS AND INOSAMINES

REFERENCES

1. Pollock and Stevens, *Dictionary of Organic Compounds*, Oxford University Press, New York, 1965.
2. Frahn and Mills, *Aust. J. Chem.*, 12, 65 (1959).
3. Dooms, Declerck, and Verachtert, *J. Chromatogr.*, 42, 349 (1969).
4. Bourne, Lees, and Weigel, *J. Chromatogr.*, 11, 253 (1963).
5. de Simone and Vicedomini, *J. Chromatogr.*, 37, 538 (1968).
6. Sawardeker, Sloneker, and Jeanes, *Anal. Chem.*, 37, 1602 (1965).
7. Whyte, *J. Chromatogr.*, 87, 163 (1973).
8. Roberts, Johnston, and Fuhr, *Anal. Biochem.*, 10, 282 (1965).
9. Dutton and Unrau, *Can. J. Chem.*, 43, 924, 1738 (1965).
10. Lindberg, *Ark. Kemi. Mineral. Geol.*, 23, A 2 (1946–1947).
11. Weatherall, *J. Chromatogr.*, 26, 251 (1967).
12. Borecký and Gasparič, *Collect. Czech. Chem. Commun.*, 25, 1287 (1960).
13. Bamberger and Landsiedl, *Monatsh. Chem.*, 21, 571 (1900).
14. Dutton, Gibney, Jensen, and Reid, *J. Chromatogr.*, 36, 152 (1968).
15. Ward, Pettijohn, Lockwood, and Coghill, *J. Am. Chem. Soc.*, 66, 541 (1944).
16. Ciamician and Silber, *Ber. Dtsch. Chem. Ges.*, 44, 1280 (1911).
17. Morell and Auernheimer, *J. Am. Chem. Soc.*, 66, 792 (1944).
18. Rubin, Lardy, and Fischer, *J. Am. Chem. Soc.*, 74, 425 (1952).
19. Bertrand, *C. R. Acad. Sci.*, 130, 1472 (1900).
20. Batt, Dickens, and Williamson, *Biochem. J.*, 77, 272 (1960).
21. Oades, *J. Chromatogr.*, 28, 246 (1967).
22. Hu, McComb, and Rendig, *Arch. Biochem. Biophys.*, 110, 350 (1965).
23. Dutton and Unrau, *J. Chromatogr.*, 20, 78 (1965).
24. Wilson and Lucas, *J. Am. Chem. Soc.*, 58, 2396 (1936).
25. Asahina and Yanagita, *Ber. Dtsch. Chem. Ges.*, 67, 799 (1934).
26. Němec, Kefurt, and Jarý, *J. Chromatogr.*, 26, 116 (1967).
27. Frèrejacque, *C. R. Acad. Sci.*, 208, 1123 (1939).
28. Onishi and Suzuki, *Agric. Biol. Chem.*, 30, 1139 (1966).
29. Richtmyer and Hudson, *J. Am. Chem. Soc.*, 73, 2249 (1951).
30. Touster and Harwell, *J. Biol. Chem.*, 230, 1031 (1958).
31. Grasshof, *J. Chromatogr.*, 14, 513 (1964).
32. Dutton, Reid, Rowe, and Rowe, *J. Chromatogr.*, 47, 195 (1970).
33. Wessely and Wang, *Monatsh. Chem.*, 72, 168 (1938).
34. Binkley and Wolfrom, *J. Am. Chem. Soc.*, 70, 2809 (1948).
35. Gregory, *J. Chromatogr.*, 36, 342 (1968).
36. Wolfrom and Kohn, *J. Am. Chem. Soc.*, 64, 1739 (1942).
37. Wells, Pittman, and Egan, *J. Biol. Chem.*, 239, 3192 (1964).
38. Horowitz and Delman, *J. Chromatogr.*, 21, 302 (1966).
39. Von Lippmann, *Ber. Dtsch. Chem. Ges.*, 60, 161 (1927).
40. Haas and Hill, *Biochem. J.*, 26, 987 (1932).
41. Jeger, Norymberski, Szpilfogel, and Prelog, *Helv. Chim. Acta*, 29, 684 (1946).
42. Richtmyer, Carr, and Hudson, *J. Am. Chem. Soc.*, 65, 1477 (1943).
43. Bertrand, *Bull. Soc. Chim. Fr. Ser. 3*, 33, 166 (1905).
44. Britton, *Biochem. J.*, 85, 402 (1962).
45. Perlin, Mazurek, Jaques, and Kavanagh, *Carbohydr. Res.*, 7, 369 (1968).
46. Braham, *J. Am. Chem. Soc.*, 41, 1707 (1919).
47. Patterson and Todd, *J. Chem. Soc.* (Lond.), p. 2876 (1929).
48. Iwate, *Chem. Zentralbl.*, 2, 177 (1929).
49. Zervas, *Ber. Dtsch. Chem. Ges.*, 63, 1689 (1930).
50. Hay, Lewis, and Smith, *J. Chromatogr.*, 11, 479 (1963).
51. Asahina, *Ber. Dtsch. Chem. Ges.*, 45, 2363 (1912).
52. Lindberg, *Acta Chem. Scand.*, 7, 1119, 1123 (1953).
53. Jones and Wall, *Nature*, 189, 746 (1961).
54. Maquenne, *Ann. Chim. Phys. Ser. 6*, 19, 5 (1890).
55. Charlson and Richtmyer, *J. Am. Chem. Soc.*, 82, 3428 (1960).
56. Buck, Foster, Richtmyer, and Zissis, *J. Chem. Soc.* (Lond.), p. 3633 (1961).

Table 1 (continued)
NATURAL ALDITOLS, INOSITOLS, INOSOSES, AND AMINO ALDITOLS AND INOSAMINES

57. Onishi and Perry, *Can. J. Microbiol.*, 11, 929 (1965).
58. Bougault and Aliard, *C. R. Acad. Sci.*, 135, 796 (1902).
59. Maclay, Hann, and Hudson, *J. Org. Chem.*, 9, 293 (1944).
60. Ackerman, *Hoppe-Seyler's Z. Physiol. Chem.*, 336, 1 (1964).
61. Von Lippmann, *Ber. Dtsch. Chem. Ges.*, 34, 1159 (1901).
62. King and Jurd, *J. Chem. Soc.* (Lond.), p. 1192 (1953).
63. Bien and Ginsburg, *J. Chem. Soc.* (Lond.), p. 3189 (1958).
64. Pilouvier, *C.R. Acad. Sci.*, 241, 983 (1955).
65. Post and Anderson, *J. Am. Chem. Soc.*, 84, 478 (1962).
66. Angyal and Bender, *J. Chem. Soc.* (Lond.), p. 4718 (1961).
67. Kubler, *Arch. Pharm.*, 246, 620 (1908).
68. Dangschat and Fischer, *Naturwissenschaften*, 27, 756 (1939).
69. DeJong, *Recl. Trav. Chim. Pays-Bas*, 27, 257 (1908).
70. Kiang and Loke, *J. Chem. Soc.* (Lond.), p. 480 (1956).
71. Angyal, Gilham, and MacDonald, *J. Chem. Soc.* (Lond.), p. 1417 (1957).
72. Ballou and Anderson, *J. Am. Chem. Soc.*, 75, 648 (1953).
73. Umezawa, Okami, Hashimoto, Suhara, Hamada, and Takeuchi, *J. Antibiot. Ser. A*, 18, 101 (1965).
74. Dzhumyrko and Shinkaxenko, *Chem. Nat. Compd.* (USSR), 7, 638 (1971).
75. Foxall and Morgan, *J. Chem. Soc.* (Lond.), p. 5573 (1963).
76. Smith, *Biochem. J.*, 57, 140 (1954).
77. Tanret, *C. R. Acad. Sci.*, 145, 1196 (1907).
78. Cosgrove, *Nature*, 194, 1265 (1962).
79. Lee and Ballou, *J. Chromatogr.*, 18, 147 (1965).
80. Adhikari, Bell, and Harvey, *J. Chem. Soc.* (Lond.), p. 2829 (1962).
81. Utkin, *Chem. Nat. Compd.* (USSR), 4, 234 (1968).
82. Angyal and McHugh, *J. Chem. Soc.* (Lond.), p. 1423 (1957).
83. Lindberg, *Acta Chem. Scand.*, 9, 1093 (1955).
84. Loewus, *Carbohydr. Res.*, 3, 130 (1966).
85. Allen, *J. Am. Chem. Soc.*, 84, 3128 (1962).
86. Cosgrove and Tate, *Nature*, 200, 568 (1963).
87. Lindberg and Wickberg, *Ark. Kemi*, 13, 447 (1959).
88. Posternak and Falbriard, *Helv. Chim. Acta*, 44, 2080 (1961).
89. Kindl, Kremlicka, and Hoffman-Ostenhof, *Monatsh. Chem.*, 97, 1783 (1966).
90. Plouvier, *C. R. Acad. Sci.*, 255, 360 (1962).
91. Plouvier, *C. R. Acad. Sci.*, 241, 765 (1955).
92. Ackermann, *Ber. Dtsch. Chem. Ges.*, 54, 1938 (1921).
93. Krzeminski and Angyal, *J. Chem. Soc.* (Lond.), p. 3251 (1962).
94. Bourne, Hutson, and Weigel, *J. Chem. Soc.* (Lond.), p. 4252 (1960).
95. Maquenne, *Ann. Chim. Phys. Ser. 6*, 22, 264 (1891).
96. Anderson, Fischer, and MacDonald, *J. Am. Chem. Soc.*, 74, 1479 (1952).
97. Pease, Reider, and Elderfield, *J. Org. Chem.*, 5, 198 (1940).
98. Plouvier, *C. R. Acad. Sci.*, 243, 1913 (1956).
99. Anderson, Takeda, Angyal, and McHugh, *Arch. Biochem. Biophys.*, 78, 518 (1958).
100. DeJong, *Recl. Trav. Chim. Pays-Bas*, 25, 48 (1906).
101. Adams, Pease, and Clark, *J. Am. Chem. Soc.*, 62, 2194 (1940).
102. Haustveit and Wold, *Carbohydr. Res.*, 29, 325 (1973).
103. Bourne, Percival, and Smestad, *Carbohydr. Res.*, 22, 75 (1972).
104. Prunier, *Ann. Chim. Phys. Ser. 5*, 15, 5 (1878).
105. McCasland, Naumann, and Durham, *Carbohydr. Res.*, 4, 516 (1967).
106. Bauer and Moll, *Arch. Pharm.*, 280, 37 (1942).
107. Plouvier, *C. R. Acad. Sci.*, 253, 3047 (1961).
108. Gorter, *Annchem*, 359, 221 (1908).
109. Haslam, Turner, Sargent, and Thompson, *J. Chem. Soc.* (Lond.), p. 1493 (1971).
110. Ervig and Koenigs, *Ber. Dtsch. Chem. Ges.*, 22, 1457 (1889).
111. Weiss, Davis, and Mingioli, *J. Am. Chem. Soc.*, 75, 5572 (1953).
112. Adlersberg and Sprinson, *Biochemistry*, 3, 1855 (1964).
113. Shyluk, Youngs, and Gamborg, *J. Chromatogr.*, 26, 268 (1967).
114. Muller, *J. Chem. Soc.* (Lond.), p. 1767 (1907).

Table 1 (continued)
NATURAL ALDITOLS, INOSITOLS, INOSOSES, AND AMINO ALDITOLS AND INOSAMINES

115. Posternak, *Helv. Chim. Acta*, 25, 746 (1942).
116. Ueno, Hasegawa, and Tsuchiya, *Carbohydr. Res.*, 29, 520 (1973).
117. Sherrard and Kurth, *J. Am. Chem. Soc.*, 51, 3139 (1929).
118. Eijkman, *Ber. Dtsch. Chem. Ges.*, 24, 1278 (1891).
119. Eijkman, *Recl. Trav. Chim. Pays-Bas*, 4, 32 (1885).
120. McCrindle, Overton, and Raphael, *J. Chem. Soc.* (Lond.), p. 1560 (1960).
121. Grewe, Buttner, and Burmeister, *Angew. Chem.*, 69, 61 (1957).
122. Salamon and Davis, *J. Am. Chem. Soc.*, 75, 5567 (1953).
123. Horii, Iwasa, Mizuta, and Kameda, *J. Antibiot. Ser. A*, 24, 59 (1971).
124. Power and Tutin, *J. Chem. Soc.* (Lond.), p. 624 (1904).
125. Angyal, Gorin, and Pitman, *J. Chem. Soc.* (Lond.), p. 1807 (1965).
126. Posternak and Schopfer, *Helv. Chim. Acta*, 33, 343 (1950).
127. Nakajima and Kurihara, *Ber. Dtsch. Chem. Ges.*, 94, 515 (1961).
128. Angyal, Gorin, and Pitman, *J. Chem. Soc.* (Lond.), p. 1807 (1965).
129. Stanacev and Kates, *J. Org. Chem.*, 26, 912 (1961).
130. Posternak, *Helv. Chim. Acta*, 19, 1333 (1936).
131. Magasanik and Chargaff, *J. Biol. Chem.*, 175, 929 (1948).
132. Post and Anderson, *J. Am. Chem. Soc.*, 84, 471 (1962).
133. Magasanik and Chargaff, *J. Biol. Chem.*, 174, 173 (1948).
134. Berman and Magasanik, *J. Biol. Chem.*, 241, 800 (1966).
135. Stevens, Gillis, French, and Haskell, *J. Am. Chem. Soc.*, 80, 6088 (1958).
136. Johnson, Gourlay, Tarbell, and Autrey, *J. Org. Chem.*, 28, 300 (1963).
137. Nakajima, Kurihara, Hasegawa, and Kurokawa, *Justus Liebigs Ann. Chem.*, 689, 243 (1965).
138. Bannister and Argoudelis, *J. Am. Chem. Soc.*, 85, 119 (1963).
139. Allen, *J. Am. Chem. Soc.*, 78, 5691 (1956).
140. Patrick, Williams, Waller, and Hutchings, *J. Am. Chem. Soc.*, 78, 2652 (1956).
141. Walker and Walker, *Biochim. Biophys. Acta*, 170, 219 (1968).
142. Carter, Clark, Lytle, and McCasland, *J. Biol. Chem.*, 175, 683 (1948).
143. Peck, Hoffhine, Peel, Graber, Holly, Mozingo, and Folkers, *J. Am. Chem. Soc.*, 68, 776 (1946).
144. Nakajima, Hasegawa, and Kurihara, *Justus Liebigs Ann. Chem.*, 689, 235 (1965).
145. Maeda, Murase, Mawatari, and Umezawa, *J. Antibiot. Ser. A*, 11, 73 (1958).
146. Neuss, Koch, Malloy, Day, Huckstep, Dorman, and Roberts, *Helv. Chim. Acta*, 53, 2314 (1970).
147. Kondo, Sezaki, Koika, and Akita, *J. Antibiot. Ser. A*, 18, 192 (1965).
148. Peck, Graber, Walti, Peel, Hoffhine, and Folkers, *J. Am. Chem. Soc.*, 68, 29 (1946).
149. Nakajima, Kurihara, and Hasegawa, *Ber. Dtsch. Chem. Ges.*, 95, 141 (1962).
150. Horii and Kameda, *J. Chem. Soc. D Chem. Commun.*, 746, 747 (1972).

Table 2
NATURAL ACIDS OF CARBOHYDRATE DERIVATION

Substance[a] (synonym) derivative	Chemical formula	Melting point °C	Specific rotation[b] $[\alpha]_D$	Reference[c]	Chromatography, R value, and referenced[d]			
					ELC	GLC	PPC	TLC
(A)	(B)	(C)	(D)	(E)	(F)	(G)	(H)	(I)
Aldonic Acids								
Glycollic acid (hydroxy-acetic acid)	$C_2H_4O_3$	80	None	1,5c	48Cl (2)			75f (4)
Acetate	$C_4H_6O_4$	66–68	None	1				
Ammonium salt	$C_4H_7NO_3$	102	None	1				
Trimethylsilyl ester ether						10.45MU (3)		
D-Glyceric acid	$C_3H_6O_4$	Gum	dextro	6			85f (8)	55f (4)

[a] In order of increasing carbon chain length in the parent compounds grouped in the classes-aldonic, uronic, aldaric, and amino sugar acids.

[b] $[\alpha]_D$ for 1–5 g solute, c, per 100 ml aqueous solution at 20–25°C, unless otherwise given.

[c] References for melting point and specific rotation data. Letter indicates the reference also has chromatographic data according to: c = column, e = electrophoresis, g = gas, p = paper, and t = thin-layer.

[d] R value times 100, given relative to that of the compound indicated by abbreviation: f = solvent front, ala = alanine, ara = arabinose, asa = ascorbic acid, Cl = chloride ion, eic = eicosane, galn = galactono-1,4-lactone, glc = glucose, glcN = glucosamine, glcU = glucuronic acid, galU = galacturonic acid, gNAc = N-acetyl-glucosamine, gNUA = glucosaminuronic acid, kdh = 3-deoxy-erythro-hexulosonic acid, kdo = 3-deoxy-manno-octulosonic acid, kgu = 2-keto-gulonic acid, mal = malonic acid, manU = mannuronic acid, myo = myo-inositol, myot = myo-inositol trimethylsilyl ether, MU = methylene standard hydrocarbon units, nana = N-acetyl-neuraminic acid, pa = picric acid, rha = rhamnose, tmg = 2,3,4,6-tetra-O-methyl glucose, and xyll = xylitol pentamethylether. Under gas chromatography (column Glc or G) numbers without code indications signify retention time in minutes. The conditions of the chromatography are correlated with the reference given in parentheses and are found in Table 5.

[e] Value is in cm/h.

[f] Equilibrates with the lactone.

[g] Data given are for the enantiomorphic isomer.

[h] The analytical elemental analysis indicates the compound is an anhydride.

[i] The enol form is L-ascorbic acid.

[j] Reference 99 terms this compound 2-deoxy-5-keto-D-gluconic acid; neither name nor structure seem definite.

[k] Value is in cm/9 h.

[l] Value is in cm/24 h.

[m] Value is in cm/1.5h.

[n] Some workers relate the formula $C_{12}H_{21}NO_{10}$ whose elemental analysis is little different from that of $C_{11}H_{19}NO_9$.

Table 2 (continued)
NATURAL ACIDS OF CARBOHYDRATE DERIVATION

Substance[a] (synonym) derivative	Chemical formula	Melting point °C	Specific rotation[b] $[\alpha]_D$	Reference[c]	Chromatography, R value, and reference[d]			
					ELC	GLC	PPC	TLC
(A)	(B)	(C)	(D)	(E)	(F)	(G)	(H)	(I)
		Aldonic Acids (continued)						
Amide	$C_3H_7NO_3$	99.5–100	−63.1 (CH₃, OH)	7				
Calcium salt	$CaC_6H_{10}O_8$		+10.9	8p		24xyll (11)		
Methyl ester methyl ether	$C_6H_{12}O_4$							
L-Glyceric acid	$C_3H_6O_4$	Gum	levo	1				
Calcium salt	$CaC_6H_{10}O_8$	134–135	−12 (30°)	9				
Trimethylsilyl ester ether						16glc (10)		
D-Lactic acid (2-hydroxy-propionic acid, 3-deoxy-D-glyceric acid)	$C_3H_6O_3$	26–27	−2.3	1,5c	42Cl (2)			
Acetate	$C_5H_8O_4$	Oil, bp 171–172	+54.3	1				
Amide	$C_3H_7NO_2$	49–51	$[\alpha]$ 18 Hg + 22.2	1				
L-Lactic acid	$C_3H_6O_3$	25–26	+3.8 (15°)	1				
Methyl ester methyl ether Trimethylsilyl ester ether	$C_7H_{10}O_3$	Oil, bp 45 (22 mm)	−95.5	1		10.65MU (3)		
D,L-Lactic acid	$C_3H_6O_3$	18	Racemic	1				
Acetate	$C_5H_8O_4$	57–60	Racemic	1				
Amide	$C_3H_7NO_2$	75.5	Racemic	1				
3-Hydroxypropionic acid (2-deoxy-glyceric acid)	$C_3H_6O_3$	Syrup	None	1				
Methyl ester methyl ether Hydroxypyruvic acid (2-keto-glyceric acid, 2-triulosonic acid)	$C_5H_{10}O_3$ $C_3H_4O_4$	Oil, bp 142–143	None None	1 12				
p-Nitrophenylhydrazone	$C_9H_9N_3O_5$	260	None	1				

Table 2 (continued)

NATURAL ACIDS OF CARBOHYDRATE DERIVATION

Substance[a] (synonym) derivative	Chemical formula	Melting point °C	Specific rotation[b] $[\alpha]_D$	Reference[c]	Chromatography, R value, and reference[d]			
					ELC	GLC	PPC	TLC
(A)	(B)	(C)	(D)	(E)	(F)	(G)	(H)	(I)
		Aldonic Acids (continued)						
Pyruvic acid (2-keto-3 deoxy-glyceric acid)	$C_3H_4O_3$	13.6	None	1	50Cl (2)			
p-Nitrophenylhydrazone								
Methyl ester	$C_9H_9N_3O_4$	220	None	1				
Trimethylsilyl ester	$C_6H_9O_3$	Oil, bp 134–137	None	1		10.91MU (3)		
D-Arabinonic acid (arabonic acid)	$C_5H_{10}O_6$	114–116	+10.5 (c6)	5c,13	8.6[e] (14)		20glc (15)	16f (16)
Phenylhydrazide	$C_{11}H_{10}N_2O_5$	208–209	–13	17				
Tetraacetate	$C_{13}H_{18}O_{10}$	135–136	+32.5	18				
Trimethylsilyl ester ether						55glc (10)		
L-Arabinonic acid	$C_5H_{10}O_6$	118–119	–9.6 → –41.7[f]	19			16f (28)	35f (32)
Amide	$C_5H_{11}NO_5$	135–136	+37.2	20				
1,4-Lactone (γ-lactone)	$C_5H_8O_5$	95–98	–71.6	21,22cp			73f (28)	40fg (16) / 75fg (23)
Lactone trimethylsilyl ether						97glc (10)		
Methyl ester methyl ether	$C_{10}H_{22}O_6$					295xyll (11)		
Phenylhydrazide	$C_{11}H_{16}N_2O_5$	215		24				
Pentulosonic acid, 3-deoxy-D-glycero-2-(2-keto-3-deoxy-D-arabonic acid)	$C_6H_8O_5$	No constants known	No constants known	29			61f (29)	62f (32)

155

Table 2 (continued)
NATURAL ACIDS OF CARBOHYDRATE DERIVATION

Substance[a] (synonym) derivative	Chemical formula	Melting point °C	Specific rotation[b] $[\alpha]_D$	Reference[c]	Chromatography, R value, and reference[d]			
					ELC	GLC	PPC	TLC
(A)	(B)	(C)	(D)	(E)	(F)	(G)	(H)	(I)
		Aldonic Acids (continued)						
2,4-Dinitrophenyl-hydrazone	$C_{11}H_{12}N_4O_8$	163		29			14f (29)	
Pentulosonic acid, D-threo-4-(4-keto-D-arabonic acid) Brucine salt	$C_5H_8O_6$	154–155	−10.3	27				
Pentulosonic acid, 3-deoxy-L-glycero-2-(2-keto-3-deoxy-L-arabonic acid)	$C_{28}H_{35}N_2O_{10}$ $C_5H_8O_6$	No constants known	−29.4 No constants known	27 28			29f (28)	
2,4-Dinitrophenyl-hydrazone	$C_{15}H_{10}N_4O_7$[h]	220–223d	−22.7 (c 0.3, dioxane)	30				
1,4-Lactone	$C_5H_6O_4$	114g					82f (28)	
L-Lyxonic acid	$C_5H_{10}O_6$	114g	+82.7g	5c,25,36 4,5p				
1,4-Lactone	$C_5H_8O_5$	108–110g	+70g					38f (32)
Phenylhydrazide	$C_{11}H_{16}N_2O_5$	163	+13.7	26cp				73f (23)
D-Ribonic acid	$C_5H_{10}O_6$	112–113	−17f	5c,31				61f (32)
Amide	$C_5H_{11}NO_5$	136–137	+17	33				
1,4-Lactone	$C_5H_8O_5$	77	+17 → +8 (13 days)	34,35p				(32)
Methyl ester methyl ether	$C_{10}H_{12}O_6$					142xyII (11)		
D-Xylonic acid	$C_5H_{10}O_6$	Syrup	−2.9 → +20.1f	5c,36	9.1e (14)			
Amide	$C_5H_{11}NO_5$	81–82	+44.5 → +23.8	37				
Brucine salt	$C_{28}H_{34}N_2O_{10}$	170–172	−37.4	38				
1,4-Lactone	$C_5H_8O_5$	98–101	+91.8 → +86.7	21				79f (23)

Table 2 (continued)
NATURAL ACIDS OF CARBOHYDRATE DERIVATION

Substance[a] (synonym) derivative (A)	Chemical formula (B)	Melting point °C (C)	Specific rotation [α]$_D$[b] (D)	Reference[c] (E)	Chromatography, R value, and reference[d]			
					ELC (F)	GLC (G)	PPC (H)	TLC (I)
Lactone trimethylsilyl ether						126glc (10) 269xyll (11) 48glc (10)		
Methyl ester methyl ether	$C_{10}H_{20}O_6$							
Trimethylsilyl ester ether								
Aldonic Acids (continued)								
L-Xylonic acid	$C_5H_{10}O_6$	No constants known	No constants known	26				
Brucine salt	$C_{29}H_{36}N_2O_{10}$	177–178	+24.3	26				
1,4-Lactone	$C_5H_8O_5$	97	−82.2	39				
Tetraacetate	$C_{13}H_{18}O_{10}$	86–88	−4.5 (c 2, C_2H_5OH)	40				
D-Altronic acid	$C_6H_{12}O_7$		+8	5c,8c,47g				
1,4-Lactone	$C_6H_{10}O_6$	110g	+35	8p			132galn (41)	
Phenylhydrazide	$C_{12}H_{18}N_2O_6$	150–152	+18.4g	42,47g				
D-Fuconic acid	$C_6H_{13}O_6$	No constants known	No constants known	43p				
1,4-Lactone	$C_6H_{10}O_5$	104g		48		438xyll (11)		
Methyl ester methyl ether	$C_{11}H_{12}O_6$							
Hexulosonic acid, 3,6-dideoxy-D-threo-2- (2-keto-3-deoxy-D-fuconic acid)	$C_6H_{10}O_5$	No constants known	No constants known	44			78f (44)	
D-Galactonic acid	$C_6H_{12}O_7$	122	−11.2 → −57.6f	49,50	8.4e (14)			38f (32)
		148	−13.6 → −17	21				
Amide	$C_6H_{13}NO_6$	175	+31.5	51			100galn (41)	78f (23)
1,4-Lactone	$C_6H_{10}O_6$	110–112, 132–133	−73 → −63.7	8,21,52				

Table 2 (continued)
NATURAL ACIDS OF CARBOHYDRATE DERIVATION

Substance[a] (synonym) derivative	Chemical formula	Melting point °C	Specific rotation[b] $[\alpha]_D$	Reference[c]	\multicolumn{4}{c}{Chromatography, R value, and reference[d]}
					ELC	GLC	PPC	TLC
(A)	(B)	(C)	(D)	(E)	(F)	(G)	(H)	(I)
		\multicolumn{2}{l}{Aldonic Acids (continued)}					
Methyl ester methyl ether	$C_{12}H_{24}O_7$					1185xyll (11)		
Pentaacetate	$C_{16}H_{22}O_{12}$	131–132	+12 (CHCl₃)	53				
Phenylhydrazide	$C_{12}H_{18}N_2O_6$	203	+10.4	24				
L-Galactonic acid	$C_6H_{12}O_7$	No constants known	No constants known	5c,8c				
Amide	$C_6H_{13}NO_6$	175	−30	54				
1,4-Lactone	$C_6H_9O_6$	110, 134–135	+77	55,56			68f (71)	
Lactone trimethylsilyl ether		Oil		57		66myo (57)		
Pentaacetate	$C_{15}H_{22}O_{12}$	132–133	−14 (28°, CHCl₃)	54				
Hexulosonic acid, D-*lyxo*-2- (2-keto-D-galactonic acid)	$C_6H_{10}O_7$	169	−5	58				
Brucine salt	$C_2H_5N_2O_{11}$	172	−22.5 (50% C₂H₅OH)	58				
Hexulosonic acid, 3-deoxy-D-*threo*-2 (2-keto-3-deoxy-D-galactonic acid)	$C_6H_{10}O_6$		+15	59cp,60			57f (61)	
Lactone phenylhydrazone	$C_{12}H_{14}N_2O_4$	213–214	−270 (c 0.5, C₅H₅N)	60				
Phenylhydrazone phenylhydrazide	$C_{18}H_{22}N_4O_4$	204–205	+13.9 (C₅H₅N)	60				
Potassium salt	$C_6H_7KO_6$	159–163d		61				
Hexulosonic acid, D-*arabino*-5- (5-keto-L-galactonic or D-tagaturonic acid)	$C_6H_{10}O_7$	108–109		62p			62galn (41)	

Table 2
NATURAL ACIDS OF CARBOHYDRATE DERIVATION

Substance[a] (synonym) derivative	Chemical formula	Melting point °C	Specific rotation[b] $[\alpha]_D$	Reference[c]	Chromatography, R value, and reference[d]			
(A)	(B)	(C)	(D)	(E)	ELC (F)	GLC (G)	PPC (H)	TLC (I)
			Aldonic Acids (continued)					
Brucine salt	$C_{23}H_{36}N_2O_{11}$	148–149, 189–190d[g]	−17[g]	62,64[g]				
Calcium salt · $5H_2O$	$CaC_{12}H_{18}O_{14} \cdot 5H_2O$		−14	63				
D-Gluconic acid	$C_6H_{12}O_7$	120–121	−6.9 → +7.3	5c,21	25Cl (2)		10glc (15)	40f (32)
Amide	$C_6H_{13}NO_6$	143–144	+31.2	20,65				
1,4-Lactone	$C_6H_{10}O_6$	133–135	+68 → +17.7	8c,21			210glc (15)	75f (23)
Lactone trimethylsilyl ether						198glc (10)		
1,5-Lactone	$C_6H_{10}O_6$	150–152	+66 → +8.8	21				
Methyl ester methyl ether	$C_{12}H_{24}O_7$					708xyll (11)		
Pentaacetate	$C_{16}H_{22}O_{12}$	110–111	+11.5 (CHCl$_3$)	40				
Trimethylsilyl ester ether						100glc (10)		
D-Gluconic acid, 6-O-(N,N-dimethylglycyl)- (pangamic acid, vitamin B$_{15}$)	$C_{10}H_{19}NO_8$	No constants known	No constants known	66				
Amide hydrochloride	$C_{10}H_{20}N_2O_7 \cdot HCl$	92–95d	+20.9 (CH$_3$OH)	66				
Lactone hydrochloride	$C_{10}H_{17}NO_7 \cdot HCl$	69–73	+32.3 (CH$_3$OH)	66				
Hexonic acid, 2-deoxy-D-arabino- (2-deoxy-D-gluconic acid)	$C_6H_{12}O_6$	142–144	+2	67,68cpt			61f (70)	
1,4-Lactone	$C_6H_{10}O_5$	93–95	+68	68,69				

Table 2 (continued)
NATURAL ACIDS OF CARBOHYDRATE DERIVATION

Substance[a] (synonym) derivative	Chemical formula	Melting point °C	Specific rotation[b] $[\alpha]_D$	Reference[c]	Chromatography, R value, and reference[d]			
					ELC	GLC	PPC	TLC
(A)	(B)	(C)	(D)	(E)	(F)	(G)	(H)	(I)
		Aldonic Acids (continued)						
Methyl ester methyl ether	$C_{11}H_{22}O_6$					353xyll (11)		
Phenylhydrazide Hexulosonic acid, D-*arabino*-2- (2-keto-D-gluconic acid)	$C_{12}H_{18}N_2O_5$, $C_6H_{10}O_7$	156	−99.6 (dil HCl)	69 5c,72	10.7e (14)		10glc (15)	18glc (73)
Brucine salt	$C_{29}H_{36}N_2O_{11}$	179–182	−59.4 (c 0.4)	74p				
Calcium salt · 3H₂O Methyl ester methyl ether	$CaC_{12}H_{18}O_{11} \cdot 3H_2O$ $C_{11}H_{20}O_7$	153d	−70.8	63,76p		348xyll (11)		
Phenylhydrazone phenylhydrazide	$C_{18}H_{22}N_4O_6$	121	−36.1 (H_2O, C_5H_5N)	72				
Hexulosonic acid, 3-deoxy-D-*erythro*-2- (2-keto-3-deoxy-D-gluconic acid)	$C_6H_{10}O_6$	119.5–120	−45.2	60,75			116galn (62)	
Calcium salt · 1/2H₂O	$CaC_{12}H_{18}O_{12} \cdot 1/2H_2O$		−29.2 (c 6)	77p				
Phenylhydrazone	$C_{12}H_{16}N_2O_5$	229d	+168 (C_5H_5N)	60				
Hexulosonic acid, D-*xylo*-5-(5-keto-D-gluconic acid)	$C_6H_{10}O_7$		−14.5	78,79	9.3e (14)		24f (80eg)	
Brucine salt	$C_{29}H_{36}N_2O_{11}$	174–175d	−24	64			79f (81)	
Calcium salt · 3H₂O	$CaC_{12}H_{18}O_{14} \cdot 3H_2O$		−11.7 (dil HCl)	79				

Table 2 (continued)
NATURAL ACIDS OF CARBOHYDRATE DERIVATION

Substance[a] (synonym) derivative (A)	Chemical formula (B)	Melting point °C (C)	Specific rotation[b] $[\alpha]_D$ (D)	Reference[c] (E)	Chromatography, R value, and reference[d]			
					ELC (F)	GLC (G)	PPC (H)	TLC (I)
Aldonic Acids (continued)								
Methyl ester methyl ether	$C_{11}H_{20}O_7$					538xyll (11)		
Hex-2,5-diulosonic acid, D-*threo*- (2,5-diketo-D-gluconic acid)	$C_6H_8O_7$	No constants known	No constants known	82p	100kgu (88)		59glc (83)	
Calcium salt · $3H_2O$ *Bis* (2,4-dinitrophenylhydrazone)	$CaC_{12}H_{14}O_{14} \cdot 3H_2O$ $C_{18}H_{16}N_4O_{13}$	156–157d	−51 ± 5 +57.2 (C_5H_5N)	82 82				
L-Gluconic acid	$C_6H_{12}O_7$	120–121g	−6.9 → +7.3g (c 8)	5c,21g,8	25Clg (2)		10glcg (15)	40fg (32)
Barium salt	$BaC_{12}H_{22}O_{14}$		−6.4	84				
Brucine salt Phenylhydrazide	$C_{29}H_{36}N_2O_{11}$ $C_{12}H_{18}N_2O_6$	181–182 203–204	−25.4 −11.7	85 85,86				
L-Gulonic acid	$C_6H_{12}O_7$	Syrup	0	5c,87				
1,4-Lactone Lactone trimethylsilyl ether	$C_6H_{10}O_6$	183–185	+55	56	47kgu (88)	70myo (57) 632xyll (11)	30f (89a) 84galn (41)	31fg (32) 53fg (32)
Methyl ester methyl ether	$C_{11}H_{24}O_7$							
Hexulosonic acid, L-xylo-2- (2-keto-L-gulonic acid)	$C_6H_{10}O_7$	170–171	−48.8	63	100kgu (88)			35glc (73)
Brucine salt · H_2O Sodium salt Trimethylsilyl ester ether	$C_{29}H_{36}N_2O_{11} \cdot H_2O$ $C_6H_9NaO_7$	114 145	−24.4	90 90		164glc (91)		
Hexulosono-1,4-lactone, L-xylo-2- (2-keto-L-gulono-γ-lactone, L-ascorbic acid)[f]	$C_6H_8O_6$	190d	+24.7	96c	25Cl (2)		90f (89b)	57f (32)

Table 2 (continued)
NATURAL ACIDS OF CARBOHYDRATE DERIVATION

Substance[a] (synonym) derivative	Chemical formula	Melting point °C	Specific rotation[b] $[\alpha]_D$	Reference[c]	Chromatography, R value, and reference[d]			
					ELC	GLC	PPC	TLC
(A)	(B)	(C)	(D)	(E)	(F)	(G)	(H)	(I)
Aldonic Acids (continued)								
Bis(phenylhydrazone) Trimethylsilyl ester ether	$C_{18}H_{15}N_4O_4$	187		1				
Hexulosono-1,4-lactone 2-sulfate, L-*xylo*-2- (ascorbic acid sulfate)	$C_6H_8O_6S$		+98.5 (pH 8.6)	96c		183glc	40f (96)	39f (97p)
Ammonium salt Hexulosonic acid, L-*xylo*-3- (3-keto-L-gulonic acid)	$C_6H_{11}NO_7,S$ $C_6H_{10}O_7$	No constants known	+202.8 No constants known	96 92				
Hexulosonic acid, D-*lyxo*-5- (5-keto-L-gulonic acid or D-fructuronic acid)	$C_6H_{10}O_7$	No constants known	No constants known	62,71	52kgu (88)		62f (41)	
Brucine salt	$C_{23}H_{35}N_2O_{11}$	195–197	–15.5	62,64			78f (81)	
Potassium salt Hex-2,3-diulosonic acid, L-*threo*- (2,3-diketo-L-gulonic acid)	$C_6H_7KO_7$ $C_6H_8O_7$	160–165 No constants known	+11 No constants known	93 94,95				
Bis(2,4-dinitro-phenylhydrazone)	$C_{18}H_{16}N_8O_{13}$	281		95				
Hexulosonic acid, 4-deoxy-D-*threo*-5 (4-deoxy-5-keto-D-idonic acid)[j]	$C_6H_{10}O_6$	No constants known	No constants known	98,99			40f (98)	

Table 2 (continued)
NATURAL ACIDS OF CARBOHYDRATE DERIVATION

Substance[a] (synonym) derivative	Chemical formula	Melting point °C	Specific rotation[b] $[\alpha]_D$	Reference[c]	Chromatography, R value, and reference[d]			
					ELC	GLC	PPC	TLC
(A)	(B)	(C)	(D)	(E)	(F)	(G)	(H)	(I)
			Aldonic Acids (continued)					
Phenylosazone	$C_{18}H_{22}N_4O_4$	113d		98				
Sodium salt	$C_6H_9NaO_6$	67–68	+5.5	98				
L-Idonic acid	$C_6H_{13}O_7$	No constants known	No constants known	5c,100	47kgu (88)			
Brucine salt	$C_{26}H_{36}N_2O_{11}$	190–192	-17	8				
1,4-Lactone	$C_6H_{10}O_6$	Syrup	+50, +4.5	8,101			111f (41)	
Phenylhydrazide	$C_{12}H_{18}N_2O_6$	115–117	+12.5	101				
Sodium salt	$C_6H_{11}NaO_7$	179	+8	102				
D-Mannonic acid	$C_6H_{12}O_7$		-15.6	5c,103	47kgu (88)		4f (104)	
Brucine salt	$C_{26}H_{36}N_2O_{11}$	203	-27.8	105				
1,4-Lactone	$C_6H_{10}O_6$	151–152	+51.5	8,21			112f (41)	62g (23)
1,5-Lactone	$C_6H_{10}O_6$	158–160	+114→ +30.3	21				
Methyl ester methyl ether	$C_{12}H_{24}O_7$					779xyil (11)		
Pentaacetate	$C_{16}H_{22}O_{12}$	68–70	+23 (CHCl₃)	106				
Phenylhydrazide	$C_{12}H_{18}N_2O_6$	212–214	+15.8	42,107				
Hex-2,5-diulosonic acid, 3-deoxy-D-glycero- (3-deoxy-2,5-diketo-D-mannonic acid)	$C_6H_8O_6$	No constants known	No constants known	108			17k (108)	
Hexulosonic acid, 2,3,6-trideoxy-D-glycero- 4-(4-keto-2,3,6-trideoxy-D-mannonic acid, 5-hydroxy-4-keto-hexanoic acid)	$C_6H_{10}O_4$		-17.9	109c			82f (110c)	

Table 2 (continued)
NATURAL ACIDS OF CARBOHYDRATE DERIVATION

Substance[a] (synonym) derivative	Chemical formula	Melting point °C	Specific rotation[b] $[\alpha]_D$	Reference[c]	Chromatography, R value, and reference[d]			
					ELC	GLC	PPC	TLC
(A)	(B)	(C)	(D)	(E)	(F)	(G)	(H)	(I)
		Aldonic Acids (continued)						
L-Mannonic acid, 6-deoxy- (L-rhamnonic acid)	$C_6H_{12}O_6$		+4 → −32.7	5c, 36,86				
Amide	$C_6H_{13}NO_5$	141–142	+27.5	111				
1,4-Lactone	$C_6H_{10}O_5$	149–151	−39.2, −51	8,21				69f (23)
1,5-Lactone	$C_6H_{10}O_5$	172–182	−100 → −35.1	21				
Methyl ester methyl ether	$C_{11}H_{20}O_5$					361xyll (11)		
Heptulosonic acid, 3-deoxy-D-*arabino*-2-	$C_7H_{12}O_7$	No constants known	No constants known	112c			23f (113)	
Ammonium salt	$C_7H_{15}NO_7$	96	+42.4	114				
1,4-Lactone	$C_7H_{10}O_6$	167	−5.8	113			39f (113)	
1,5-Lactone	$C_7H_{10}O_6$		+33	115				
Methyl ester glycoside	$C_9H_{14}O_6$	148	+78.2 (CH_3OH)	115				
7-Phosphate	$C_7H_{13}O_{10}P$						49f (112)	
Octulosonic acid, 3-deoxy-D-*manno*-2-	$C_8H_{14}O_8$	No constants known	No constants known	116c	100kdo (117)		52kdh (116)	
Ammonium salt · H_2O	$C_8H_{17}NO_8 \cdot H_2O$	125–126	+41.3	118c			25ara (116)	
1,4-Lactone	$C_8H_{12}O_7$	192–194	+31.8	118c				
Pentaacetate	$C_{18}H_{24}O_{13}$	98–103		118c				63f (118)
8-Phosphate	$C_8H_{15}O_{11}P$						51f (119)	

Table 2 (continued)
NATURAL ACIDS OF CARBOHYDRATE DERIVATION

Substance[a] (synonym) derivative	Chemical formula	Melting point °C	Specific rotation[b] $[\alpha]_D$	Reference[c]	Chromatography, R value, and reference[d]			
					ELC	GLC	PPC	TLC
(A)	(B)	(C)	(D)	(E)	(F)	(G)	(H)	(I)
Uronic Acids								
Glyoxylic acid	$C_2H_2O_3$	98	None	1,5c	57Cl (2)			30f (16)
Methyl ester	$C_3H_4O_3$	53	None	1				
Phenylhydrazone	$C_9H_8N_2O_2$	144,137d	None	1				
Trimethylsilyl ester								
Malonic semi-aldehyde (2-deoxy-glyceruronic acid, formylacetic acid)	$C_3H_4O_3$	No constants known	No constants known	8		12.65MU (3)		
Semicarbazone	$C_4H_7N_3O_3$	116d		1				
Glyceruronic acid (tartronic semialdehyde)	$C_3H_4O_4$	No constants known	No constants known	8				
D-Lyxuronic acid	$C_5H_8O_6$	No constants known	No constants known	120				
Calcium salt · 2H₂O	$CaC_{10}H_{14}O_{12} \cdot 2H_2O$		−23→	120				
Methyl ester	$C_6H_{10}O_6$	140g	−53 −37.7→ −23g	121				
Phenylosazone salt	$C_{17}H_{18}N_4O_4$	164d		122				
α-D-Galacturonic acid · H₂O	$C_6H_{10}O_7 \cdot H_2O$	159—160 (110—115s)	+97.9→ +50.9	123	7.9e (14)	85f (41)	32f (32)	
p-Bromophenylhydrazone salt	$Br_2C_{18}H_{14}N_4O_6$	145—146	+9 ± 2 (c 0.7, CH₃OH)	124				
2,3,4-Tri-O-methyl ether	$C_{11}H_{12}O_7$	160	+27→	123			67tmg (138a)	

Table 2 (continued)
NATURAL ACIDS OF CARBOHYDRATE DERIVATION

Substance[a] (synonym) derivative	Chemical formula	Melting point °C	Specific rotation[b] $[\alpha]_D$	Reference[c]	Chromatography, R value, and reference[d]			
					ELC	GLC	PPC	TLC
(A)	(B)	(C)	(D)	(E)	(F)	(G)	(H)	(I)
			Uronic Acids (continued)					
β-D-Galacturonic acid	$C_6H_{10}O_7$	160	+27→ +55.6	123			18glc (153,141c)	
p-Bromophenylhydrazone	$BrC_{13}H_{15}N_2O_6$	150–151	+11.5 ± 2 (CH_3OH)	124				
Brucine salt	$C_{23}H_{36}N_2O_{11}$	180	−7.7	123				
Methyl ester β-methyl pyranoside	$C_8H_{14}O_7$	194–196	−49 (CH_3OH)	125pt				
β-D-Glucuronic acid	$C_6H_{10}O_7$	156	+11.7→ +36.3	126,127	9.3e (14)		46f (41)	13f (4)
Brucine salt · H_2O	$C_{23}H_{36}N_2O_{11} \cdot H_2O$	156–157	−15.1	128				
Phenylhydrazide phenylhydrazone	$C_{18}H_{23}N_4O_5$	182		129				
2,3,4-Tri-O-methyl ether	$C_{12}H_{22}O_7$					372tmg (156) 7	84tmg (138a)	
Trimethylsilyl ether						(154)		
D-Glucurono-3,6-lactone	$C_6H_8O_6$	163–165, 180	+18.6	130,131			125f (41)	58f (32)
D-Glucuronic acid, 3-O-methyl-p-Bromophenylosazone salt	$C_7H_{12}O_7$ $Br_3C_{15}H_{35}N_6O_5$	Syrup 157	+6 −104→ −14	132,133 134				
Methyl ester α-methyl pyranoside	$C_9H_{16}O_7$	88.5–89	+150 (CH_3OH)	135ct				
D-Glucuronic acid, 4-O-methyl-	$C_7H_{12}O_7$	Syrup	+48,+82	136p,137p	9.2e (14)		145galu (138b)	
Amide α-methyl-pyranoside	$C_8H_{15}NO_6$	232	+143 (c0.7)	139				
Methyl ester	$C_7H_{14}O_7$	123–124	+41	140				
Methyl ester α-methyl pyranoside	$C_9H_{16}O_7$	203–216	+145.5 (CH_3OH, 15°)	140				

Table 2 (continued)
NATURAL ACIDS OF CARBOHYDRATE DERIVATION

Substance[a] (synonym) derivative	Chemical formula	Melting point °C	Specific rotation[b] $[\alpha]_D$	Reference[c]	Chromatography, R value, and reference[d]			
					ELC	GLC	PPC	TLC
(A)	**(B)**	**(C)**	**(D)**	**(E)**	**(F)**	**(G)**	**(H)**	**(I)**
			Uronic Acids (continued)					
L-Glucuronic acid	$C_6H_{10}O_7$		−33.3 (c 0.5)	141c			40asc (141a) 310glcu (141b)	
3,6-Lactone	$C_6H_8O_6$	174–176	−19	142pt				
Lactone 1,2,5-triacetate	$C_{12}H_{16}O_9$	195–196	−85.4 ($CHCl_3$)	142				
L-Guluronic acid	$C_6H_{10}O_7$	Syrup		143,147cp	81manu (144)	28glc (153,141c)	28glc (153,141c)	53glc (145)
3,6-Lactone	$C_6H_8O_6$	141–142	+81.7	146ct			377glcu (141b) 26l (141b)	150glc (145)
Hexulosuronic acid, 4-deoxy-L-erythro-5-(4-deoxy-5-keto-D-mannuronic acid)	$C_6H_8O_6$	No constants known	No constants known	148c			26l (148)	
Hexulosuronic acid, 4-deoxy-L-threo-5-(4-deoxy-5-keto-L-iduronic acid)	$C_6H_8O_6$	No constants known	No constants known	108c			26l (1480)	
Methyl ester β-methyl glucoside	$C_8H_{12}O_8$		+192.5 (CH_3OH)	125				30f (125)
Methyl ester α-methyl glycoside	$C_8H_{12}O_8$		−67 (CH_3OH)	125			76f (149)	
L-Iduronic acid	$C_6H_{10}O_7$	131–133	+37→ +33	150,151	79glcu (152)		65glc (131,141c)	
3,6-Lactone	$C_6H_8O_6$	Syrup	+30 (18°)	131			85glc (131,141c) 264glcu (141c)	
Sodium salt	$C_6H_9NaO_7$							
Trimethylsilyl ether						5 (154)		

Table 2 (continued)
NATURAL ACIDS OF CARBOHYDRATE DERIVATION

Substance[a] (synonym) derivative	Chemical formula	Melting point °C	Specific rotation[b] $[\alpha]_D$	Reference[c]	Chromatography, R value, and reference[d]			
					ELC	GLC	PPC	TLC
(A)	(B)	(C)	(D)	(E)	(F)	(G)	(H)	(I)
		Uronic Acids (continued)						
α-D-Mannuronic acid · H_2O	$C_6H_{10}O_7 \cdot H_2O$	120–130 (110s)	+16→ -6.1 (c 6.8)	155	100manu (144)		22f (80)	36f (32)
3,6-Lactone	$C_6H_8O_6$	140–141	+89.3	155				
β-D-Mannuronic acid	$C_6H_{10}O_7$	165–167	-47.9→ -23.9	155			52f (153)	53f (32)
p-Bromophenylhydrazone salt	$Br_2C_{18}H_{24}N_4O_6$	143–144d	+48.5 ± 1 (CH_3OH)	124				
		Aldaric Acids						
Oxalic acid	$C_2H_2O_4$	189–190	None	1	70Cl (2)			88f (4)
Dihydrate	$C_2H_2O_4 \cdot 2H_2O$	102, 150–160s	None	1				
Diamide	$C_2H_4N_2O_2$	320d	None	1				
Dimethyl ester	$C_4H_6O_4$	54	None	1				
Trimethylsilyl ester						11.14MU (3)		
Malonic acid (deoxy tartronic acid)	$C_3H_4O_4$	135–136	None	1	63Cl (2)			
Diamide	$C_3H_6N_2O_2$	170	None	1				
Dimethyl ester	$C_5H_8O_4$	Bp 181	None	1				
Trimethylsilyl ester						12.MU (3)		
Tartronic acid	$C_3H_4O_5$	141–142	None (meso)	1	57Cl (2)			73f (4)
Diamide	$C_3H_6N_2O_3$	198	None	1				
Dimethyl ester	$C_5H_8O_5$	44–45	None	1				
Trimethylsilyl ester ether						28glc (10)		

Table 2 (continued)
NATURAL ACIDS OF CARBOHYDRATE DERIVATION

Substance[a] (synonym) derivative	Chemical formula	Melting point °C	Specific rotation[b] $[\alpha]_D$	Reference[c]	Chromatography, R value, and reference[d] ELC	GLC	PPC	TLC
(A)	(B)	(C)	(D)	(E)	(F)	(G)	(H)	(I)
Aldaric Acids (continued)								
D-Threaric acid (*l*-tartaric)	$C_4H_6O_6$	170	−15	157	59Cl (2)			58f (4)
Trimethylsilyl ester ether						16.8MU (3)		
L-Threaric acid (*d*-tartaric)	$C_4H_6O_6$	170	+15 (15°)	158,159				
Diamide	$C_4H_8N_2O_4$	195	+106.5	160				
Dimethyl ester	$C_6H_{10}O_6$	48, 61.5	+2.7	161−163				
L-Malic acid (hydroxy succinic acid, deoxy-tartaric acid)	$C_4H_6O_5$	100	−2.3 (c 8.4)	164,165	57Cl (2)		56f (166a)	60f (166b)
Acetate	$C_8H_8O_6$	132	−37.9	167				
Diamide	$C_4H_8N_2O_3$	156−157	+6	168				
Dimethyl ester	$C_6H_{10}O_5$			1				
Trimethylsilyl ester ether						15MU (3)		
Oxalosuccinic acid (hydroxy maleic acid, keto-succinic acid)	$C_4H_4O_5$	No constants known	No constants known					
Diamide	$C_4H_8N_2O_3$			1				
Dimethyl ester	$C_6H_8O_5$			1	48Cl (2)			
Trimethylsilyl ester ether						15.65MU (3)		
Allaric acid (*allo*-mucic acid)	$C_6H_{10}O_8$	188−192d		169				
D-Galactaric acid (mucic acid)	$C_6H_{10}O_8$	215d	None (meso)	170	200pa (171cp)		90mal (170)	
Dimethyl ester	$C_8H_{14}O_8$	184−186	None	171				
Bis(phenylhydrazide)	$C_{18}H_{22}N_4O_6$	242	None	170				
D-Glucaric acid (saccharic acid)	$C_6H_{10}O_8$	125−126	+6.9 → +20.6	172	10.8[e] (14)		2f (89b)	59f (4)

Table 2 (continued)
NATURAL ACIDS OF CARBOHYDRATE DERIVATION

Substance[a] (synonym) derivative	Chemical formula	Melting point °C	Specific rotation[b] [α]D	Reference[c]	Chromatography, R value, and reference[d]			
					ELC	GLC	PPC	TLC
(A)	(B)	(C)	(D)	(E)	(F)	(G)	(H)	(I)
Aldaric Acids (continued)								
Diamide	$C_6H_{11}N_3O_4$	172–173	+13.3	20				
1,4-Lactone · H_2O	$C_6H_8O_7 \cdot H_2O$	90–95		173				
6,3-Lactone	$C_6H_8O_7$	143–145		173			23f (173)	43f (32)
Bis(phenylhydrazide)	$C_{18}H_{22}N_4O_6$	209–210	+3.5–	173			30f (173)	85f (32)
D-Mannaric acid (D-mannosaccharic acid)	$C_6H_{10}O_8$	128.5	+48.7	174				
Diamide	$C_6H_{12}N_2O_6$	188–189.5	−24.4	20				
Bis(phenylhydrazide)	$C_{18}H_{22}N_4O_6$	214–216d		175				
Amino Sugar Acids								
Glycine (aminoacetic acid, amino deoxyglycollic acid)	$C_2H_5NO_2$	233–236d	None	176	150ala (177)		32f (178)	22f (179)
Amide	$C_2H_6N_2O$	65–67	None	1				
Hydrochloride	$C_2H_5NO_2 \cdot HCl$	185	None	1				
Methyl ester	$C_3H_7NO_2$	Bp 54 (50 mm)	None	1				
N,N-Trimethylsilyl amine ester						13.18MU (3)		
Sarcosine (N-methylamino-acetic acid)	$C_3H_7NO_2$	212–213d	None	1				
Hydrochloride N-Trimethylsilyl amine ester	$C_3H_7NO_2 \cdot HCl$	168–170	None	1		11.43MU (3)		

Table 2 (continued)

NATURAL ACIDS OF CARBOHYDRATE DERIVATION

Substance[a] (synonym) derivative	Chemical formula	Melting point °C	Specific rotation[b] $[\alpha]_D$	Reference[c]	Chromatography, R value, and reference[d]			
					ELC	GLC	PPC	TLC
(A)	(B)	(C)	(D)	(E)	(F)	(G)	(H)	(I)
		Amino Sugar Acids (continued)						
L-Serine (2-amino-2-deoxy-L-glyceric acid, 2-amino-3-hydroxy-propionic acid)	$C_3H_7NO_3$	228dg	−7.3 (c 5.5, 26°)	1,180p	215ala (177)		28f (178)	47f (179)
Methyl ester hydrochloride N-Trimethylsilyl amine ester ether	$C_4H_9NO_3 \cdot HCl$	167		1		13.8MU (3)		
L-Alanine (2-amino-2,3-di-deoxy-L-glyceric acid, deoxy-L-serine, 2-amino-propionic acid)	$C_3H_7NO_2$	297d	+2.7	1	100ala (177)		49f (178)	26f (179)
Amide	$C_3H_8N_2O$	72		1				
Hydrochloride N-Trimethylsilyl amine ester	$C_3H_7NO_2 \cdot HCl$	204	+10.4	1		11.05MU (3)		
Acetoacetic acid, 2-amino-	$C_4H_7NO_3$	No constants known	No constants known	1				
Ethyl ester hydrochloride	$C_6H_{11}NO_3 \cdot HCl$	95d		1				
L-Xylonic acid, 2-amino-2-deoxy (polyoxamic acid)	$C_5H_{11}NO_6$	171−173d	+2.8	181				
N-Acetyl 1,4-lactone	$C_7H_{11}NO_5$	150−152		181				
L-Xylonic acid, 2-amino-2-deoxy-5-O-carbamoyl-	$C_6H_{13}N_2O_6$	226−232d	+1.3	181				
L-Xylonic acid, 2-amino-2,3-dideoxy-	$C_5H_{11}NO_4$	Syrup	+11	181				
L-Xylonic acid, 2-amino-carbamoyl-	$C_6H_{13}N_3O_5$	215−216d	+5.8	181				

Table 2 (continued)
NATURAL ACIDS OF CARBOHYDRATE DERIVATION

Substance[a] (synonym) derivative	Chemical formula	Melting point °C	Specific rotation[b] $[\alpha]_D$	Reference[c]	Chromatography, R value, and reference[d]			
					ELC	GLC	PPC	TLC
(A)	(B)	(C)	(D)	(E)	(F)	(G)	(H)	(I)
Amino Sugar Acids (continued)								
N-Acetyl 1,4-lactone D-Galactonic acid, 2-amino-2-deoxy- (D-galactosaminic acid, chondrosaminic acid)	$C_6H_{12}N_2O_5$ $C_6H_{13}NO_6$	181–191 198–203d	–5 (c 0.6)	181 60				
N-Acetyl acid · H_2O	$C_6H_{13}NO_6 \cdot H_2O$	102–103	–33.8 → –16 (3 days)	182pt				
N-Acetyl 1,4-lactone	$C_6H_{13}NO_6$	165		183				
D-Alluronic acid, 3-acetamido-3-deoxy-	$C_8H_{13}NO_7$	182–183		184				
3-Amino-3-deoxy-D-allose · hydrochloride	$C_6H_{13}NO_5 \cdot HCl$	157–160d	+25 (c 0.7)	199				
D-Alluronic acid, 5-amino-5-deoxy-	$C_6H_{11}NO_6$	No constants known	No constants known	181				
D-Galacturonic acid, 2-amino-2-deoxy- (D-galactosaminuronic acid)	$C_6H_{11}NO_6$	160d	+84 (pH 2, HCl)	186p	68gNUA (192a)		46f (185)	
α-D-Galactosamine · HCl	$C_6H_{13}NO_5 \cdot HCl$	185	+121 → +80	187			69f (194)	
β-D-Galactosamine · HCl	$C_6H_{13}NO_5 \cdot HCl$	187	+44 →	187				
D-Glucuronic acid, 2-amino-2-deoxy- (D-glucosaminuronic acid)	$C_6H_{11}NO_6$	120–172d	+55	188,189	7.2^m (188cp)		57f (185)	

Table 2 (continued)
NATURAL ACIDS OF CARBOHYDRATE DERIVATION

Substance[a] (synonym) derivative	Chemical formula	Melting point °C	Specific rotation[b] $[\alpha]_D$	Reference[c]	Chromatography, R value, and reference[d]			
					ELC	GLC	PPC	TLC
(A)	(B)	(C)	(D)	(E)	(F)	(G)	(H)	(I)
		Amino Sugar Acids (continued)						
α-D-Glucosamine	$C_6H_{13}NO_5$	88	+100 → +47	190	9^m (188cp)		76f (194)	
β-D-Glucosamine	$C_6H_{13}NO_5$	110–111	+28 → +47	190				
Methyl α-glycoside	$C_7H_{13}NO_6$	203–207 (196s)	+126.3	189			90glcN (189)	
N-Acetyl furanurono-1,4-lactone	$C_8H_{11}NO_6$	177–178	+43.6	191			38f (191)	
D-Guluronic acid, 2-amino-2-deoxy- (D-gulosaminuronic acid)	$C_6H_{11}NO_6$	No constants known	No constants known	193c	71gNUA (193a)		43glcN (193b)	
D-Gulosamine · HCl	$C_6H_{13}NO_5 \cdot HCl$	150–170d	+34 → -19	200,201			77f (194)	
Hexuronic acid, 2-amino-2-deoxy- N-Trimethylsilyl amine ester ether	$C_6H_{11}NO_6$		+11.5	192c	40gNUA (192a)	128eic (192c)	27glcN (192b)	
Hex-2-ene-uronic acid, 4-amino-2,3,4-trideoxy-D-erythro	$C_6H_9NO_4$	No constants known	No constants known	195				
Methyl α-pyranoside	$C_7H_{11}NO_4$	>270d	+30.5 (c 0.3)	196				
N-Acetyl methyl α-pyranoside methyl ester	$C_{10}H_{15}NO_5$	145–146	+87 (CHCl$_3$)	196				

Table 2 (continued)
NATURAL ACIDS OF CARBOHYDRATE DERIVATION

Substance[a] (synonym) derivative	Chemical formula	Melting point °C	Specific rotation[b] $[\alpha]_D$	Reference[c]	Chromatography, R value, and reference[d]			
					ELC	GLC	PPC	TLC
(A)	(B)	(C)	(D)	(E)	(F)	(G)	(H)	(I)
Amino Sugar Acids (continued)								
D-Mannuronic acid, 2-amino-2-deoxy- (D-mannosaminuronic acid)	$C_6H_{11}NO_6$	92–94	-9.9 (c 0.6)	197,198	115gNUA (193a)		49glcN (193b)	
D-Mannosamine hydrochloride	$C_6H_{13}NO_5 \cdot HCl$	178–180d	-3	202			80f (194)	
Destomic acid	$C_7H_{15}NO_7$	207–209d	+1.9 / -12.1 → -30.6 (2 N HCl)	211 / 211				
Methyl ester · HCl	$C_8H_{17}NO_6 \cdot HCl$	150–151d	+165→	211	13glcN (210a)		76f (194)	
Muramic acid (2-amino-3-O-(D-1-carboxyethyl)-2-deoxy-D-glucose)	$C_9H_{17}NO_7$	155	+123 (3 h)	203cp, 204cp				
N-Acetyl muramic acid	$C_{11}H_{19}NO_8$	122–124	+59 → / +39 (6 h)	205	194gNAc (210b)		100glcN (205)	
N-Acetyl trimethylsilyl ether glycoside						152myot (206a)		
N-Acetyl muramic acid 6-acetate · 1/2 H₂O	$C_{13}H_{21}NO_9 \cdot 1/2\ H_2O$	176	+56 (c 0.6)	206,207			245gNAc (206b)	
N-Acetyl 6-acetate trimethylsilyl ether glycoside						175myot (206a)		
N-Glycolyl muramic acid · H₂O	$C_{11}H_{19}NO_9 \cdot H_2O$		+56 (50% C₂H₅OH)	208	13glcN (210a)		130gNAc (208a)	62gNAc (208b)
manno-Muramic acid [2-amino-3-O-(D-1-carboxyethyl)-2-deoxy-D-mannose]	$C_9H_{17}NO_7$		+21 (c 0.6, 79% C₂H₅OH)	209c			180glcN (209a)	25f (209b)

Table 2 (continued)
NATURAL ACIDS OF CARBOHYDRATE DERIVATION

Substance[a] (synonym) derivative	Chemical formula	Melting point °C	Specific rotation[b] $[\alpha]_D$	Reference[c]	Chromatography, R value, and reference[d]			
					ELC	GLC	PPC	TLC
(A)	(B)	(C)	(D)	(E)	(F)	(G)	(H)	(I)
		Amino Sugar Acids (continued)						
N-Acetyl *muramic* acid	$C_{11}H_{19}NO_8$	No constants known	No constants known		189gNAc (210b)		160gNAc (209a)	
N-Acetyl trimethylsilyl ether glycoside						19.6 (209c)		
Nonulosonic acid, 5-acetamino-3,5-dideoxy-D-*glycero*-D-*galacto*- (N-acetyl neuraminic acid, gynaminic acid, lactaminic acid, sialic acid)	$C_{11}H_{19}NO_9{}^n$	183–186d	–31.7	212,213			14f (212)	17f (214)
Quinoxaline deriv.	$C_{17}H_{23}N_3O_7$	204–205	–100 (c 0.3, 1:1 H_2O, CH_3SOCH_3)	215				
Methyl glycoside tetratrifluoroacetate						80–82 (216)		
N-Acetyl neuraminic acid 4-acetate	$C_{13}H_{21}NO_{10}$	200d	–62±1	217			233nana (217)	
N-Acetyl neuraminic acid 7-acetate · H_2O	$C_{13}H_{21}NO_{10} \cdot H_2O$	138–140d	+6.2±2	217			466nana (217)	
N-Acetyl neuraminic acid 7,8(9)-diacetate · CH_3OH	$C_{15}H_{23}NO_{11} \cdot CH_3OH$	130–131d	+9.2±2	217				
N-Glycolyl neuraminic acid	$C_{11}H_{19}NO_{10}$	189–191d	–33.6	218c,220ep			30f (218)	47nana (219c)

Table 2 (continued)
NATURAL ACIDS OF CARBOHYDRATE DERIVATION

Substance[a] (synonym) derivative	Chemical formula	Melting point °C	Specific rotation[b] $[\alpha]_D$	Reference[c]	Chromatography, R value, and reference[d]				
					ELC	GLC	PPC	TLC	
(A)	(B)	(C)	(D)	(E)	(F)	(G)	(H)	(I)	
			Amino Sugar Acids (continued)						
Methyl glycoside tetratrifluoroacetate						86–88 (216)			
N-Acetoglycolyl-4-C methyl-4,9-dideoxy-neuraminic acid	$C_{14}H_{23}NO_9$	No constants known	No constants known					144nana (219c)	
N-Glycolyl sialic acid 4-acetate	$C_{13}H_{21}NO_{11}$	No constants known	No constants known				123nana (221ct) 25–35f (222)		
N-Glycolyl-8-O-methyl-neuraminic acid	$C_{12}H_{21}NO_{10}$	No constants known	No constanst known						
Hf-Neuraminic acid	Unknown	No constants known	No constants known				31f (223cgt)		

Compiled by George G. Maher.

Table 2 (continued)
NATURAL ACIDS OF CARBOHYDRATE DERIVATION

REFERENCES

1. Pollock and Stevens, *Dictionary of Organic Compounds,* Oxford University Press, New York, 1965.
2. Gross, *Chem. Ind.,* p. 1219 (1959).
3. Butts, *Anal. Biochem.,* 46, 187 (1972).
4. Baraldi, *J. Chromatogr.,* 42, 125 (1969).
5. Carlsson and Samuelson, *Anal. Chim. Acta,* 49, 248 (1970).
6. Frankland and McGregor, *J. Chem. Soc.* (Lond.), p. 513 (1893).
7. Frankland, Wharton, and Aston, *J. Chem. Soc.* (Lond.), p. 269 (1901).
8. Isherwood, Chen, and Mapson, *Biochem. J.,* 56, 1, 15 (1954).
9. Wolfrom and DeWalt, *J. Am. Chem. Soc.,* 70, 3148 (1948).
10. Verhaar and de Wilt, *J. Chromatogr.,* 41, 168 (1969).
11. Whyte, *J. Chromatogr.,* 87, 163 (1973).
12. Hough and Jones, *J. Chem. Soc.* (Lond.), p. 4052 (1952).
13. Robbins and Upson, *J. Am. Chem. Soc.,* 62, 1074 (1940).
14. Theander, *Sven. Kem. Tidskr.,* 70, 393 (1958).
15. Bourne, Hutson, and Weigel, *J. Chem. Soc.* (Lond.), p. 5153 (1960).
16. Wolfrom, Patin, and Lederkremer, *J. Chromatogr.,* 17, 488 (1965).
17. Hardegger, Kreiss, and El Khadem, *Helv. Chim. Acta,* 35, 618 (1952).
18. Robbins and Upson, *J. Am. Chem. Soc.,* 62, 1074 (1940).
19. Rehorst, *Ber. Dtsch. Chem. Ges.,* 63, 2280 (1930).
20. Hudson and Komatsu, *J. Am. Chem. Soc.,* 41, 1141 (1919).
21. Isbell and Frush, *J. Res. Nat. Bur. Stand.,* 11, 649 (1933).
22. Assarson, Lindberg, and Vorbrueygen, *Acta Chem. Scand.,* 13, 1395 (1959).
23. Němec, Kefurt, and Jarý, *J. Chromatogr.,* 26, 116 (1967).
24. Bates, *Polarimetry, Saccharimetry and the Sugars,* Nat. Bur. Stand. Circ. C440, U.S. Govt. Print. Off., Washington, D.C., 1942, 790.
25. Gardner and Wenis, *J. Am. Chem. Soc.,* 73, 1855 (1951).
26. Kanfer, Ashwell, and Burns, *J. Biol. Chem.,* 235, 2518 (1960).
27. Liebster, Kulhanek, and Tadra, *Chem. Listy,* 47, 1075 (1953).
28. Weimberg, *J. Biol. Chem.,* 234, 727 (1959).
29. Palleroni and Doudoroff, *J. Biol. Chem.,* 223, 499 (1956).
30. Kurata and Sakurai, *Agric. Biol. Chem.,* 32, 1250 (1968).
31. Ladenberg, Tishler, Wellmann, and Babson, *J. Am. Chem. Soc.,* 66, 1217 (1944).
32. Hay, Lewis, and Smith, *J. Chromatogr.,* 11, 479 (1963).
33. Wolfrom, Bennett, and Crum, *J. Am. Chem. Soc.,* 80, 944 (1958).
34. Steiger, *Helv. Chim. Acta,* 19, 189 (1936).
35. Hough, Jones, and Mitchell, *Can. J. Chem.,* 36, 1720 (1958).
36. Rehorst, *Justus Liebigs Ann. Chem.,* 503, 143, 154 (1933).
37. Weerman, *Recl. Trav. Chim. Pays-Bas,* 37, 15, 40, (1917).
38. Menzinsky, *Ber. Dtsch. Chem. Ges.,* 68, 822 (1935).
39. Heyns and Stein, *Justus Liebigs Ann. Chem.,* 558, 194 (1947).
40. Major and Cook, *J. Am. Chem. Soc.,* 58, 2474, 2477 (1936).
41. Hickman and Ashwell, *J. Biol. Chem.,* 241, 1424 (1966).
42. Hickman and Ashwell, *J. Biol. Chem.,* 235, 1566 (1960).
43. Dahms and Anderson, *J. Biol. Chem.,* 247, 2222, 2228 (1972).
44. Dahms and Anderson, *J. Biol. Chem.,* 247, 2233 (1972).
45. Isbell, *J. Res. Nat. Bur. Stand.,* 29, 227 (1942).
46. Gorin and Perlin, *Can. J. Chem.,* 34, 693 (1956).
47. Humoller, McManus, and Austin, *J. Am. Chem. Soc.,* 58, 2479 (1936).
48. Mortensson-Egnund, Schöyen, Howe, Lee, and Harboe, *J. Bacteriol.,* 98, 924 (1969).
49. Kiliani, *Ber. Dtsch. Chem. Ges.,* 55, 75 (1922).
50. Pryde, *J. Chem. Soc.* (Lond.), p. 1808 (1923).
51. Glattfeld and MacMillan, *J. Am. Chem. Soc.,* 56, 2481 (1934).
52. Levene and Meyer, *J. Biol. Chem.,* 46, 307 (1921).
53. Hurd and Sowden, *J. Am. Chem. Soc.,* 60, 235 (1938).
54. Wolfrom, Berkebile, and Thompson, *J. Am. Chem. Soc.,* 71, 2360 (1949).
55. Fukunaga and Kubata, *Bull. Chem. Soc. Jap.,* 13, 272 (1938).

Table 2 (continued)
NATURAL ACIDS OF CARBOHYDRATE DERIVATION

56. Wolfrom and Anno, *J. Am. Chem. Soc.*, 74, 5583 (1952).
57. Loewus, *Carbohydr. Res.*, 3, 130 (1966).
58. Ettel, Liebster, and Tadra, *Chem. Listy*, 46, 45 (1952).
59. Claus, *Biochem. Biophys. Res. Commun.*, 20, 745 (1965).
60. Kuhn, Weiser, and Fischer, *Justus Liebigs Ann. Chem.*, 628, 207 (1959).
61. Ley and Doudoroff, *J. Biol. Chem.*, 227, 745 (1957).
62. Ashwell, Wahba, and Hickman, *J. Biol. Chem.*, 235, 1559 (1960).
63. Regna and Caldwell, *J. Am. Chem. Soc.*, 66, 243, 244, 246 (1944).
64. Hart and Everett, *J. Am. Chem. Soc.*, 61, 1822 (1939).
65. Wolfrom, Thompson, and Evans, *J. Am. Chem. Soc.*, 67, 1793 (1945).
66. Yurkevich, Vereikina, Dolgikh, and Preobrazheuskii, *J. Gen. Chem. USSR*, 37, 1201 (1967).
67. Hughes, Overend, and Stacey, *J. Chem. Soc.*, (Lond.), p. 2846 (1949).
68. Bauer and Biely, *Collect. Czech. Chem. Commun.*, 33, 1165 (1968).
69. Fischer and Dangschat, *Helv. Chim. Acta*, 20, 705 (1937).
70. Williams and Egan, *J. Bacteriol.*, 77, 167 (1959).
71. Kilgore and Starr, *Biochim. Biophys. Acta*, 30, 652 (1958).
72. Ohle and Berend, *Ber. Dtsch. Chem. Ges.*, 60, 1159 (1927).
73. Waldi, *J. Chromatogr.*, 18, 417 (1965).
74. Cirelli and de Lederkremer, *Chem. Ind.*, p. 1139 (1971).
75. Paerels, *Recl. Trav. Chim. Pays-Bas*, 80, 985 (1961).
76. Henderson, *J. Am. Chem. Soc.*, 79, 5304 (1957).
77. Merrick and Roseman, *J. Biol. Chem.*, 235, 1274 (1960).
78. Boutroux, *Ann. Chim. Phys. Ser. 6*, 21, 565 (1890).
79. Barch, *J. Am. Chem. Soc.*, 55, 3656 (1933).
80. Strobel, *J. Biol. Chem.*, 245, 32 (1970).
81. Rosenthal, Spaner, and Brown, *J. Chromatogr.*, 13, 152 (1964).
82. Wakisaka, *Agric. Biol. Chem.*, 28, 819 (1964).
83. Katznelson, Tanenbaum, and Tatum, *J. Biol. Chem.*, 204, 43 (1953).
84. Hudson, *J. Am. Chem. Soc.*, 73, 4498 (1951).
85. Upson, Sands, and Whitnah, *J. Am. Chem. Soc.*, 50, 519 (1928).
86. Barber and Hassid, *Bull. Res. Counc. Isr. Sect. A.*, 11, 249 (1963).
87. Burns, *J. Am. Chem. Soc.*, 79, 1257 (1957).
88. Okazaki, Kanzaki, Sasajima, and Terada, *Agric. Biol. Chem.*, 33, 207 (1969).
89. Puhakainen and Hänninen, *Acta Chem. Scand.*, 26, 3599 (1972).
90. Heyns, *Justus Liebigs Ann. Chem.*, 558, 177 (1947).
91. deWilt, *J. Chromatogr.*, 63, 379 (1971).
92. Grollman and Lehninger, *Arch. Biochem. Biophys.*, 69, 458 (1957).
93. Okazaki, Kanzaki, Doi, Nara, and Motizuki, *Agric. Biol. Chem.*, 32, 1250 (1968).
94. Smiley and Ashwell, *J. Biol. Chem.*, 236, 357 (1961).
95. Penney and Zilva, *Biochem. J.*, 37, 403 (1943).
96. Mead and Finamore, *Biochemistry*, 8, 2652 (1969).
97. Mumma and Verlangieri, *Biochim. Biophys. Acta*, 273, 249 (1972).
98. Berman and Magasanik, *J. Biol. Chem.*, 241, 807 (1966).
99. Anderson and Magasanik, *J. Biol. Chem.*, 246, 5653, 5662 (1971).
100. Takagi, *Agric. Biol. Chem.*, 26, 717 (1962).
101. Hamilton and Smith, *J. Am. Chem. Soc.*, 76, 3543 (1954).
102. Kanzaki and Okazaki, *Agric. Biol. Chem.*, 34, 432 (1970).
103. Levene, *J. Biol. Chem.*, 59, 123 (1924).
104. Phillips and Criddle, *J. Chem. Soc.* (Lond.), p. 3404 (1960).
105. Pervozvanski, *Microbiology* (USSR), 8, 915 (1939).
106. Wolfrom, Konigsberg, and Weisblat, *J. Am. Chem. Soc.*, 61, 576 (1939).
107. Gakhokidge and Gvelukashvili, *J. Gen. Chem. USSR*, 22, 143 (1952).
108. Preiss and Ashwell, *J. Biol. Chem.*, 238, 1571, 1577 (1963).
109. Bloom and Westerfeld, *Biochemistry*, 5, 3204 (1966).
110. Hirabayashi and Harada, *Agric. Biol. Chem.*, 33, 276 (1969).
111. Kuhn, Bister, and Dafeldecker, *Justus Liebigs Ann. Chem.*, 617, 115 (1958).
112. Srinivasan and Sprinson, *J. Biol. Chem.*, 234, 716 (1959).
113. Paerels and Geluk, *Recl. Trav. Chim. Pays-Bas*, 89, 813 (1970).

Table 2 (continued)
NATURAL ACIDS OF CARBOHYDRATE DERIVATION

114. Charon and Szabo, *J. Chem. Soc.* (Lond.), Perk I, p. 1175 (1973).
115. Adlersberg and Sprinson, *Biochemistry*, 3, 1855 (1964).
116. Ghalambor, Levine, and Heath, *J. Biol. Chem.*, 241, 3207 (1966).
117. Droge, Lehmann, Luderitz, and Westphal, *Eur. J. Biochem.*, 14, 175 (1970).
118. Hershberger, Davis, and Binkley, *J. Biol. Chem.*, 243, 1578, 1585 (1968).
119. Levin and Racker, *J. Biol. Chem.*, 234, 2532 (1959).
120. Ameyama and Kondo, *Bull. Agric. Chem. Soc. Jap.*, 22, 271, 380 (1958).
121. Hulyalkar and Perry, *Can. J. Chem.*, 43, 3241 (1965).
122. Bergmann, *Ber. Dtsch. Chem. Ges.*, 54, 1362 (1921).
123. Ehrlich and Schubert, *Ber. Dtsch. Chem. Ges.*, 62, 1987, 2022 (1929).
124. Niemann, Schoeffal, and Link, *J. Biol. Chem.*, 101, 337 (1933).
125. Kováč, Hirsch, and Kováčik, *Carbohydr. Res.*, 32, 360 (1974).
126. Winmann, *Ber. Dtsch. Chem. Ges.*, 62, 1637 (1929).
127. Ehrlich and Rehorst, *Ber. Dtsch. Chem. Ges.*, 58, 1989 (1925).
128. Ehrlich and Rehorst, *Ber. Dtsch. Chem. Ges.*, 62, 628 (1929).
129. Bergmann and Wolff, *Ber. Dtsch. Chem. Ges.*, 56, 1060 (1923).
130. Goebel and Babers, *J. Biol. Chem.*, 100, 573, 743 (1933).
131. Fischer and Schmidt, *Ber. Dtsch. Chem. Ges.*, 92, 2184 (1954).
132. Das Gupta and Sarkar, *Text. Res. J.*, 24, 705, 1071 (1954).
133. Marsh, *J. Chem. Soc.*, (Lond.), p. 1578 (1952).
134. Levene and Meyer, *J. Biol. Chem.*, 60, 173 (1924).
135. Kováč, *Carbohydr. Res.*, 31, 323 (1973).
136. Currie and Timell, *Can. J. Chem.*, 37, 922 (1959).
137. Jones and Painter, *J. Chem. Soc.* (Lond.), p. 669 (1957).
138. Tyler, *J. Chem. Soc.* (Lond.), p. 5288, p. 5300 (1965).
139. Jones and Nunn, *J. Chem. Soc.* (Lond.), p. 3001 (1955).
140. Wacek, Leitinger, and Hochbahn, *Monatsh. Chem.*, 90, 555, 562 (1959).
141. Charalampous and Lyras, *J. Biol Chem.*, 228, 1 (1957).
142. Sowa, *Can. J. Chem.*, 47, 3931 (1969).
143. Sutter and Reichstein, *Helv. Chim. Acta*, 21, 1210 (1938).
144. Haug and Larsen, *Acta Chem. Scand.*, 15, 1395 (1961).
145. Gunther and Schweiger, *J. Chromatogr.*, 34, 498 (1968).
146. Fischer and Dörfel, *Hoppe-Seyler's Z. Physiol. Chem.*, 302, 186 (1955).
147. Whistler and Schweiger, *J. Am. Chem. Soc.*, 80, 5701 (1958).
148. Preiss and Ashwell, *J. Biol. Chem.*, 237, 309, 317 (1962).
149. Heim and Neukom, *Helv. Chim. Acta*, 45, 1737 (1962).
150. Cifonelli, Ludowieg, and Dorfman, *J. Biol. Chem.*, 233, 541 (1958).
151. Shafizadeh and Wolfrom, *J. Am. Chem. Soc.*, 77, 2568 (1955).
152. St. Cyr, *J. Chromatogr.*, 47, 284 (1970).
153. Fischer and Dörfel, *Hoppe-Seyler's Z. Physiol. Chem.*, 301, 224 (1955).
154. Lehtonen, Kärkkäinen, and Haahti, *Anal. Biochem.*, 16, 526 (1966).
155. Schoeffel and Link, *J. Biol. Chem.*, 100, 397 (1933).
156. Stephen, Kaplan, Taylor, and Leisegang, *Tetrahedron Suppl.*, 7, 233 (1966).
157. Pasteur, *Ann. Chim. Phys.*, Ser. 3, 28, 71 (1850).
158. Walden, *Ber. Dtsch. Chem. Ges.*, 29, 1701 (1896).
159. Fandolt, *Ber. Dtsch. Chem. Ges.*, 6, 1075 (1873).
160. Frankland and Slater, *J. Chem. Soc.* (Lond.), 83, 1354 (1903).
161. Anschütz and Pictet, *Ber. Dtsch. Chem. Ges.*, 13, 1176 (1880).
162. Patterson, *J. Chem. Soc.* (Lond.), 85, 765 (1904).
163. Frankland and Wharton, *J. Chem. Soc.* (Lond.), 69, 1310 (1896).
164. Pasteur, *Justus Liebigs Ann. Chem.*, 82, 331 (1852).
165. Schneider, *Ber. Dtsch. Chem. Ges.*, 13, 620 (1880).
166. Walczyk and Burczyk, *Chem. Anal.* (Warsaw), 17, 404 (1972).
167. Anschütz and Bennert, *Justus Liebigs Ann. Chem.*, 254, 165 (1889).
168. Lutz, Dissertation, University of Rostock (1899); *Chem. Zentralbl.*, II, 1013 (1900).
169. Bond, D., *J. Chem. Soc. D*, p. 338 (1969).
170. Anet and Reynolds, *Nature*, 174, 930 (1954).
171. Kessler, Neufeld, Feingold, and Hassid, *J. Biol. Chem.*, 236, 308 (1961).

Table 2 (continued)
NATURAL ACIDS OF CARBOHYDRATE DERIVATION

172. Rehorst, *Ber. Dtsch. Chem. Ges.*, 61, 163 (1928).
173. Marsh, *Biochem. J.*, 86, 77 (1963); 87, 82 (1963); 89, 108 (1963).
174. Rehorst, *Ber. Dtsch. Chem. Ges.*, 65, 1476 (1932).
175. Matsui, Okada, and Ishidata, *J. Biochem.* (Tokyo), 57, 715 (1965).
176. Tobie and Ayres, *J. Am. Chem. Soc.*, 64, 725 (1942).
177. Katz and Lewis, *Anal. Biochem.*, 17, 306 (1966).
178. Wright, Jr., Burton, and Berry, Jr., *Arch Biochem. Biophys.*, 86, 94 (1960).
179. Frei, Fukui, Lieu T., and Frodyma, *Chemia* (Aarau), 20, 24 (1966).
180. Fusari, Haskell, Frohardt, and Bartz, *J. Am. Chem. Soc.*, 76, 2881 (1954).
181. Isono, Asahi, and Suzuki, *J. Am. Chem. Soc.*, 91, 7490 (1969).
182. Zissis, Diehl, and Fletcher, Jr., *Carbohydr. Res.*, 28, 327 (1973).
183. Karrer and Mayer, *Helv. Chim. Acta*, 20, 407 (1937).
184. Iwasaki, *Yakugaku Zasshi*, 82, 1380 (1962); *Chem. Abstr.*, 59, 758 (1963).
185. Heyns, Kiessling, Lindenberg, and Paulsen, *Ber. Dtsch. Chem. Ges.*, 92, 2435 (1959).
186. Heyns and Beck, *Ber. Dtsch. Chem. Ges.*, 90, 2443 (1957).
187. Levene, *J. Biol. Chem.*, 57, 337 (1923).
188. Williamson and Zamenhof, *J. Biol. Chem.*, 238, 2255 (1963).
189. Heyns and Paulsen, *Ber. Dtsch. Chem. Ges.*, 88, 188 (1955).
190. Westphal and Holzmann, *Ber. Dtsch. Chem. Ges.*, 75, 1274 (1942).
191. Weidmann, Fauland, Helbig, and Zimmerman, *Justus Liebigs Ann. Chem.*, 694, 183 (1966).
192. Romanowska and Reinhold, *Eur. J. Biochem.*, 36, 160 (1973).
193. Torii, Sakakibara, and Kuroda, *Eur. J. Biochem.*, 37, 401 (1973).
194. Crumpton, *Biochem. J.*, 72, 479 (1959).
195. Ōtake, Takeuchi, Endō, and Yonehara, *Tetrahedron Lett.*, 1405 (1965).
196. Watanabe, Goody, and Fox, *Tetrahedron*, 26, 3883 (1970).
197. Kundu, Crawford, Prajsnar, Reed, and Rosenthal, *Carbohydr. Res.*, 12, 225 (1970).
198. Perkins, *Biochem. J.*, 86, 475 (1963); 89, 104P (1963).
199. Koto, Kawakatsu, and Zen, *Bull. Chem. Soc. Jap.*, 46, 876 (1973).
200. Tarasiejska and Jeanloz, *J. Am. Chem. Soc.*, 79, 2660 (1957).
201. Kuhn and Bister, *Justus Liebigs Ann. Chem.*, 617, 92 (1958).
202. Lemieux and Nagabhushan, *Can. J. Chem.*, 46, 401 (1968).
203. Strange and Kent, *Biochem. J.*, 71, 333 (1959).
204. Lambert and Zilliken, *Ber. Dtsch. Chem. Ges.*, 93, 2915 (1960).
205. Flowers and Jeanloz, *J. Org. Chem.*, 28, 1564, 2983 (1963).
206. Osawa, Sinay, Halford, and Jeanloz, *Biochemistry*, 8, 3369 (1969).
207. Ghuysen and Strominger, *Biochemistry*, 2, 1119 (1963).
208. Sinay, *Carbohydr. Res.*, 16, 113 (1971).
209. Sinay, Halford, Choudhary, Gross, and Jeanloz, *J. Biol. Chem.*, 247, 391 (1972).
210. Hoshino, Zehavi, Sinay, and Jeanloz, *J. Biol. Chem.*, 247, 381 (1972).
211. Kondo, Akita, and Sezaki, *J. Antibiot.* (Tokyo) *Ser. A*, 19, 137 (1966).
212. Faillard, *Hoppe-Seyler's Z. Physiol. Chem.*, 307, 62 (1957).
213. Zilliken and McGlick, *Naturwissenschaften*, 43, 536 (1956).
214. Khorlin and Privalova, *Chem. Nat. Compd.* (U S S R), 3, 159 (1967).
215. Kuhn and Baschang, *Justus Liebigs Ann. Chem.*, 659, 156 (1962).
216. Zanetta, Breckenridge, and Vincendon, *J. Chromatogr.*, 69, 291 (1972).
217. Blix and Lindberg, *Acta Chem. Scand.*, 14, 1809 (1960).
218. Faillard and Blohm, *Hoppe-Seyler's Z. Physiol. Chem.*, 341, 167 (1965).
219. Hotta, Kurokawa, and Isaka, *J. Biol. Chem.*, 245, 6307 (1970).
220. Brunetti, Jourdian, and Roseman, *J. Biol. Chem.*, 237, 2447 (1962).
221. Hakomori and Saito, *Biochemistry*, 8, 5082 (1969).
222. Warren, *Biochim. Biophys. Acta*, 83, 129 (1964).
223. Isemura, Zahn, and Schmid, *Biochem. J.*, 131, 509 (1973).

Table 3
NATURAL ALDOSES

Substance[a] (synonym) derivative	Chemical formula	Melting point °C	Specific rotation[b] $[\alpha]_D$	Reference[c]	Chromatography, R value, and reference[d] ELC	GLC	PPC	TLC
(A)	(B)	(C)	(D)	(E)	(F)	(G)	(H)	(I)
Acetaldehyde (deoxy-glycolaldehyde)	C_2H_4O	Liquid, bp 21	None	1				
2,4-Dinitrophenyl-hydrazone	$C_8H_8N_4O_4$	146, 163.5.—164.5	None	1		0.6 (2)		52f (3)
D-Glyceraldehyde (glycerose)	$C_3H_6O_3$	Syrup	+13.5±0.5	4	<10sor (5)		310f (6)	58f (7)
Dimethione	$C_{15}H_{22}O_6$	199–201	+197.5 (c 0.7, C_2H_5OH)	8				
2,4-Dinitrophenyl-hydrazone Trimethylsilyl ether	$C_9H_{18}N_4O_6$	155–156		8		48glct (9)		10f (3)
D-Glyceraldehyde, 3,3-bis-(C-hydroxymethyl)-(D-apiose)	$C_5H_{10}O_5$	138–139	–29 (CH_3OH) +5.6 (c 10)(15°)	10 11,12				

[a] In alphabetical order of parent sugar names within groups of increasing carbon chain length in the parent compounds.

[b] $[\alpha]_D$ for 1–5 g solute, c, per 100 ml aqueous solution at 20–25°C, unless otherwise given.

[c] References for melting point and specific rotation data. Letter indicates that the reference also has chromatographic data as follows: c = column, e = electrophoresis, g = gas, p = paper, and t = thin layer.

[d] R value times 100, given relative to that of the compound indicated by abbreviation: f = solvent front, aco = acovenose, amgl = tetraacetyl dimethyl glucitol, aral = arabinitol penta-acetate, cym = cymarose, cymo = cymaronolactone, damg = methyl 4,6-di-O-acetyl-2,3-di-O-methyl-α-D-lucopyranoside, digx = digitoxose, dmxyl = 2,3-di-O-methyl-xylitol triacetate, drho = 2-deoxy-rhamnonolactone, erya = erythritol tetraacetate, fuc = fucose, gal = galactose, gals = galactose 6-sulfate, glc = glucose, glca = glucitol hexaacetate, glcl = glucitol, glcs = glucitol trimethylsilyl ether, glct = glucose trimethylsilyl ether, hep = D-glycero-D-manno-heptonolactone, manl = mannitol hexaacetate, mant = mannose trimethylsilyl ether, mfuc = methyl α-fucopyranoside, mmt = methyl α-mannopyranose trimethylsilyl ether, ole = oleandrose, rha = rhamnose, rib = ribose, sor = sorbitol, temg = 2,3,4,6-tetra-O-methyl-glucose, αtemg = methyl 2,3,4,5-tetra-O-methyl-α-glucoside, βtemg = methyl 2,3,4,5-tetra-O-methyl-β-glucoside, temga = 2,3,4,6-tetra-O-methyl-glucitol diacetate, temgt = 2,3,4,6-tetra-O-methyl-galactose trimethylsilyl ether, βtrma = methyl 2,3,4-tri-O-methyl-β-D-arabinoside, trma = 2,3,4-tri-O-methyl-L-arabinose, trmal = 2,3,4-tri-O-methyl-L-arabinitol, xyl = xylose, and xyll = xylitol pentaacetate. Under gas chromatography (column GLC or G), numbers without code indication signify retention time in min. The conditions of the chromatography are correlated with the reference given in parentheses and are found in Table 5.

[e] As the methyl furanoside.

[f] Data are for the enanthiomorphic isomer.

[g] By inference from the enanthiomorphic isomer.

[h] Value is in cm/3.75 hr.

Table 3 (continued)
NATURAL ALDOSES

Substance[a] (synonym) derivative	Chemical formula	Melting point °C	Specific rotation[b] $[\alpha]_D$	Reference[c]	Chromatography, R value, and reference[d]			
					ELC	GLC	PPC	TLC
(A)	(B)	(C)	(D)	(E)	(F)	(G)	(H)	(I)
Benzylphenylhydrazone	$C_{18}H_{22}N_2O_4$	137–138	$[\alpha]_{570}$ −78.5 (C₅H₅N)	11,12				
Di-O-iso-propylidene ether	$C_{11}H_{20}O_5$		+54±1 (c 0.55, C₂H₅OH)	13c,p				
2,3,4-Tri-O-methyl ether	$C_9H_{16}O_5$		−1.7 (CH₃OH)	14		234αtemg (14a)	91temg (14b)	91temg (14c)
D-Glyceraldehyde, 3,3-bis-(C-hydroxymethyl)-3-deoxy- (cordycepose)	$C_7H_{10}O_4$	Syrup	−26 (c 0.6, C₂H₅OH)	15				
Cordyceponic acid phenyl hydrazide	$C_{11}H_{16}N_2O_4$	151	+26±3 (c 0.3, C₂H₅OH)	15				
β-D-Arabinose	$C_5H_{10}O_5$	155	−175→−103	16,411c	<10sor (5)		130f (6)	
Benzylphenylhydrazone	$C_{18}H_{22}N_2O_4$	177–178	+14.4 (CH₃OH)(16°)	18				

iNot, however, anomeric with aldgaroside A. Reference 88 assigns a 4-deoxy-β-D-*ribo*-hexopyranose or 4-deoxy-D-allose structure.

jValue is in cm/5 hr.

kAs the methyl pyranoside.

lThe reference is not clear as to D or L configuration.

mReference 202 structures this as a glycoside, not an ester; but it may be an ester in view of the recent comparative isolates of Reference 58 under D-ribose, C-hydroxymethyl-.

nThe inference is that olivomycose *iso*-butyrate exists in the parent antibiotic.

oValue is in cm/17 hr.

pValue is in cm/23 hr.

qReference 95 has the definitive names for tyvelose and abequose reversed from those of References 265 and 300.

rAlthough rhodinose is the L-isomer, it is not clear whether the sugar form in ydginic acid is D or L.

sEarly work had supported an L-*xylo*-configuration,[333] but additional study has established the L-*ribo*-.[320-322]

tA recent publication gives the reverse sign to the glycoside's optical rotation.

uA more recent publication has tentatively assigned the L-rhamnose configuration to the natural compound and called it nogalose.[349]

wThough never proved, some evidence exists for this sugar, or for L-altrose, in the polysaccharide varianose.

vAs data here are meager, see those for the enanthiomorphic isomer.

xColumn was at 210° instead of 140°.

yValue is for the D-*glycero*-L-*hexo*- isomer.

zThese may well be D-*glycero*-D-*manno*-, D-*glycero*-L-*manno*-, and L-*glycero*-D-*manno*- for References 404, 405, and 406, respectively; Reference 407 remains uncertain.

Table 3 (continued)
NATURAL ALDOSES

Substance[a] (synonym) derivative	Chemical formula	Melting point °C	Specific rotation[b] $[\alpha]_D$	Reference[c]	Chromatography, R value, and reference[d]			
					ELC	GLC	PPC	TLC
(A)	(B)	(C)	(D)	(E)	(F)	(G)	(H)	(I)
2,3,5-Tri-O-methyl ether	$C_7H_{14}O_5$	Syrup	+40 (CH_3OH)	20		39[e]temg (19b)	97temg (19a)	38,51f (40)[e]
Trimethylsilyl ether	$C_6H_{12}O_5$	Syrup	−102±3	21,22	42temg (19c)	33glct (9)	16f (19d)	56trma (23a)[f]
D-Arabinose, 2-O-methyl-								
2-O-Methyl-D-arabinitol	$C_6H_{14}O_5$	98—99	−11 (CH_3OH)	24				32trmal (23a)[f]
Methyl β-pyranoside	$C_7H_{14}O_5$	113	+55.4→+105	25				
Phenylhydrazone	$C_{12}H_{18}N_2O_4$	Amorphous, 158		26				
α-L-Arabinose	$C_6H_{10}O_5$	160	+190.6→+104.5	27		56βtrma (27a)		
β-L-Arabinose		181	+22.6 (1:1, C_5H_5N, C_2H_5OH)	31	30rib (28)		21f (29)	31f (30a)
p-Nitrophenylhydrazone	$C_{11}H_{15}N_3O_6$	97	+42.5 ($CHCl_3$)	32				
α-Pyranoside tetraacetate	$C_{13}H_{18}O_9$	86	+147.2 ($CHCl_3$)	32				
β-Pyranoside tetraacetate	$C_{13}H_{18}O_9$							
2,3,5-Tri-O-methyl ether	$C_9H_{16}O_5$	Syrup	0	33		7.07 (34)		167trma (23a)
Trimethylsilyl ether	$C_6H_{10}O_8S$	105	+75 (c 0.6)	35	118gals (35a)		83gal (35b)	46f (37)[f]
L-Arabinose 3-sulfate	$C_6H_{10}O_5$		+5.8→+13.5	36,411c	42rib (28)[f]		25f (29)	
α-L-Lyxose	$BrC_{11}H_{11}N_2O_4$	157—158	−30.1→−10 (C_5H_5N)	38				
p-Bromophenylhydrazone	$C_{11}H_{15}N_3O_6$	172		36				
p-Nitrophenylhydrazone	$C_{13}H_{18}O_9$	93—94	+25 ($CHCl_3$)[g]	39		26glct (9)		
α-Pyranoside tetraacetate								
Trimethylsilyl ether								
L-Lyxose, 5-deoxy-3-C-formyl- (streptose)	$C_6H_{10}O_5$	Syrup	−18	41				
Streptosonolactone	$C_6H_8O_5$	146—148	−37 (c 0.7)	42				
L-Lyxose, 5-deoxy-3-C-hydroxymethyl- (dihydrostreptose)	$C_6H_{12}O_6$	Syrup	−24	41,43				
Dihydrostreptosonolactone	$C_6H_{10}O_5$	140.5—142.5	−32	41				

Table 3 (continued)
NATURAL ALDOSES

Substance[a] (synonym) derivative (A)	Chemical formula (B)	Melting point °C (C)	Specific rotation[b] $[\alpha]_D$ (D)	Reference[c] (E)	Chromatography, R value, and reference[d]			
					ELC (F)	GLC (G)	PPC (H)	TLC (I)
L-Lyxose, 3-C-formyl-(hydroxystreptose)	$C_6H_{10}O_6$	No constants known	No constants known	44				
3-Hydroxy-2-hydroxy-methyl-1,4-pyrone	$C_6H_6O_4$	152–153		44				
L-Lyxose, 2-O-methyl-	$C_6H_{12}O_5$	120–121	+6	45				
Pyranoside triacetate	$C_{12}H_{18}O_8$	Syrup	−10.5 (CHCl₃)	46				
2,3,4-Tri-O-methyl ether	$C_9H_{18}O_5$	Syrup	−21.6	46				
Pentose, 4,5-anhydro-5-deoxy-D-erythro-	$C_5H_8O_3$	No constants known	No constants known	47ce			75f (47)	
Pentose, 2-deoxy-D-erythro- (2-deoxy-D-ribose)	$C_5H_{10}O_4$	96–98	−91→−58	4?	<10sor (5)		40f (49)	266glc (50)
p-Nitrophenylhydra-zone	$C_{11}H_{15}N_3O_6$	160	−11.1 (c 0.1, C₂H₅OH)(14°)	51				
Pyranoside triacetate	$C_{11}H_{16}O_7$	98	−171.8 (c 0.5, CHCl₃)	51				
Tetra-O-acetyl-2-deoxy-D-ribitol Trimethylsilyl ether	$C_{13}H_{18}O_8$					57xyll (52)		
D-Ribose	$C_5H_{10}O_5$	87	−23.7	53,411c	40sor (5)	6.53 (34)	25f (49)	39f (30a)
p-Bromophenylhydra-zone	$BrC_{11}H_{15}N_2O_4$	164–165	+10.3 (C₂H₅OH)	54				
α-Pyranoside tetra-acetate	$C_{13}H_{18}O_9$	Syrup	+46.1 (CH₃OH)	55				
β-Pyranoside tetra-acetate	$C_{13}H_{18}O_9$	110	−54.5 (CH₃OH)	55				
2,3,4-Tri-O-methyl ether	$C_8H_{16}O_5$	88.5–91		56		32glct (9)	62f (56)	
Trimethylsilyl ether D-Ribose, 2-C-hydroxy-methyl- (D-hamamelose)	$C_6H_{12}O_6$	110–111	+7.7→−7.0	57			18f (57)[f]	57f (59a)
Ammonium D-hamamel-onate	$C_6H_{15}NO_7$	152	$[\alpha]_{578}$ −3.9 (c 10)	57				

Table 3 (continued)
NATURAL ALDOSES

Substance[a] (synonym) derivative	Chemical formula	Melting point °C	Specific rotation[b] $[\alpha]_D$	Reference[c]	Chromatography, R value, and reference[d]			
					ELC	GLC	PPC	TLC
(A)	(B)	(C)	(D)	(E)	(F)	(G)	(H)	(I)
Hamamelonolactone	$C_9H_{10}O_6$	Syrup						
p-Nitrophenylhydrazone	$C_{15}H_{17}N_3O_7$	165–166	$[\alpha]_{578}$ +144 (C_5H_5N)	57			30f (57)[f]	
D-Ribose, 1',5-di-O-galloyl-2-C-hydroxymethyl- (hamamelitannin)	$C_{20}H_{20}O_{14}$	145–147.5	+31.3	58t			26f (58)	
Methyl α-furanoside	$C_{11}H_{22}O_{14} \cdot H_2O$	147–150	+33 (C_2H_5OH)	58				
Methyl α-furanoside hexamethyl ether	$C_{27}H_{34}O_{14}$	94–95	+43 (c 0.5, C_2H_5OH)	58			49f (58)	
Methyl β-furanoside	$C_{11}H_{22}O_{14} \cdot H_2O$	206–208	-30.6 (C_2H_5OH)	58				
Methyl β-furanoside hexamethyl ether	$C_{27}H_{34}O_{14}$	162.5–163.5	-28.5 (acetone)	58			54f (58)	
Ribose, 5-deoxy-5-S-methyl-5-thio- (5-methylthioribose)	$C_6H_{12}O_4S$	Syrup	+41.9 (CH_3OH)(30°)	60e,61			71f (60a)	55f (60b)
Trimethylsilyl ether						11.75 (60c)		
α-D-Xylose	$C_5H_{10}O_5$	145	+93.6→+18.8	62,63,411c	17rib (28)		15f (49)	33f (30a)
p-Bromophenylhydrazone	$BrC_{11}H_{15}N_2O_4$	128	-20.7	64,65				
α-Pyranoside tetraacetate	$C_{13}H_{18}O_9$	59	+89.3 ($CHCl_3$)	66				84f (69)
β-Pyranoside tetraacetate	$C_{13}H_{18}O_9$	128	-24.7 ($CHCl_3$)	66				
2,3,4-Tri-O-methyl ether	$C_8H_{16}O_5$	84–86	+45.5→+22 (c 0.7)	68		44,59[kβ] temg (67)	97temg (68)	28f (69)
Trimethylsilyl ether						8.47 (34)		57f (59a)
D-Xylose, 5-deoxy-	$C_5H_{10}O_4$	69–70d	+16	70				
p-Bromophenylhydrazone	$BrC_{11}H_{15}N_2O_3$		-26.1 (C_5H_5N)	71				
Triacetate Bis-Trimethylsilyl ether	$C_{11}H_{16}O_7$		+60.9 ($CHCl_3$)	71		4.5 (72)[e]		
D-Xylose, 2-O-methyl-	$C_6H_{12}O_5$	132–133	+37±6 (c 0.27)	73	6.8[h] (77)		38temg (74)	

Table 3 (continued)
NATURAL ALDOSES

Substance[a] (synonym) derivative	Chemical formula	Melting point °C	Specific rotation[b] $[\alpha]_D$	Reference[c]	Chromatography, R value, and reference[d]			
					ELC	GLC	PPC	TLC
(A)	(B)	(C)	(D)	(E)	(F)	(G)	(H)	(I)
Methyl glycosides	$C_7H_{14}O_6$	111–112 (β-anomer)	−67.7 (CHCl$_3$)(β-anomer)	75		411,623^{k}βtemg (80) 189dmxyl (76a)		
2-O-Methyl xylitol tetraacetate	$C_{14}H_{22}O_9$							
D-Xylose, 3-O-methyl-	$C_6H_{12}O_5$	95	+45→+19	77cp,78	13.6^h (77)		136xyl (82a)	
3-O-Methyl xylitol tetraacetate	$C_{14}H_{22}O_9$					189dmxyl (76a)		
3-O-Methyl-D-xylono-lactone	$C_6H_{10}O_5$	90	+72→+40 (c 0.9)	79cep				
Methyl glycosides	$C_7H_{14}O_5$					355,557^{k}βtemg (80)		
Phenylosazone	$C_{18}H_{22}N_4O_4$	172	+9±2	83				
D-Xylose, 4-O-methyl-	$C_6H_{12}O_5$	Syrup		81,82		233dmxyl (76b)	126xyl (82a)	
4-O-Methyl-D-xylose diethyl dithioacetal triacetate								
4-O-Methyl xylitol tetraacetate	$C_{14}H_{22}O_9$					54xyll (82c)		
Methyl glycosides	$C_7H_{14}O_5$	95 (β-anomer)	−69 (β-anomer) +25→0 (C$_2$H$_5$OH; C$_5$H$_5$N)	81		435^{k}βtemg (80)		
Phenylosazone	$C_{18}H_{22}N_4O_4$	158–158.5	−18	84				
L-Xylose, 3-O-methyl-	$C_6H_{12}O_5$			85		292temga (85c)	120rha (85a)	112rha (85b)
3-O-Methyl xylitol tetraacetate	$C_{14}H_{22}O_9$							
Methyl β-furanoside	$C_7H_{14}O_5$	No constants known	No constants known	87		14.61^f (86)		
Aldarose A (a dideoxy-C-hydroxyethylhexose carbonate)	$C_9H_{16}O_6$							
Methyl aldaroside A	$C_{10}H_{18}O_6$	91–94		87				
Aldarose B (a dideoxy-C-hydroxyethylhexose carbonate)	$C_9H_{16}O_6$	No constants known	No constants known	87				
Methyl aldaroside B'	$C_{10}H_{18}O_6$	175–177	−41 (CH$_3$OH)	87,88				

Table 3 (continued)
NATURAL ALDOSES

Substance[a] (synonym) derivative (A)	Chemical formula (B)	Melting point °C (C)	Specific rotation[b] $[\alpha]_D$ (D)	Reference[c] (E)	Chromatography, R value, and reference[d]			
					ELC (F)	GLC (G)	PPC (H)	TLC (I)
D-Allose	$C_6H_{12}O_6$	130–132	+14.5±0.3	89,90,411c	75rib (28)			
Allitol	$C_6H_{14}O_6$	150–151		90	92rib (28)			
Allitol hexaacetate							110glc (91a)	
Allonolactone	$C_6H_{10}O_6$	145–147	−6.7 (C_2H_5OH)	92		88manl (91b)	109f (383)	
p-Bromophenylhydra-zone	$BrC_{12}H_{17}N_2O_5$							
β-Pyranoside penta-acetate	$C_{16}H_{22}O_{11}$	93–93.5	−13.7 ($CHCl_3$)	93				
Trimethylsilyl ether						81glct (9)		
D-Allose, 6-deoxy-	$C_6H_{12}O_5$	132–135, 151–152	−4→+1.2	94	127rha (96a)		100rha (95)	44rha (96b)
p-Bromophenylhydra-zone	$BrC_{13}H_{17}N_2O_4$	138–140, 145–146	−21.9→−11.8 (C_5H_5N)	96,97				
6-Deoxy-D-allitol pentaacetate	$C_{16}H_{14}O_{10}$					55aral (98p)		
Pyranoside tetra-acetate	$C_{16}H_{20}O_9$	109–110	+10.4 ($CHCl_3$)	99,100				
D-Allose, 6-deoxy-2-O-methyl- (javose)	$C_7H_{14}O_5$	112–114	−54→−40,−8.2	94,101	8j (94a)		50aco (94b)	28f (102 ep)
Methyl α-pyranoside	$C_8H_{16}O_5$	Syrup	+90±3 ($CHCl_3$)	101				
Methyl β-pyranoside	$C_8H_{16}O_5$	97–98	−82.8±1 (CH_3OH)	102				
D-Allose, 6-deoxy-3-O-methyl-	$C_7H_{14}O_5$	122–123	+9 (30°)	103	16.5j (94a)		52aco (94b)	41f (102)
Methyl α-pyranoside	$C_8H_{16}O_5$	110–111	+195±5 (c 0.7, CH_3OH)	103t				129rha (96b, ep)
Methyl β-pyranoside	$C_8H_{16}O_5$	153–154	−37.1±2 (CH_3OH)	104c				
D-Allose, 6-deoxy-2,3-di-O-methyl- (mycinose)		102–106	−46→−29	105,411c				
Methyl α-pyranoside	$C_9H_{18}O_5$	88–88.5	+140 (c 0.7, $CHCl_3$), −36 ($CHCl_3$)(27°)	106t				
Methyl β-pyranoside	$C_9H_{18}O_5$	101–103	+32 (c 0.4, $CHCl_3$)	105,107t				
β-Pyranoside diacetate	$C_{13}H_{20}O_7$			106				
D-Altrose, 6-deoxy-	$C_6H_{12}O_5$	Syrup	+16.2	108	164rha (96a)		110rha (95)	128rha (96b)

Table 3 (continued)
NATURAL ALDOSES

Substance[a] (synonym) derivative	Chemical formula	Melting point °C	Specific rotation[b] $[\alpha]_D$	Reference[c]	Chromatography, R value, and reference[d]			
					ELC	GLC	PPC	TLC
(A)	(B)	(C)	(D)	(E)	(F)	(G)	(H)	(I)
p-Bromophenylhydrazone	$BrC_{12}H_{17}N_2O_4$	155. 177		109,110	104glcl (312)			
6-Deoxy-D-altritol (1-deoxy-D-talitol)	$C_6H_{14}O_5$							
6-Deoxy-D-altritol pentaacetate	$C_{16}H_{24}O_{10}$					61aral (98p)		
Methyl α-pyranoside	$C_7H_{14}O_5$	Syrup	+118 (CH₃OH)(16°)	109				
D-Altrose, 6-deoxy-3-O-methyl- (D-vallarose)	$C_7H_{14}O_5$	111–113	+8.6→+22.3 (c 0.6) (18°)	111,112				
Methyl α-pyranoside	$C_8H_{16}O_5$		+133±2	112				
α-Pyranoside triacetate	$C_{13}H_{20}O_8$	112–113	+14.8±2 (15°) (CHCl₃)	112				
β-Pyranoside triacetate	$C_{13}H_{20}O_8$	79	-96.5±2 (15°) (CHCl₃)	112				
D-Altrose, 6-deoxy-4-O-methyl- (sordarose)	$C_7H_{14}O_5$	Syrup	+29 (c 0.45)	113				139rha (113)
Methyl α-pyranoside	$C_8H_{16}O_5$		+153 (CH₃OH)	113t				
Methyl β-pyranoside	$C_8H_{16}O_5$		-12 (CH₃OH)	113t				
L-Altrose, 6-deoxy-	$C_6H_{12}O_5$	Gum	-16.1±2	114pt				
L-Altrose, 6-deoxy-3-O-methyl- (L-vallarose)	$C_7H_{14}O_5$	106–110	-17.2±2 (c 0.9)	115	20j (94a)		75aco (94b)	154rha (96b, cp)
α-Pyranoside triacetate	$C_{13}H_{20}O_8$	112–113s, 122–123	-12±1 (CHCl₃)	116t				
Antiarose	$C_6H_{12}O_5$	Syrup	levo	117,118				
Antiaronolactone	$C_6H_{10}O_5$	Syrup	-30	117,118				
Antiaronic acid phenylhydrazide	$C_{12}H_{18}N_2O_5$	143–145		117,118				
α-D-Galactose	$C_6H_{12}O_6$	167	+150.7→+80.2	119	28rib (28)		6f (49)	21f (30a)
Pyranose tetramethyl ether	$C_{10}H_{20}O_6$	71–73	+149.4→+116.9	120			92temg (68)	78f (30b)
α-Pyranoside pentaacetate	$C_{16}H_{22}O_{11}$	96	+106.7 (CHCl₃)	122				
Trimethylsilyl ether					8.94 (34)		66f (59)	

Table 3 (continued)
NATURAL ALDOSES

Substance[a] (synonym) derivative	Chemical formula	Melting point °C	Specific rotation[b] $[\alpha]_D$	Reference[c]	Chromatography, R value, and reference[d]			
					ELC	GLC	PPC	TLC
(A)	(B)	(C)	(D)	(E)	(F)	(G)	(H)	(I)
α-D-Galactopyranoside, ethyl-	$C_8H_{16}O_6$	143	+185	121			35f (150)	
β-D-Galactose	$C_6H_{12}O_6$	143–145	+52.8→+80.2	119,411c				
p-Nitrophenylhydrazone	$C_{12}H_{17}N_3O_7$	192	+70 (c 0.3, C_5H_5N-C_2H_5OH)	31				
β-Pyranoside penta-acetate	$C_{16}H_{22}O_{11}$	142	+25 (CHCl$_3$)	122				81f (69)
Dimethyl acetal						108glct (9)		54f (59)
D-Galactose, 3,6-anhydro-	$C_6H_{10}O_5$		+12,+21.3 (10°)	123–125				
Trimethylsilyl ether	$C_6H_6O_5$		+29 (17°)	125			170rha (124)	
Diphenylhydrazone	$C_{18}H_{20}N_2O_4$	153–155	+34.5→+23.6 (CH$_3$OH) (14°)	124				
Methyl α-pyranoside	$C_7H_{12}O_5$	109, 139–140	+80,+175 (10°)	123,124				
D-Galactose, 4,6-O-(1-carboxyethylidene)-	$C_9H_{14}O_8$	No constants known	No constants known	126				
Ammonium salt	$C_9H_{17}NO_8$		+51 (c 0.43)	127			20gal (127)	
Ethanolate	$C_9H_{14}O_8 \cdot C_2H_5OH$		+49	126				
4,6-O-ethylidene methyl ester)-D-galactitol	$C_{10}H_{18}O_8$	104–105	−18 (c 0.6, CH$_3$OH)	126				
Methyl α-pyranoside methyl ester	$C_{11}H_{18}O_8$	Syrup	+133 (CHCl$_3$)	128				
α-D-Galactose, 6-deoxy-(D-fucose, rhodeose)	$C_6H_{12}O_5$	140–145	+120→+76.3 (c 10)	129,412c			19f (49)	25f (130)
Benzylphenylhydrazone	$C_{19}H_{24}N_2O_4$	178–179	−14.9 (c 0.4, CH$_3$OH)	129				
6-Deoxy-D-galactitol	$C_6H_{14}O_5$				100sor (132)			
Fucitol pentaacetate	$C_{16}H_{24}O_{10}$					7.7 (131)		
α-Pyranoside tetra-acetate	$C_{14}H_{22}O_9$	92–93	+129 (CHCl$_3$)	133				
Trimethylsilyl ether						6.2.7.1 (59b)	180fuc (135)	61.69f (59a)
D-Galactose, 6-deoxy-2-O-methyl-	$C_7H_{14}O_5$	155–161	+73→+87	134				

Table 3 (continued)
NATURAL ALDOSES

Substance[a] (synonym) derivative	Chemical formula	Melting point °C	Specific rotation[b] $[\alpha]_D$	Reference[c]	Chromatography, R value, and reference[d]			
					ELC	GLC	PPC	TLC
(A)	(B)	(C)	(D)	(E)	(F)	(G)	(H)	(I)
Methyl α-pyranoside	$C_8H_{16}O_6$	Syrup	+173.6	136			180mfuc (136)	
Methyl β-pyranoside	$C_8H_{16}O_6$	98.5–99.5	+3.5 (CH₃OH)	136				
D-Galactose, 6-deoxy-3-O-methyl- (digitalose)	$C_7H_{14}O_5$	106, 119	+106	137	12.5^j (94a)		30aco (94b)	104rha (96b, ep)
Digitalonolactone	$C_7H_{12}O_6$	137–138	−83	137			217mfuc (136)	
Methyl α-pyranoside	$C_8H_{16}O_5$	98.5–100	+198 (c 0.7, CH₃OH)	136			163mfuc (136)	
Methyl β-pyranoside	$C_8H_{16}O_5$	108–110	+9.9 (c 0.3, CH₃OH)	136			142mfuc (136)	
D-Galactose, 6-deoxy-4-O-methyl- (curacose)	$C_7H_{14}O_5$	131–132	+102.6→+80.6 (c 0.9)	38,138			52f (38)	
Methyl β-pyranoside p-Tolylsulfonylhydrazone	$C_8H_{16}O_5$ / $C_{14}H_{22}N_2O_6S$	144–145 / 134	−14.6 (c 0.9, CH₃OH) / −16→−3 (C₅H₅N)	138 / 138				
D-Galactose, 6-deoxy-2,3-di-O-methyl-	$C_8H_{16}O_5$	75–76	+73,+105	136,139			267fuc (135)	
Methyl α-pyranoside	$C_8H_{16}O_5$	Syrup	+190 (acetone)	135,136			85temg (136)	
Methyl β-pyranoside	$C_8H_{16}O_5$	Syrup	+0.7 (acetone)	135,136			97temg (136)	
Onic acid phenylhydrazide	$C_{14}H_{22}N_2O_6$	99–103	+21.5±3 (c 0.7, CH₃OH)	135				
D-Galactose, 6-deoxy-2,4-di-O-methyl- (labilose)	$C_8H_{16}O_5$	129	+82 (c 0.5)(27°)	140cp			275fuc (135)	
Labilitol	$C_8H_{18}O_5$		+37.4 (c 0.5, CHCl₃) (30°)	140				17f (140a)
Methyl α-pyranoside	$C_9H_{18}O_5$	85	+176 (CHCl₃)(30°)	140				13f (140b)
Methyl β-pyranoside	$C_9H_{18}O_5$	111	−20.9 (CHCl₃)(30°)	140				18f (140b)
Methyl α-D-fucopyranoside trimethyl ether	$C_{13}H_{24}O_5$	96	+213 (c 0.3)	140		4.6 (140c)		28f (140b)
Methyl β-D-fucopyranoside trimethyl ether	$C_{13}H_{24}O_5$	93–98	+11.2	173				

Table 3 (continued)
NATURAL ALDOSES

Substance[a] (synonym) derivative	Chemical formula	Melting point °C	Specific rotation[b] $[\alpha]_D$	Reference[c]	Chromatography, R value, and reference[d]			
					ELC	GLC	PPC	TLC
(A)	(B)	(C)	(D)	(E)	(F)	(G)	(H)	(I)
D-Galactose, 2-O-methyl-								
Methyl α-pyranoside	$C_7H_{14}O_6$	148–149	+84.9 (c 0.5)(16°)	141			35temg (68)	
Methyl β-pyranoside	$C_7H_{14}O_6$	Syrup	+180 (CH₃OH)	142				
2-O-Methyl-N-phenyl-D-galactosylamine	$C_{13}H_{18}O_6$	131–132	+1.69	142,143				
2-O-Methyl-D-galactitol trimethylsilyl ether	$C_{13}H_{19}NO_5$	164–164		141		289temgt (144)		
D-Galactose, 3-O-methyl- (madurose)	$C_7H_{14}O_6$	144–147	+150→+108	145,146			73rib (145a)	2f (30b)
Methyl β-pyranoside	$C_8H_{16}O_6$	Syrup	+31.9	146				
3-O-Methyl-D-galactitol trimethylsilyl ether Trimethylsilyl ether						294temgt (144)		
D-Galactose, 4-O-methyl-								
4-O-Methyl-D-galactitol trimethylsilyl ether	$C_7H_{14}O_6$	207, 218	+62→+92	147–149		16 (145b)	31f (150)	2f (30b)
						294temgt (144)		
4-O-Methyl-N-phenyl-D-galactosylamine Trimethylsilyl ether	$C_{13}H_{19}NO_5$	167–168	−84→−39 (CH₃OH)	148		19,26 (149)		
D-Galactose, 6-O-methyl-								
6-O-Methyl-D-galactitol trimethylsilyl ether	$C_7H_{14}O_6$	119–120	+76 (17°)	141		299temgt (144)	85rib (145a)	
Methyl α-pyranoside	$C_6H_{14}O_6$	137–138	+165	151		200βtemg (67)		6f (69)
Methyl pyranoside tetramethyl ether	$C_{13}H_{23}O_6$							21,28f (40)
Phenylhydrazone	$C_{13}H_{20}N_2O_5$	181.5–182.5	+52 (as Ba salt)	152	100glcs (153a)			
D-Galactose 2-sulfate	$C_6H_{12}O_9S$		+64 (c 0.5)(as NH₄ salt)	153	104glc (155a)		24gal (153b)	
D-Galactose 4-sulfate	$C_6H_{12}O_9S$		+58.4 (16°)(as Na salt)	154			27f (155b)	
				155				

Table 3 (continued)
NATURAL ALDOSES

Substance[a] (synonym) derivative	Chemical formula	Melting point °C	Specific rotation[b] [α]_D	Reference[c]	Chromatography, R value, and reference[d]			
					ELC	GLC	PPC	TLC
(A)	(B)	(C)	(D)	(E)	(F)	(G)	(H)	(I)
D-Galactose 6-sulfate	$C_6H_{11}O_9S$		+49 (c 0.33)(as NH_4 salt); +47 (16°)(as Na salt)	154	132glc (155a)			
L-Galactose	$C_6H_{12}O_6$	163–165	−78	155			13f (155b)	
Phenylhydrazone	$C_{12}H_{18}N_2O_5$	158–160		156				
L-Galactose, 3,6-anhydro-	$C_6H_{10}O_5$		+21.6	157				
Dimethyl acetal	$C_8H_{16}O_6$		−39.4→−25.2; −16.2	158; 159cgp				50f (159a)
3,6-Anhydro-L-dulcitol	$C_6H_{12}O_5$	138.5–140	−10	160gpt				
Methyl α-pyranoside	$C_7H_{12}O_5$	118	−77 (c 0.9)(19°)	161				
Methyl β-pyranoside	$C_7H_{12}O_5$		−113.5	162				
L-Galactose, 3,6-anhydro-2-O-methyl-	$C_7H_{12}O_5$		−14.3 (c 0.6)(12°)	153,163				
Dimethyl acetal	$C_9H_{18}O_6$		−20.4	159cgp				60f (159a)
3,6-Anhydro-2-O-methyl-dulcitol	$C_7H_{14}O_5$		−13	160gpt				
3,6-Anhydro-2-O-methyl-L-galactonic acid	$C_7H_{12}O_6$	141–142	−70.3 (c 0.8)(12°)	158				
Methyl α-pyranoside	$C_8H_{14}O_5$						49f (160)	70f (159b)
Methyl β-pyranoside	$C_8H_{14}O_5$							80f (159b)
α-L-Galactose, 6-deoxy- (L-fucose)	$C_6H_{12}O_5$	145	−124.1→−76.4	163	22rib (28)		83rha (95)	49f (37)
6-Deoxy-L-galactitol (L-fucitol)	$C_6H_{14}O_5$						94rha (95)	
L-Fucitol pentaacetate	$C_{16}H_{24}O_{10}$	126.5–127.5		52		73xyll (52)		
L-Fucitol trimethylsilyl ether						8.33 (167)		
Methyl α-pyranoside	$C_7H_{14}O_5$	158–159	−191 (18°)	164			53temg (164)	
Methyl β-pyranoside	$C_7H_{14}O_5$	126–127	+10.5 (18°)	164			48temg (164)	

Table 3 (continued)
NATURAL ALDOSES

Substance[a] (synonym) derivative	Chemical formula	Melting point °C	Specific rotation[b] $[\alpha]_D$	Reference[c]	Chromatography, R value, and reference[d]			
					ELC	GLC	PPC	TLC
(A)	(B)	(C)	(D)	(E)	(F)	(G)	(H)	(I)
α-Pyranoside tetraacetate	$C_{14}H_{20}O_9$	92–93	-113 (CHCl$_3$)	165				
β-Pyranoside tetraacetate	$C_{14}H_{20}O_9$	172	-39 (CHCl$_3$)	166	—			
Trimethylsilyl ether						7.2 (34)	60temg (164)	
L-Galactose, 6-deoxy-2-O-methyl-	$C_7H_{14}O_5$	149–150	-68→-85 (18°)	164,168				
Methyl α-pyranoside	$C_8H_{16}O_5$	Syrup	-179 (26°) (CH$_3$OH)	136			180mfuc (136)	
Methyl β-pyranoside	$C_8H_{16}O_5$	98–99	+17.2 (c 0.5) (CH$_3$OH)	136			217mfuc (136)	
L-Galactose, 6-deoxy-3-O-methyl- (L-digitalose)	$C_7H_{14}O_5$	110	-97	164,170gpt			45glc (169)	
Phenyl osazone	$C_9H_{16}O_5$ / $C_{19}H_{24}N_4O_3$	76–78, 130–132 / 178–179d	-200,-173 (c 0.4)	169,170pt / 169			92temg (164)	
2,3,4-Tri-O-methyl-L-fucose	$C_9H_{18}O_5$	36–37	-184→-128	172				
Methyl α-L-fucopyranoside trimethyl ether	$C_{10}H_{18}O_5$	97–98	-209	164,172			72βtemg (80)	
Methyl β-L-fucopyranoside trimethyl ether	$C_{10}H_{18}O_5$	101.5–102.5	-21.1	172				
L-Galactose, 6-deoxy-, 4-sulfate	$C_9H_{18}O_5S$		-55	174g	100gals (175a)		81glc (175b)	
L-Galactose, 2-O-methyl-	$C_7H_{14}O_6$		-75 (c 0.5)(18°)	153ep				
2-O-Methyl-L-galactonolactone	$C_7H_{12}O_6$		+17 (18°)	153				
L-Galactose, 3-O-methyl-	$C_7H_{14}O_6$			159p	74xyl (159c)			
L-Galactose, 4-O-methyl-	$C_7H_{14}O_6$	203–206	-84 (17°)	141gp				
4-O-Methyl-N-phenyl-L-galactopyranosyl amine	$C_{13}H_{19}NO_6$	167–168		176				

Table 3 (continued)
NATURAL ALDOSES

Substance[a] (synonym) derivative	Chemical formula	Melting point °C	Specific rotation[b] $[\alpha]_D$	Reference[c]	ELC	GLC	PPC	TLC
(A)	(B)	(C)	(D)	(E)	(F)	(G)	(H)	(I)
						Chromatography, R value, and reference[d]		
L-Galactose, 6-O-methyl[l]	$C_7H_{14}O_6$			159	92xyl (159c)			
L-Galactose 3-sulfate	$C_6H_{12}O_9S$	Syrup	-32 (c 0.56)(as NH_4 salt)	127			75gal (127)	
L-Galactose 6-sulfate	$C_6H_{12}O_9S$	Syrup	-43 (c 0.56)(as NH_4 salt)	127			56gal (127)	
			-47 (c 0.2)(as Na salt)	177				
α-D-Glucopyranoside, ethyl-	$C_8H_{16}O_6$	113-114	+150.3	1,180c			60f (180a)	
Tetra-p-nitrobenzoate	$C_{34}H_{23}N_4O_{18}$	110-115		1				
Trifluoroacetate								
β-D-Glucopyranoside, ethyl-	$C_8H_{16}O_6$	98-100	-37.9	1,180c		6.2 (180b)		
Tetraacetate	$C_{16}H_{24}O_{10}$	101-108	+16.2 ($CHCl_3$)	1				78f (69)
Tetra-p-nitrobenzoate	$C_{34}H_{23}N_4O_{18}$	215-216	+28 (18°)(acetone)	1				
Trifluoroacetate								
Trimethylsilyl ether						10.1 (180b) 195mmt (192)		
β-D-Glucopyranoside, methyl-	$C_7H_{14}O_6$	102-104	-32	181	6rib (28)		24f (150)	61f (30c)
Tetraacetate	$C_{15}H_{22}O_{10}$	104-105	-18.7 ($CHCl_3$)	182,183		358damg (184)		76f (69)
2,3,4,6-Tetramethyl ether[k]	$C_{11}H_{22}O_6$	40-41	-17.3	185		100, 143βtemg (80)		46f (40)
Trimethylsilyl ether						49, 107glct (9)		
α-D-Glucose	$C_6H_{12}O_6$	146	+112→+52.7	186,411c	16rib (28)		8f (49)	25f (30a)
Methyl α-pyranoside	$C_7H_{14}O_6$	166	+158.9	186	9rib (28)		20f (49)	29f (130)
Methyl α-pyranoside tetramethyl ether	$C_{11}H_{22}O_6$	Syrup	+144 (acetone)	194,195		6.9 (189)		29f (40)
Monohydrate	$C_6H_{12}O_6 \cdot H_2O$	83		186				
Pentaacetate	$C_{16}H_{22}O_{11}$	114	+101.6 ($CHCl_3$)	182,187			27f (188a)	68f (188b)
2,3,4,6-Tetra-O-methyl-D-glucopyranose							82f (150)	86f (30b)
Trimethylsilyl ether	$C_{10}H_{20}O_6$	96	+92→+84	193	0 (5, 28)	100glct (9)		66f (59)

Table 3 (continued)
NATURAL ALDOSES

Substance[a] (synonym) derivative (A)	Chemical formula (B)	Melting point °C (C)	Specific rotation[b] [α]$_D$ (D)	Reference[c] (E)	Chromatography, R value, and reference[d] — ELC (F)	GLC (G)	PPC (H)	TLC (I)
β-D-Glucose	C$_6$H$_{12}$O$_6$	148–150	+18.7→+52.7	186				
p-Nitrophenylhydra-zone	C$_{12}$H$_{17}$N$_3$O$_7$	189	+21.5 (C$_2$H$_5$N, C$_2$H$_5$OH)	65,191				
			−88 (c 0.5)	31				
Pentaacetate	C$_{16}$H$_{22}$O$_{11}$	135	+3.8 (c 7, CHCl$_3$)	182,190			21f (188a)	81f (69)
Trimethylsilyl ether						157glct (9)	28temg (197)	56f (59)
D-Glucose 6-acetate	C$_8$H$_{14}$O$_7$	133–135	+48	196,197				
Phenylhydrazone	C$_{14}$H$_{20}$N$_2$O$_6$	136	−13	197				
Tetrabenzoate	C$_{35}$H$_{30}$O$_{11}$	183–184	+30.2 (CHCl$_3$)	198				
D-Glucose 6-acetate, 2,3,4-tri-O-[(+)-3-methyl-valeryl]-	C$_{26}$H$_{44}$O$_{10}$	104–106		199c				
D-Glucose 1-benzoate (periplanetin)	C$_{13}$H$_{16}$O$_7$	193	−26.8	178p, 179				
Tetraacetate	C$_{23}$H$_{34}$O$_{11}$	140–141		178				
D-Glucose 6-benzoate	C$_{13}$H$_{16}$O$_7$	Amorphous	+48 (C$_2$H$_5$OH)	200				
Monohydrate	C$_{13}$H$_{16}$O$_7$ · H$_2$O	104–106		178				
β-Pyranoside tetra-acetate	C$_{21}$H$_{24}$O$_{11}$	132	+32.9 (CHCl$_3$)	201				
D-Glucose 4-gallate[m]	C$_{13}$H$_{16}$O$_{10}$	211–212	−25.6 (18°)	202[m]				
Heptaacetate	C$_{27}$H$_{30}$O$_{17}$	125–126	−24.3 (acetylene tetrachloride)	202				
D-Glucose 1-γ-hydroxy-α-methylene-butyrate (1-tuliposide A)	C$_{11}$H$_{18}$O$_8$		+64	203			312glc (203)	
D-Glucose 6-γ-hydroxy-α-methylene-butyrate (6-tuliposide A)	C$_{11}$H$_{18}$O$_8$	No constants known	No constants known	203				
D-Glucose 1-β,γ-di hydroxy-α-methylene-butyrate (1-tuliposide B)	C$_{11}$H$_{18}$O$_8$		+56	203			149glc (203)	

Table 3 (continued)
NATURAL ALDOSES

Substance[a] (synonym) derivative (A)	Chemical formula (B)	Melting point °C (C)	Specific rotation[b] $[\alpha]_D$ (D)	Reference[c] (E)	Chromatography, R value, and reference[d] — ELC (F)	GLC (G)	PPC (H)	TLC (I)
D-Glucose ? (tuliposide C)	?	No constants known	No constants known	203			100glc (203)	
D-Glucose 3-malonate	$C_9H_{14}O_9$	No constants known	No constants known	212p				
D-Glucose di-β-nitro-propionate (endecaphyllin D)	$C_{12}H_{18}N_2O_{12}$	145–146		204t				
(endecaphyllin E)	$C_{12}H_{18}N_2O_{12}$	132–134, 138		204,205			27temg (205)	
D-Glucose tri-β-nitro-propionate (endecaphyllin A, karakin)	$C_{15}H_{21}N_3O_{15}$	120–122	+4.5	204,205p				
Monoacetate	$C_{17}H_{23}N_3O_{16}$	125.5–126.5		204				
Diacetate	$C_{19}H_{25}N_3O_{17}$	103		205				
(endecaphyllin B)	$C_{15}H_{21}N_3O_{15}$	125–126.5		204				
(endecaphyllin C)	$C_{15}H_{21}N_3O_{15}$	150–152.5		204				
D-Glucose tetra-β-nitro-propionate (endecaphyllin X, hiptagin)	$C_{18}H_{24}N_4O_{18}$	104–105.5		204,206				
D-Glucose, 4,6-O-(1'-carboxyethylidene)	$C_9H_{14}O_8$	No constants known	No constants known	207				
α-D-Glucose, 6-deoxy- (chinovose, epirhamnose, quinovose)	$C_6H_{12}O_5$	139–140	+73.3→+29.7 (c 8)	208,411c	148rha (96a)		96rha (96c)	99rha (96b)
6-Deoxy-D-glucitol (1-deoxy-L-gulitol)	$C_6H_{14}O_5$				94glc (312)			
D-Glucomethylonic acid lactone	$C_6H_{10}O_5$	151–152	+66.9→+5.4	209				
Methyl α-pyranoside trimethylsilyl ether						3.4 (210a)		
Methyl β-pyranoside trimethylsilyl ether						3.6 (210a)		
Methyl α- or β-pyranoside	$C_7H_{14}O_5$							48f (210b)
Pyranoside tetraacetate	$C_{14}H_{20}O_9$	145	+23 (CHCl₃)	211				

Table 3 (continued)
NATURAL ALDOSES

Substance[a] (synonym) derivative	Chemical formula[b]	Melting point °C	Specific rotation[b] $[\alpha]_D$	Reference[c]	Chromatography, R value, and reference[d]			
(A)	(B)	(C)	(D)	(E)	ELC (F)	GLC (G)	PPC (H)	TLC (I)
α-D-Glucose, 6-deoxy-3-O-methyl- (D-thevetose)	$C_7H_{14}O_5$	116, 126	+84→+33	213,214 cp	15.5ʲ (94a)		50aco (94b)	
Methyl α-pyranoside	$C_8H_{16}O_5$	86–87	+148±2	215				
Methyl α-pyranoside triacetate	$C_{13}H_{20}O_8$	105	+122 (acetone)	213				
Methyl β-pyranoside	$C_8H_{16}O_5$	116–117	-44±2	215				
Methyl β-pyranoside triacetate	$C_{13}H_{20}O_8$	121	+6 (acetone)	213				
D-Glucose, 6-deoxy-2,3-di-O-methyl-	$C_8H_{16}O_5$	Syrup	+40.4±2	216ep				
Methyl β-pyranoside	$C_9H_{18}O_5$	76–78	-49 (CHCl₃)	216				
D-Glucose, 6-deoxy-6-sulfonic acid (6-sulfoquinovose)	$C_6H_{13}O_8S$	No constants known	No constants known	217				
Allyl α-pyranoside cyclohexylamine salt	$C_{15}H_{29}NO_6S$	151.5–153	$[\alpha]Na_{589}$ +86	217			39f (217)	
Methyl α-pyranoside cyclohexylamine salt	$C_{13}H_{27}NO_5S$	173–174	+87	217				
α-D-Glucose, 3-O-methyl-	$C_7H_{14}O_6$	162–167	+98→+59.5 (c 0.4)	218c	13rib (28)		184glc (219a)	22f (219c)
Methyl α-pyranoside	$C_8H_{16}O_6 \cdot \tfrac{1}{2}H_2O$	80–81	+164±2 (c 0.9)	220				
Methyl α-pyranoside triacetate	$C_{14}H_{22}O_9$					180damg (184)		
Trimethylsilyl ether						3.46 (219b)		
β-D-Glucose, 3-O-methyl-	$C_7H_{14}O_6$	130–132	+31.9→+55.1	221	90glc (223)			4f (30b)
3-O-Methyl-N-phenyl-D-glucopyranoside	$C_{13}H_{19}NO_5$	152–153	-108→-46±2 (c 0.5, CH₃OH)	223				
Methyl β-pyranoside	$C_8H_{16}O_6$	Syrup	-26 (c 5.5)	222		266damg (184)		
Methyl β-pyranoside triacetate	$C_{14}H_{22}O_9$							
Penta-O-acetyl-3-O-methyl-D-glucitol	$C_{17}H_{26}O_{11}$					181amgl (184)		
β-Pyranoside tetraacetate	$C_{15}H_{22}O_{10}$	95–96	-5.2 (CHCl₃)	224				

Table 3 (continued)
NATURAL ALDOSES

Substance[a] (synonym) derivative	Chemical formula	Melting point °C	Specific rotation[b] $[\alpha]_D$	Reference[c]	Chromatography, R value, and reference[d]			
(A)	(B)	(C)	(D)	(E)	ELC (F)	GLC (G)	PPC (H)	TLC (I)
D-Glucose, 6-O-methyl-	$C_7H_{14}O_6$	139–141	+57.5	225	87glc (219d)		176glc (219a)	22f (219c)
Methyl α-pyranoside	$C_8H_{16}O_6$	Syrup	+127.9	226				
Methyl α-pyranoside triacetate	$C_{14}H_{22}O_9$	133–135	-27	227		110damg (184)		
Methyl β-pyranoside	$C_8H_{16}O_6$							
Methyl β-pyranoside triacetate	$C_{14}H_{22}O_9$					139damg (184)		
α-Pyranoside tetraacetate	$C_{15}H_{22}O_{10}$	119–120	+111.8 (CHCl₃)	228				
β-Pyranoside tetraacetate	$C_{15}H_{22}O_{10}$	91–93	+20.9 (CHCl₃)	228				
Trimethylsilyl ether α-D-Glucose, 2,3-di-O-methyl-	$C_8H_{18}O_6$	85–87	+81.9→+48.3 (acetone)	135,221		3.76 (219b)	211fuc (135)	
Methyl α-pyranoside	$C_7H_8O_6$	80–82	+142.6	221				13f (69)
Methyl α-pyranoside diacetate	$C_{11}H_{12}O_8$					15 (184)		
Tetra-O-acetyl-2,3-di-O-methyl-D-glucitol	$C_{14}H_{26}O_{10}$					29 (184)		
β-D-Glucose, 2,3-di-O-methyl-	$C_8H_{16}O_6$	108–110, 121	+5.9→+50.9 (acetone)	221,229	20.6glc (19c)		57lemg (19a)	
2,3-Di-O-methyl-N-phenyl-D-glucopyranosylamine	$C_{14}H_{21}NO_5$	134	-83 (CHCl₃)	230				
Methyl β-pyranoside	$C_7H_8O_6$	62–64	-36.6	222				
Methyl β-pyranoside diacetate	$C_{11}H_{12}O_8$					72.5damg (184)		
α-L-Glucose	$C_6H_{12}O_6$	141–143 143–145	-95.5→-51.4 -84.7→-30.1	231 232,233				
L-Glucose, 6-deoxy- (*epi*-rhamnose)	$C_6H_{12}O_5$						97rha (95)	
Diethyl mercaptal	$C_{10}H_{22}O_4S_2$	97–98	+47.1	233				
L-Glucose, 6-deoxy-3-O-methyl- (L-thevetose)	$C_7H_{14}O_5$	126–129	-36.9±2	234	99rha (96a)		247rha (96c)	153rha (96b)

Table 3 (continued)
NATURAL ALDOSES

Substance[a] (synonym) derivative	Chemical formula	Melting point °C	Specific rotation[b] $[\alpha]_D$	Reference[c]	Chromatography, R value, and reference[d]			
					ELC	GLC	PPC	TLC
(A)	(B)	(C)	(D)	(E)	(F)	(G)	(H)	(I)
α-Pyranoside triacetate	$C_{13}H_{20}O_8$	103–104	−113 (CH₃OH)	235,236				
β-Pyranoside triacetate	$C_{13}H_{20}O_8$	118–119	−7.5±2 (acetone)	234				
D-Gulose, 6-deoxy- (antiarose)	$C_6H_{12}O_5$	130–131	−38	71,237	115rha (96a)		106rha (96c)	43rha (96b)
p-Bromophenylhydrazone	$BrC_{12}H_{17}N_2O_4$	135–136	−49→−34.7 (C_5H_5N)	71				
6-Deoxy-D-gulono-lactone	$C_6H_{10}O_5$	180–181		71				
6-Deoxy-D-gulitol pentaacetate	$C_{16}H_{24}O_{10}$					83aral (238a)		
Tetra-O-acetylglycoside	$C_{14}H_{20}O_9$	137–139	+5.2 (CHCl₃)	239	53^{f}rib (28)		13^f (49)	
L-Gulose	$C_6H_{12}O_6$		+21.3	240,241, 411c				
L-Gulono-γ-lactone	$C_6H_{10}O_6$	183–185	+55	242				
Methyl α-pyranoside	$C_7H_{14}O_6$	77^f	+109.4^f	186				
Methyl α-pyranoside tetraacetate	$C_{15}H_{22}O_{10}$	96–97	−96.5 (c 0.8, CHCl₃)	240				
Methyl β-pyranoside	$C_7H_{14}O_6$	176^f	−83.3^f	186				
Methyl β-pyranoside tetraacetate	$C_{15}H_{22}O_{10}$	64–66.5	+33 (CHCl₃)	240				
Methyl pyranoside tetramethyl ether	$C_{11}H_{22}O_6$	No constants known	No constants known			1.37 (243)		
Trimethylsilyl ether						66, 74glct (9)		91rha (244a)
L-Gulose, 6-deoxy-	$C_6H_{12}O_5$	135–137	+13±2 (C_2H_5OH)	244				
p-Bromophenylhydrazone	$BrC_{12}H_{17}N_2O_4$			244	98glcl (312)			
6-Deoxy-L-gulitol (1-deoxy-D-glucitol)	$C_6H_{14}O_5$							
Methyl α-pyranoside triacetate	$C_{13}H_{20}O_8$	Syrup	+35 (CHCl₃)	244				73f (244b)
Methyl β-pyranoside triacetate	$C_{13}H_{20}O_8$	Syrup	−55 (CHCl₃)	244				62f (244b)

Table 3 (continued)
NATURAL ALDOSES

Chromatography, R value, and reference[d] (columns F–I)

Substance[a] (synonym) derivative (A)	Chemical formula (B)	Melting point °C (C)	Specific rotation[b] $[\alpha]_D$ (D)	Reference[c] (E)	ELC (F)	GLC (G)	PPC (H)	TLC (I)
Methyl 6-deoxy-L-guloside	$C_7H_{14}O_5$	Syrup	None (meso)	245		4 (244c)		
Hexodialdose, D-*galacto*-	$C_8H_{10}O_6$							
Methyl β-pyranoside	$C_7H_{12}O_6$	206–108	+41.6 (CHCl$_3$)	246c			60f (245)	46f (246)
Methyl β-pyranoside dimer hexaacetate	$C_{26}H_{36}O_{18}$	184d		247				
Tetraacetate	$C_{14}H_{18}O_{10}$			246				
Hexodialdo-1,5-pyranose, 4-deoxy-4-ene-L-*threo*-	$C_6H_8O_5$	No constants known	No constants known					
2,4-Dinitrophenyl-hydrazone	$C_{12}H_{12}N_4O_8$	148–152	+32 (c 6.1, CH$_3$OH)	246				75f (246)
Methyl α-pyranoside diacetate	$C_{11}H_{14}O_7$		+309 (CHCl$_3$)	248t				
Methyl β-pyranoside diacetate	$C_{11}H_{14}O_7$			248t				
Hexopyranose, 1,1'-anhydro-2,6-dideoxy-4-C-(1'-hydroxyethyl)-	$C_8H_{14}O_4$	153–154	−144	249				
3,5-Dinitrobenzoate	$C_{15}H_{16}N_2O_9$	167–168		249				
Hexose, 2-deoxy-D-*arabino*- (2-deoxy-D-glucose)	$C_6H_{12}O_5$	146	+38.3→+45.9 (c 0.5) (18°)	250	<10sor (5)		97rha (95)	68f (37)
2-Deoxy-D-glucitol	$C_6H_{14}O_5$				100sor (132)		22f (49)	
2-Deoxy-D-glucitol pentaacetate	$C_{16}H_{24}O_{10}$					15 (131)		
2-Deoxy-N-phenyl-D-*arabino*-hexopyranosylamine	$C_{12}H_{17}NO_4$	193–194	−138→−106 (C$_5$H$_5$N)	250				
α-Pyranoside tetraacetate	$C_{14}H_{20}O_9$	91	+12.3 (c 0.3, C$_2$H$_5$OH)	250				35f (252)
β-Pyranoside tetraacetate	$C_{14}H_{20}O_9$	109.7–110.7 75–78	+107.7 (CHCl$_3$) +30 (c 0.2, C$_2$H$_5$OH)	251 250				33f (252)
Trimethylsilyl ether		92.2–93.2	−2.8 (CHCl$_3$)	251		64glct (9)		

Table 3 (continued)
NATURAL ALDOSES

Substance[a] (synonym) derivative	Chemical formula	Melting point °C	Specific rotation[b] $[\alpha]_D$	Reference[c]	Chromatography, R value, and reference[d]			
					ELC	GLC	PPC	TLC
(A)	(B)	(C)	(D)	(E)	(F)	(G)	(H)	(I)
Hexose, 4-deoxy-D-*arabino*- (4-deoxy-D-altrose or idose)	$C_6H_{12}O_5$	No constants known	No constants known	253			168glc (253a)	127glc (253a)
Dibenzylmercaptal	$C_{20}H_{26}O_4S_2$	103–105	+146 (c 0.2, C_2H_5OH)	254				
4-Deoxy-D-*arabino*-hexitol			+97	253		190xyll (253b)	128glc (253a)	
4-Deoxy-D-*arabino*-hexitol pentaacetate								
Hexose, 2,6-dideoxy-D-*arabino*- (canarose, chromose C, olivose)	$C_6H_{12}O_4$	86–98 / 100–103	+19.6, +25 (H_2O) / +95.9, +110 (acetone) / +31	256, 257 / 256, 257 / 258			54f (258a)	14f (258b)
2,4-Dinitrophenylhydrazone	$C_{13}H_{16}N_4O_7$	132–132.5		256				
Methyl α-pyranoside	$C_8H_{16}O_4$		+131 (c 0.7, C_2H_5OH)	258			75f (268)	38f (258c)
Methyl β-pyranoside	$C_8H_{16}O_4$	84	−85 (C_2H_5OH)	258			70f (268)	27f (258c)
Hexose, 2,6-dideoxy-3-O-carbamoyl-D-*arabino*-	$C_7H_{13}NO_5$	No constants known	No constants known	259				
Methyl α-pyranoside	$C_8H_{15}NO_5$	146–149	+137 (acetone)	259				28f (259a)
Methyl α-pyranoside acetate	$C_{10}H_{17}NO_6$	100–110		259				
Olivose	$C_6H_{12}O_4$		+19.9 (H_2O), +60.8 (acetone)	259				30f (259b)
Hexose, 2,6-dideoxy-3-C-methyl-D-*arabino*- (D-3-epimycarose, evermicose)	$C_7H_{14}O_4$	108–112	+20.7 (24h)	260t				
1,4-Diacetate	$C_{11}H_{18}O_6$	73	+39.5 ($CHCl_3$)	260				

Table 3 (continued)
NATURAL ALDOSES

Substance[a] (synonym) derivative	Chemical formula	Melting point °C	Specific rotation[b] $[\alpha]_D$	Reference[c]	Chromatography, R value, and reference[d]			
					ELC	GLC	PPC	TLC
(A)	(B)	(C)	(D)	(E)	(F)	(G)	(H)	(I)
Hexose, 2,6-dideoxy-3-O-methyl-D-arabino-(D-oleandrose)	$C_7H_{14}O_4$	62–63	−12.5	261,262			77f (262)	
Hexonolactone	$C_7H_{12}O_4$	Syrup	+12.8±2 (acetone) (14°)	261			85cymo (263a)	44f (263b)
Hexonic acid phenyl-hydrazide	$C_{13}H_{20}N_2O_4$	134–135	−20.6± (16°)(c 0.8, CH_3OH)	261				
Hexose, 3,6-dideoxy-D-arabino- (D-tyvelose)	$C_6H_{12}O_4$	95–99, 143–144	+24±2	264–266	122rha (273)		129rha[q] (265)	33f (266)
3,6-Dideoxy-D-arabino-hexitol	$C_6H_{12}O_4$	113–115	−35±2 (c 0.7)	265			107rha (304)	
Methyl α-pyranoside	$C_7H_{14}O_4$	84.5–85.5	$[\alpha]_{5461}$ +137±2 (CH_3OH)	267t				
Methyl β-pyranoside	$C_7H_{14}O_4$	Oil	$[\alpha]_{5461}$ −72±2 (CH_3OH)	267t				40f (266)
Hexose, 2,6-dideoxy-3-C-methyl-L-arabino- (olivomycose)	$C_7H_{14}O_4$	103–106	−13→−22 (26°) 1.5h	258,268			58f (268)	
Methyl α-pyranoside	$C_8H_{16}O_4$	Syrup	−147 (C_2H_5OH)	268c			77f (268)	
Methyl α-pyranoside iso-butyrate[n]	$C_{12}H_{22}O_5$	Syrup	−123 (c 0.6, C_2H_5OH)	268				
Methyl β-pyranoside	$C_8H_{16}O_4$	93–94	+50 (C_2H_5OH)	268			73f (268)	
Methyl β-pyranoside iso-butyrate[n]	$C_{12}H_{22}O_5$	Syrup	+29 (C_2H_5OH)	268				
Hexose, 4-O-acetyl-2,6-dideoxy-3-C-methyl-L-arabino- (chromose B)	$C_9H_{16}O_5$	Syrup	−24	269p			80f (258a)	
Hexose, 4-O-iso-butyryl-2,6-dideoxy-3-C-methyl-L-arabino-	$C_{11}H_{20}O_5$	Syrup	−43→−33.5 (c 0.5)	258			84f (258a)	
Hexose, 2,6-dideoxy-3-O-methyl-L-arabino- (L-oleandrose)	$C_7H_{14}O_4$	62–63	+11.9±2.5	270			14p (290)	
2,4-Dinitrophenyl-hydrazone	$C_{13}H_{18}N_4O_7$	155–160		271				

Table 3 (continued)
NATURAL ALDOSES

Substance[a] (synonym) derivative	Chemical formula	Melting point °C	Specific rotation[b] $[\alpha]_D$	Reference[c]	Chromatography, R value, and reference[d]			
					ELC	GLC	PPC	TLC
(A)	(B)	(C)	(D)	(E)	(F)	(G)	(H)	(I)
Hexonic acid phenyl-hydrazide	$C_{13}H_{20}N_2O_4$	135–136	+21.1±3 (c 0.8 CH₃OH)	270				
Methyl α-pyranoside	$C_8H_{16}O_4$	Syrup	-125.6 (C₂H₅OH)	272ct				
Methyl β-pyranoside	$C_8H_{16}O_4$	74–78	+71.5 (C₂H₅OH)	272ct				
Hexose, 3,6-dideoxy-L-arabino- (ascarylose, L-tyvelose)	$C_6H_{12}O_4$	Syrup	-25	265,273	122rha (273)		129rha (265)	
Ascarylitol	$C_6H_{14}O_4$	112–113	+38±3 (CH₃OH)	273			107rha (304)	
Hexose, 3-C-methyl-4-O-methyl-3-nitro-2,3,6-trideoxy-L-arabino- (evernitrose)	$C_8H_{15}NO_5$	88–92	-4.9→-19.4 (C₂H₅OH)	274				
Evernitronolactone	$C_8H_{13}NO_5$	63–64	-70	274				
Monoacetate	$C_9H_{15}NO_5$	58–59	-20.5 (C₂H₅OH)	274				
Hexose, 2,3,6-trideoxy-D-erythro- (erythro-amicitose)	$C_6H_{12}O_3$	Oil, bp 65–70	+28.6 (CHCl₃)	275				
2,4-Dinitrophenyl-hydrazone	$C_{12}H_{16}N_4O_6$	137.5–138, 152–153	-10 (c 0.9, C₅H₅N)	275,276	0.1 (276a)		79f (276b)	
Methyl α-pyranoside	$C_7H_{14}O_3$	Syrup	+142±1 (18°)	277				33f (277)
Methyl β-pyranoside	$C_7H_{14}O_3$	Syrup	-21.9 (c 0.8, CHCl₃)	278				32f (278)
Hexose, 2,6-dideoxy-D-lyxo- (2-deoxy-D-fucose, oliose)	$C_6H_{12}O_4$	Syrup	+46, +53	269c,279p			35f (269)	35f (280b)
3,4-Di-O-methyl-D-oliose	$C_8H_{12}O_4$	61–64	+117 (30°)(c 0.5, CHCl₃)	280				37f (280c)
Methyl α-pyranoside	$C_7H_{14}O_4$	70–72	+122 (16°)(CHCl₃)	281				
Methyl α-pyranoside	$C_7H_{16}O_4$	Syrup	+115, +133 (C₂H₅OH)	280			67f (279)	67f (280d)
3,4-di-O-methyl ether								
Hexose, 3-O-acetyl-2,6-dideoxy-D-lyxo- (chromose D)	$C_8H_{14}O_5$	115–116.5	+100→+78 (29°)	279,281t				38f (280e)
Methyl α-pyranoside	$C_7H_{16}O_5$	Syrup	+142 (16°)(CHCl₃)	281				59f (281a)

Table 3 (continued)
NATURAL ALDOSES

Substance[a] (synonym) derivative	Chemical formula	Melting point °C	Specific rotation[b] [α]_D	Reference[c]	Chromatography, R value, and reference[d]			
					ELC	GLC	PPC	TLC
(A)	(B)	(C)	(D)	(E)	(F)	(G)	(H)	(I)
Methyl α-pyranoside 4-O-methyl ether	$C_{10}H_{18}O_5$	Syrup	+104 (15°)(CHCl$_3$)	281				82f (281b)
Hexose, 2,6-dideoxy-3-O-methyl-D-lyxo- (diginose)	$C_7H_{14}O_4$	90–92	+56±4	283,284			11.4P (290)	
Diginonolactone	$C_7H_{12}O_4$	Syrup	−30 (14°)(acetone)	283			87cymo (263a)	50f (263b)
Hexose, 2,6-dideoxy-4-O-methyl-D-lyxo- (chromose A, olivomose)	$C_7H_{14}O_4$	158–162	+98.5→+89 (c 0.5)	268,285			65f (258a)	
2,4-Dinitrophenyl-hydrazone	$C_{13}H_{18}N_4O_7$	146–147		286				
Methyl α-pyranoside	$C_8H_{16}O_5$	98	+150 (c 0.4, C$_2$H$_5$OH)(26°)	268,286				61f (258c)
Methyl β-pyranoside	$C_8H_{16}O_4$	152–153	−37.4 (c 0.4, C$_2$H$_5$OH)(26°)	268,286				54f (258c)
Olivomose 3-acetate	$C_8H_{16}O_5$		+69 (c 0.4)	280				42f (280a)
Hexose, 2,6-dideoxy-L-lyxo-	$C_6H_{12}O_4$	103–106	−90.4→−61.6	287,288pt			10.7° (289)	
2,6-Dideoxy-L-lyxo-hexonolactone	$C_6H_{10}O_4$		+31.2±2 (acetone)	263			55drho (263c)	
Hexonic acid phenyl-hydrazide	$C_{12}H_{18}N_2O_4$	167–169	−8.5±2	263				
Hexose, 2,6-dideoxy-3-O-methyl-L-lyxo- (L-diginose)	$C_7H_{14}O_4$	78–85	−65	290			11.4P (290)	
Hexose, 2,6-dideoxy-D-ribo- (digitoxose)	$C_6H_{12}O_4$	110	+46.4	291			128rha (95)	94f (292)
2,6-Dideoxy-D-ribo-hexitol trimethylsilyl ether						46.5glcs (294)		

Table 3 (continued)
NATURAL ALDOSES

Substance[a] (synonym) derivative	Chemical formula	Melting point °C	Specific rotation[b] $[\alpha]_D$	Reference[c]	Chromatography, R value, and reference[d]			
					ELC	GLC	PPC	TLC
(A)	(B)	(C)	(D)	(E)	(F)	(G)	(H)	(I)
Digitoxonolactone	$C_6H_{10}O_4$		−29.5±2 (c 0.6, acetone)	263			63drho (263c)	
Digitoxonic acid phenylhydrazide	$C_{12}H_{18}N_2O_4$	123−125	−17.8±2 (c 0.4)	263				
Methyl α-pyranoside	$C_7H_{14}O_4$	Bp 98−100 (10⁻¹ torr)	+178.4 (CHCl₃)	293				
Phenylhydrazone	$C_{12}H_{18}N_2O_3$	204−209	+215 (C₂H₅OH, C₅H₅N)	307				
Trimethylsilyl ether						18glct (9)		
Hexose, 2,6-dideoxy-3-O-methyl-D-ribo- (cymarose)	$C_7H_{14}O_4$	83−90, 93	+55	295,296			83f (150)	100 (410)
Cymaronolactone	$C_7H_{12}O_4$	Syrup	−25	263			100 (263a)	54f (263b)
Cymaronic acid phenylhydrazide	$C_{13}H_{20}N_2O_4$	155−156	+1.4 (c 0.7, CH₃OH) (16°)	263,297				
Methyl α-pyranoside	$C_8H_{16}O_4$	34−36	+210 (14°)(CH₃OH)	298				
Hexose, 3,6-dideoxy-D-ribo- (paratose)	$C_6H_{12}O_4$	Syrup	+10±2 (c 0.9)	273,299p	138rha (273)		125rha (300)	
Methyl α-pyranoside	$C_7H_{14}O_4$	Syrup	$[\alpha]_{578}$ +170 (CHCl₃)	301				33f (301)
Methyl β-pyranoside	$C_7H_{14}O_4$	63−65	−60 (CH₃OH)	266p				
Paratitol	$C_6H_{14}O_4$	67−68	−18±2 (c 0.9)	299			71f (299)	
Hexose, 4,6-dideoxy-3-O-methyl-D-ribo- (chalcose, lancavose)	$C_7H_{14}O_4$	96−99	+120→+76	302,303t			71f (305a)	10f (305b)
4,6-Dideoxy-D-ribo-hexose	$C_6H_{12}O_4$							
Methyl α-pyranoside	$C_8H_{16}O_4$		+184.5 (CHCl₃)	305			65f (302)	
Methyl β-pyranoside	$C_8H_{16}O_4$	101.5−102	−21 (27°)(CHCl₃)	302	47glc (320a)		65f (320b)	30f (305b)
Hexose, 2,6-dideoxy-3-C-methyl-L-ribo- (L-mycarose)[e]	$C_7H_{14}O_4$	128−129	−31.1	319				

Table 3 (continued)
NATURAL ALDOSES

Substance[a] (synonym) derivative	Chemical formula	Melting point °C	Specific rotation[b] $[\alpha]_D$	Reference[c]	Chromatography, R value, and reference[d]			
					ELC	GLC	PPC	TLC
(A)	(B)	(C)	(D)	(E)	(F)	(G)	(H)	(I)
3,4-Di-*O*-methyl mycarose	$C_9H_{18}O_4$	83–86	−20 (CHCl$_3$)	321				
Methyl α-pyranoside[f]	$C_8H_{16}O_4$	Syrup	+22, +54 (CHCl$_3$)	319,324	48glc (320a)			
Methyl β-pyranoside[f]	$C_8H_{16}O_4$	62	−155 (CHCl$_3$)	319,324	37glc (320a)			
Mycaronolactone	$C_7H_{12}O_4$	108–109	−35	319				
1,3,4-Triacetate	$C_{13}H_{20}O_7$	133–135	−61.3 (26°) (C$_2$H$_5$OH)	325				
Mycarose 4-*O*-acetate	$C_9H_{16}O_5$	Bp 65 (1.5 mm)		327				
Methyl α-pyranoside	$C_{10}H_{18}O_5$	Bp 88–99 (2 mm)	−148 (CHCl$_3$)	326				
Methyl β-pyranoside	$C_{10}H_{18}O_5$	Bp 104–106 (1.5 mm)	+25 (CHCl$_3$)	326				
Mycarose 4-*O*-*n*-butyrate	$C_{11}H_{20}O_5$	No constants known	No constants known	326				
Methyl α-pyranoside	$C_{12}H_{22}O_5$	Bp 112–122 (3 mm)	−137 (CHCl$_3$)	326				
Methyl β-pyranoside	$C_{12}H_{22}O_5$	Bp 118–119 (2 mm)	+16.9 (CHCl$_3$)	326				
Mycarose 4-*O*-*iso*-valerate	$C_{12}H_{22}O_5$	No constants known	No constants known	326				
Methyl α-pyranoside	$C_{13}H_{24}O_5$	Bp 115–116 (2 mm)	−135.5 (CHCl$_3$)	326				
Methyl β-pyranoside	$C_{13}H_{24}O_5$	Bp 117–118 (0.7 mm)	+13.5 (CHCl$_3$)	326				
Mycarose 4-*O*-*n*-propionate	$C_{10}H_{18}O_5$	No constants known	No constants known	326				
Methyl α-pyranoside	$C_{11}H_{20}O_5$	Bp 98–100 (2 mm)	−145 (CHCl$_3$)	326				
Methyl β-pyranoside	$C_{11}H_{20}O_5$	Bp 109–110 (2 mm)	+20 (CHCl$_3$)	326				
Hexose, 2,6-dideoxy-3-C-methyl-3-*O*-methyl-L-*ribo*- (cladinose)[g]	$C_8H_{16}O_4$	Bp 120–132 (0.25 mm)	−23.1	328	0glc (320a)		74f (320b)	

Table 3 (continued)
NATURAL ALDOSES

Substance[a] (synonym) derivative	Chemical formula	Melting point °C	Specific rotation[b] $[\alpha]_D$	Reference[c]	ELC	GLC	PPC	TLC
(A)	(B)	(C)	(D)	(E)	(F)	(G)	(H)	(I)
Cladinitol	$C_6H_{14}O_4$		-25 (27°)(95% C_2H_5OH)	329			160ole (329)	
Cladinose diacetate	$C_{12}H_{20}O_6$	66–67	-36 (CH_3OH)	323				
Cladinonolactone 3,5-dinitrobenzoate	$C_{13}H_{14}N_2O_9$	123–125		330				
Methyl α-pyranoside	$C_9H_{18}O_4$	27.5–28.5[f]	-6.9	322,328				
Hexose, 2,6-dideoxy-3-O-methyl-L-ribo- (L-cymarose)	$C_7H_{14}O_4$	87–91	-53.6±2	295				
L-Cymaronic acid phenylhydrazide	$C_{13}H_{20}N_2O_4$	153–154	0.3±3 (c 0.7, CH_3OH)	295				
Hexose, 2,3,6-trideoxy-D-threo- (threo-amicitose)	$C_6H_{12}O_3$	Syrup	+10.2 (acetone)	306	2.3 (276a)			116digx (306)
2,4-Dinitrophenylhydrazone	$C_{12}H_{16}N_4O_6$	105–106, 121–122	+13.7 (c 0.9, C_5H_5N)	276,306				
Hexose, 2,3,6-trideoxy-L-threo- (L-threo-amicitose, rhodinose)	$C_6H_{12}O_3$	Syrup	-11±1.6	307,308[r]			71f (307a)	73f (307b)
2,4-Dinitrophenylhydrazone	$C_{13}H_{16}N_4O_6$	121–122	-14.9 (c 0.5, C_5H_5N)	306,309				
Hexose, 2-deoxy-D-xylo- (2-deoxy-D-gulose or idose)	$C_6H_{12}O_5$	Syrup	+12±2	310,311			47digx (310)	
2-Deoxy-D-xylo-hexonolactone	$C_6H_{10}O_5$	Syrup	-56.6±2 (acetone)	311				
2-Deoxy-D-xylo-hexonic acid phenylhydrazide	$C_{12}H_{18}N_2O_5$	124–126	-8.1±2 (CH_3OH)	311				
2-Deoxy-xylo-hexitol	$C_6H_{14}O_5$	96–98	-3.9→+3.9±2 (18°)	313	107glcf (312)			
Hexose, 2,6-dideoxy-D-xylo- (boivinose)	$C_6H_{12}O_4$		-14 (acetone)	238			176digx (310)	
Methyl α-pyranoside	$C_7H_{14}O_4$	Syrup	+108.7±2 (CH_3OH)	313			522 gal (238b)	
Hexose, 2,6-dideoxy-3-O-methyl-D-xylo- (sarmentose)	$C_7H_{14}O_4$	78–79	+12→+15.8	314			75cym (315)	

Chromatography, R value, and reference[d]

Table 3 (continued)
NATURAL ALDOSES

Substance[a] (synonym) derivative	Chemical formula	Melting point °C	Specific rotation[b] $[\alpha]_D$	Reference[c]	Chromatography, R value, and reference[d]			
					ELC	GLC	PPC	TLC
(A)	(B)	(C)	(D)	(E)	(F)	(G)	(H)	(I)
Methyl α-pyranoside	$C_6H_{12}O_4$	33–36	+156±1 (acetone)	316				
Methyl β-pyranoside	$C_6H_{12}O_4$	46–45	−39.4±1.5 (acetone)	316				
Sarmentonolactone	$C_7H_{12}O_4$						66cymo (263a)	42f (263b)
Hexose, 3,6-dideoxy-D-xylo- (abequose)	$C_6H_{12}O_4$	138–139	−3.2±0.6	264,265			117rha (95)q	
3,6-Dideoxy-D-xylo-hexitol	$C_6H_{14}O_4$	92–93	+51±2	265				
Methyl α-pyranoside	$C_7H_{14}O_4$	Syrup	$[\alpha]_{5461}$ +102±5 (CH₃OH)	267				
Methyl β-pyranoside	$C_7H_{14}O_4$	Syrup	$[\alpha]_{5461}$ −90±3 (CH₃OH)	267				
Hexose, 2,6-dideoxy-4-C-[1'-hydroxyethyl]-L-xylo-	$C_8H_{16}O_5$	No constants known	No constants known	317				
Methyl α-pyranoside (?) (glycoside A2)	$C_9H_{18}O_5$		+15 (c 0.5, CHCl₃)	317			31f (317a)	25f (317b)
Methyl β-pyranoside (?) (glycoside A1)	$C_9H_{18}O_5$		−104 (c 0.7, CHCl₃)	317				48f (317b)
Hexose, 2,6-dideoxy-3-C-methyl-L-xylo- (axenose)	$C_7H_{14}O_4$	111–112	−28.5	318				
Methyl α-pyranoside	$C_8H_{16}O_4$	101–103	−142	318				
Methyl β-pyranoside	$C_8H_{16}O_4$	122–123	+38	318				
Hexose, 2,6-dideoxy-3-C-methyl-3-O-methyl-L-xylo- (arcanose)	$C_8H_{16}O_4$	96–98	−20.9 (C₂H₅OH)	303				
Arcanitol	$C_8H_{18}O_4$	bp 110 (0.05 torr)	−2.0 (C₂H₅OH)	303				
Arcanose 4-acetate	$C_{10}H_{18}O_5$	Oil	−52.3 (C₂H₅OH)	303				93f (303)
Methyl pyranoside acetate	$C_{11}H_{20}O_5$	Oil	−24.3 (c 6.5, C₂H₅OH)	303				

Table 3 (continued)
NATURAL ALDOSES

Substance[a] (synonym) derivative	Chemical formula	Melting point °C	Specific rotation[b] $[\alpha]_D$	Reference[c]	Chromatography, R value, and reference[d]			
					ELC	GLC	PPC	TLC
(A)	**(B)**	**(C)**	**(D)**	**(E)**	**(F)**	**(G)**	**(H)**	**(I)**
Hexose, 2,6-dideoxy-4-C-[1'-oxoethyl]-L-xylo-	$C_8H_{14}O_5$	No constants known	No constants known	317				
Methyl α-pyranoside (?) (glycoside B2)	$C_9H_{16}O_5$		+46 (c 0.18, CHCl₃)	317			70f (317a)	57f (317c)
Methyl β-pyranoside (?) (glycoside B1)	$C_9H_{16}O_5$		-60 (c 0.12, CHCl₃)	317				70f (317c)
Hexose, 3,6-dideoxy-L-xylo- (colitose)	$C_6H_{12}O_4$	Syrup	+4	265,331			116rha (265)	
Colititol	$C_6H_{14}O_4$	92–94	-51±2	265				
p-Nitrophenylsulfonyl-hydrazone	$C_{10}H_{21}N_3O_5S$	141		331				
Everninose (a deoxy-O-methyl-hexose)	$C_7H_{14}O_5$	186–188	-69	255			56f (255)	
p-Tolylsulfonyl-hydrazone	$C_{14}H_{22}N_2O_5S$	135–137	+36.2 (C₅H₅N)	255				
Variose (a dideoxy-C-methyl-hexose)	$C_7H_{14}O_4$		+54 (c 0.5)	333c				45f (333)
Vinelose (a 6-deoxy-3-C-methyl-2-O-methyl-hexose)	$C_8H_{16}O_5$	Oil	$[\alpha]_{546}$ +12 (14.5°)	334	62glc (334c)		454rha (334a)	
Diacetate	$C_{12}H_{20}O_7$	Oil	$[\alpha]_{546}$ -6.4 (19.8°) (CHCl₃)	334		120erya (282)		
Vinelitol	$C_8H_{18}O_5$	Oil	$[\alpha]_{546}$ -45.7 (CHCl₃)	334				
Vinelitol triacetate	$C_{14}H_{24}O_8$			334				
Vinelose, O-[2'-O-methyl-glycolyl]-	$C_{11}H_{20}O_7$	Oil	-26.5 (c 0.9, CHCl₃)	334	0glc (334c)		76f (334b)	
D-Idose[v]	$C_6H_{12}O_6$	Syrup See Table 1 also	+15.8±1 See Table 1 also	335,336			9f[f] (49)	
D-Iditol	$C_6H_{14}O_6$						80glc (91a)	
Methyl α-pyranoside	$C_7H_{14}O_6$	67–68	+99.8±1	336				
Methyl β-pyranoside	$C_7H_{14}O_6$	Syrup	-81.1±1	336				
Pentaacetate	$C_{16}H_{22}O_{11}$	91–92	+54.3±2 (CHCl₃)	336				
Trimethylsilyl ether						50glct (9)		

Table 3 (continued)
NATURAL ALDOSES

Substance[a] (synonym) derivative	Chemical formula	Melting point °C	Specific rotation[b] $[\alpha]_D$	Reference[c]	Chromatography, R value, and reference[d]			
					ELC	GLC	PPC	TLC
(A)	(B)	(C)	(D)	(E)	(F)	(G)	(H)	(I)
L-Idose	$C_6H_{12}O_6$	Syrup	−17.4	339p	115rib[f] (28) 100glcf (312)		172glc (337)	
L-Iditol	$C_6H_{14}O_6$	See Table 1 also	See Table 1 also					
Methyl α-pyranoside	$C_7H_{14}O_6$	Syrup	−98 (CH_3OH)	338		75glc (9)	57f (338)	
Methyl α-pyranoside trimethylsilyl ether								
Methyl β-pyranoside	$C_7H_{14}O_6$	Syrup	+61 (27°)(CH_3OH)	338		64glc (9)	63f (338)	
Methyl β-pyranoside trimethylsilyl ether								
L-Idopyranose, 1,6-anhydro-	$C_6H_{10}O_5$	128–129	+113 (acetone)	337			265glc (337)	
β-Triacetate	$C_{12}H_{16}O_8$	85–86	+75.5 (c 0.7, ($CHCl_3$)	337c				
β-Trimethyl ether	$C_9H_{16}O_5$	39–40	+88 (19°)($CHCl_3$)	338c	35rib (28)		8f (49)	30f (30)
α-D-Mannose	$C_6H_{12}O_6$	133	+29.3→+14.5	340	17rib (28)		42f (49)	2f (69)
Methyl α-pyranoside	$C_7H_{14}O_6$	193–194	+79.2	186				
Methyl α-pyranoside tetramethyl ether	$C_{11}H_{22}O_6$	38–39	+69 (CH_3OH)	341gt		154αtemg (67)	98temg (341)	54f (69)
Pentaacetate	$C_{16}H_{22}O_{11}$	64	+55 ($CHCl_3$)	182				
2,3,4,6-Tetra-O-methyl-D-mannose	$C_{10}H_{20}O_6$	50–52	+7.4→+2.4	186				
Trimethylsilyl ether							100temg (342)	
β-D-Mannose	$C_6H_{12}O_6$	132	−17→+14.6	343,411c	<10sor (5)	70glc (9)		56f (59)
Methyl β-pyranoside	$C_7H_{14}O_6$	202–203	+56 (C_5H_5N, C_2H_5OH)	64,65,191, 344				
p-Nitrophenylhydrazone	$C_{12}H_{17}N_3O_7$	117–118	−25.3 ($CHCl_3$)	182,343				
Pentaacetate	$C_{16}H_{22}O_{11}$							
Trimethylsilyl ether						108glc (9)		54f (59)
D-Mannose, 3-O-carbamoyl-	$C_7H_{13}NO_7$	No constants known	No constants known	240				
Methyl α-pyranoside	$C_8H_{15}NO_7$	Amorphous	+49 (CH_3OH)	345cg				
Methyl α-pyranoside triacetate	$C_{14}H_{19}NO_{10}$	142.5	+35.8 ($CHCl_3$)	345t				40f (244 b,g)

Table 3 (continued)
NATURAL ALDOSES

Substance[a] (synonym) derivative	Chemical formula	Melting point °C	Specific rotation[b] $[\alpha]_D$	Reference[c]	Chromatography, R value, and reference[d]			
					ELC	GLC	PPC	TLC
(A)	(B)	(C)	(D)	(E)	(F)	(G)	(H)	(I)
Methyl α-pyranoside tribenzoate	$C_9H_{27}NO_{10}$	Glass	-19.5 (c 0.9, $CHCl_3$)	345				33f (345)
D-Mannose, 4,6-O-(1-carboxy-ethylidene)-	$C_9H_{14}O_8$	No constants known	No constants known	346gpt				
D-Mannose, 6-deoxy- (D-rhamnose)	$C_6H_{12}O_5$	86-90	-7.0	347,411c			100rha (347)	37f (130)
D-Rhamnitol	$C_6H_{14}O_5$				100glc (312)		97rha[f] (95)	38f (197)
Rhamnitol pentaacetate	$C_{16}H_{24}O_{10}$					7.1 (131)		
Rhamnitol pentamethyl ether	$C_{11}H_{24}O_5$					7.1 (353)		
D-Mannose, 6-deoxy-3-C-methyl- (D-evalose)	$C_7H_{14}O_5$	Glass	-4.7→-5.2	348b				
2,3,4-Tri-O-methyl-D-evalose (D-nogalose)[u]	$C_{10}H_{20}O_5$	115-120	+18.3→+6.3 (CH_3OH) 24h	348				
D-Mannose, 6-deoxy-2-O-methyl-	$C_7H_{14}O_5$		-22	350cg	32glc (350a)		137rha (350b)	
D-Mannose, 6-deoxy-3-O-methyl- (D-acofriose)	$C_7H_{14}O_5$		-27 (c 0.9)	350	56glc (350a)		132rha (350b)	
D-Mannose, 6-deoxy-2,3-di-O-methyl-	$C_8H_{16}O_5$		w	351			192rha (352e)	
D-Mannose, 6-deoxy-3,4-di-O-methyl-	$C_8H_{16}O_5$	86-88	w	351			198rha (352e)	
2,3,4-Tri-O-methyl-D-rhamnose	$C_9H_{18}O_5$		w				232rha (352)	
Methyl 2,3,4-tri-O-methyl-α-pyranoside	$C_{10}H_{20}O_5$		w			31atemg (350c)		
2,3,4-Tri-O-methyl-D-rhamnonic acid phenylhydrazide	$C_{16}H_{25}N_2O_5$	181-183	-36.3 (c 0.14, C_2H_5OH)	350				
D-Mannose, 3-O-methyl-	$C_7H_{14}O_6$	133-134	+14→+3 (c 0.6)	354,355	48glc (354a)		94rha (354b)	176glc (356p)
D-Mannose, 2,6-di-O-methyl- (D-curamicose)	$C_8H_{16}O_6$	Syrup	+10.3, +22.4	357,358ep	0 (357c)		72glc (357a)	

Table 3 (continued)
NATURAL ALDOSES

Substance[a] (synonym) derivative	Chemical formula	Melting point °C	Specific rotation[b] $[\alpha]_D$	Reference[c]	Chromatography, R value, and reference[d]			
					ELC	GLC	PPC	TLC
(A)	(B)	(C)	(D)	(E)	(F)	(G)	(H)	(I)
Curamicitol (1,5-di-O-methyl-L-mannitol)	$C_8H_{18}O_6$	Syrup	+18.5 (c 0.5)	357				
Curamiconolactone	$C_8H_{14}O_6$	Syrup	+58	357		368αtemg (357b)		
2,6-Di-O-methyl-D-mannonic acid phenylhydrazide	$C_{14}H_{22}N_2O_6$	130	-40 (c 0.5)	357				
Methyl α-pyranoside Trimethylsilyl ether	$C_9H_{18}O_6$					324αtemg (357b) 77,96αtemg (357b)		
α-L-Mannose, 6-deoxy- (L-rhamnose)	$C_6H_{12}O_5 \cdot H_2O$	93–94	-8.6→+8.2	63,359	100rha (96a)		100rha (96c)	100rha (96b)
Methyl α-pyranoside	$C_7H_{14}O_5$	109–110	-62.5	362		44βtemg (67)	76f (360a)	
Methyl α-pyranoside trimethyl ether	$C_{10}H_{20}O_5$	Syrup	-15.1	361				
Rhamnitol trimethylsilyl ether						66glcs (294)		
2,3,4,-Tri-O-methyl-L-rhamnose	$C_9H_{18}O_5$	Syrup	+26	361		30glct (9)	102temg (68)	
Trimethylsilyl ether								
β-L-Mannose, 6-deoxy-	$C_6H_{12}O_5$	123–125	+38.4→+8.9	363	32rib (28)		53digx (310)	46f (30)
Methyl β-pyranoside	$C_7H_{14}O_5$	138–140	+95.4	364				
p-Nitrophenylhydrazone	$C_{13}H_{17}N_3O_6$	190–191	-50→-8.5 (C_5H_5N, C_2H_5OH)	64				
L-Rhamnonolactone	$C_6H_{10}O_5$	98–99	+13.9 (c 15, $C_2H_5Cl_2$)	364				
Tetraacetate	$C_{14}H_{20}O_9$		+15.5 (H_2O)					
L-Mannose, 6-deoxy-3-C-methyl-2,3,4-tri-O-methyl- (nogalose)	$C_{10}H_{20}O_5$	115–121	-10.6 (CH_3OH)	332				69f (17)
Methyl pyranoside	$C_{11}H_{22}O_5$	41–43	-48.4 (CH_3OH)	349				
Nogalitol	$C_{10}H_{22}O_5$	Oil	-13 (CH_3OH)	349				
Nogalonolactone	$C_{10}H_{18}O_5$	Bp 76 (0.1 mm)	+15.9 ($CHCl_3$) +6.7 (CH_3OH)	349 332				

Table 3 (continued)
NATURAL ALDOSES

Substance[a] (synonym) derivative	Chemical formula	Melting point °C	Specific rotation[b] $[\alpha]_D$	Reference[c]	Chromatography, R value, and reference[d] ELC	GLC	PPC	TLC
(A)	(B)	(C)	(D)	(E)	(F)	(G)	(H)	(I)
L-Mannose, 6-deoxy-5-C-methyl-4-O-methyl- (noviose, 5,5-di-C-methyl-4-O-methyl-L-lyxose)	$C_8H_{16}O_5$	133–134	+22.6 (50% C_2H_5OH)	365				
Methyl α-pyranoside	$C_9H_{18}O_5$	68–70	−62±2 (C_2H_5OH)	366				
Methyl β-pyranoside	$C_9H_{18}O_5$	61–68	+113.8	367				
Noviono-γ-lactone	$C_8H_{14}O_5$	111–113	−35 (0.1N HCl)	368				
Noviose, 3-O-carbamoyl-	$C_9H_{17}NO_6$	124–126	+45.3 (C_2H_5OH)	367				
Methyl α-pyranoside	$C_{10}H_{19}NO_6$	194–195	−24.7 (C_2H_5OH)	367				
Methyl β-pyranoside	$C_{10}H_{19}NO_6$	117–118	+124±4 (C_2H_5OH)	366				
L-Mannose, 6-deoxy-2-O-methyl-	$C_7H_{14}O_5$	113–114	+31 (27°)	134,352, 369			148rha (352)	
6-Deoxy-2-O-methyl-N-phenyl-L-mannopyranosylamine	$C_{13}H_{19}NO_4$	152	+43 (C_5H_5N)	370				
6-Deoxy-2-O-methyl-L-mannonolactone	$C_7H_{12}O_5$	116–117	−62	370				
Methyl pyranoside	$C_8H_{16}O_5$	139–140		134	72rha (96a)		212rha (96c)	135rha (96b)
L-Mannose, 6-deoxy-3-O-methyl- (L-acofriose)	$C_7H_{14}O_5$	112–116	+37.3±2	115				
Acofrionolactone	$C_7H_{12}O_5$	Syrup	−20 (15°)	371				
Methyl glycoside	$C_8H_{16}O_5$	128–130	+57 (C_5H_5N-C_2H_5OH)	372		486βtemg (67)		
Phenylosazone	$C_{19}H_{22}N_4O_5$			372				
L-Mannose, 6-deoxy-2,3-di-O-methyl-	$C_8H_{16}O_5$	Syrup	+47.6	372,373	2glc (375a)		83glc (373)	
6-Deoxy-2,3-di-O-methyl-N-phenyl-L-mannopyranosylamine	$C_{14}H_{21}NO_4$	136–137	+147.8→+42.8 (c 0.4, C_2H_5OH) 70h	374,357				
2,4-Dinitrophenyl-hydrazone	$C_{14}H_{20}N_4O_8$	168d	+45.4 (c 0.6, dioxane)	375				
Methyl α-pyranoside	$C_9H_{18}O_5$	Syrup	−6, −14	373,374				

Table 3 (continued)
NATURAL ALDOSES

Substance[a] (synonym) derivative	Chemical formula	Melting point °C	Specific rotation[b] $[\alpha]_D$	Reference[c]	Chromatography, R value, and reference[d]			
					ELC	GLC	PPC	TLC
(A)	(B)	(C)	(D)	(E)	(F)	(G)	(H)	(I)
L-Mannose, 6-deoxy-2,4-di-O-methyl-	$C_9H_{18}O_5$	82, 91–93	+42 (CH$_3$OH) −19 (16°), +10.6	377cp 352,375, 376	2glc (375a)		87glc (375b)	
6-Deoxy-2,4-di-O-methyl-N-phenyl-L-mannopyranoosylamine	$C_{14}H_{21}NO_4$	133–134 141–142	+137 (c 0.7, CH$_3$OH) +110→+7 (c 0.4, C$_2$H$_5$OH)	377p 376				
6-Deoxy-2,4-di-O-methyl-L-mannono-lactone	$C_8H_{14}O_5$	Syrup	+47 (15°)(c 0.9)	376				
2,4-Dinitrophenyl-hydrazone	$C_{14}H_{20}N_4O_8$	164–165d	+39 (dioxane)	375				
Methyl α-pyranoside	$C_8H_{16}O_5$	Syrup 98–100	−68 (CH$_3$OH) +85 (c 0.5, CH$_3$OH)	375				
Methyl β-pyranoside	$C_8H_{16}O_5$	98–99	+18.5 (c 0.5)	375				
L-Mannose, 6-deoxy-3,4-di-O-methyl-	$C_8H_{16}O_5$			378,379	40glc (375a)		88glc (375b)	
2,4-Dinitrophenyl-hydrazone	$C_{14}H_{20}N_4O_8$	170	−75.6 (dioxane)	375				
Methyl glycoside	$C_8H_{16}O_5$							
D-Talose	$C_6H_{12}O_6$	128–132 143–144	+16.9	380,411c 380	70sor (5)	110étemg (67)	19glc (379)	36f (17)
Methylphenylhydra-zone	$C_{13}H_{20}N_2O_5$							
α-Pyranoside penta-acetate	$C_{16}H_{22}O_{11}$	106–107	+70.2 (CHCl$_3$)	381				
Talitol	$C_6H_{14}O_6$				138rib (28)		110sor (382)	31f (17)
Talitol hexaacetate	$C_{18}H_{26}O_{12}$					102manl (91b)	107f (383)	68f (17)
Talonolactone	$C_6H_{10}O_6$							
Trimethylsilyl ether						86glct (9)		
D-Talose, 6-deoxy- (D-talomethylose)	$C_6H_{12}O_5$	129–131	+20.6	347			124rha (351)	
6-Deoxy-D-talitol (1-deoxy-D-altritol)	$C_6H_{14}O_6$				98glc (312)			
6-Deoxy-D-talitol pentaacetate	$C_{16}H_{24}O_{10}$					41xyll (82c)		
Methyl α-pyranoside triacetate	$C_{13}H_{20}O_8$	91–91.5	+76 (26°)(CH$_2$OH)	384				

Table 3 (continued)
NATURAL ALDOSES

Substance[a] (synonym) derivative (A)	Chemical formula (B)	Melting point °C (C)	Specific rotation[b] $[\alpha]_D$ (D)	Reference[c] (E)	Chromatography, R value, and reference[d]			
					ELC (F)	GLC (G)	PPC (H)	TLC (I)
Phenylosazone	$C_{18}H_{22}N_4O_3$	176–178	+53 (C_5H_5N:C_2H_5OH, 2:3)	347				
D-Talose, 6-deoxy-3-O-methyl- (D-acovenose)	$C_7H_{14}O_5$	Syrup	+16.5	82	106rha (82b)		163xyl (82a)	
6-Deoxy-3-O-methyl-D-talitol tetraacetate	$C_{15}H_{24}O_9$					31xyll (82c)		
L-Talose, 6-deoxy- (L-talomethylose)	$C_6H_{12}O_5$	126–127	-20.5±1.4	385cp 360ep		113rha (96a)	189rha (96c)	49rha (96b)
p-Bromophenylhydrazone	$BrC_{13}H_{17}N_2O_4$	145–147	-10→+4 (16°)(c 0.8, C_2H_5OH)	386				
6-Deoxy-L-talonolactone	$C_6H_{10}O_5$	134–135	+33±2 (18°)	386				
Methylphenylhydrazone	$C_{13}H_{20}N_2O_4$	136–137	-12 (17°)(c 0.8, C_2H_5OH)	386				
Methyl α-pyranoside	$C_7H_{14}O_5$	63–65	-104	360	39glc (360b)		81f (360a)	
Methyl α-pyranoside triacetate	$C_{13}H_{20}O_8$	91–92	-73.3 (c 1.2, CH_3OH)	360				
L-Talose, 6-deoxy-3-O-methyl- (L-acovenose)	$C_7H_{14}O_5$	Amorphous	-19.4	351,387	103rha (96a)		385rha (96c)	94rha (96b)
L-Acovenonolactone	$C_7H_{12}O_5$	167–168	+29.4±2 (16°)(CH_3OH)	387,388pt				
Heptose, D-glycero-D-galacto-	$C_7H_{14}O_7$	139–140	+47→+64 (c 0.5)	389ep, 392cp 389	40sor (5)		15f (391)	
2,5-Dichlorophenyl-hydrazone	$C_{13}Cl_2H_{18}N_2O_6$	203–204						
Heptitol, D-glycero-D-galacto-	See Table 1 for this compound							
β-Hexaacetate	$C_{19}H_{26}O_{13}$	109–110	+30.4 (CHCl$_3$)	390				
Trimethylsilyl ether						427^{x}glct (9)		
Heptose, D-glycero-D-gluco-	$C_7H_{14}O_7$	156–157	+17→+46.2 (6h)	394cp	20^{y}sor (5)		80glc (393)	
Heptitol, D-glycero-D-gluco-	See Table 1 for this compound							
α-Hexaacetate	$C_{19}H_{26}O_{13}$	180–182	+105 (CCl$_4$H$_2$)	394				
β-Hexaacetate	$C_{19}H_{26}O_{13}$	133–134	+19.6 (CHCl$_3$)	394				

Table 3 (continued)
NATURAL ALDOSES

Substance[a] (synonym) derivative	Chemical formula	Melting point °C	Specific rotation[b] $[\alpha]_D$	Reference[c]	Chromatography, R value, and reference[d]			
					ELC	GLC	PPC	TLC
(A)	(B)	(C)	(D)	(E)	(F)	(G)	(H)	(I)
Heptose, D-*glycero*-D-*manno*-	$C_7H_{14}O_7$		+21 (CH_3OH)	395–397 egpt	80[y]sor (5)		85glc (398a)	
Heptonolactone, D-*glycero*-D-*manno*-	$C_7H_{12}O_7$	164–165	+48 (*c* 0.2)	395cp			100hep (395)	
Heptitol, D-*glycero*-D-*manno*-	See Table 1 for this compound							
D-*glycero*-D-*manno*-heptitol heptaacetate	$C_{21}H_{30}O_{14}$	Syrup	+34 (*c* 0.4, $CHCl_3$)	397g		198glca (398b)		
α-Hexaacetate	$C_{19}H_{26}O_{13}$	139–140	+65 ($CHCl_3$)	396cp				
Methyl pyranoside	$C_8H_{16}O_7$	Syrup	+47 (CH_3OH)	396				
p-Nitrophenylhydrazone	$C_{13}H_{19}N_3O_8$	176–177		396				
Trimethylsilyl ether						338mant (398b)		
Heptose, L-*glycero*-D-*manno*-	$C_7H_{14}O_7 \cdot H_2O$	179–181	+14 (*c* 0.9)	397–399	80glc (397)		64glc (398a)	
L-*glycero*-D-*manno*-heptitol heptaacetate	$C_{21}H_{30}O_{14}$	116	−11 ($CHCl_3$)	397g		229glca (398b)		
Heptose diethyl dithioacetal	$C_{11}H_{24}O_6S_2$	201–202	+9.9 (C_5H_5N)	400				
Hexabenzoate	$C_{49}H_{38}O_{13}$	100	−32 ($CHCl_3$)	397				
Trimethylsilyl ether						461mant (398b)		
Heptose, 7-deoxy-L-*glycero*-D-*manno*-	$C_7H_{14}O_6$	No constants known	No constants known	401				
Heptononitrile acetate						16.9 (401a)		
Potassium heptonate trimethylsilyl ether						14.2 (401b)		
Heptose, 6-deoxy-D-*manno*-	$C_7H_{14}O_6$		+30±5	402,403			ca. 10 (402a)	
6-Deoxy-D-*manno*-heptitol hexaacetate	$C_{19}H_{28}O_{12}$					125glca (402b)		
Methyl α-pyranoside	$C_8H_{16}O_6$		+80 (*c* 0.5)	403 egp				
Methyl α-pyranoside tetraacetate	$C_{16}H_{24}O_{10}$	77–78	+62 (*c* 0.4, $CHCl_3$)	403				

Table 3 (continued)
NATURAL ALDOSES

Substance[a] (synonym) derivative	Chemical formula	Melting point °C	Specific rotation[b] $[\alpha]_D$	Reference[c]	Chromatography, R value, and reference[d]			
					ELC	GLC	PPC	TLC
(A)	(B)	(C)	(D)	(E)	(F)	(G)	(H)	(I)
Heptose, unidentified		No constants known	No constants known	404–407[z]			68glc (406a) 99glc (406b)	
Octose, 6-amino-6,8-dideoxy-7-O-methyl-D-erythro-D-galacto-(celestose)	$C_9H_{19}NO_6$	No constants known	No constants known	408				
Pentaacetate	$C_{19}H_{29}NO_{11}$	215–216t, 234–234.5		409				

Compiled by George G. Maher.

Table 3 (continued)
NATURAL ALDOSES

REFERENCES

1. Pollock and Stevens, *Dictionary of Organic Compounds*, Oxford University Press, New York, 1965.
2. Williams and Tucknott, *J. Sci. Food Agric.*, 22, 264 (1971).
3. Bloem, *J. Chromatogr.*, 35, 108 (1968).
4. Wohl and Momber, *Ber. Dtsch. Chem. Ges.*, 50, 456 (1917).
5. Bourne, Hutson, and Weigel, *J. Chem. Soc.* (Lond.), p. 4252 (1960).
6. Bourne, Hutson, and Weigel, *J. Chem. Soc.* (Lond.), p. 5153 (1960).
7. Bancher, Scherz, and Kaindl, *Mikrochim. Acta*, p. 1043 (1964).
8. Fischer and Baer, *Helv. Chim. Acta*, 17, 622 (1934).
9. Sweeley, Bentley, Makita, and Wells, *J. Am. Chem. Soc.*, 85, 2497 (1963).
10. Williams and Jones, *Can. J. Chem.*, 42, 69 (1964).
11. Vongerichten, *Justus Liebigs Ann. Chem.*, 321, 71 (1902).
12. Schmidt, *Justus Liebigs Ann. Chem.* 483, 115 (1930).
13. Duff, *Biochem. J.*, 94, 768 (1965).
14. Hulyalkar, Jones, and Perry, *Can. J. Chem.*, 43, 2085 (1965).
15. Bentley, Cunningham, and Spring, *J. Chem. Soc.* (Lond.), p. 2301 (1951).
16. Hockett and Hudson, *J. Am. Chem. Soc.*, 56, 1632 (1934).
17. Němec, Kefurt, and Jarý, *J. Chromatogr.*, 26, 116 (1967).
18. Fischer, Bergmann, and Schotts, *Ber. Dtsch. Chem. Ges.*, 53, 522 (1920).
19. Misaki and Yukawa, *J. Biochem.* (Tokyo), 59, 511 (1966).
20. Haworth, Peat, and Whetstone, *J. Chem. Soc.* (Lond.) p. 1975 (1938).
21. Halliburton and McIlroy, *J. Chem. Soc.* (Lond.), p. 299 (1949).
22. Lynch, Olney, and Wright, *J. Sci. Food Agric.*, 9, 56 (1958).
23. Williams and Jones, *Can. J. Chem.*, 45, 275 (1967).
24. Sowden, Oftedahl, and Kirkland, *J. Org. Chem.*, 27, 1791 (1962).
25. Jones, Kent, and Stacey, *J. Chem. Soc.* (Lond.), p. 1341 (1947).
26. Vogel, *Helv. Chim. Acta*, 11, 1210 (1928).
27. Montgomery and Hudson, *J. Am. Chem. Soc.*, 56, 2074 (1934).
28. Frahn and Mills, *Aust. J. Chem.*, 12, 65 (1959).
29. Phillips and Criddle, *J. Chem. Soc.* (Lond.), p. 3404 (1960).
30. Wolfrom, Patin, and de Lederkremer, *J. Chromatogr.*, 17, 488 (1965).
31. Whistler and Kirby, *J. Am. Chem. Soc.*, 78, 1755 (1956).
32. Hudson and Dale, *J. Am. Chem. Soc.*, 40, 995 (1918).
33. Jones, *J. Chem. Soc.* (Lond.), p. 1055 (1947).
34. Roberts, Johnston, and Fuhr, *Anal. Biochem.*, 10, 282 (1965).
35. Mackie and Percival, *Biochem. J.*, 91, 5P (1964).
36. Alberda van Ekenstein, *Chem. Weekbl.*, 11, 189 (1914).
37. Adachi, *J. Chromatogr.*, 17, 295 (1965).
38. Galmarini and Deulofeu, *Tetrahedron*, 15, 76 (1961).
39. Levene and Wolfrom, *J. Biol. Chem.*, 78, 525 (1928).
40. Gee, *Anal. Chem.*, 35, 354 (1963).
41. Dyer, McGonigal, and Rice, *J. Am. Chem. Soc.*, 87, 654 (1965).
42. Kuehl, Jr., Flynn, Brink, and Folkers, *J. Am. Chem. Soc.*, 68, 2679 (1946).
43. Tatsuoka, Kusaka, Miyake, Inone, Hitomi, Shiraishi, Iwasaki, and Imanishi, *Pharm. Bull.*, 5, 343 (1957).
44. Stodola, Shotwell, Borud, Benedict, and Riley, Jr., *J. Am. Chem. Soc.*, 73, 2290, 5912 (1951).
45. Brimacombe and Mofti, *J. Chem. Soc. D Chem. Commun.*, p. 241 (1971).
46. Ganguly, Sarre, and Morton, *J. Chem. Soc. D Chem. Commun.*, p. 1488 (1969).
47. Hogenkamp and Barker, *J. Biol. Chem.*, 236, 3097 (1961).
48. Deriaz, Overend, Stacey, Teece, and Wiggins, *J. Chem. Soc.* (Lond.), p. 1879 (1949).
49. Bourne, Lees, and Weigel, *J. Chromatogr.*, 11, 253 (1963).
50. Lombard, *J. Chromatogr.*, 26, 283 (1967).
51. Allerton and Overend, *J. Chem. Soc.* (Lond.), p. 1480 (1951).
52. Oades, *J. Chromatogr.*, 28, 246 (1967).
53. Phelps, Isbell, and Pigman, *J. Am. Chem. Soc.*, 56, 747 (1934).
54. Levene and Tipson, *J. Biol. Chem.*, 115, 731 (1936).
55. Zinner, *Ber. Dtsch. Chem. Ges.*, 86, 817 (1953).
56. Barker and Smith, *J. Chem. Soc.* (Lond.), p. 1323 (1955).

Table 3 (continued)
NATURAL ALDOSES

57. Burton, Overend, and Williams, *J. Chem. Soc.* (Lond.), pp. 3433, 3446 (1965).
58. Ezekial, Overend, and Williams, *Carbohydr. Res.*, 11, 233 (1969).
59. Kärkkainen, Haohti, and Lehtonen, *Anal. Chem.*, 38, 1316 (1966).
60. Schroeder, Barnes, Bohinski, Mumma and Mallette, *Biochim. Biophys. Acta*, 273, 254 (1972).
61. Levene and Sobotka, *J. Biol. Chem.*, 65, 55 (1925).
62. Hudson and Yanovsky, *J. Am. Chem. Soc.*, 39, 1013 (1917).
63. Isbell and Pigman, *J. Res. Natl. Bur. Stand.*, 18, 141 (1937).
64. Alberda van Ekenstein and Blanksma, *Recl. Trav. Chim. Pays-Bas*, 22, 434 (1903).
65. Reclaire, *Ber. Dtsch. Chem. Ges.*, 41, 3665 (1908).
66. Hudson and Johnson, *J. Am. Chem. Soc.*, 37, 2748 (1915).
67. Stephen, Kaplan, Taylor, and Leisegang, *Tetrahedron*, Suppl. 7, 233 (1966).
68. Tyler, *J. Chem. Soc.* (Lond.), pp. 5288, 5300 (1965).
69. Hay, Lewis, and Smith, *J. Chromatogr.*, 11, 479 (1963).
70. Gorin, Hough, and Jones, *J. Chem. Soc.* (Lond.), p. 2140 (1953).
71. Levene and Compton, *J. Biol. Chem.*, 111, 325 (1935).
72. Ryan, Arzoumanian, Acton, and Goodman, *J. Am. Chem. Soc.*, 86, 2497 (1964).
73. Andrews and Hough, *Chem. Ind*, p. 1278 (1956).
74. Alam and McIlroy, *J. Chem. Soc. Sect. C Org. Chem.*, p. 1579 (1967).
75. Robertson and Speedie, *J. Chem. Soc.* (Lond.), p. 824 (1934).
76. Lance and Jones, *Can. J. Chem.*, 45, 1995 (1967).
77. Laidlaw, *J. Chem. Soc.* (Lond.), p. 752 (1954).
78. Aspinall and McKay, *J. Chem. Soc.* (Lond.), p. 1059 (1958).
79. Laidlaw and Percival, *J. Chem. Soc.* (Lond.), p. 528 (1950).
80. Aspinall, *J. Chem. Soc.* (Lond.), p. 1676 (1963).
81. Hough and Jones, *J. Chem. Soc.* (Lond.), p. 4349 (1952).
82. Weckesser, Mayer, and Fromme, *Biochem. J.*, 135, 293 (1973).
83. Percival and Willox, *J. Chem. Soc.* (Lond.), p. 1608 (1949).
84. Wintersteiner and Klingsberg, *J. Am. Chem. Soc.*, 71, 939 (1949).
85. Weckesser, Rosenfelder, Mayer, and Lüderitz, *Eur. J. Biochem.*, 24, 112 (1971).
86. Anderle, Kováč and Anderlová, *J. Chromatogr.*, 64, 368 (1972).
87. Kunstmann, Mitscher, and Bohonos, *Tetrahedron Lett.*, p. 839 (1966).
88. Paulsen and Redlich, *Angew. Chem. Int. Ed.*, 11, 1021 (1972).
89. Beylis, Howard, and Perold, *J. Chem. Soc. D Chem. Commun.*, p. 597 (1971).
90. Steiger and Reichstein, *Helv. Chim. Acta*, 19, 184 (1936).
91. Scher and Ginsburg, *J. Biol. Chem.*, 243, 2385 (1968).
92. Levene and Jacobs, *Ber. Dtsch. Chem. Ges.*, 43, 3141 (1910).
93. Lerner and Kohn, *J. Med. Chem.*, 7, 655 (1964).
94. Muhlradt, Weiss, and Reichstein, *Justus Liebigs Ann. Chem.*, 685, 253 (1965).
95. MacLennan and Randall, *Anal. Chem.*, 31, 2020 (1959).
96. Kaufmann, Mühlradt, and Reichstein, *Helv. Chim. Acta*, 50, 2287 (1967).
97. Keller and Reichstein, *Helv. Chim. Acta*, 32, 1607 (1949).
98. Perry and Daoust, *Carbohydr. Res.*, 31, 131 (1973).
99. Levene and Compton, *J. Biol. Chem.*, 117, 37 (1937).
100. Iselin and Reichstein, *Helv. Chim. Acta*, 27, 1203 (1944).
101. Brimacombe and Husain, *Chem. Commun.*, 630 (1966).
102. Hoffman, Weiss, and Reichstein, *Helv. Chim. Acta*, 49, 2209 (1966).
103. Brimacombe and Portsmouth, *J. Chem. Soc. Sect. C Org. Chem.*, p. 499 (1966).
104. Krasso and Weiss, *Helv. Chim. Acta*, 49, 1113 (1966).
105. Dion, Woo, and Bartz, *J. Am. Chem. Soc.*, 84, 880 (1962).
106. Brimacombe, Ching, and Stacey, *J. Chem. Soc. Sect. C Org. Chem.*, p. 197 (1969).
107. Brimacombe, Stacey, and Tucker, *J. Chem. Soc.* (Lond.), p. 5391 (1964).
108. Jäger, *Dissertation* (Basel) (1959).
109. Gut and Prins, *Helv. Chim. Acta*, 29, 1555 (1946).
110. Iwadare, *Bull. Chem. Soc. Jap.*, 17, 296 (1942).
111. Krauss, *Dissertation* (Basel) (1959).
112. Grob and Prins, *Helv. Chim. Acta*, 28, 840 (1945).
113. Hauser and Sigg, *Helv. Chim. Acta*, 54, 1178 (1971).
114. Ellwood and Kirk, *Biochem. J.*, 122, 14P (1971).

Table 3 (continued)
NATURAL ALDOSES

115. Kaufmann, *Helv. Chim. Acta*, 48, 83 (1965).
116. Brimacombe, Da'aboul, and Tucker, *J. Chem. Soc. Sec. C Org. Chem.*, p. 3762 (1971).
117. Kiliani, *Ber. Dtsch. Chem. Ges.*, 46, 667 (1913).
118. Kiliani, *Arch. Pharm.*, 234, 449 (1896); *Chem. Zentralbl.*, 67, II, 591 (1896).
119. Ruber, Minsaas, and Lyche, *J. Chem. Soc.* (Lond.), p. 2173 (1929).
120. Charlton, Haworth, and Hickinbottom, *J. Chem. Soc.* (Lond.), p. 1527 (1927).
121. Nottbohm and Mayer, *Vorratspflege Lebensmittelforsch.*, 1, 243 (1938).
122. Hudson and Parker, *J. Am. Chem. Soc.*, 37, 1589 (1915).
123. O'Neill, *J. Am. Chem. Soc.*, 77, 2837 (1955).
124. Araki and Hirase, *Bull. Chem. Soc. Jap.*, 29, 770 (1956).
125. Clingman and Nunn, *J. Chem. Soc.* (Lond.), p. 493 (1959).
126. Gorin and Spencer, *Can. J. Chem.*, 42, 1230 (1964).
127. Nunn, Parolis, and Russell, *Carbohydr. Res.*, 29, 281 (1973).
128. Gorin and Ishikawa, *Can. J. Chem.*, 45, 521 (1967).
129. Votoček and Valentin, *Collect. Czech. Chem. Commun.*, 2, 36 (1930).
130. Lato, Brunelli, Ciuffini, and Mezzetti, *J. Chromatogr.*, 34, 26 (1968).
131. Shaw and Moss, *J. Chromatogr.*, 41, 350 (1969).
132. Bourne, Hutson, and Weigel, *J. Chem. Soc.* (Lond.), p. 35 (1961).
133. Levvy and McAllan, *Biochem. J.*, 80, 433 (1961).
134. MacPhillamy and Elderfield, *J. Org. Chem.*, 4, 150 (1939).
135. Khare, Schindler, and Reichstein, *Helv. Chim. Acta*, 45, 1534 (1962).
136. Springer, Desai, and Kolechi, *Biochemistry*, 3, 1076 (1964).
137. Lamb and Smith, *J. Chem. Soc.* (Lond.), p. 422 (1936).
138. Gros, *Carbohydr. Res.*, 2, 56 (1966).
139. Schmidt and Wernicke, *Justus Liebigs Ann. Chem.*, 556, 179 (1944).
140. Akita, Maeda, and Umezawa, *J. Antibiot.* (Tokyo) Ser. A, 71, 200 (1964).
141. Nunn and Parolis, *Carbohydr. Res.*, 6, 1 (1968); 8, 361 (1968).
142. Bell and Williamson, *J. Chem. Soc.* (Lond.), p. 1196 (1938).
143. Oldham and Bell, *J. Am. Chem. Soc.*, 60, 323 (1938).
144. Freeman, Stephan, and Van der Bijl, *J. Chromatogr.*, 73, 29 (1972).
145. Lechevalier and Gerber, *Carbohydr. Res.*, 13, 451 (1970).
146. Reber and Reichstein, *Helv. Chim. Acta*, 28, 1164 (1945).
147. Hirst and Jones, *J. Chem. Soc.* (Lond.), p. 506 (1946).
148. Jeanloz, *J. Am. Chem. Soc.*, 76, 5684 (1954).
149. Itasaka, *J. Biochem.* (Tokyo), 60, 52 (1966).
150. Kocourek, Tichà, and Koštiv, *J. Chromatogr.*, 24, 117 (1966).
151. Goldstein, Hamilton, and Smith, *J. Am. Chem. Soc.*, 79, 1190 (1957).
152. Hassid and Su, *Biochemistry*, 1, 468 (1962).
153. Bowker and Turvey, *J. Chem. Soc.* (Lond.), p. 983, 989 (1968).
154. Love and Percival, *J. Chem. Soc.* (Lond.), p. 3338 (1964).
155. Turvey and Williams, *J. Chem. Soc.* (Lond.), p. 2119 (1962); p. 2242 (1963).
156. Anderson, *J. Biol. Chem.*, 100, 249 (1933).
157. Fischer and Hertz, *Ber. Dtsch. Chem. Ges.*, 25, 1247 (1892).
158. Araki and Hirase, *Bull. Chem. Soc. Jap.*, 26, 463 (1953); 33, 291 (1960).
159. Kochetkov, Usov, and Miroshnikova, *J. Gen. Chem. USSR Engl. Ed.*, 40, 2457, 2461 (1970).
160. Usov, Lotov, and Kochetkov, *J. Gen. Chem. USSR Engl. Ed.*, 41, 1156 (1971).
161. Nunn and von Holdt, *J. Chem. Soc.* (Lond.), p. 1094 (1957).
162. Duff and Percival, *J. Chem. Soc.* (Lond.), p. 830 (1941).
163. Minsaas, *Recl. Trav. Chim. Pays-Bas*, 50, 424 (1933).
164. Gardiner and Percival, *J. Chem. Soc.* (Lond.), p. 1414 (1958).
165. Levvy and McAllan, *Biochem. J.*, 80, 433 (1961).
166. Westphal and Feier, *Ber. Dtsch. Chem. Ges.*, 89, 582 (1956).
167. Horowitz and Delman, *J. Chromatogr.*, 21, 302 (1966).
168. Anderson, Andrews, and Hough, *Chem. Ind.*, p. 1453 (1957).
169. Conchie and Percival, *J. Chem. Soc.* (Lond.), p. 827 (1950).
170. Percival and Young, *Carbohydr. Res.*, 32, 195 (1974).
171. Dejter-Juszynski and Flowers, *Carbohydr. Res.*, 28, 61 (1973).
172. Schmidt, Mayer, and Distelmaier, *Justus Liebigs Ann. Chem.*, 555, 26 (1943).

Table 3 (continued)
NATURAL ALDOSES

173. James and Smith, *J. Chem. Soc.* (Lond.), p. 739, 746 (1945).
174. Katzman and Jeanloz, *J. Biol. Chem.*, 248, 50 (1973).
175. Anno, Seno, and Ota, *Carbohydr. Res.*, 13, 167 (1970).
176. Araki, Arai, and Hirasi, *Bull. Chem. Soc. Jap.*, 40, 959 (1967).
177. Turvey and Rees, *Nature*, 189, 831 (1961).
178. Quilico, Piozzi, Pavan, and Mantia, *Tetrahedron*, 5, 10 (1959).
179. Zervas, *Ber. Dtsch. Chem. Ges.*, 64, 2289 (1931).
180. Imanari and Tamura, *Agric. Biol. Chem.*, 35, 321 (1971).
181. Plouvier, *C.R. Acad. Sci.*, 256, 1397 (1963).
182. Hudson and Dale, *J. Am. Chem. Soc.*, 37, 1264, 1280 (1915).
183. Harris, Hirst, and Wood, *J. Chem. Soc.* (Lond.), p. 2108 (1932).
184. Jones and Jones, *Can. J. Chem.*, 47, 3269 (1969).
185. Purdie and Irvine, *J. Chem. Soc.* (Lond.), p. 1049 (1904).
186. Bates, *Polarimetry, Saccharimetry and the Sugars: National Bureau of Standards Circular C440*, U.S. Gov. Print. Off., Washington, D.C., 1942.
187. Georg, *Helv. Chim. Acta*, 12, 261 (1929).
188. Micheel and Berendes, *Mikrochim. Acta*, 519 (1963).
189. Brennan, *J. Chromatogr.*, 59, 231 (1971).
190. Brigl and Scheyer, *Hoppe-Seyler's Z. Physiol. Chem.*, 160, 214 (1926).
191. Alberda van Ekenstein and Blanksma, *Recl. Trav. Chim. Pays-Bas*, 24, 33 (1905).
192. Yoshida, Honda, Iino, and Kato, *Carbohydr. Res.*, 10, 333 (1969).
193. Irvine and Oldham, *J. Chem. Soc.* (Lond.), p. 1744 (1921).
194. Purdie and Irvine, *J. Chem. Soc.* (Lond.), p. 1049 (1904).
195. Irvine and Moodie, *J. Chem. Soc.* (Lond.), p. 1578 (1906).
196. Duff, *J. Chem. Soc.* (Lond.), p. 4730 (1957).
197. Duff, Webley, and Farmer, *Biochem. J.*, 65, 21P (1957).
198. Josephson, *Ber. Dtsch. Chem. Ges.*, 62, 317 (1929).
199. Schumacher, *Carbohydr. Res.*, 13, 1 (1970).
200. Ohle, *Biochem. Z.*, 131, 611 (1922).
201. Brigl and Grüner, *Justus Liebigs Ann. Chem.*, 495, 60 (1932).
202. Fischer and Bergmann, *Ber. Dtsch. Chem. Ges.*, 51, 1760, 1804 (1918).
203. Tschesche, Kämmerer, and Wulff, *Tetrahedron Lett.*, p. 701 (1968).
204. Finnegan, Mueller, and Morris, *Proc. Chem. Soc. London*, p. 182 (1963).
205. Carter, *J. Sci. Food Agric.*, 2, 54 (1951).
206. Finnegan and Stephani, *J. Pharm. Sci.*, 57, 353 (1968).
207. Sloneker and Orentas, *Can. J. Chem.*, 40, 2188 (1962).
208. Fischer and Lieberman, *Ber. Dtsch. Chem. Ges.*, 26, 2415 (1893).
209. Fischer and Zach, *Ber. Dtsch. Chem. Ges.*, 45, 3761 (1902).
210. Evans, Long, Jr., and Parrish, *J. Chromatogr.*, 32, 602 (1968).
211. Staněk and Tajmr, *Chem. Listy*, 52, 551 (1958).
212. Ebert and Zenk, *Arch. Mikrobiol.*, 54, 276 (1966).
213. Frèrejacque, *C.R. Acad. Sci.*, 230, 127 (1950).
214. Korte, *Ber. Dtsch. Chem. Ges.*, 88, 1527 (1955).
215. Reyle and Reichstein, *Helv. Chim. Acta*, 35, 195 (1956).
216. Allgeier, Weiss, and Reichstein, *Helv. Chim. Acta*, 50, 456 (1967).
217. Miyano and Benson, *J. Am. Chem. Soc.*, 84, 59 (1962).
218. Chanley, Ledeen, Wax, Nigrelli, and Sobotka, *J. Am. Chem. Soc.*, 81, 5180 (1959).
219. Saier, Jr. and Ballou, *J. Biol. Chem.*, 243, 992 (1968).
220. Jeanloz and Gut, *J. Am. Chem. Soc.*, 76, 5793 (1954).
221. Irvine and Scott, *J. Chem. Soc.* (Lond.), p. 571, 575, 582 (1913).
222. Oldham, *J. Am. Chem. Soc.*, 56, 1360 (1934).
223. Jeanloz, Rapin, and Hakomori, *J. Org. Chem.*, 26, 3939 (1961).
224. Levene and Raymond, *J. Biol. Chem.*, 88, 513 (1930).
225. Lee and Ballou, *J. Biol. Chem.*, 239, 3602 (1964).
226. Helferich, Klein, and Schafer, *Ber. Dtsch. Chem. Ges.*, 59, 79 (1926).
227. Helferich and Himmen, *Ber. Dtsch. Chem. Ges.*, 62, 2136, 2141 (1929).
228. Helferich and Gunther, *Ber. Dtsch. Chem. Ges.*, 64, 1276 (1931).
229. White and Rao, *J. Am. Chem. Soc.*, 75, 2617 (1953).

Table 3 (continued)
NATURAL ALDOSES

230. Christensen and Smith, *J. Am. Chem. Soc.*, 79, 4492 (1957).
231. Fischer, *Ber. Dtsch. Chem. Ges.*, 23, 2618 (1890).
232. Makarevich and Kolesnikov, *Chem. Nat. Compd., (USSR)*, 5, 164 (1969).
233. Zissis, Richtmyer, and Hudson, *J. Am. Chem. Soc.*, 73, 4714 (1951).
234. Blindenbacher and Reichstein, *Helv. Chim. Acta*, 31, 1669 (1948).
235. Frèrejacque and Hasenfratz, *C.R. Acad. Sci.*, 222, 815 (1946).
236. Frèrejacque and Durgeat, *C.R. Acad. Sci.*, 228, 1310 (1949).
237. Doebel, Schlittler, and Reichstein, *Helv. Chim. Acta*, 31, 688 (1948).
238. Perry and Daoust, *Can. J. Chem.*, 51, 3039 (1973).
239. Capek, Tikal, Jary, and Masojidková, *Collect. Czech. Chem. Commun.*, 36, 1973 (1971).
240. Takita, Maeda, Umezawa, Omoto, and Umezawa, *J. Antibiot. (Tokyo) Ser. A*, 22, 237 (1969).
241. Evans and Parrish, *Carbohydr. Res.*, 28, 359 (1973).
242. Wolfrom and Anno, *J. Am. Chem. Soc.*, 74, 5583 (1952).
243. Cooke and Percival, *Carbohydr. Res.*, 32, 383 (1974).
244. Ohashi, Kawabe, Kono, and Ito, *Agric. Biol. Chem.*, 37, 2379 (1973).
245. Avigad, Amaral, Asensio, and Horecker, *J. Biol. Chem.*, 237, 2736 (1962).
246. Maradufer and Perlin, *Carbohydr. Res.*, 32, 127 (1974).
247. Wolfrom and Usdin, *J. Am. Chem. Soc.*, 75, 4318 (1953).
248. Perlin, Mackie, and Dietrich, *Carbohydr. Res.*, 18, 185 (1971).
249. Webb, Broschard, Cosulich, Mowat, and Lancaster, *J. Am. Chem. Soc.*, 84, 3183 (1962).
250. Overend, Stacey, and Staněk, *J. Chem. Soc.* (Lond.), p. 2841 (1949).
251. Bonner, *J. Org. Chem.*, 26, 908 (1961).
252. Wirz and Hardegger, *Helv. Chim. Acta*, 54, 2017 (1971).
253. Keleti, Mayer, Fromme, and Lüderitz, *Eur. J. Biochem.*, 16, 284 (1970).
254. Černy, Pacák, and Staněk, *Chem. Ind.*, p. 945 (1961).
255. Herzog, Meseck, Delorenzo, Murawski, Charney, and Rosselet, *Appl. Microbiol.*, 13, 515 (1965).
256. Zorbach and Ciaudelli, *J. Org. Chem.*, 30, 451 (1965).
257. Studer, Panavaram, Gavilanes, Linde, and Meyer, *Helv. Chim. Acta*, 46, 23 (1963).
258. Berlin, Esipov, Kiseleva, and Kolosov, *Chem. Nat. Compd., (USSR)*, 3, 280 (1967).
259. Brufani, Keller-Schierlein, Löffler, Mansperger, and Zähner, *Helv. Chim. Acta*, 51, 1293 (1968).
260. Ganguly and Sarre, *J. Chem. Soc. D Chem. Commun.*, p. 1149 (1969).
261. Vischer and Reichstein, *Helv. Chim. Acta*, 27, 1332 (1944).
262. Tschesche and Buschauer, *Justus Liebigs Ann. Chem.*, 603, 59 (1957).
263. Allgeier, *Helv. Chim. Acta*, 51, 311, 668 (1968).
264. Westphal, Lüderitz, Fromme, and Joseph, *Angew. Chem.*, 65, 555 (1953).
265. Fouquey, Lederer, Lüderitz, Polonsky, Staub, Stirm, Tirelli, and Westphal, *C.R. Acad. Sci.*, 246, 2417 (1958).
266. Williams, Szarek, and Jones, *Can. J. Chem.*, 49, 796 (1971).
267. Stirm, Lüderitz, and Westphal, *Justus Liebigs Ann. Chem.*, 696, 180 (1966).
268. Berlin, Esipov, Kolosov, Shemyakin, and Brazhnikova, *Tetrahedron Lett.*, p. 1323 (1964).
269. Miyamoto, Kawamatsu, Shinohara, Nakadaira, and Nakanishi, *Tetrahedron*, 22, 2785 (1966).
270. Blindenbacher and Reichstein, *Helv. Chim. Acta*, 31, 2061 (1948).
271. Hesse, *Ber. Dtsch. Chem. Ges.*, 70, 2264 (1937).
272. Celmer and Hobbs, *Carbohydr. Res.*, 1, 137 (1965).
273. Davies, *Nature*, 191, 43 (1961).
274. Ganguly, Sarre, and Reimann, *J. Am. Chem. Soc.*, 90, 7129 (1968).
275. Stevens, Nagarajan, and Haskell, *J. Org. Chem.*, 27, 2991 (1962).
276. Stevens, Cross, and Toda, *J. Org. Chem.*, 28, 1283 (1963).
277. Albano and Horton, *J. Org. Chem.*, 34, 3519 (1969).
278. Williams, Szarek, and Jones, *Carbohydr. Res.*, 20, 49 (1971).
279. Berlin, Esipov, Kolosov, and Shemyakin, *Tetrahedron Lett.*, p. 1431 (1966).
280. Berlin, Borisova, Esipov, Kolosov, and Kirvoruchko, *Chem. Nat. Compd., (USSR)*, 5, 89, 94 (1969).
281. Brimacombe and Portsmouth, *Carbohydr. Res.*, 1, 128 (1965); *Chem. Ind.*, p. 468 (1965).
282. Howarth, Szarek, and Jones, *Can. J. Chem.*, 46, 3375 (1968).
283. Shoppe and Reichstein, *Helv. Chim. Acta*, 25, 1611 (1942).
284. Tamm and Reichstein, *Helv. Chim. Acta*, 31, 1630 (1948).
285. Brimacombe, Portsmouth, and Stacey, *J. Chem. Soc.* (Lond.), p. 5614 (1965).
286. Miyamoto, Kawamatsu, Shinohara, Asahi, Nakedaira, Kakisawa, Nakanishi, and Bhacca, *Tetrahedron Lett.*, p. 693 (1963).

Table 3 (continued)
NATURAL ALDOSES

287. Iselin and Reichstein, *Helv. Chim. Acta*, 27, 1200 (1944).
288. Brockmann and Waehneldt, *Naturwissenschaften*, 48, 717 (1961).
289. Wyss, Jäger, and Schindler, *Helv. Chim. Acta*, 43, 664 (1960).
290. Renkonen, Schindler, and Reichstein, *Helv. Chim. Acta*, 42, 182 (1959); 39, 1490 (1956).
291. Kilani, *Arch. Pharm.*, 234, 486 (1896).
292. Stahl and Kaltenbach, *J. Chromatogr.*, 5, 351 (1961).
293. Haga, Chonan, and Tejima, *Carbohydr. Res.*, 16, 486 (1971).
294. El-Dash and Hodge, *Carbohydr. Res.*, 18, 259 (1971).
295. Krasso, Weiss, and Reichstein, *Helv. Chim. Acta*, 46, 1691 (1963).
296. Jacobs, *J. Biol. Chem.*, 88, 519 (1930).
297. Bolliger and Ulrich, *Helv. Chim. Acta*, 35, 93 (1952).
298. Prins, *Helv. Chim. Acta*, 29, 378 (1949).
299. Fouquey, Polonsky, Lederer, Westphal, and Lüderitz, *Nature*, 182, 944 (1958).
300. Davies, Staub, Fromme, Lüderitz, and Westphal, *Nature*, 181, 822 (1958).
301. Ekborg and Svensson, *Acta Chem. Scand.*, 27, 1437 (1973).
302. Woo, Dion, and Bartz, *J. Am. Chem. Soc.*, 83, 3352 (1961).
303. Keller-Schierlein and Roncari, *Helv. Chim. Acta*, 45, 138 (1962); 49, 705 (1966).
304. Westphal and Lüderitz, *Angew. Chem.*, 72, 881 (1960).
305. Kochetkov and Usov, *Bull. Acad. Sci. USSR Engl. Ed.*, p. 471 (1965).
306. Stevens, Blumbergs, and Wood, *J. Am. Chem. Soc.*, 86, 3592 (1964).
307. Brockmann and Waehneldt, *Naturwissenschaften*, 50, 43 (1963).
308. Rinehart, Jr. and Borders, *J. Am. Chem. Soc.*, 85, 4037 (1963).
309. Haines, *Carbohydr. Res.*, 21, 99 (1972).
310. Kowalewski, Schindler, Jäger, and Reichstein, *Helv. Chim. Acta*, 43, 1214, 1280 (1960).
311. Golab and Reichstein, *Helv. Chim. Acta*, 44, 616 (1961).
312. Angus, Bourne, and Weigel, *J. Chem. Soc.* (Lond.), p. 22 (1965).
313. Bolliger and Reichstein, *Helv. Chim. Acta*, 36, 302 (1953).
314. Jacobs and Bigelow, *J. Biol. Chem.*, 96, 355 (1932).
315. Abisch, Tamm, and Reichstein, *Helv. Chim. Acta*, 42, 1014 (1959).
316. Hauenstein and Reichstein, *Helv. Chim. Acta*, 33, 446 (1950).
317. Matern, Grisebach, Karl, and Achenbach, *Eur. J. Biochem.*, 29, 1, 5 (1972).
318. Arcamone, Barbieri, Franceschi, Penco, and Vigevani, *J. Am. Chem. Soc.*, 95, 2008 (1973).
319. Regna, Hochstein, Wagner, and Woodward, *J. Am. Chem. Soc.*, 75, 4625 (1953).
320. Hofheinz, Grisebach, and Friebolin, *Tetrahedron*, 18, 1265 (1962).
321. Lemal, Pacht, and Woodward, *Tetrahedron*, 18, 1275 (1962).
322. Flaherty, Overend, and Williams, *J. Chem. Soc., Sect. C, Org. Chem.*, p. 398 (1966).
323. Foster, Inch, Lehmann, Thomas, Webber, and Wyer, *Proc. Chem. Soc. London*, p. 254 (1962); *Chem. Ind.*, p. 1619 (1962).
324. Paul and Tchelitcheff, *Bull. Soc. Chim. Fr.*, p. 443 (1957).
325. Jaret, Mallams, and Reimann, *J. Chem. Soc. (Lond.) Perk. I*, p. 1374 (1973).
326. Omura, Katagiri, and Hata, *J. Antibiot.* (Tokyo), 21, 272 (1968).
327. Watanabe, Fujii, and Satake, *J. Biochem.* (Tokyo), 50, 197 (1961).
328. Flynn, Sigal, Wiley, and Gerzon, *J. Am. Chem. Soc.*, 76, 3121 (1954).
329. Corcoran, *J. Biol. Chem.*, 236, PC27 (1961).
330. Wiley and Weaver, *J. Am. Chem. Soc.*, 77, 3422 (1955); 78, 808 (1956).
331. Lüderitz, Staub, Stirm, and Westphal, *Biochem. Z.*, 330, 193 (1958).
332. Wiley, Mackellar, Carron, and Kelly, *Tetrahedron Lett.*, p. 663 (1968).
333. Zhdanovich, Lokshin, Kuzovkov, and Rudaya, *Chem. Nat. Compd.*, *(USSR)*, 7, 625 (1971).
334. Okuda, Suzuki, and Suzuki, *J. Biol. Chem.*, 242, 958 (1967); 243, 6353 (1968).
335. Haworth, Raistrick, and Stacey, *Biochem. J.*, 29, 2668 (1935).
336. Sorkin and Reichstein, *Helv. Chim. Acta*, 28, 1, 662 (1945).
337. Stoffyn and Jeanloz, *J. Biol. Chem.*, 235, 2507 (1960).
338. Baggett, Stoffyn, and Jeanloz, *J. Org. Chem.*, 28, 1041 (1963).
339. Vargha, *Ber. Dtsch. Chem. Ges.*, 87, 1351 (1954).
340. Levene, *J. Biol. Chem.*, 57, 329 (1923); 59, 129 (1924).
341. Bishop, Perry, Blank, and Cooper, *Can. J. Chem.*, 43, 30 (1965).
342. Hamilton, Partlow, and Thompson, *J. Am. Chem. Soc.*, 82, 451 (1960).
343. Levine, Hansen, and Sell, *Carbohydr. Res.*, 6, 382 (1968).

Table 3 (continued)
NATURAL ALDOSES

344. Butler and Cretcher, *J. Am. Chem. Soc.*, 53, 4358, 4363 (1931).
345. Omoto, Takita, Maeda, and Umezawa, *Carbohydr. Res.*, 30, 239 (1973).
346. Dutton and Yang, *Can. J. Chem.*, 50, 2382 (1972).
347. Markovitz, *J. Biol. Chem.*, 237, 1767 (1962).
348. Ganguly and Saksena, *J. Chim. Soc. D Chem. Commun.*, p. 531 (1973).
349. Wiley, Duchamp, Hsiung, and Chidester, *J. Org. Chem.*, 36, 2670 (1971).
350. Morrison, Young, Perry, and Adams, *Can. J. Chem.*, 45, 1987 (1967).
351. MacLennan, *Biochem. J.*, 82, 394 (1962).
352. MacLennan, Smith, and Randell, *Biochem. J.*, 74, 3P (1960); 80, 309 (1961).
353. Ovodov and Evtushenko, *J. Chromatogr.*, 31, 527 (1967).
354. Caudy and Baddiley, *Biochem. J.*, 98, 15 (1966).
355. Aspinall and Zweifel, *J. Chem. Soc.* (Lond.), p. 2271 (1957).
356. Scheer, Terai, Kulkami, Conant, Wheat, and Plowe, *J. Bacteriol.*, 103, 525 (1970).
357. Perry and Webb, *Can. J. Chem.*, 47, 31 (1969).
358. Gros, Deulofeu, Galmarini, and Frydman, *Experientia*, 24, 323 (1968).
359. Behrend, *Ber. Dtsch. Chem. Ges.*, 11, 1353 (1878).
360. Collins and Overend, *J. Chem. Soc.* (Lond.), p. 1912 (1965).
361. Purdie and Young, *J. Chem. Soc.* (Lond.), p. 89, 1194 (1906).
362. Fischer, *Ber. Dtsch. Chem. Ges.*, 28, 1158 (1895).
363. Fischer, *Ber. Dtsch. Chem. Ges.*, 29, 324 (1896).
364. Fischer, Bergmann, and Rabe, *Ber. Dtsch. Chem. Ges.*, 53, 2362 (1920).
365. Vaterlaus, Kiss, and Spieglberg, *Helv. Chim. Acta*, 47, 381 (1964).
366. Barker, Homer, Keith, and Thomas, *J. Chem. Soc.* (Lond.), p. 1538 (1963).
367. Hinman, Caron, and Hoeksema, *J. Am. Chem. Soc.*, 79, 3789 (1957).
368. Walton, Rodin, Stammer, Holly, and Folkers, *J. Am. Chem. Soc.*, 80, 5168 (1958).
369. Young and Elderfield, *J. Org. Chem.*, 7, 241 (1942).
370. Andrews, Hough, and Jones, *J. Am. Chem. Soc.*, 77, 125 (1955).
371. Hirst, Percival, and Williams, *J. Chem. Soc.* (Lond.), p. 1942 (1958).
372. Schmidt, Plankenhorn, and Kubler, *Ber. Dtsch. Chem. Ges.*, 75, 579 (1942).
373. Brown, Hough, and Jones, *J. Chem. Soc.* (Lond.), p. 1125 (1950).
374. Percival and Percival, *J. Chem. Soc.* (Lond.), p. 690 (1950).
375. Butler, Lloyd, and Stacey, *J. Chem. Soc.* (Lond.), pp. 1531, 1537 (1955).
376. Charalambous and Percival, *J. Chem. Soc.* (Lond.), p. 2443 (1954).
377. Geerdes and Smith, *J. Am. Chem. Soc.*, 77, 3572 (1955).
378. Chaput, Michel, and Lederer, *Experientia*, 17, 107 (1961).
379. Hirst, Hough, and Jones, *J. Chem. Soc.* (Lond.), pp. 928, 3145 (1949).
380. Wiley and Sigal, *J. Am. Chem. Soc.*, 80, 1010 (1958).
381. Pigman and Isbell, *J. Res. Natl. Bur. Stand.*, 19, 189 (1937).
382. Britton, *Biochem. J.*, 85, 402 (1962).
383. Hickman and Ashwell, *J. Biol. Chem.*, 241, 1424 (1966).
384. Stevens, Glinski, and Taylor, *J. Org. Chem.*, 33, 1586 (1968).
385. MacLennon, *Biochim. Biophys. Acta*, 48, 600 (1961).
386. Schmutz, *Helv. Chim. Acta*, 31, 1719 (1948).
387. Von Euw and Reichstein, *Helv. Chim. Acta*, 33, 485 (1950).
388. Kapur and Allgeier, *Helv. Chim. Acta*, 51, 89 (1968).
389. Sephton and Richtmyer, *J. Org. Chem.*, 28, 1691 (1963).
390. Strobach and Szabo, *J. Chem. Soc.* (Lond.), p. 3970 (1963).
391. Isherwood and Jermyn, *Biochem. J.*, 48, 515 (1951).
392. MacLennon and Davies, *Biochem. J.*, 66, 562 (1957).
393. Davies, *Biochem. J.*, 67, 253 (1957).
394. Begbie and Richtmyer, *Carbohydr. Res.*, 2, 272 (1966).
395. Richtmyer and Charlson, *J. Am. Chem. Soc.*, 82, 3428 (1960).
396. Hulyalkar, Jones, and Perry, *Can. J. Chem.*, 41, 1490 (1963).
397. Young and Adams, *Can. J. Chem.*, 43, 2929 (1965).
398. Adams, Quadling, and Perry, *Can. J. Microbiol.*, 13, 1605 (1967).
399. Teuber, Bevill, and Osborn, *Biochemistry*, 7, 3303 (1969).
400. Weidell, *Hoppe-Seyler's Z. Physiol. Chem.*, 299, 253 (1955).
401. Varma, Varma, Allen, and Wardi, *Carbohydr. Res.*, 32, 386 (1974).

Table 3 (continued)
NATURAL ALDOSES

402. Hellerqvist, Lindberg, Samuelson, and Brubaker, *Acta Chem. Scand.*, 26, 1389 (1972).
403. Boren, Eklind, Garegg, Lindberg, and Pilotti, *Acta Chem. Scand.*, 26, 4143 (1972).
404. Davies, *Nature*, 180, 1129 (1957).
405. Missale, Colajacomo, and Bologna, *Boll. Soc. Ital. Biol. Sper.*, 36, 1885 (1960); *Chem. Abstr.*, 55, 24869 (1961).
406. Kuriki and Kurahashi, *J. Biochem.* (Tokyo), 58, 308 (1965).
407. Fraenkel, Osborn, Horecker, and Smith, *Biochem. Biophys. Res. Commun.*, 11, 423 (1963).
408. Hoeksema, *J. Am. Chem. Soc.*, 90, 755 (1968).
409. Hoeksema and Hinman, *J. Am. Chem. Soc.*, 86, 4979 (1964).
410. Tschesche and Kohl, *Tetrahedron*, 24, 4359 (1968).
411. Martinsson and Samuelson, *J. Chromatogr.*, 50, 429 (1970).
412. Walborg, Jr. and Kondo, *Anal. Biochem.*, 37, 323 (1970).

Table 4
NATURAL KETOSES

Substance[a] (synonym) derivative	Chemical formula	Melting point °C	Specific rotation[b] $[\alpha]_D$	Reference[c]	Chromatography, R value, and reference[d]			
					ELC	GLC	PPC	TLC
(A)	(B)	(C)	(D)	(E)	(F)	(G)	(H)	(I)
Triosulose, 3-deoxy-(3-deoxy-2-keto-glyceraldehyde, methyl glyoxal, pyruvic aldehyde)[e]	$C_5H_4O_3$	Oil, bp 72	None	1		6.3, 26.6 (3)		75f (2)
bis-2,4-Dinitrophenylhydrazone	$C_{15}H_{12}N_8O_8$	308–309	None	1			88f (7)	113 for (17)
p-Nitrophenylhydrazone	$C_9H_9N_3O_5$	217	None	1				
Triulose (2-keto-glyceritol, dihydroxyacetone)	$C_3H_6O_3$	80 (dimer)	None	1			55f (4)	40f (2)
Diacetate	$C_7H_{10}O_5$	46–47	None	1			0f (8)	

[a] In alphabetical order by parent sugar names within groups of increasing carbon chain length in the parent compounds.

[b] $[\alpha]_D$ for 1–5 g solute, c, per 100 ml aqueous solution at 20–25°C, unless otherwise given.

[c] References for m.p. and specific rotation data. Letter indicates that the reference also has chromatographic data as follows: c = column, e = electrophoresis, g = gas, p = paper, and t = thin-layer.

[d] R value times 100, given relative to that of the compound indicated by abbreviation: f = solvent front, for = formaldehyde 2,4-dinitrophenylhydrazone, fru = fructose, glc = glucose, glc1 = glucitol, glct = glucose trimethylsilyl ether, manh = *manno*-heptulose, rha = rhamnose, rib = ribose, sed = sedoheptulose, sor = sorbitol, van = vanillin, xyl = xylose. Under gas chromatography (column GLC or G), numbers without code indication signify retention time in minutes. The conditions of the chromatography are correlated with the reference given in parentheses and are found in Table 5.

[e] A possible finding of glyoxal as a component in ethanol distillery streams exists, retention time of 29.9 min, but the identification needs other evidence.[3]

[f] There is no clear evidence that the configuration is D- or L.

[g] Value is in cm/3 hr.

[h] Data are for the enanthiomorphic isomer.

[i] The $1/2H_2O$ and $2H_2O$ forms also exist.

[j] From cured tobacco and animal products fructose and amino acid combinations, which are probably rearranged glycoside compounds and hence not included here, have been isolated; see References 71 and 72.

[k] This is an early structural name. The modern, preferred one is 3-hydroxy-2-furyl methyl ketone.** While perhaps not carbohydrates in a strict sense, this group of pyranose compounds is included because of their intimate relationship.

[l] A hemihydrate of lower melting point forms from the anhydrous anhydro sugar upon aging.

Table 4 (continued)
NATURAL KETOSES

Substance[a] (synonym) derivative	Chemical formula	Melting point °C	Specific rotation[b] [α]_D	Reference[c]	Chromatography, R value, and reference[d]			
					ELC	GLC	PPC	TLC
(A)	(B)	(C)	(D)	(E)	(F)	(G)	(H)	(I)
bis-2,4-Dinitrophenylhydrazone	$C_{16}H_{12}N_8O_9$	277–278	None	1				
p-Nitrophenylhydrazone	$C_9H_{11}N_5O_4$	160	None	1				
Trimethylsilyl ether	Dimer					82glct (5)		
Triulose, 1-amino-1,3-dideoxy- (aminoacetone)	C_3H_7NO	No constants known	No constants known	1				
Hydrochloride	$C_3H_7NO \cdot HCl$	75	None	1				
Triulose, dideoxy- (acetone)	C_3H_6O	Liquid, bp 56	None	1	1.6 (6)			73f (14)
2,4-Dinitrophenyl-hydrazone	$C_9H_{10}N_4O_4$	128	None	1			93f (7)	
p-Nitrophenylhydrazone	$C_9H_{11}N_5O_2$	149	None	1				
Tetradiulose, 1,4-dideoxy- (2,3-butane-dione, diacetyl, di-methylglyoxal)	$C_4H_6O_2$	Liquid, bp 88	None	None	1, 6		4.1 (3)	82f (9)
bis-2,4-Dinitro-phenylhydrazone	$C_{16}H_{14}N_8O_8$	252–254	None	1				
erythro-Butane-2,3-diol	$C_4H_{10}O_2$	23.4	None (meso)	1	6rib (10)	See also Table I	0f (8)	
D,L-threo-Butane-2,3-diol	$C_4H_{10}O_2$	7.6	None (racemic)	1	33rib (10)	See also Table I		
Tetrulose, L-glycero- (L-erythrulose, keto-erythritol, L-treulose)	$C_4H_8O_4$	Syrup	+12	11,12			225glc (13)	
o-Nitrophenylhydra-zone	$C_{10}H_{13}N_3O_6$	152–153	+48 (C_2H_5OH) (18°)	15				

Table 4 (continued)
NATURAL KETOSES

Substance[a] (synonym) derivative	Chemical formula	Melting point °C	Specific rotation[b] $[\alpha]_D$	Reference[c]	Chromatography, R value, and reference[d]			
					ELC	GLC	PPC	TLC
(A)	(B)	(C)	(D)	(E)	(F)	(G)	(H)	(I)
Tetrulose, 1,4-dideoxy-D-*glycero*-(acetoin, 3-hydroxybutan-2-one)	$C_4H_8O_2$	Liquid, bp 143	−1.4 (neat), −105 (H_2O)	1,6,16		24 (3)	91f (9)	
2,4-Dinitrophenyl-hydrazone	$C_{10}H_{12}N_4O_4$	114–116	−12 (CHCl_3)	1				
Pentodiulose, 1,3,5-trideoxy-2,4-(acetyl-acetone, 2,4-pentane-dione)	$C_5H_8O_2$	Liquid bp 139 (746 mm)	None	1		17.3 (3)		
2,4-Dinitrophenyl-hydrazone	$C_{11}H_{12}N_4O_8$	122	None	22				
o-Nitrophenylhydra-zone	$C_{11}H_{13}N_3O_3$	100s, 135m	None	23				
erythro-Pentane-2,4-diol	$C_5H_{12}O_3$				0rib (10)			
threo-Pentane-2,4-diol	$C_5H_{12}O_2$				0rib (10)			
Pentosulose, 3-deoxy-D-(3-deoxy-D-pento-sone)	$C_5H_8O_4$	Oil	+7	17–10	250van (10a)		430glc (19b)	
bis-2,4-Dinitro-phenylhydrazone	$C_{17}H_{16}N_8O_{10}$	259	+294 (dioxane)	18, 19ct		16.5, 18.5 (19c)		66 for (17)
3-Deoxy-pentitol acetates	$C_{15}H_{16}O_8$							
Pentosulose, D-*threo*-[f] (xylosone, xylosulose)	$C_5H_8O_5$	No constants known	No constants known	17				
bis-2,4-Dinitro-phenylhydrazone	$C_{17}H_{17}N_8O_{11}$	231	+187 (c 0.36, dioxane)	17				
Methyl β-pyranoside	$C_6H_{10}O_6$	No constants known	No constants known		100van (20a)		162glc (20b)	
Pentulose, 4-*C*-methyl 1,3,5-trideoxy- (dl-acetone alcohol, 4-hydroxy-4-methyl-2-pentanone)	$C_6H_{12}O_2$	Liquid, bp 164	None	1		37.8 (3)		

Table 4 (continued)
NATURAL KETOSES

Substance[a] (synonym) derivative	Chemical formula	Melting point °C	Specific rotation[b] $[\alpha]_D$	Reference[c]	Chromatography, R value, and reference[d] ELC	GLC	PPC	TLC
(A)	(B)	(C)	(D)	(E)	(F)	(G)	(H)	(I)
2,4-Dinitrophenylhydrazone	$C_{13}H_{16}N_4O_8$	198–199	None	1				
Pentulose, D-erythro- (adonose, D-ribulose)	$C_5H_{10}O_5$	Syrup	−15	24,25cp	209rib (10)		38f (26)	
o-Nitrophenylhydrazone	$C_{11}H_{15}N_3O_6$	165–166.5	−52 ± 5 (CH_3OH)	27				
Trimethylsilyl ether						25, 33, 35glct (28)		
Pentulose, L-erythro- (L-ribulose)	$C_5H_{10}O_5$	Syrup	+16.6	27p, 29			68f (30c)	
o-Nitrophenylhydrazone	$C_{11}H_{15}N_3O_6$	162–163	+47.4 (c 0.3, CH_3OH)	30				
Pentulose, erythro-3-	$C_5H_{10}O_5$		None (meso)	31cp	9.1g (31)			
2,5-Dichlorophenylhydrazone	$C_{11}Cl_3H_{14}N_2O_4$	126–127	None	32cp				
Pentulose, D-threo- (D-xylulose)	$C_5H_{10}O_5$	Syrup	−33	24p	194rib (10)	43f (26)		
p-Bromophenylhydrazone	$BrC_{11}H_{15}N_2O_4$	126–128	+24.1→−31 (C_5H_5N) 7d	24, 33				
2,4-Dinitrophenylhydrazone	$C_{11}H_{14}N_4O_8$	175–176		32				
Pentulose, 5-deoxy-D-threo- (5-deoxy-D-xylulose)	$C_5H_{10}O_4$	−5 ± 1 (CH_3OH) 34c				153rha (34)		
1-Deoxy-D-arabinitol	$C_5H_{12}O_4$				103glct (43)			
1-Deoxy-L-xylitol	$C_5H_{12}O_4$				96glct (43)h			
Phenylosazone	$C_{17}H_{20}N_4O_2$	174–175	+74→+7 (C_5H_5N-C_2H_5OH)	34			45f (44)	
Pentulose, L-threo- (L-xylulose, L-xyloketose, xyloketose)	$C_5H_{10}O_5$	Syrup	+33.3	25p,35,36			65f (30c)	117 xyl (36)
p-Bromophenylhydrazone	$BrC_{11}H_{15}N_2O_4$	128–129	−26→+31.9 (C_6H_5N)	35				

Table 4 (continued)
NATURAL KETOSES

Substance[a] (synonym) derivative (A)	Chemical formula (B)	Melting point °C (C)	Specific rotation[b] $[\alpha]_D$ (D)	Reference[c] (E)	ELC (F)	GLC (G)	PPC (H)	TLC (I)
						Chromatography, R value, and reference[d]		
Phenylosazone	$C_{17}H_{20}N_4O_3$	162–164	No constants known	25				
Hexodiulose, 6-deoxy-D-erythro-2,5-	$C_6H_{10}O_5$	No constants known		37				
1-Deoxy-L-altritol	$C_6H_{14}O_6$	106–108	−2.6 (18°)	58	98glcl (43)[h]		36f (44)[h]	
1-Deoxy-D-galactitol	$C_6H_{14}O_5$				100glcl (43)[h]		31f (44)	
1-Deoxy-D-talitol	$C_6H_{14}O_6$	157–159,			104glcl (43)			
Hexodiulose, D-threo-2,5-(5-keto-fructose)	$C_6H_{10}O_6$	172–174	−85	38,39p			70fru (38)	
bis-Phenylhydrazone	$C_{18}H_{22}N_4O_4$	133–135, 141	−164 (C_5H_5N)	38,39				
Hexos-2,3-diulose, 4,6-dideoxy- (actinospectose)	$C_6H_{10}O_4$	No constants known	No constants known	40				
Hexosulose, D-arabino- (D-glucosone)	$C_6H_{10}O_6$	Syrup	−10.6 → +7.9 (c 8.5) (15°)	41,42			25glc (45)	
2,4-Dinitrophenyl-osazone	$C_{18}H_{18}N_8O_{12}$	253d		46				10 for (17)
Phenylosazone	$C_{18}H_{22}N_4O_4$	206–208	−75→−41 (c 0.7, C_5H_5N-C_2H_5OH, 2:3)	45				
Tetraacetate · H_2O	$C_{14}H_{18}O_{10} \cdot H_2O$	112	+14.7→+53.7 (20% C_2H_5OH) 96h	47				
Hexos-5-ulose, 6-deoxy-D-arabino-	$C_6H_{10}O_5$		−4.3 (CH_3OH) (12°)	48,49			38f (49)	
bis-(p-Nitrophenyl-	$C_{18}H_{20}N_6O_8$	211d	+1.1 (c 0.6, C_5H_5N) (15°)	49				
See also 1-Deoxy-D-galactitol and -D-talitol under Hexodiulose, 6-deoxy-D-erythro-2,5- above								
Hexosulose, 3-deoxy-D-erythro- (3-deoxy-2-	$C_6H_{10}O_5$		−2.5→+1.5 (c 6) (27°)	17,46,50			200–270, 137 / 106 glc (51)	

Table 4 (continued)
NATURAL KETOSES

Substance[a] (synonym) derivative	Chemical formula	Melting point °C	Specific rotation[b] $[\alpha]_D$	Reference[c]	Chromatography, R value, and reference[d]			
					ELC	GLC	PPC	TLC
(A)	(B)	(C)	(D)	(E)	(F)	(G)	(H)	(I)
2,4-Dinitrophenyl-osazone	$C_{18}H_{18}N_8O_{11}$	251d, 265d	+86 (c 0.09, DMSO)	46,51,52				37 for (17)
Hexos-4-ulose, 3,6-dideoxy-D-erythro-	$C_6H_{10}O_4$	No constants known	No constants known	53t				
iso-Propylidene ether	$C_9H_{14}O_4$	Oil, bp 47–49 (0.3 mm)	+166.3 (27°)	53				
Hexos-4-ulose, 3,6-dideoxy-L-erythro-	$C_6H_{10}O_4$	No constants known	No constants known	54				
Hexos-4-ulose, 2,3,6-trideoxy-L-glycero- (cinerulose A)	$C_6H_{10}O_3$			55				
Methyl α-pyranoside	$C_7H_{12}O_3$	158–159	+310±2 (CHCl$_3$)[h]	56				70f (56)[h]
Methyl α-pyranoside p-nitrophenylhy-drazone	$C_{13}H_{17}N_3O_4$		+347±2 (c 0.6, CHCl$_3$)[h]	56				
Hexos-5-ulose, D-lyxo-	$C_6H_{10}O_6$	157–158	-86.6	57p				
bis-(p-Nitrophenyl-hydrazone)	$C_{18}H_{20}N_6O_9$	173–174		57				
bis-Phenylhydrazone	$C_{18}H_{22}N_4O_4$	123–124	-138.5 (c 0.25, C$_5$H$_5$N)	57				
Hexosulose, 6-deoxy-L-lyxo- (angustose, 2-keto-fucose)	$C_6H_{10}O_5$	115–116	+18 (C$_2$H$_5$OH)	58c			36f (58)	
Methyl pyranoside dimethyl acetal	$C_9H_{16}O_6$		-19.3 (CH$_3$OH)	58				
Methyl pyranoside	$C_{11}H_{22}O_6$	77–78	-53.3 (C$_2$H$_5$OH) (18°)	58				
6-Deoxy-L-talitol (1-deoxy-L-altritol)	$C_6H_{14}O_5$	106–108	-2.6 (18°)	58	98glcl (43)[h]		36f (44)[h]	
Hexos-3-ulose, D-ribo- (3-keto-D-glucose)	$C_6H_{10}O_6 \cdot 5H_2O$	58–60	+14.8 (26°)	59			116fru (59)	
Methyl α-pyranoside trimethyl ether	$C_{10}H_{18}O_6$	82.5–83.5	$[\alpha]_{1,78}$ +164 (c 0.9, CHCl$_3$)	60t				

Table 4 (continued)
NATURAL KETOSES

Substance[a] (synonym) derivative	Chemical formula	Melting point °C	Specific rotation[b] $[\alpha]_D$	Reference[c]	Chromatography, R value, and reference[d]			
					ELC	GLC	PPC	TLC
(A)	(B)	(C)	(D)	(E)	(F)	(G)	(H)	(I)
Methyl β-pyranoside trimethyl ether	$C_{10}H_{18}O_6$	117.5–119.5	$[\alpha]_{578}$ −24 (CHCl₃)	60t				
Hexos-3-ulose, 6-deoxy-L-ribo-, 2-acetate	$C_8H_{12}O_6$	No constants known	No constants known	61				
Hexulose, β-D-arabino-β-D-fructose, levulose)[j]	$C_6H_{12}O_6{}^l$	102–104	−133.5→−92	62,63	75rib (10)		38f (4)	28f (64)
β-Furanoside tetrabenzoate	$C_{34}H_{28}O_{10}$	174–175	−165 (CHCl₃)	65				87f (66)
Methyl α-pyranoside tetramethyl ether	$C_{11}H_{22}O_6$							23f (67)
Methyl β-pyranoside tetramethyl ether	$C_{11}H_{22}O_6$							16f (67)
p-Nitrophenylhydrazone	$C_{12}H_{17}N_3O_7$	176		68				
β-Pyranoside tetraacetate	$C_{14}H_{20}O_{10}$	131–132	−91.6 (CHCl₃)	69,70				
Trimethylallyl ether	$C_{21}H_{55}O_6Si_5$		−73.8 (hexane)	106		69glct (28)		
Hexulose, 6-deoxy-D-arabino-(D-rhamnulose)	$C_6H_{12}O_5$	Syrup	−6±1,−13±2	73,74			120rha (74)	
1-Deoxy-L-gulitol 1-Deoxy-D-mannitol	$C_6H_{14}O_5$ $C_6H_{14}O_5$			73	94glct (43) 100glct (43)			
o-Nitrophenylhydrazone	$C_{12}H_{17}N_3O_6$	136–137	+40±3 (C₂H₅OH)	73				
Hexulose, D-lyxo- (D-tagatose)	$C_6H_{12}O_6$	131–132	+2,7→−4	75	103rib (10)		38f (4)	46f (64)
Phenylosazone	$C_{18}H_{22}N_4O_4$	186–187		76				
Pyranose pentaacetate	$C_{16}H_{22}O_{11}$	132	$[\alpha]_{578}$ +30.2 (CHCl₃)	77,78				

Table 4 (continued)
NATURAL KETOSES

Substance[a] (synonym) derivative	Chemical formula	Melting point °C	Specific rotation[b] $[\alpha]_D$	Reference[c]	Chromatography, R value, and reference[d]			
					ELC	GLC	PPC	TLC
(A)	(B)	(C)	(D)	(E)	(F)	(G)	(H)	(I)
Tagaturonic acid Trimethylsilyl ether	See Table 2							
Hexulose, 6-deoxy-L-lyxo-(L-fuculose)	$C_6H_{12}O_5$	68–69	+3.4±1	80		varied 60–159 glct (79)	50f (81)	
o-Nitrophenylhydrazone	$C_{12}H_{17}N_3O_6$	162–163		81				
See also 1-Deoxy-D-galacitol and -L-altritol under Hexodiulose, 6-deoxy-D-erythro-2,5-, above								
Hexulose, D-ribo- (D-allulose, D-psicose)	$C_6H_{12}O_6$	Amorphous	+3.2, +4.7	82,83	188rib (10)		145glc (84)	
Methyl glycoside tetramethyl ether	$C_{11}H_{22}O_6$	104 (2 mm)	-28.3 (C_2H_5OH) (18°)	82				
Phenylosazone Pyranose pentaacetate	$C_{18}H_{22}N_4O_4$ $C_{16}H_{22}O_{11}$	159–163 63–65	-74→-68 (C_5H_5N) -21.5 ($CHCl_3$) (29°)	85p 86c				
Hexulose, L-xylo- (L-sorbose)	$C_6H_{12}O_6$	159–161	-43.1	87	73rib (10)		33f (4)	43f (64)
α-Pyranoside pentaacetate	$C_{16}H_{22}O_{11}$	97	-56.5 ($CHCl_3$)	88				
β-Pyranoside pentaacetate	$C_{16}H_{22}O_{11}$	113.8	+74.4 ($CHCl_3$)	88				
Trimethylsilyl ether	$C_{21}H_{52}O_6Si_5$		-16.4 (hexane)	106		85glct (28)		
Hexulose, 6-deoxy-L-xylo- (6-deoxy-L-sorbose)	$C_6H_{12}O_5$	88	-25±2 (c 0.7)	74			134rha (74)	
1-Deoxy-D-glucitol Phenylosazone	$C_6H_{14}O_5$ $C_{18}H_{22}N_4O_3$	184–185		89	98glcl (43)			

Table 4 (continued)
NATURAL KETOSES

Substances[a] (synonym) derivative	Chemical formula	Melting point °C	Specific rotation[b] $[\alpha]_D$	Reference[c]	Chromatography, R value, and reference[d]			
					ELC	GLC	PPC	TLC
(A)	(B)	(C)	(D)	(E)	(F)	(G)	(H)	(I)
Pyran-4-one, 3,5-dihydroxy-2-hydroxymethyl- (iso-kojic acid, hydroxy-kojic acid, oxy-kojic acid)	$C_6H_6O_5$	187	None	90			46f (91)	
3,5-Di-O-methyl ether	$C_8H_{10}O_5$	115.5–117	None	90				
2,4-Dinitrophenyl-hydrazone	$C_{12}H_{11}N_4O_8$	118.5–119.5	None	90				
Pyran-4-one, 3,5-dihydroxy-2-methyl- (5-hydroxy-maltol, oxy-maltol)	$C_6H_6O_4$	156–156.5, 184–184.5	None	90,92		67.5 (92a)	72f (91)	43f (92b)
3,5-Di-O-methyl ether	$C_8H_{10}O_4$	98	None	90				
Pyran-4-one, 2,3-dihydro-3,5-dihydroxy-6-methyl- (dihydrohydroxymaltol)	$C_6H_8O_4$	67–70	None	92		65 (92a)		38f (92b)
Pyran-4-one, 5-hydroxy-2-hydroxymethyl- (kojic acid)	$C_6H_6O_4$	150–152	None	91			61f (91)	
Diacetate	$C_{10}H_{10}O_6$	101–103	None	93				
2,4-Dinitrophenyl hydrazone	$C_{12}H_{14}N_8O_{10}$	221–224	None	94				
Phenylosazone	$C_{18}H_{18}N_4O_3$	169–170	None	92				
Pyran-4-one, 3-hydroxy-2-methyl- (maltol)	$C_6H_6O_3$	161–162	None	95,96,98p		44 (92a)		45f (92b)
Benzoate	$C_{13}H_{10}O_4$	114–115	None	95				
Methyl ether	$C_7H_8O_3$	Liquid, bp 78–79 (4 mm)						
Phenylurethane	$C_{13}H_{11}NO_4$	152–153	None	95				

Table 4 (continued)
NATURAL KETOSES

Substance[a] (synonym) derivative	Chemical formula	Melting point °C	Specific rotation[b] [α]$_D$	Reference[c]	Chromatography, R value, and reference[d]			
					ELC	GLC	PPC	TLC
(A)	(B)	(C)	(D)	(E)	(F)	(G)	(H)	(I)
Trimethylsilyl ether						4.6 (100)		
Pyran-4-one, 3-hydroxy-5-methyl[k] (iso-maltol)	$C_6H_6O_3$	101±2	None	97		21 (92a)		75f (92b)
Benzoate	$C_{13}H_{16}O_4$	100–101	None	97				
2,4-Dinitrophenyl-hydrazone	$C_{13}H_{16}N_4O_6$	216	None	97				
Methyl-ether	$C_7H_8O_3$	101.5–103	None	92,97				50f (92b)
Heptulose, D-*allo*-	$C_7H_{14}O_7$	128–130	+52.8 (c 0.2)	101c,122	100rib (10)		99fru (101)	
D-*glycero*-D-*allo*-Heptitol	$C_7H_{16}O_7$	144.5–146	None (meso)	122				
D-*glycero*-D-*altro*-Heptitol	$C_7H_{16}O_7$	125–128	−0.3±0.4	107,122	144rib (10)			
Phenylosazone	$C_{19}H_{22}N_4O_5$	164–167	+2.5 (c 10)	101			41f (103)	
Heptulose, D-*altro*-, (sedoheptose, sedo-heptulose)	$C_7H_{14}O_7$	Amorphous		101,102				
See D-*glycero*-D-*gluco*- and D-*glycero*-D-*talo*-Heptitols in Table 1								
2,7-Anhydro-β-pyranose (sedo-heptulosan)	$C_7H_{12}O_6$	155–156	−145	101			73f (103)	
Pyranose hexa-acetate	$C_{19}H_{26}O_{13}$	98–99.5	+59 (CHCl$_3$)	105				
Sedoheptulosan hydrate	$C_7H_{12}O_6 \cdot H_2O$	101–102 (91s)	−132	104		112glct (28)		
Sedoheptulosan trimethylsilyl ether								
Trimethylsilyl ether	$C_{25}H_{62}O_7Si_6$		+18 (hexane)	106		166glct (106)		

Table 4 (continued)
NATURAL KETOSES

Substance[a] (synonym) derivative	Chemical formula	Melting point °C	Specific rotation[b] $[\alpha]_D$	Reference[c]	Chromatography, R value, and reference[d]			
					ELC	GLC	PPC	TLC
(A)	(B)	(C)	(D)	(E)	(F)	(G)	(H)	(I)
Heptulose, D-altro-3-coriose)	$C_7H_{14}O_7$	169–171	+20	101,107gp			99fru (101)	
See D-glycero-D-altro-Heptitol above and D-glycero-D-talo-Heptitol in Table 1								
Pentabenzoate	$C_{42}H_{34}O_{12}$	100–102		107				
Heptulose, L-galacto- (perseulose)	$C_7H_{14}O_7 \cdot \frac{1}{2}H_2O$	100–115	−80, −90	108,109			88manh (110)	
See L-glycero-manno-Heptitol (D-glycero-D-galacto-Heptitol) in Table 1								
L-glycero-D-gluco-Heptitol	$C_7H_{14}O_7$				176rib (10)h			
Phenylosazone	$C_{19}H_{23}N_4O_6$	198–199	−90→−45	110				
Pyranose hexaacetate	$C_{19}H_{26}O_{13}$	112	−113 (CHCl₃)	111				
Heptulose, L-gluco-	$C_7H_{14}O_7$	171–172	−68	110	100sor (116)h		93manh (110)	
L-glycero-L-gulo-Heptitol	$C_7H_{16}O_7$		None (meso)	3	160rib (10)			
L-glycero-L-ido-Heptitol	$C_7H_{16}O_7$	129–130	−0.8	114	168rib (10)h			
Phenylosazone	$C_{19}H_{25}N_4O_6$	181–182d	+6−−35.3 (C₅H₅N-C₂H₅OH,2:3) 96h	114				
Trimethylsilyl ether	$C_{25}H_{62}O_7Si_6$		+36 (hexane)h	106		206glct (106)h		
Heptulose, L-gulo-	$C_7H_{14}O_7$	Syrup	−28	112			53f (118)	
See L-glycero-D-gluco-Heptitol above and D-glycero-D-gluco-Heptitol in Table 1								

Table 4 (continued)
NATURAL KETOSES

Substance[a] (synonym) derivative	Chemical formula	Melting point °C	Specific rotation[b] $[\alpha]_D$	Reference[c]	Chromatography, R value, and reference[d]			
					ELC	GLC	PPC	TLC
(A)	(B)	(C)	(D)	(E)	(F)	(G)	(H)	(I)
2,7-Anhydro-L-gulo-heptulose (gulo-heptulosan)	$C_7H_{12}O_6$	113–115[l]	–39.7	112			65f (118)	
Phenylosazone	$C_{19}H_{26}N_4O_5$	197–200d	+111→+65 (C_5H_5N) 47h	112				
Heptulose, D-ido- See D-glycero-D-ido-Heptitol in Table 1	$C_7H_{14}O_7$		–20	104			50f (118)	
D-glycero-L-ido-Heptitol	$C_7H_{16}O_7$		None (meso)		182rib (10)			
Anhydro-D-ido-heptulose (idoheptulosan)	$C_7H_{12}O_6$	172	–34±8 (c 0.3)	113			86rib (113)	
Phenylosazone	$C_{19}H_{24}N_4O_6$	178–179	+11.6→–43.4 (C_5H_5N) 72h	104				
Heptulose, D-manno- See D-glycero-D-galacto- and D-glycero-D-talo-Heptitols in Table 1	$C_7H_{14}O_7$	152	+29.4	101c,115	40sor (116)		102glc (117)	
Phenylosazone	$C_{19}H_{24}N_4O_6$	200	+74→+35	110,119				
Pyranose hexaacetate	$C_{19}H_{26}O_{13}$	110	+39 ($CHCl_3$)	120				
Trimethylsilyl ether	$C_{25}H_{62}O_7Si_6$		+30.4 (hexane)	106		194glct (106)		
Heptulose, D-talo- See D-glycero-D-altro-Heptitol above D-glycero-L-altro-Heptitol	$C_7H_{14}O_7$	135–137	+47.4→+12.9 (6h)	121,122			138manh (110)	
	$C_7H_{16}O_7$		None (meso)	3				
Octulose, D-glycero-L-galacto	$C_8H_{16}O_8$	Syrup	–57, –43.3→–13.4 (c 0.6)	123cp, 124cp			42sed (101)	
2,5-Dichlorophenyl-hydrazone	$C_{14}Cl_2H_{20}N_2O_7$	178–180		123				

Table 4 (continued)
NATURAL KETOSES

Substance[a] (synonym) derivative (A)	Chemical formula (B)	Melting point °C (C)	Specific rotation[b] $[\alpha]_D$ (D)	Reference[c] (E)	Chromatography, R value, and reference[d]			
					ELC (F)	GLC (G)	PPC (H)	TLC (I)
Octulose, D-glycero-D-manno-	$C_8H_{16}O_8$	Syrup	+20, +25 (CH_3OH)	101c,121p			46sed (101)	
2,5-Dichlorophenyl-hydrazone	$C_{14}Cl_2H_{20}N_2O_7$	169–170		121			80glc (117)	
Phenylosazone	$C_{20}H_{26}N_4O_6$	188–189d		121				
Heptulose, D-ido- See D-glycero-D-ido-Heptitol in Table 1	$C_7H_{14}O_7$		−20	104			50f (118)	
D-glycero-L-ido-Heptitol	$C_7H_{16}O_7$		None (meso)		182rib (10)			
Anhydro-D-ido-heptulose (idoheptulosan)	$C_7H_{12}O_6$	172	−34±8 (c 0.3)	113			86rib (113)	
Phenylosazone	$C_{19}H_{23}N_4O_5$	178–179	+11.6→−43.4 (C_5H_5N) 72h	104				
Heptulose, D-manno- See D-glycero-D-galacto- and D-glycero-D-talo-Heptitols in Table 1	$C_7H_{14}O_7$	152	+29.4	101c,115	40sor (116)		102glc (117)	
Phenylosazone	$C_{19}H_{22}N_4O_5$	200	+74→+35	110,119				
Pyranose hexaacetate	$C_{19}H_{26}O_{13}$	110	+39 $(CHCl_3)$	120				
Trimethylsilyl ether	$C_{25}H_{62}O_7Si_6$		+30.4 (hexane)	106		194glct (106)		
Heptulose, D-talo- See D-glycero-D-altro-Heptitol above	$C_7H_{14}O_7$	135–137	+47.4→+12.9 (6h)	121,122			138manh (110)	
D-glycero-L-altro-Heptitol	$C_7H_{16}O_7$		None (meso)	3				
Octulose, D-glycero-L-galacto	$C_8H_{16}O_8$	Syrup	−57, −43.4→−13.4 (c 0.6)	123cp, 124cp, 123			42sed (101)	
2,5-Dichlorophenyl-hydrazone	$C_{14}Cl_2H_{20}N_2O_7$	178–180						

Table 4 (continued)
NATURAL KETOSES

Substance[a] (synonym) derivative	Chemical formula	Melting point °C	Specific rotation[b] $[\alpha]_D$	Reference[c]	Chromatography, R value, and reference[d]			
					ELC	GLC	PPC	TLC
(A)	(B)	(C)	(D)	(E)	(F)	(G)	(H)	(I)
Octulose, D-glycero-D-manno-	$C_8H_{16}O_8$	Syrup	+20, +25 (CH₃OH)	101c,121p			46sed (101) 80glc (117)	
2,5-Dichlorophenyl-hydrazone	$C_{14}Cl_2H_{18}N_2O_7$	169–170		121				
Phenylosazone See D-erythro-D-galacto-Octitol in Table 1	$C_{20}H_{26}N_4O_6$	188–189d		121				
D-erythro-D-talo-Octitol	$C_8H_{18}O_8$		None (meso)	3				
Nonulose, D-erythro-L-galacto-	$C_9H_{18}O_9$	Syrup	−9.7, −37 (H₂O) −36.2 (95% CH₃OH)	101cp,125 cp				
2,5-Dichlorophenyl-osazone	$C_{21}Cl_4H_{14}N_4O_7$	238–240		125				
D-arabino-D-gluco-Nonitol	$C_9H_{20}O_9$	180–181		125				
D-arabino-D-manno-Nonitol	$C_9H_{20}O_9$	192–193		125				
Trimethylsilyl ether						18.2 (125)		
Nonulose, D-erythro-L-gluco-	$C_9H_{18}O_9$	Syrup	−40 (c 0.6)	126p				
2,5-Dichlorophenyl-osazone	$C_{21}Cl_4H_{14}N_4O_7$	248–250d		126				

Compiled by George G. Maher.

Table 4 (continued)
NATURAL KETOSES

REFERENCES

1. Pollock and Stevens, *Dictionary of Organic Compounds,* Oxford University Press, New York, 1965.
2. Bancher, Scherz, and Kaindl, *Mikrochim. Acta,* 1043 (1964).
3. Maher, unpublished data.
4. Adachi, *Anal. Biochem.,* 9, 224 (1964).
5. Verhaar and de Wilt, *J. Chromatogr.,* 41, 168 (1969).
6. Williams and Tucknott, *J. Sci. Food Agric.,* 22, 264 (1971).
7. Bush and Hockaday, *J. Chromatogr.,* 8, 433 (1962).
8. Gasparic and Vecera, *Collect. Czech. Chem. Commun.,* 22, 1426 (1957).
9. Reio, *J. Chromatogr.,* 1, 338 (1958).
10. Frahn and Mills, *Aust. J. Chem.,* 12, 65 (1959).
11. Bertrand, *Bull. Soc. Chim. Fr. Ser. 3,* 23, 681 (1904).
12. Hu, McComb, and Rendig, *Arch. Biochem. Biophys.,* 110, 350 (1965).
13. Batt, Dickens, and Williamson, *Biochem. J.,* 77, 272 (1960).
14. Bloehm, *J. Chromatogr.,* 35, 108 (1968).
15. Müller, Montigel, and Reichstein, *Helv. Chim. Acta,* 20, 1468 (1937).
16. Blom, *J. Am. Chem. Soc.,* 67, 494 (1945).
17. Kato, Tsusaka, and Fujimaki, *Agric. Biol. Chem.,* 34, 1541 (1970).
18. Kurata and Sakurai, *Agric. Biol. Chem.,* 31, 170, 177 (1967).
19. Humphries and Theander, *Acta Chem. Scand.,* 25, 883 (1971).
20. Brimacombe, Brimacombe, and Lindberg, *Acta Chem. Scand.,* 14, 2236 (1960).
21. Theander, *Acta Chem. Scand.,* 11, 717 (1957).
22. Spence and Degering, *J. Am. Chem. Soc.,* 66, 1624 (1944).
23. Schöpf and Ross, *Justus Liebigs Ann. Chem.,* 546, 30 (1941).
24. Hickman and Ashwell, *J. Am. Chem. Soc.,* 78, 6209 (1956).
25. Futterman and Roe, *J. Biol. Chem.,* 215, 257 (1955).
26. Uehara and Takeda, *J. Biochem. (Tokyo),* 56, 42 (1964).
27. Horecker, Smyrniotis, and Seegmiller, *J. Biol. Chem.,* 193, 383 (1951).
28. Sweeley, Bentley, Makita, and Wells, *J. Am. Chem. Soc.,* 85, 2497 (1963).
29. Reichstein, *Helv. Chim. Acta,* 17, 996 (1934).
30. Simpson, Wolin, and Wood, *J. Biol. Chem.,* 230, 457 (1958).
31. Ashwell and Hickman, *J. Am. Chem. Soc.,* 77, 1062 (1955).
32. Stankovič, Linek, and Fedoroňko, *Carbohydr. Res.,* 10, 579 (1969).
33. Ashwell and Hickman, *J. Biol. Chem.,* 226, 65 (1957).
34. Gorin, Hough, and Jones, *J. Chem. Soc.* (Lond.), p. 2140 (1953).
35. Levene and LaForge, *J. Biol. Chem.,* 18, 319 (1914).
36. Wolfrom and Bennett, *J. Org. Chem.,* 30, 458 (1965).
37. Chassy, Sugimori, and Suhadolnik, *Biochim. Biophys. Acta,* 130, 12 (1966).
38. Avigad and England, *J. Biol. Chem.,* 240, 2290, 2297, 2302 (1965).
39. Whiting and Coggins, *Chem. Ind.,* p. 1925 (1963).
40. Hoeksema, Argoudelis, and Wiley, *J. Am. Chem. Soc.,* 84, 3212 (1962).
41. Bean and Hassid, *Science,* 124, 171 (1956).
42. Bayne, Collie, and Fewster, *J. Chem. Soc.* (Lond.), p. 2766 (1952).
43. Angus, Bourne, and Weigel, *J. Chem. Soc.* (Lond.), p. 22 (1965).
44. Bourne, Lees, and Weigel, *J. Chromatogr.,* 11, 253 (1963).
45. Walton, *Can. J. Chem.,* 47, 3483 (1969).
46. Kato, *Agric. Biol. Chem.,* 27, 461 (1963).
47. Maurer, *Ber. Dtsch. Chem. Ges.,* 63, 25 (1930).
48. Mann and Woolf, *J. Am. Chem. Soc.,* 79, 120 (1957).
49. Takahashi and Nakajima, *Tetrahedron Lett.,* p. 2285 (1967).
50. Együd, *Carbohydr. Res.,* 23, 307 (1972).
51. Fodor, Sachetto, Szent-Györgyi, and Együd, *Proc. Natl. Acad. Sci. U.S.A.,* 57, 1644 (1967).
52. El Khadem, Horton, Meshreki, and Nashed, *Carbohydr. Res.,* 17, 183 (1971).
53. Stevens, Schultze, Smith, Pillai, Rubenstein, and Strominger, *J. Am. Chem. Soc.,* 95, 5767 (1973).
54. Richle, Winkler, Hawley, Dobler, and Keller-Schierlein, *Helv. Chim. Acta,* 55, 467 (1972).
55. Keller-Schierlein and Richle, *Chimia,* 24, 35 (1970).
56. Albano and Horton, *Carbohydr. Res.,* 11, 485 (1969).
57. Weidenhagen and Bernsee, *Angew. Chem.,* 72, 109 (1960).

Table 4 (continued)
NATURAL KETOSES

58. Yünsten, *J. Antibiot. Ser. A*, 11, 77, 233 (1958).
59. Fukui and Hochster, *J. Am. Chem. Soc.*, 85, 1697 (1963).
60. Kenne, Larm, and Svensson, *Acta Chem. Scand.*, 26, 2473 (1972).
61. Kupchan, Sigel, Guttman, Restivo, and Bryan, *J. Am. Chem. Soc.*, 94, 1353 (1972).
62. Hudson and Brauns, *J. Am. Chem. Soc.*, 38, 1216 (1916).
63. Hudson and Yanovsky, *J. Am. Chem. Soc.*, 39, 1025 (1917).
64. Adachi, *J. Chromatogr.*, 17, 295 (1965).
65. Brigl and Schinle, *Ber. Dtsch. Chem. Ges.*, 66, 325 (1933).
66. Hay, Lewis, and Smith, *J. Chromatogr.*, 11, 479 (1963).
67. Gee, *Anal. Chem.*, 35, 350 (1963).
68. Reclaire, *Ber. Dtsch. Chem. Ges.*, 41, 3665 (1908).
69. Pacsu and Rich, *J. Am. Chem. Soc.*, 55, 3018 (1933).
70. Barry and Honeyman, *Adv. Carbohydr. Chem.*, 7, 60, 85 (1952).
71. Tomita, Noguchi, and Tamaki, *Agric. Biol. Chem.*, 29, 515, 959 (1965).
72. Yamamoto and Noguchi, *Agric. Biol. Chem.*, 37, 2185, (1973).
73. Morgan and Reichstein, *Helv. Chim. Acta*, 21, 1023 (1938).
74. Hough and Jones, *J. Chem. Soc.* (Lond.), p. 4052 (1952).
75. Reichstein and Bosshard, *Helv. Chim. Acta*, 17, 753 (1934).
76. Adachi, *J. Agric. Chem. Soc. Jap.*, 32, 309 (1958).
77. Khouvine and Tomoda, *C. R. Acad. Sci.*, 205, 736 (1937).
78. Khouvine, Arragon, and Tomoda, *Bull. Soc. Chim. Fr. Ser. 5*, 6, 354 (1939).
79. Tesařík, *J. Chromatogr.*, 65, 295 (1972).
80. Barnett and Reichstein, *Helv. Chim. Acta*, 21, 913 (1938).
81. Green and Cohen, *J. Biol. Chem.*, 219, 557 (1956).
82. Yüngsten, *J. Antibiot. (Tokyo) Ser. A*, 11, 244 (1958).
83. Wolfrom, Thompson, and Evans, *J. Am. Chem. Soc.*, 67, 1793 (1945).
84. Bourne, Percival, and Smestad, *C. R. Acad. Sci.*, 260, 999 (1965)
85. Strecker, Gouret, and Montreuil, *Compt. Rend.*, 260, 999 (1965).
86. Binkley and Wolfrom, *J. Am. Chem. Soc.*, 70, 3940 (1948).
87. Schlubach and Vorwerk, *Ber. Dtsch. Chem. Ges.*, 66, 1251 (1933).
88. Schlubach and Graefe, *Justus Liebigs Ann. Chem.*, 532, 211 (1937).
89. Müller and Reichstein, *Helv. Chim. Acta*, 21, 263 (1938).
90. Terada, Suzuki, and Kinoshita, *Agric. Biol. Chem.*, 25, 802, 939 (1961).
91. Sato, Yamada, Aida, and Uemura, *Agric. Biol. Chem.*, 33, 1606 (1969).
92. Shaw, Tatum, and Berry, *Carbohydr. Res.*, 16, 207 (1971).
93. Chittenden, *Carbohydr. Res.*, 11, 424 (1969).
94. Corbett, *J. Chem. Soc. (Lond.)*, p. 3213 (1959).
95. Schenck and Spielman, *J. Am. Chem. Soc.*, 67, 2276 (1945).
96. Spielman and Freifelder, *J. Am. Chem. Soc.*, 69, 2908 (1947).
97. Hodge and Nelson, *Cereal Chem.*, 38, 207 (1961).
98. Potter and Patton, *J. Dairy Sci.*, 39, 978 (1956).
99. Fisher and Hodge, *J. Org. Chem.*, 29, 776 (1964).
100. Gunner, Hand, and Sahasrabudhe, *J. Assoc. Of. Anal. Chem.*, 51, 959 (1968).
101. Begbie and Richtmyer, *Carbohydr. Res.*, 2, 272 (1966).
102. LaForge and Hudson, *J. Biol. Chem.*, 30, 61 (1917).
103. Wood, *J. Chromatogr.*, 35, 352 (1968).
104. Pratt, Richtmyer, and Hudson, *J. Am. Chem. Soc.*, 74, 2203, 2210 (1952).
105. Richtmyer and Pratt, *J. Am. Chem. Soc.*, 78. 4717 (1956).
106. Okuda and Konishi, *J. Chem. Soc. D Chem. Commun.*, p. 796 (1969).
107. Okuda and Konishi, *Tetrahedron*, 24, 6907 (1968).
108. Bertrand, *Bull. Soc. Chim. Fr. Ser. 4*, 51, 629 (1909).
109. Hann and Hudson, *J. Am. Chem. Soc.*, 61, 336 (1939).
110. McComb and Rendig, *Arch. Biochem. Biophys.*, 95, 316 (1961); 97, 562 (1962).
111. Khouvine and Arragon, *C. R. Acad. Sci.*, 206, 917 (1938).
112. Stewart, Richtmyer, and Hudson, *J. Am. Chem. Soc.*, 74, 2206 (1952).
113. Gorin and Jones, *J. Chem. Soc.* (Lond.), p. 1537 (1953).
114. Maclay, Hann, and Hudson, *J. Am. Chem. Soc.*, 64, 1606 (1942).
115. Bevenne, White, Secor, and Williams, *J. Assoc. Of. Agric. Chem.*, 44, 265 (1961).

Table 4 (continued)
NATURAL KETOSES

116. Bourne, Hutson, and Weigel, *J. Chem. Soc.* (Lond.), p. 4252 (1960).
117. Rendig, McComb, and Hu, *J. Agric. Food Chem.*, 12, 421 (1964).
118. Noggle, *Arch. Biochem. Biophys.*, 43, 238 (1953).
119. LaForge, *J. Biol. Chem.*, 28, 511 (1917).
120. Montgomery and Hudson, *J. Am. Chem. Soc.*, 61, 1654 (1939).
121. Charlson and Richtmyer, *J. Am. Chem. Soc.*, 82, 3428 (1960).
122. Pratt and Richtmyer, *J. Am. Chem. Soc.*, 77, 6326 (1955).
123. Sephton and Richtmyer, *J. Org. Chem.*, 28, 1691 (1963).
124. Jones and Sephton, *Can. J. Chem.*, 38, 753 (1960).
125. Sephton and Richtmyer, *Carbohydr. Res.*, 2, 289 (1966).
126. Sephton and Richtmyer, *J. Org. Chem.*, 28, 2388 (1963).

TABLE 5
CHROMATOGRAPHIC CONDITIONS FOR CHROMATOGRAPHY DATA IN TABLES 1—4

Reference[a]	Conditions[b]
(A)	(B)

For Table 1

(2) Whatman® No. 4 paper, pH 9.6 Na_2HAsO_3 (as 19.8 g $As_2O_3/1$ and NaOH added), 90-min runs at 20—25 V/cm, 20—25° using 18—20° cooling water.

(3) Polypak 1 (120—200 mesh), 0.5 or 1 m by 6 mm O.D. glass column, N_2 gas at 32.5 ml/min, 250° isothermic or programmed 150—250° at 4°/min.

(4) Whatman No. 1 paper, EtAc-HAc-H_2O (9:2:2 v/v), front moves 30 cm in 3—4 h, descending.

(5) Silica Gel H, 0.25 mm thick, 30 min 110° activation, EtOH-32% NH_3-H_2O (21:2:3.5).

(6) Chromosorb® W (80—100 mesh) with 10% Carbowax® 20 M terminated with terephthalic acid, 4 ft by 0.25 in. O.D. copper column, He gas at 85 ml/min, 190°.

(7) Gas-Chrom® Q with 3% QF-1 (w/w), 180 cm by 0.45 cm O.D. coiled hardened aluminum column, N_2 gas at 60 ml/min, 110°.

(8) Chromosorb W (60—80 mesh) with 20% diethylene glycol succinate, 6 ft by 0.25 in. O.D. aluminum column, He gas at 55 ml/min, programmed 70—220° at 15°/min.

(11) Silanized Celite® (60—80 mesh) with 15% LAC-2R-446 diethylene glycol adipate cross-linked with pentaerythritol, 20 ft by 0.37 in. O.D. copper column, H_2 gas at 300 ml/min, 175°.

(12) Whatman No. 3 paper, water-saturated, EtAc descending.

(14) Diatoport® S (60—80 mesh) with 20% SF96, 8 ft by 0.25 in. O.D. coiled copper column, He gas at 88 ml/min, 130° for 6 min and programmed to 220° at 3°/min.

(20) Whatman No. 1 paper, EtAc-Pyr-H_2O (12:5:4), descending.

(21) Chromosorb W coated by hexamethyldisilazane (60—80 mesh) with 10% LAC-IR-296 diethylene glycol adipate, 1.84 m by 0.32 cm I.D. glass column, N_2 gas at 30—50 ml/min, programmed 170—220° at 0.8°/min.

(26) Silica Gel G (240—270 μm), 2 mm thick, dried at room temperature and 55—60° relative humidity 1—3 days, MeC(O)Et-HAc-H_2O (60:20:20).

(31) Magnesium silicate, air-dried plates with no chamber saturation, PrOH-H_2O (5:5 v/v).

(32) Diatoport S (80—100 mesh) with 10% SF-96, 8 ft by 0.25 in. O.D. copper column, He gas, 190°.

(35g) Silanized Diatomate C (85—100 mesh) with 3.5% SE 52, 5 ft glass column, gas (not specified) flow rate at 45 ml/min.

(35t) Merck® Silica Gel F 254, C_6H_6.

(38) Celite AW (80—100 mesh) with 10% butanediol succinate polyester, 6 ft by 0.25 in. O.D. glass column, He gas at 28 ml/min, programmed 125—215° at 4°/min.

(44) Whatman No. 1 paper, AmOH-Pyr-H_2O (4:3:2 v/v).

(50a) Silica Gel G, dried overnight at 135°, upper phase of C_6H_6-EtOH-H_2O-0.8 sp gr NH_4OH (200:47:15:1 v/v).

(50b) Same as (50a) but solvent is BuOH-HAc-EtOEt-H_2O (9:6:3:1 v/v).

(55a) Whatman No. 1 paper, BuOH-EtOH-H_2O (40:11:19), descending.

(55b) Whatman No. 1 paper, EtAc-HAc-HC(O)OH-H_2O (18:3:1:4), descending.

(57p) Whatman No. 1 paper, EtAc-Pyr-H_2O (10:4:3 v/v), descending.

(57g) Chromosorb (80—100 mesh) with 10% neopentylglycol sebacate polyester, 120 cm by 0.5 cm I.D. glass column, Ar gas at 150 ml/min, 205°.

(60) Whatman No. 1 paper, BuOH-HAc-H_2O (4:1:1), descending (?).

(66) Whatman No. 1 paper, BuOH-Pyr-H_2O (6:4:3).

(70) Whatman No. 1 paper, BuOH-EtOH-H_2O (4:1:5 v/v) upper phase, descending.

(72) Whatman No. 1 paper, MeC(O)Me-H_2O (95:5 v/v), descending.

(74) Paper not described, BuOH-MeC(O)Me-H_2O (4:1:5).

(79) Anakrom® ABS (100—110 mesh) with 5% QF-1, 5 ft by 0.13 in. O.D. column (material of construction not given), N_2 gas at 20 ml/min, 150°.

(80) Whatman® No. 3 paper, 0.05 M $Na_2B_4O_7$, 15 h run at 10 V/cm, room temperature.

[a]The reference number correlates with the same reference number in the respective preceding tables.
[b]Abbreviations used in developing solvent compositions: Ac = $CH_3C(O)O$, Am = n-amyl, Bu = n-butyl, DMF = dimethylformamide, DMSO = dimethylsulfoxide, Et = ethyl, Me = methyl, Pr = n-propyl, Pyr = pyridine. For trade names of support and liquid phase materials, one is referred to an adequate chemical supply house catalog of chromatographic materials, or to *Handbook of Chromatography*, Vol. 2, Zweig, G. and Sherma, J., Eds., CRC Press, Cleveland, Ohio, 1972, 255.

Table 5 (continued)
CHROMATOGRAPHIC CONDITIONS FOR CHROMATOGRAPHY DATA IN TABLES 1–4

Reference[a]	Conditions[b]
(A)	(B)

For Table 1 (continued)

(81) Whatman No. 1 paper, MeC(O)Me-BuOH-H$_2$O (3:1:1), ascending.

(82) Whatman No. 1 paper, 0.15 *M* Na$_2$B$_4$O$_7$, 10 V/cm, room temperature.

(84) Gas-Chrom Q (100–120 mesh) with 3% silicone polymer JXR, 1.8 m by 4 mm O.D. coilied glass column, N$_2$ gas at 60 ml/min, 140° for 2 min and programmed to 210° at 3°/min.

(87a) pH 10 Borate buffer solvent, only detail given.

(87b) Whatman No. 1 paper, MeC(O)Me-aq 10% HAc (4:1).

(87c) Whatman No. 1 paper impregnated with DMSO; *iso*-propylether solvent.

(89) Breite, Macherey, Nagel, and Company No. MN847 paper, BuOH-Pyr-H$_2$O (10:3:3 v/v).

(93) Embacel kieselguhr (60–100 mesh) with 1.5% polyester resin LAQ 1-R-296, 115 cm by 4.5 mm I.D. glass column, N$_2$ gas at 30 ml/min, 215°.

(94) Whatman No. 3 MM paper, aq Na$_2$MoO$_4$ · 2H$_2$O (25 g/1,200 ml) made to pH 5 with H$_2$SO$_4$, 2-h run at 30–60 V/cm, cooled.

(103) Whatman No. 1 paper, EtAc-HAc-HC(O)OH-H$_2$O (18:3:1:4), descending.

(109) Whatman No. 1 paper, *sec*-BuOH-HAc-H$_2$O (14:1:5).

(113) Anachrom ABS with 10% XE-60, 24 in. by 0.19 in. O.D. stainless steel column, He gas at 70 ml/min, 170°.

(128) Acid-alkali-washed Celite with 1.5% LAC 1-R-296 polyester, N$_2$ gas at 30–40 ml/min, 210°.

(132) Whatman No. 1 paper, MeC(O)Me-H$_2$O (9:1 v/v), descending.

(134) Whatman No. 3 MM paper, EtAc-HAc-H$_2$O (3:1:3), descending.

(145) Toyo No. 50 paper, BuOH-HAc-H$_2$O (4:2:1 v/v).

(149) Whatman No. 1 paper, Pyr-EtAc-HAc-H$_2$O (5:5:1:3), descending (?).

For Table 2

(2) Whatman No. 3 MM paper, ca. 0.1 *M* (NH$_4$)$_2$CO$_3$ (7.9 g/l) at pH 8.9, 25-min run at 80 V/cm, 8°.

(3) Chromosorb W(HP) (80–100 mesh) with 3% OV-1, 1.9 m by 4 mm I.D. glass column, He gas at 80 ml/min, programmed 70–325° at 10°/min.

(4) Cellulose MN300HR, 350 μm thick, dried 24 h at room temperature, *iso*-PrOH-EtAc-H$_2$O (23.5:65:11.5).

(8) Whatman No. 1 paper, PrOH-conc NH$_3$ (7:3 v/v), descending.

(10) Chromosorb G-AW-DMCS (60–80 mesh) with 3% polypenyl ether-5 ring, 4.5 m by 0.13 in. O.D. AlSl 321 stainless steel coiled column, Ar gas at 20 ml/min, 200°.

(11) Gas-Chrom Q with 3% QF-1 (w/w), 180 cm, by 0.45 cm O.D. coiled hardened aluminum column, N$_2$ gas at 60 ml/min, 110°.

(14) Whatman No. 1 paper, 0.05 *M* acetate buffer at pH 4, 1-h run at 35 V/cm.

(15) Whatman No. 1 paper, BuOH-EtOH-H$_2$O (4:1:5 v/v) upper phase, descending.

(16) Avirin® microcrystalline cellulose, dried 30–60 min at 80°, EtAc-HAc-HC(O)OH-H$_2$O (18:3:1:4).

(23) Silica Gel G (240–270 μm), 2 mm thick, dried at room temperature and 55–60° relative humidity 1–3 days, MeC(O)Et-HAc-H$_2$O (60:20:20).

(28) Whatman No. 1 paper, BuOH-Pyr-H$_2$O (6:4:3), ascending.

(29) Paper not described, PrOH-HC(O)OH-H$_2$O (6:3:1) for the acid, BuOH saturated with aq 3% conc NH$_3$ for the hydrazone.

(32) Silica Gel G, dried overnight at 135°, BuOH-HAc-H$_2$O (2:1:1 v/v).

(41) Whatman No. 1 paper, EtAc-HAc-H$_2$O (3:1:3), upper phase (?).

(44) Whatman No. 1 paper, BuOH-Pyr-H$_2$O (6:4:3).

(57) Gas-Chrom Q (100–200 mesh) with 3% silicone polymer JXR, 1.8 m by 4 mm O.D. coiled glass column, N$_2$ gas at 60 ml/min, 140° for 2 min and programmed at 210° at 3°/min.

(61) Whatman No. 1 paper, acid-washed, PrOH-HC(O)OH-H$_2$O (6:3:1), descending.

(62) Whatman No. 1 paper, EtAc-HAc-H$_2$O (3:1:3), upper phase (?).

(70) Whatman No. 1 paper, BuOH-HAc-H$_2$O (4:1:1), descending (?).

(71) Whatman No. 1 paper, Pyr-EtAc-HAc-H$_2$O (5:5:1:3), descending (?).

(73) Kieselgur G, phosphate-impregnated, air-dried overnight, BuOH-MeC(O)Me-phosphate buffer (40:50:10).

(80) Whatman No. 1 paper, BuOH-HAc-H$_2$O (4:1:5), descending.

(81) Whatman No. 1 paper, BuOH-HAc-H$_2$O (4.4:1.6:4.0), descending.

(83) Whatman No. 1 paper, water-saturated isobutyric acid, descending.

(88) Paper not described, 0.1 *M* formate buffer at pH 3, 45-min run at 50 V/cm.

(89a) Whatman P20 phosphocellulose paper, PrOH-EtAc-25% NH$_3$-H$_2$O (5:1:1:3), descending.

Table 5 (continued)

CHROMATOGRAPHIC CONDITIONS FOR CHROMATOGRAPHY DATA IN TABLES 1—4

Reference[a]	Conditions[b]
(A)	(B)

For Table 2 (continued)

(89b)	Whatman No. 1 paper, EtAc-Pyr-H$_2$O (80:34:12), descending.
(91)	Chromosorb G (HP) (80—100 mesh) with 1% OV-17, 3 m by 3 mm I.D. stainless steel column, He gas at 35 ml/min, 130—190°.
(96)	Whatman No. 1 paper, BuOH-HAc-H$_2$O (5:2:3 v/v), descending.
(97)	Silica Gel Supelcosil 12B, 0.5 mm thick, CHCl$_3$-MeOH-HAc-H$_2$O (65:50:2:12 v/v).
(98)	Whatman No. 3HR paper, EtAc-HAc-H$_2$O (3:1:3), descending.
(104)	Whatman No. 1 paper, BuOH-HAc-H$_2$O (4:1:5), descending.
(108)	Whatman No. 1 paper, EtAc-HAc-HC(O)OH-H$_2$O (18:3:1:4), descending.
(110)	Toyo-Roshi No. 52 paper, BuOH-HAc-H$_2$O (4:1:5 v/v), descending.
(112)	Whatman No. 1 paper, acid-washed, tert-AmOH-98% HC(O)OH-H$_2$O (3:3:1), descending.
(113)	Schleicher & Schüll No. 2043 paper, washed 2 days with developing solvent, BuOH-HAc-H$_2$O (4:1:1 v/v).
(116)	Whatman No. 1 paper, BuOH-Pyr-0.1 N HCL (5:3:2), descending.
(117)	Pyr-HAc-H$_2$O (100:40:860 v/v, pH 5.3), only details given.
(118)	Whatman Chromedia SG-41, 0.20 mm thick, MeOH-CHCl$_3$ (2:98), ascending.
(119)	Whatman No. 3 paper, EDTA-washed, EtOH-HAc-H$_2$O (70:1:29), ascending.
(125)	Silica Gel G, CHCl$_3$-MeC(O)Me (4:1).
(138a)	Whatman No. 1 paper, BuOH-HAc-H$_2$O (4:1:5), descending.
(138b)	Whatman No. 1 paper, Pyr-EtAc-HAc-H$_2$O (5:5:1:3), descending (?).
(141a)	Whatman No. 1 paper, BuOH-HAc-H$_2$O (100:21:50), ascending.
(141b)	Whatman No. 1 paper, EtAc-Pyr-H$_2$O (40:11:6), descending.
(141c)	Whatman No. 1 paper, Pyr-EtAc-HAc-H$_2$O (5:5:1:3), descending (?).
(144)	Schleicher & Schüll No. 2043b paper, 0.01 M borax sol 0.007 M with CaCl$_2$, pH 9.2, 0.5 mA/cm.
(145)	Cellulose Pulver MN300HR, 0.5 mm thick, iso-PrOH-Pyr-HAc-H$_2$O (8:8:1:4).
(148)	Whatman No. 1 paper, BuOH-HAc-H$_2$O (50:12:25), descending.
(149)	Whatman No. 1 paper, EtAc-HAc-HC(O)OH-H$_2$O (18:3:1:4), descending.
(152)	Whatman No. 1 paper, 0.1 M cadmium acetate, 90-min run at 20 V/cm.
(153)	Whatman No. 1 paper, EtAc-Pyr-H$_2$O (40:11:6), descending.
(154)	Siliconized Gas-Chrom P (100—140 mesh) with 1% SE-30, column not detailed, N$_2$ gas at 30 cc/min, 140°.
(156)	Chromosorb W (80—100 mesh) with 14% ethylene glycol succinate polyester, 3 ft column, He gas at 23 psi, 155°.
(166a)	Whatman No. 1 paper, BuOH-HAc-H$_2$O (4:1:1), descending (?).
(166b)	Silica Gel (Merck), BuOH-HAc-H$_2$O (4:1:1), thickness not given.
(170)	Whatman No. 1 paper, EtOH-0.88d. NH$_3$-H$_2$O (80:5:15), descending.
(171)	0.2 M NH$_4$Ac buffer, pH 5.8, only detail given.
(173)	Whatman No. 1 paper, BuOH-HAc-H$_2$O (4:1:5), descending.
(177)	Chromedia® CC 41 binder free cellulose, 0.01 M NH$_3$ and 0.0033 M HAc, pH 10.2, 16-min run at 4.5 kV.
(178)	Whatman No. 1 paper, sec-BuOH-90% HC(O)OH-H$_2$O (15:3:2), ascending.
(179)	Silica Gel G (Merck), BuOH-HAc-H$_2$O (3:1:1).
(185)	Paper not described, DMF-iso-PrOH-MeC(O)Et-H$_2$O (10:25:45:20).
(188)	Whatman No. 1 paper, 0.05 M acetate pH 4.5 buffer, 90-min run at 20 V/cm.
(189)	Paper not described, BuOH-HAc-H$_2$O (7:7:2.3).
(191)	Whatman No. 1 paper, BuAc-HAc-EtOH-H$_2$O (3:2:1:1).
(192a)	Whatman No. 3 MM paper, aq Na$_2$MoO$_4$ · 2H$_2$O (25 g/1,200 ml) made to pH 5 with H$_2$SO$_4$, 2 h-run at 30—60 V/cm, cooled.
(192b)	Whatman No. 1 paper, BuOH-Pyr-H$_2$O (6:4:3).
(192c)	Glass beads (120—140 mesh) with 0.05% OV-11, 150 cm by 0.3 cm I.D. stainless steel column, gas not described, programmed from 80° at 10°/min.
(193a)	Toyo No. 51A paper with the buffer of (192a) above.
(193b)	Toyo No. 51A paper, EtAc-Pyr-HAc-H$_2$O (5:5:1:3 v/v), descending.
(194)	Whatman No. 1 paper, phenol-aq NH$_3$, only detail given.
(205)	Whatman No. 1 paper, BuOH-Pyr-H$_2$O (6:4:3).
(206a)	Gas-Chrom A (60—80 mesh) with 3% OV-17, 300 cm by 0.3 cm I.D. stainless steel column, gas not described, programmed from 120° at 5°/min.

Table 5 (continued)
CHROMATOGRAPHIC CONDITIONS FOR CHROMATOGRAPHY DATA IN TABLES 1–4

Reference[a]	Conditions[b]
(A)	(B)

For Table 2 (continued)

(206b)	Whatman No. 1 paper, BuOH-HAc-H_2O (6:1:1 v/v), descending.
(208a)	Cellulose MN 300, 0.25 mm thick, BuOH-Pyr-H_2O (6:4:3).
(208b)	Whatman No. 1 paper, BuOH-HAc-H_2O (50:12:25), descending.
(209a)	Whatman No. 1 paper, BuOH-HAc-H_2O (5:2:2 v/v), descending.
(209b)	Cellulose Sigmacell, BuOH-HAc-H_2O (5:1:2 v/v), thickness not given.
(209c)	Gas-Chrom A (60–80 mesh) with 3% OV-17, 300 cm by 0.3 cm I.D. stainless steel column, gas not described, programmed from 120° at 5°/min.
(210a)	Whatman No. 3 MM paper, water-washed, BuOH-Pyr-HAc-H_2O (40:5:1:954), pH 5.8, 75-min run at 35 V/cm.
(210b)	Whatman No. 1 paper, 0.2 M pyridine acetate buffer pH 6.5, time not given, 57 V/cm.
(212)	Schleicher & Schüll No. 2043b paper, BuOH-HAc-H_2O (4:1:5).
(214)	KSK Silica Gel (150–200 mesh), PrOH-H_2O (7:3), thickness not given.
(216)	Varaport 30 with 5% OV-210, 2 m by 2 mm I.D. Pyrex® U glass column, N_2 gas at 7.5 ml/min, programmed from 90° at 1°/min.
(217)	Whatman No. 1 paper, BuOH-Pyr-H_2O (6:4:3).
(218)	Schleicher & Schüll No. 2043b paper, BuOH-PrOH-0.1 N HCl (1:2:1).
(219)	Silica Gel F_{245} (Merck) impregnated with 0.2 M NaH_2PO_4, thickness not given, BuOH-EtOH-H_2O (2:1:1).
(221)	Whatman No. 3 MM paper, BuOH-HAc-H_2O (4:1:5).
(222)	Whatman No. 17 paper, EtOH-H_2O (70:30 v/v).
(223)	Whatman No. 3 MM paper, BuOH-PrOH-0.1 N HCl (1:2:1 v/v).

For Table 3

(2)	Chromosorb W (60–80 mesh) with 10% Carbowax 20M, 12 ft by 0.125 in. I.D. column, N_2 gas at 40 ml/min, programmed 65–210° at 8°/min.
(3)	Silica Gel G (Merck 7731) with 0.3 parts Carbowax 4000 and 0.0035 parts Tinopol WG (w/w), 0.3 mm thick, dried 30 min at 80°, benzene-heptane (65:35 v/v).
(5)	Whatman No. 3 MM paper, aq $Na_2MoO_4 \cdot 2H_2O$ (25 g/1,200 ml) made to pH 5 with H_2SO_4, 2-h run at 30–60 V/cm, cooled.
(6)	Whatman No. 1 paper, BuOH-EtOH-H_2O (4:1:5 v/v) organic phase.
(7)	Kieselgel G (Merck), BuOH-HAc-H_2O (4:1:5).
(9)	Acid-washed and silanized Chromosorb W (80–100 mesh) with 3% SE-52, 6 ft by 0.25 in. O.D. coiled stainless steel column, unspecified gas at 75 ml/min, 140°.
(14a)	Chromosorb W (80–100 mesh) with 10% Carbowax 6000, 120 cm by 0.5 cm I.D. glass column, no gas or temperature data.
(14b)	Whatman No. 1 paper, BuOH-EtOH-H_2O (10:3:3 v/v), descending.
(14c)	Silica Gel G, dried 10 h at 110°, solvent as in (14b).
(17)	Silica Gel G (240–270 μm), 2 mm thick, dried at room temperature and 55–60° relative humidity 1–3 days, MeC(O)Et-HAc-H_2O (60:20:20).
(19a)	Whatman No. 1 paper, BuOH-EtOH-H_2O (4:1:5 v/v) upper phase, descending.
(19b)	Neosorb NC with 15% butanediol succinate polyester, 100 cm by 0.4 cm I.D. stainless steel column, He gas at 40 ml/min, 200°.
(19c)	Whatman No. 1 paper, 0.1 M borate buffer at pH 9.6, 400 V, 3.5 h.
(19d)	Whatman No. 1 paper, MeC(O)Et-H_2O azeotrope.
(23a)	Silica Gel G, 0.25 mm thick, MeC(O)Et-H_2O azeotrope (85:7 v/v).
(23b)	Chromosorb W (100–120 mesh) with 15% LAC-4R-886, 120 cm by 0.5 cm I.D. glass column, unspecified gas at 20 ml/min, 200°.
(28)	Whatman No. 4 paper, pH 9.6 Na_2HAsO_3 (as 19.8 g As_2O_3/l and NaOH added), 90-min runs at 20–25 V/cm, 20–25° using 18–20° cooling water.
(29)	Whatman No. 1 paper (?), BuOH-HAc-H_2O (4:1:5), descending.
(30a)	Avirin microcrystalline cellulose, dried 30–60 min at 80°, BuOH-HAc-H_2O (3:1:1).
(30b)	Avirin microcrystalline cellulose, dried 30–60 min at 80°, MeC(O)Et-water azeotrope.
(30c)	Avirin microcrystalline cellulose, dried 30–60 min at 80°, Pyr-EtAc-HAc-H_2O (5:5:1:3).
(34)	Chromosorb W (60–80 mesh) with 20% diethylene glycol succinate, 6 ft by 0.25 in. O.D. aluminum column, He gas at 55 ml/min programmed 70–220° at 15°/min.

Table 5 (continued)
CHROMATOGRAPHIC CONDITIONS FOR CHROMATOGRAPHY DATA IN TABLES 1—4

Reference[a]	Conditions[b]
(A)	(B)

For Table 3 (continued)

(35a)	Whatman 3 MM paper, 0.05 M Pyr-HAc buffer, pH 6.
(35b)	Whatman 3 MM paper, EtAc-Pyr-H$_2$O (10:4:3 v/v).
(37)	"Kieselgel nach Stahl" (Merck), with 0.1 M sodium bisulfite, 0.25 mm thick, dried 1 h at 110—120°, EtAc-HAc-MeOH-H$_2$O (6:1.5:1.5:1).
(38)	Whatman No. 1 paper, BuOH-EtOH-H$_2$O (4:1:5 v/v) upper phase, descending.
(40)	Silica Gel G (Merck), 0.25 mm thick, dried 0.5 h at 100°, EtOEt-toluene (2:1 v/v).
(47)	Whatman No. 1 paper, BuOH-EtOH-H$_2$O (52.5:32:15.5), descending.
(49)	Whatman No. 1 paper, EtAc-HAc-H$_2$O (9:2:2 v/v), front moves 30 cm in 3—4 h, descending.
(50)	Kieselgel G (Merck) with 0.15 M phosphate buffer, pH 8, 0.25 mm thick, dried overnight, phenol-H$_2$O (75:25 w/v), ascending.
(52)	Chromosorb W coated by hexamethyldisilazane (60—80 mesh) with 10% LAC-IR-296 diethylene glycol adipate, 1.84 m by 0.32 cm I.D. glass column, N$_2$ gas at 30—50 ml/min, programmed 170—220° at 0.8°/min.
(56)	Whatman No. 1 paper, water-saturated BuOH.
(57)	Whatman No. 1 paper, BuOH-EtOH-H$_2$O (4:1:5 v/v) upper phase, descending.
(58)	Whatman No. 1 paper, BuOH-EtOH-H$_2$O (4:1:5 v/v) upper phase, descending.
(59a)	Kieselgel G (Merck), 0.25 mm thick, dried 2 h at 120°, activated 15 min at 120°, benzene.
(59b)	Acid-washed, siliconized Gas-Chrom P (100—140 mesh) with 1% SE-30, 6 ft by 4 mm glass U column treated with hexamethyldisilazane, N$_2$ gas at 40—60 ml/min, 150°.
(60a)	Whatman No. 1 paper, EtAc-HAc-H$_2$O (3:1:1 v/v), descending.
(60b)	Silica Gel G, 0.5 mm thick, CHCl$_3$-MeOH-H$_2$O (65:25:4 v/v).
(60c)	Unspecified support with 3% SE-30 (methyl silicone), 5 ft by 0.125 in. unspecified column, He gas at 25 ml/min, 150°.
(67)	Chromosorb W (80—100 mesh) with 14% ethylene glycol succinate polyester, 3 ft column, He gas at 23 psi, 155°.
(68)	Whatman No. 1 paper, BuOH-EtOH-H$_2$O (4:1:5 v/v) upper phase, descending.
(69)	Silica Gel G, dried overnight at 135°, upper phase of C$_6$H$_6$-EtOH-H$_2$O-0.8 sp gr NH$_4$OH (200:47:15:1 v/v).
(72)	Acid-washed Chromosorb W (80—100 mesh) with 20% butanediol succinate, 1.5 m by 0.375 cm unspecified column, He gas at 120 ml/min, 145°.
(74)	Whatman No. 1 paper, BuOH-EtOH-H$_2$O (4:1:5 v/v) upper phase, descending.
(76a)	Acid-washed Chromosorb W (100—120 mesh) with 2% octylphenoxypoly (oxyethylene) ethanol, 115 cm by 3.8 mm unspecified U column purged 1 d at 180°, He gas at 50 ml/min, 165°.
(76b)	Support of (76a) with 5% LAC-4R-886 polyester wax, purged 1 d at 200°, He gas at 100 ml/min, 190°.
(77)	Whatman No. 1 paper, borate buffer, pH 10, 400 V.
(80)	Acid-washed Celite (80—100 mesh) with 15% butanediol succinate, 120 cm by 0.5 cm unspecified column, unspecified gas at 80—100 ml/min, 175°.
(82a)	Whatman No. 1 paper, BuOH-Pyr-H$_2$O (6:4:3).
(82b)	Whatman No. 3 paper, borate buffer, pH 10.4, 26.3 V/cm, 4.25-h run.
(82c)	ECNSS-M liquid phase in a glass column at 155—165° only data given.
(85a)	Whatman No. 1 paper, BuOH-Pyr-H$_2$O (6:4:3).
(85b)	Substrate not given, BuOH-Pyr-H$_2$O (6:4:3 v/v).
(85c)	Glass column at 155—165° only detail, see *Angew. Chem.*, 82, 643 (1970).
(86)	Embacel AW (60—70 mesh) with 5% XE-60, 6 ft by 0.25 in. O.D. unspecified column, N$_2$ gas at 39 ml/min, programmed 100—220° at 10°/min.
(91a)	Whatman No. 1 paper, EtAc-Pyr-H$_2$O (3.6:1:1.15), descending.
(91b)	Unspecified support with 3% ECNSS-M (ethylene glycol succinate combined with cyanoethylsilicone), 10 ft by 0.25 in. unspecified column, N$_2$ gas at 60 ml/min, 175°.
(94a)	Whatman No. 3 paper, borate buffer, pH 10.4, 30 V/cm, 5-h run.
(94b)	Whatman No. 1 paper, toluol-BuOH (1:2)/H$_2$O.
(95)	Whatman No. 1 paper, BuOH-Pyr-H$_2$O (6:4:3).
(96a)	Whatman No. 3 paper, borate buffer, pH 10.4, 26.3 V/cm, 4.25-h run.
(96b)	Kieselgel G (Merck), activated 1 h at 120°, EtAc-iso-PrOH-MeOH (70:15:15).
(96c)	Whatman No. 1 paper, toluol-BuOH (1:2)/H$_2$O.

Table 5 (continued)
CHROMATOGRAPHIC CONDITIONS FOR CHROMATOGRAPHY DATA IN TABLES 1–4

Reference[a]	Conditions[b]
(A)	(B)

For Table 3 (continued)

(98)	Gas-Chrom Q (100–120 mesh) with 3% ECNSSM, 1.3 m by 3 mm I.D. glass U column, gas and temperature
(102)	Kieselgel G (Merck), activated 1 h at 120°, EtAc-*iso*-PrOH-MeOH (70:15:15).
(113)	Kieselgel G (Merck), activated 1 h at 120°, EtAc-*iso*-PrOH-MeOH (70:15:15).
(124)	Whatman No. 1 paper, BuOH-EtOH-H_2O (40:11:19).
(127)	Whatman No. 1 paper, EtAc-Pyr-H_2O (10:4:3 v/v), descending.
(130)	T1C grade silica gel (Fluka DO) with 0.03 M H_3BO_3, 0.3 mm thick, dried at room temperature 24 h, activated 1 h at 110°, BuOH-HAc-H_2O (4:1:5).
(131)	Chromosorb W (60–80 mesh) with 2% EGSS-X, 2.74 mm by 3.16 mm I.D. glass column, N_2 gas at 40 ml/min, 199°.
(135)	Whatman No. 1 paper, BuOH-H_2O (1:1?), descending.
(136)	Whatman No. 1 paper, MeC(O)Et-H_2O (4:1).
(140a)	Silica Gel, C_6H_6-MeC(O)Me (1:1).
(140b)	Silica Gel, C_6H_6-MeC(O)Me (5:1).
(140c)	Shimazer Gaschromatograph apparatus, NGS, 136°, only details given.
(144)	Chromosorb W (60–80 mesh) with 3% OV-101, 1.8 m by 6.25 mm O.D. glass column, He gas at 60 ml/min, 140°.
(145a)	Whatman No. 1 paper, EtAc-HAc-H_2O (3:1:3), upper phase (?).
(145b)	Diatoport W (60–80 mesh) with 10% SE-30, 6 ft by 0.25 in. column, He gas at 46 ml/min, 190°.
(149)	Chromosorb W (HMDS) with 5% Ucon LB 55OX, 2 m by 3 mm stainless steel column, undescribed gas and temperature.
(150)	Whatman No. 3 paper, BuOH-HAc-H_2O (10:1:3), descending.
(153a)	Whatman 3 MM paper, 0.05 M Pyr-HAc buffer, pH 6, 40 V/cm.
(153b)	Whatman No. 54 paper, EtAc-HAc-H_2O (6:3:2).
(155a)	Whatman 3 MM paper, 0.1 M borate buffer, pH 10, 40 V/cm., 1-h run.
(155b)	Whatman No. 1 paper, BuOH-EtOH-H_2O (5:1:4), descending.
(159a)	Silica Gel (KSK), $CHCl_3$-MeC(O)Me (6:4).
(159b)	Silica Gel (KSK), water-saturated cyclohexanol.
(159c)	Volodarskii M paper, 0.2 M borate buffer, pH 9.2, 8.5 V/cm, 5-h run.
(160)	Volodarskii C paper, EtAc-HAc-HC(O)OH-MeC(O)Et-H_2O (17:3:1:15:5), descending.
(164)	Whatman No. 1 paper, BuOH-EtOH-H_2O (4:1:5 v/v) upper phase, descending.
(167)	Celite AW (80–100 mesh) with 10% butanediol succinate polyester, 6 ft by 0.25 in. O.D. glass column, He gas at 28 ml/min, programmed 125–215° at 4°/min.
(169)	Whatman No. 1 paper, BuOH-EtOH-H_2O (4:1:5 v/v) upper phase, descending.
(175a)	Toyo No. 51 paper, 0.1 M HAc-Pyr buffer, pH 6.5, 3000 V, 30-min run.
(175b)	Toyo No. 51 paper, BuOH-HAc-H_2O (50:12:25) descending.
(180a)	Toyo-Roshi No. 51A paper, BuOH-Pyr-H_2O (6:4:3), descending.
(180b)	Gas-Chrom P with 2% XF-1105, 1.8 m by 4 mm I.D. glass column, N_2 gas at 70 ml/min 140°.
(184)	Chromosorb W (60–80 mesh) 15% LAC-4R-886, 120 cm by 0.5 cm I.D. glass column, unspecified gas at 190 ml/min and 190°.
(188a)	Ederol 208 paper impregnated with 40% dimethylformamide in acetone, cyclohexane-benzene-dimethyl-formamide (7:2:1 v/v).
(188b)	Kieselgel G (Merck), 0.25 mm thick, cyclohexane-diisopropyl ether-Pyr (4:4:2 v/v).
(189)	Chromosorb W (100–125 mesh) with 10% diethylene glycol succinate, column not given, N_2 gas at 45 ml/min, 175°.
(192)	Chromosorb W (60–80 mesh) with 1.5% SE-30, 1.5 m by 3 mm I.D. stainless steel column, N_2 gas at undisclosed flow, 170°.
(197)	Whatman No. 1 paper, water-saturated BuOH.
(203a)	Whatman No. 1 paper, EtAc-Pyr-H_2O (3.6:1:1.15), descending, (?).
(203b)	Kieselgel G (Merck), C_6H_6-MeC(O)Me (2:1).
(205)	BuOH-HAc-H_2O only detail given.
(210a)	Chromosorb W (80–100 mesh) with 10% Carbowax 6000, 6 ft by 0.25 in. unspecified column, N_2 gas at 120 ml/min, 145°.

Table 5 (continued)

CHROMATOGRAPHIC CONDITIONS FOR CHROMATOGRAPHY DATA IN TABLES 1-4

Reference[a]	Conditions[b]
(A)	**(B)**

For Table 3 (continued)

(210b)	Silica Gel G (nach Stahl), EtAc-EtOH-H$_2$O (15:2:1 v/v).
(217)	Whatman No. 4 paper, phenol-H$_2$O, 20°.
(219a)	Whatman No. 1 paper, BuOH-Pyr-H$_2$O (10:3:3 v/v), descending.
(219b)	Aeropak 30 with 10% Carbowax, 5 ft by 0.125 in. stainless steel column, N$_2$ gas at 15-20 ml/min, 170°.
(219c)	Silica Gel H, EtAc-HAc-HC(O)OH-H$_2$O (18:3:1:4 v/v), ascending.
(219d)	Whatman No. 1 paper, borate buffer, pH 10, 1,250 V, 2-h run.
(223)	Whatman No. 3 paper, borate buffer, pH 10, 1,500 V.
(238a)	Gas-Chrom Q (100-200 mesh) with 3% ECNSSM, 1.3 m by 3 mm I.D. glass U column, gas and temperature not given.
(238b)	Whatman No. 1 paper, Pyr-EtAc-H$_2$O (2:5:5: v/v), upper layer, descending.
(241)	Whatman No. 4 paper, 0.05 M sodium tetraborate, 90-min runs at 20-25 V/cm, 20-25° using 18-20° cooled water.
(243)	Acid-washed Celite (80-100 mesh) with 10% m-bis(m-phenoxyphenoxy) benzene, 120 cm by 0.5 cm unspecified column, unspecified gas at 80-100 ml/min, 175°.
(244a)	Silica Gel G (Merck), MeC(O)Et saturated with H$_2$O.
(244b)	Silica Gel G (Merck), EtAc-toluene (2:1).
(244c)	Chromosorb W with SE-30, 150 cm by 0.3 cm stainless steel column, N$_2$ gas at 70 ml/min, programmed 110-170° at 4°/min.
(245)	Whatman No. 1 paper, PrOH-HAc-H$_2$O (6:1:2 v/v), descending.
(246)	Silica Gel G, PrOH-EtAc-H$_2$O (3:2:1 v/v).
(252)	Kieselgel G (Merck), activated at 140°, EtOEt-cyclohexane (5:1).
(253a)	Cellulose MN 300, 0.25 mm thick, BuOH-Pyr-H$_2$O (6:4:3), (?).
(253b)	Chromosorb G (80-100 mesh) with 3% ECNSS-M, 200 cm by 0.318 cm column, only details given.
(255)	Whatman No. 1 paper, BuOH-EtOH-H$_2$O (4:1:5 v/v) upper phase, descending.
(258a)	Whatman No. 2 paper, BuOH-EtOH-H$_2$O (4:1:5 v/v) upper phase, descending.
(258b)	Silica gel as aqueous silicic acid (activity grade IV); < 150 mesh, 0.5 mm thick, C$_6$H$_6$-MeC(O)Me (1:1).
(258c)	Neutral alumina (Al$_2$O$_3$, activity grade V), 0.5 mm thick, C$_6$H$_6$-MeC(O)Me (1:1).
(259a)	Kieselgel F254 Fertigplatten (Merck), activated at 140°; EtAc.
(259b)	EtAc-MeOH (8:2), only detail.
(262)	Schliecher and Schüll No. 2043b paper, EtAc-Pyr-H$_2$O (2:1:2).
(263a)	Whatman No. 1 paper, toluene-BuOH (9:1), 6-h run.
(263b)	Kieselgel G (Merck), EtAc-MeOH (9:1), 45-min run.
(263c)	Whatman No. 1, paper toluene-BuOH-Pyr-H$_2$O, 18-h run.
(265)	Whatman No. 1 paper, BuOH-Pyr-H$_2$O (6:4:3).
(266)	Silica Gel G, EtAc-MeOH (19:1) or (9:1).
(268)	Whatman No. 2 paper, BuOH-EtOH-H$_2$O (4:1:5 v/v) upper phase, descending.
(269)	Whatman No. 1 paper, water-saturated BuOH, ascending.
(273)	Borate buffer in the method of Foster, *Chem. Ind.*, 828, 1050 (1952).
(276a)	Spinco No. 300-846 or Schleicher and Schüll No. 2043 A gl paper, 0.083 M borax at pH 9.2, 380 V, 2 h and 10 min run.
(276b)	Paper not given, MeOH saturated with heptane.
(277)	Silica Gel G, 0.25 mm thick, activated at 120°, CH$_2$Cl$_2$-EtOEt (1:1).
(278)	Silica Gel G, EtAc-petroleum ether (3:2 v/v).
(279)	Whatman No. 2 paper, BuOH-EtOH-H$_2$O (4:1:5 v/v) upper phase, descending.
(280a)	Neutral alumina (Al$_2$O$_3$, activity grade V), 0.5 mm thick, C$_6$H$_6$ MeC(O)Me (3:1).
(280b)	Silica Gel as aqueous silica acid (activity grade IV); < 150 mesh, 0.5 mm thick, CHCl$_3$-MeC(O)Me (1:2).
(280c)	Neutral alumina (AlCO$_3$, activity grade V); 0.5 mm thick, C$_6$H$_6$-MeC(O)Me (2:1).
(280d)	Silica Gel as aqueous silica acid (activity grade IV); < 150 mesh, 0.5 mm thick, EtAc-heptane (3:1).
(280e)	Silica Gel as aqueous silicic acid (activity grade IV); < 150 mesh, 0.5 mm thick, C$_6$H$_6$-MeC(O)Me (1:1).

Table 5 (continued)
CHROMATOGRAPHIC CONDITIONS FOR CHROMATOGRAPHY DATA IN TABLES 1–4

Reference[a]	Conditions[b]
(A)	(B)

For Table 3 (continued)

(281a)	Silica Gel (Merck), EtAc.
(281b)	Silica Gel (Merck), EtAc-CHCl$_3$ (1:1 v/v).
(289)	Whatman No. 1 paper, water-saturated BuOH, 17 h.
(290)	Whatman No. 1 paper, toluene-BuOH (4:1)/H$_2$O, 18-h run.
(292)	Kieselgur G, EtAc-65% *iso*-PrOH (65:35 v/v).
(294)	Chromosorb W (80–100 mesh) with 3% SE-52 silicone gum, 6 ft by 0.125 in. O.D. stainless steel column, unspecified gas, programmed from 120° at 2°/min.
(299)	Whatman No. 3 paper, BuOH-Pyr-H$_2$O (6:4:3).
(300)	Whatman No. 3 paper, BuOH-Pyr-H$_2$O (6:4:3).
(301)	Kieselgel F254 Fertigplatten (Merck), activated at 140°; EtAc, (?).
(302)	*tert*-BuOH-HAc-H$_2$O (2:2:1), only detail given.
(303)	Silica Gel (Merck), EtAc.
(304)	Whatman No. 1 paper, BuOH-Pyr-H$_2$O (6:4:3).
(305a)	Lenigrad factory N$_2$ "M" paper, BuOH-HAc-H$_2$O (4:1:1), ascending.
(305b)	Alumina with Brockmann activity of II-III, C$_6$H$_6$-MeOH (9:1).
(306)	Silica Gel G, CHCl$_3$-MeC(O)Me (1:7).
(307a)	Silica Gel G, CHCl$_3$-MeC(O)Me (1:7).
(307b)	Whatman No. 1 paper, BuOH-HAc-H$_2$O (4:1:1), descending (?).
(310)	Whatman No. 1 paper, BuOH-MeC(O)Et (1:1)/borate buffer 50%, descending.
(312)	Whatman No. 3 MM paper, aq Na$_2$MoO$_4$ · 2H$_2$O (25 g/1,200 ml) made to pH 5 with H$_2$SO$_4$, 2-h run at 30–60 V/cm, cooled.
(315)	Toluene-MeC(O)Et (1:1)/H$_2$O, descending, 23-h run.
(317a)	Schleicher and Schüll No. 2043b paper, BuOH-borate buffer.
(317b)	Silica thin-layer foil (Merck, Kieselgel-Fertigfolien), CH$_2$Cl$_2$-MeOH (100:5 v/v).
(317c)	Silica thin-layer foil (Merck, Kieselgel-Fertigfolien), CH$_2$Cl$_2$-MeOH (100:3 v/v).
(320a)	Paper not given, 0.1 *M* sodium borate buffer, pH 10, 1,600 V, 0°.
(320b)	Paper not given, BuOH-H$_2$O, [see *J. Chromatogr.*, 3, 63 (1960)].
(329)	Whatman No. 1 paper, solvent as in (315) above.
(333)	Silica Gel as aqueous silicic acid (activity grade IV); < 150 mesh, 0.5 mm thick, C$_6$H$_6$-MeC(O)Me (1:1).
(334a)	Toyo No. 51A paper, toluene-BuOH-H$_2$O (1:1:2), descending.
(334b)	Toyo No. 51A paper, EtAc-HAc-H$_2$O (3:1:3), descending.
(334c)	Toyo No. 51A paper, 0.1 *M* sodium borate pH 9.5, 30 V/cm, 70-min run.
(337)	Whatman No. 1 paper, BuOH-EtOH-H$_2$O (4:1:1).
(338)	Schleicher and Schüll No. 589 green paper, *tert*-AmOH-PrOH-H$_2$O (3:1:1), descending.
(341)	Whatman No. 1 paper, MeC(O)Et saturated with H$_2$O, descending.
(342)	Whatman No. 1 paper, MeC(O)Et-H$_2$O (10:1 v/v).
(345)	Silica Gel, C$_6$H$_4$-EtAc (7:1).
(347)	Whatman No. 1 paper, MeC(O)Et saturated with H$_2$O, descending.
(350a)	Whatman No. 3 MM paper, 0.05 *M* sodium tetraborate, 25 V/cm, 2–3-h run.
(350b)	Whatman No. 1 paper, BuOH-Pyr-H$_2$O (6:4:3).
(350c)	Chromosorb W (80–100 mesh) with 10% neopentylglycol sebacate polyester, 120 cm by 0.5 cm I.D. glass column, Ar gas at 150 ml/min, 205°.
(352)	Whatman No. 1 paper, BuOH-EtOH-H$_2$O (4:1:5 v/v) upper phase, descending.
(354a)	0.05 *M* Sodium tetraborate, only detail given.
(354b)	Whatman No. 1 paper, BuOH-EtOH-H$_2$O (4:1:5 v/v) upper phase, descending.
(356)	Cellulose Sigmacell, BuOH-HAc-H$_2$O (5:1:2 v/v), thickness not given.
(357a)	Whatman No. 1 paper, Pyr-EtAc-H$_2$O (2:5:5 v/v), upper layer, descending.
(357b)	Chromosorb W (80–100 mesh) with 10% neopentylglycol sebacate polyester, 120 cm by 0.5 cm I.D. glass column, Ar gas at 150 ml/min, 205°.
(357c)	0.05 *M* Sodium tetraborate, only detail given.
(360a)	Whatman No. 1 paper, EtAc-PrOH-H$_2$O (5:3:2).
(360b)	Whatman No. 4 paper, pH 9.6 Na$_2$HAsO$_3$ (as 19.8 g As$_2$O$_3$/l and NaOH added), 90-min runs at 20–25 V/cm, 20–25° using 18–20° cooling water.

Table 5 (continued)
CHROMATOGRAPHIC CONDITIONS FOR CHROMATOGRAPHY DATA IN TABLES 1—4

Reference[a]	Conditions[b]
(A)	(B)

For Table 3 (continued)

(373) Whatman No. 1 paper, BuOH-EtOH-H$_2$O-NH$_3$ (40:10:49:1).
(375a) Borate buffer in the method of Foster, *Chem. Ind.*, 828, 1050 (1952).
(375b) Whatman No. 1 paper, BuOH-EtOH-H$_2$O (4:1:5 v/v) upper phase, descending.
(379) Whatman No. 1 paper, BuOH-EtOH-H$_2$O-NH$_3$ (40:10:49:1).
(382) Whatman No. 1 paper, AmOH-Pyr-H$_2$O (4:3:2 v/v).
(383) Whatman No. 1 paper, EtAc-HAc-H$_2$O (3:1:3), upper phase (?).
(391) Whatman No. 1 paper, EtAc-Pyr-H$_2$O (2:1:2) water-poor phase, descending.
(393) Whatman No. 1 paper, BuOH-Pyr-H$_2$O (6:4:3).
(395) Whatman No. 1 paper, EtAc-HAc-HC(O)OH-H$_2$O (18:3:1:4), descending.
(397) Whatman No. 3 MM paper, 0.1 *M* sodium tetraborate, 25 V/cm, 2—3-h run.
(398a) Whatman No. 1 paper, MeC(O)Me-H$_2$O (95:5 v/v), descending.
(398b) Chromosorb W (80—100 mesh) with 10% neopentylglycol sebacate polyester, 120 cm by 0.5 cm I.D. glass
    column, Ar gas at 150 ml/min, 204° for acetates and ·165° for ethers.
(401a) Acid-washed Chromosorb W (100—200 mesh) with 10% LAC-4R-886 polyester wax, 5 ft by 0.125 in. coiled
    metal column, N$_2$ gas at 75 ml/min, 190°.
(401b) Acid-washed, siliconized Gas-Chrom P (100—400 mesh) with 15% SE-30, same column as (401a), N$_2$ gas at
    60 ml/min, 180°.
(402a) Whatman No. 1 paper, EtAc-HAc-H$_2$O (9:2:2 v/v), front moves 30 cm in 3—4 h, descending.
(402b) ECNSS-M, only data given; glass column at 155—165° assumed.
(406a) Whatman No. 1 paper, MeC(O)Me-H$_2$O (95:5 v/v), descending.
(406b) Whatman No. 1 paper, *iso*-BuOH-Pyr-H$_2$O (10:3:3 v/v).
(410) Kieselgel G (Merck), C$_6$H$_6$-MeC(O)Me (2:1).

For Table 4

(2) Kieselgel G (Merck), BuOH-HAc-H$_2$O (4:1:5).
(3) Gas-Chrom Z (60—80 mesh) with 20% Carbowax 20M, 7 ft by 0.25 in. O.D. stainless steel U column, He gas
    at 80 ml/min, 90°.
(4) Toyo No. 51 paper, *n*-PrOH-EtAc-H$_2$O (7:1:2), ascending.
(5) Chromosorb G-AW-DMCS (60—80 mesh) with 3% polypenyl ether-5 ring, 4.5 m by 0.13 in. O.D. AISI 321
    stainless steel coiled column, Ar gas at 20 ml/min, 200°.
(6) Chromosorb W (60—80 mesh) with 10% Carbowax 20M, 12 ft by 0.125 in. I.D. column, N$_2$ gas at 40 ml/min,
    programmed 65—210° at 8°/min.
(7) Whatman No. 3 MM paper, *n*-BuOH-0.5 *M* NH$_3$ in H$_2$O (1:1 v/v), descending.
(8) Whatman No. 4 paper dipped in 25% solution of DMF in EtOH, dried 10—15 min, cyclohexane.
(9) Whatman No. 1 paper, *iso*-BuC(O)Me-HC(O)OH-H$_2$O (1,000:4:96 v/v), descending.
(10) Whatman No. 4 paper, pH 9.6 Na$_2$HAsO$_3$ (as 19.8 g As$_2$O$_3$/l and NaOH added), 90-min runs at 20—25 V/cm,
    20—25° using 18—20° cooling water.
(13) Whatman No. 1 paper, EtAc-Pyr-H$_2$O (12:5:4), descending.
(14) Silica Gel G (Merck 7731) with 0.3 parts Carbowax 4000 and 0.0035 parts Tinopol WG (w/w), 0.3 mm
    thick, dried 30 min at 80°, benzene-heptane (65:35 v/v).
(17) Silica Gel G (Merck), after Stahl, 0.5 mm thick, toluene-EtAc (2:1 v/v).
(19a) Whatman No. 3 paper, bisulphite buffer, pH 4.7, 12—18 V/cm, 50°.
(19b) Whatman No. 1 paper, BuOH-EtOH-H$_2$O (4:1:5 v/v) upper phase, descending.
(19c) 3% ECNSS containing column, 150°, only details given.
(20a) Whatman No. 3 paper, bisulphite buffer, pH 4.7, 12—18 V/cm, 50°, (see also Reference 21).
(20b) Whatman No. 1 paper, EtAc-HAc-H$_2$O (3:1:3), upper phase (?).
(26) Toyo-Roshi No. 50 paper, *iso*-PrOH-H$_2$O (6:1), ascending.
(28) Acid-washed and silanized Chromosorb W (80—100 mesh) with 3% SE-52, 6 ft by 0.25 in. O.D. coiled
    stainless steel column, unspecified gas at 75 ml/min, 140°.
(30) Whatman No. 4 paper, water-saturated phenol, descending.
(31) Paper not given, 0.05 *M* borate buffer, pH 10, 500 V, 3-h run.
(34) Whatman No. 1 paper, BuOH-EtOH-H$_2$O (40:11:19).

Table 5 (continued)
CHROMATOGRAPHIC CONDITIONS FOR CHROMATOGRAPHY DATA IN TABLES 1–4

Reference[a]	Conditions[b]
(A)	(B)

For Table 4 (continued)

(36)	Microcrystalline cellulose (Avirin), BuOH-EtOH-H_2O (40:11:19 v/v), ascending.
(38)	Whatman No. 1 paper, BuOH-EtOH-H_2O (5:2:2 v/v), descending.
(43)	Whatman No. 3 MM paper, aq $Na_2MoO_4 \cdot 2H_2O$ (25 g/1,200 ml) made to pH5 with H_2SO_4. 2-h run at 30–60 V/cm, cooled.
(44)	Whatman No. 1 paper, EtAc-HAc-H_2O (9:2:2: v/v), front moves 30 cm in 3–4 h, descending.
(45)	Paper not given, phenol-H_2O (4:1).
(49)	Whatman No. 1 paper, water-saturated BuOH.
(51)	Whatman No. 1 paper, BuOH-HAc-H_2O (4:1:1), descending (?).
(56)	Silica Gel G, 0.25 mm thick, activated at 120°, CH_2Cl_2-EtOEt (1:1).
(58)	Paper not given, BuOH-HAc-H_2O (4:5:1).
(59)	Whatman No. 1 paper, MeC(O)Me-aq 10% HAc (4:1).
(64)	"Kieselgel nach Stahl" (Merck), with 0.1 M sodium bisulfite, 0.25 mm thick, dried 1 h at 110–120°. EtAc-HAc-MeOH-H_2O (6:1.5:1.5:1).
(66)	Silica Gel G, dried overnight at 135°, upper phase of C_6H_6-EtOH-H_2O-0.8 sp gr NH_4OH (200:47:15:1 v/v).
(67)	Silica Gel G (Merck), 0.25 mm thick, dried 0.5 h at 100°, EtOEt-toluene (2:1 v/v).
(74)	Whatman No. 1 paper, BuOH-EtOH-H_2O (40:11:19).
(79)	3–10% XE-60 on silanized glass capillary, 28 m by 0.17 mm I.D., N_2 gas flow not given, 130–170°.
(81)	Whatman No. 1 paper, MeC(O)Et-EtC(O)OH-H_2O (75:25:30 v/v), ascending.
(84)	Whatman No. 1 paper, BuOH-EtOH-H_2O (40:11:19).
(91)	Toyo-Roshi No. 50 paper, PrOH-H_2O (4:1 v/v).
(92a)	Gas-Chrom P (60–80 mesh) with 20% Carbowax 20M, 9 ft by 0.25 in O.D. stainless steel column, He gas at 180 ml/min, 80°, programmed irregularly at 215° in 76 min.
(92b)	Bio Sil A, dried overnight at 135°, upper phase of C_6H_6-EtOH-H_2O-0.8 sp gr NH_4OH (200:47:15:1 v/v).
(100)	Diatoport A (80–100 mesh) with 10% UCW 98, 6 ft by 0.125 in. O.D. stainless steel column, He gas at 120 ml/min, 130°.
(101)	Whatman No. 1 paper, EtAc-HAc-HC(O)OH-H_2O (18:3:1:4), descending.
(103)	Whatman No. 1 paper, phenol-H_2O (80:10 w/v).
(106)	Chromosorb W with 1.5% SE-30, 225 cm by 4 mm stainless steel column.
(110)	Whatman No. 1 paper, EtAc-Pyr-H_2O (8:2:1 v/v), descending.
(113)	Whatman No. 1 paper, EtAc-HAc-H_2O (9:2:2 v/v), front moves 30 cm in 3–4 h, descending.
(116)	Whatman No. 3 MM paper, aq $Na_2MoO_4 \cdot 2H_2O$ (25 g/1,200 ml) made to pH5 with H_2SO_4, 2-h run at 30–60 V/cm, cooled.
(117)	Whatman No. 1 paper, EtAc-Pyr-H_2O (8:2:1 v/v), descending.
(118)	Whatman No. 1 paper, water saturated phenol, pH 5.5, descending.
(125)	Gas-Chrom A with 3% SE-52, 183 cm by 0.6 cm column, N_2 gas at 100 ml/min, programmed 75–280° at 11°/min.

Compiled by George G. Maher.

Table 6
CARBOHYDRATE PHOSPHATE ESTERS

Substance[a] (synonym) (A)	Constant[b] $k \times 10^3$ (B)	Hydrolysis Temperature °C (C)	Hydrolysis Medium (D)	Ester group form[c] (E)	Specific rotation[d] (F)	Concentration[e] solvent (G)	Melting point, °C (H)	Reference (I)
2-Aminoethanol 1-phosphate	—	—	—	FA	—	—	236–238	1
D-Glycerol 1-phosphate (α-L-glycerophosphate, L-glycerin 3-phosphate)	0.15	80	Water pH 6.3	Ag	+1.0	6.5	—	2–4
D-Erythritol 4-phosphate	—	—	—	FA	−2.6, +2.6	—	183–186	5, 6
				dcha	−2.3	—	—	6
L-Erythritol 4-phosphate	—	—	—	dcha	+2.3	—	186–190	6
L-Ribitol 1-phosphate (D-ribitol 5-phosphate)	< 5[f]	100	N HCl	FA	—	—	—	7
D-myo-Inositol 1-phosphate (myo-inositol 3-phosphate)	—	—	—	dcha	+9.3	pH 2.0	210–215d	8, 9, 10
	—	—	—	dcha	−3.2	pH 9.0	—	8
L-myo-Inositol 1-phosphate (myo-inositol 3-phosphate)	—	—	—	B	—	—	238	11
L-myo-Inositol 2-phosphate	0.99	100	Water pH 2.0	FA	−9.8	pH 2.0	194–203	12
	—	—	—	dcha	+3.4	pH 9.0	244–247	12
	—	—	—	FA	0 (meso)	—	202–205	12
	—	—	—	B	—	—	215–220d	13
	—	—	—	cha	—	—	186–197d	13
	—	—	—	dcha	—	—	182–183d	9
myo-Inositol 1,4-diphosphate	—	—	—	trcha	—	—	—	14
myo-Inositol 4,5-diphosphate	—	—	—	trcha	—	—	—	14
myo-Inositol hexaphosphate (phytic acid)	—	—	—	d CH₃ ester	—	—	247–249	125
D-Mannitol 1-phosphate	< 0.5[f]	100	N HCl	FA	—	—	—	15
Shikimic acid 5-phosphate	—	—	—	K · H₂O	−107.6	(29°)	—	16
Bis(2,3-dihydroxypropyl) hydrogen phosphate (α,α-diglycerophosphate)	150[f]	100	N HNO₃	FA	—	—	—	17

[a] In order of increasing carbon chain-length in the parent compounds, grouped in the classes: alditols, acids, aldoses, ketoses, and disaccharides. The term phosphate ester denotes a carbohydrate dihydrogen phosphate wherein the two acidic groups of the acid ester are combined with suitable cations.

[b] For the ester group that is farthest in the carbon chain structure from the asymetric center which determines the D or L configuration of the parent compound.

[c] FA = free acid, Ag = silver salt, Ba = barium salt, K = potassium salt, Na = sodium salt, B = brucine salt, cha = cyclohexylammonium salt, d = di, tr = tri, and t = tetra.

[d] $[\alpha]_D$ at the sodium D line, 5876 A, unless indicated otherwise in parentheses.

[e] In grams per 100 ml of solution at 20–25°C. Other temperatures are in parentheses. Unless otherwise indicated, the concentration is 1–5 g in water.

[f] Calculated by the contributors from the data of the reference cited, using $k = 0.30$/time in min for 50% hydrolysis of the ester linkage.

[g] For the pyrophosphate group.

[h] For the second ester group.

[i] Both ester linkages hydrolyze equally.

[j] D-Mannonic acid 6-phosphate and 2-deoxy-D-arabino-hexose 6-phosphate have been reported as skin metabolites in unnatural environments (see Reference 123).

Table 6 (continued)
CARBOHYDRATE PHOSPHATE ESTERS

Substance[a] (synonym) (A)	Hydrolysis Constant[b] $k \times 10^3$ (B)	Hydrolysis Temperature °C (C)	Hydrolysis Medium (D)	Ester group form[c] (E)	Specific rotation[d] (F)	Concentration[e] solvent (G)	Melting point, °C (H)	Reference (I)
2,3-Dihydroxypropyl *myo*-inositol hydrogen phosphate (1-*O*-glycerophosphoryl-*myo*-inositol)	15^f	100	*N* HCl	F A	—	—	—	18
		—	—	cha	-14	6, pH 3.5	115–117d	18, 126
D-Glyceric acid 2-phosphate	—	—	—	F A	+24.3, +13	*N* HCl	—	19, 20
					-68, +5	$(NH_4)_2 MoO_4$		19, 21
D-Glyceric acid 3-phosphate	1.8^f	125	*N* HCl	Ba	-14.5, +14	*N* HCl	—	19, 20
				Ba	-725	$MoO_4^=$		21
					+5	$(NH_4)_2 MoO_4$		19
								23
D-Glyceric acid 1,3-diphosphate	26	38	Water	F A	very small	6–17, *N* HNO_3	—	24, 25
D-Glyceric acid 2,3-diphosphate	—	—	—	Ba	-2, -4	6–28	—	24–26
				Na	-4, +4.6	—		27
3-Hydroxypyruvic acid phosphate (2-deoxy-2-keto-glyceric acid phosphate)	15^f	90	*N* HCl	trcha	-20	—	—	28, 29
D-Erythronic acid 4-phosphate	—	—	—	d Benzyl ester	+12.2	$CHCl_3$	84.5–86	127, 128
D-Galacturonic acid 1-phosphate	—	—	—	—	—	—	—	
methyl ester triacetate								
D-Gluconic acid 6-phosphate	0.21	100	*N* HCl	F A	+0.2 (5461)	—	—	30, 31
				F A lactone	+18 (5461)	—	—	31
D-*arabino*-Hexulosonic acid 6-phosphate (2-keto-D-gluconic acid)	3^f	94	*N* H_2SO_4	K	+3.3	—	—	32
3-Deoxy-D-*erythro*-hexulosonic acid 6-phosphate (3-deoxy-2-keto-D-gluconic acid)	$5–6^f$	100	*N* HCl	F A	—	—	—	33
D-Glucuronic acid 1-phosphate	—	—	—	K	+53.6	(19°)	—	34
L-*xylo*-Hexulosonic acid diphosphate (2-keto-L-gulonic acid)	No constants	—	—	—	—	—	—	35
D-Glyceraldehyde 3-phosphate	37.5	100	*N* HCl	F A	+12	—	—	36–39
D-Erythrose 4-phosphate	15	100	*N* H_2SO_4	F A	0	—	—	40
D-Arabinose 5-phosphate	3^f	100	*N* H_2SO_4	F A	+16.9	—	—	41, 42
L-Arabinofuranosyl phosphate	—	—	—	F A	+48.2	—	—	22
				Ba	—	—	—	22
L-Arabinopyranosyl phosphate	—	—	—	dcha (α-anomer)	+30.8	(26°)	144–150	44
				dcha (β-anomer)	+91	(26°)	155–161	44
α-D-Ribofuranosyl phosphate	1.25^f	20	0.01 *N* HCl	F A	+40.3	—	—	43
		—	—	dcha	—	—	—	45

Table 6 (continued)
CARBOHYDRATE PHOSPHATE ESTERS

| Substance[a] (synonym) | Hydrolysis | | | Ester group form[c] | Specific rotation[d] | Concentration[e] solvent | Melting point, °C | Reference |
| | Constant[b] $k \times 10^3$ | Temperature °C | Medium | | | | | |
(A)	(B)	(C)	(D)	(E)	(F)	(G)	(H)	(I)
β-D-Ribofuranosyl phosphate	0.63[f]	20	0.01 N HCl	Ba	−9.3	—	—	43
		—		dcha	−13.6	Ethanol	—	45
D-Ribopyranosyl phosphate	1.25[f]	20	0.1 N HCl	Ba	−47.1	5% Acetic acid	—	43
D-Ribose 2-phosphate	—	—	—	Ba	−6.8	—	—	46
	—	—	—	dB	−27.5	H₂O:C₅H₅N, 1:1	112–114d	46
D-Ribose 3-phosphate	—	—	—	Ba	−6.8	—	—	46
	—	—	—	dB	−35, −28	H₂O:C₅H₅N, 1:1	114–117d	46, 47
D-Ribose 5-phosphate	4.5	100	0.25 N HCl	Na	−9.7	—	—	48, 49
	0.5	100	0.25 N HCl	FA	18 ± 2	0.2, 1 N HCl	—	50, 51
				Ba	+6	—	—	48, 52
α-D-Ribofuranose 1,5-diphosphate	1.66	70	0.01 N HCl	FA	+20.8	0.43	—	53, 54
	—	—	—	tcha	—	—	—	53
D-Ribofuranose 5-phosphate 1-pyro-phosphate	30[g]	65	Acetate pH 4 buffer	—	—	—	—	55
2-Deoxy-α-D-erythro-pentosyl phosphate (2-deoxy-D-ribosyl phosphate)	—	—	—	cha	+34.5	—	—	56
2-Deoxy-β-D-erythro-pentosyl phosphate (2-deoxy-β-D-ribosyl phosphate)	13–17[f]	—	Acetate pH 4.5 buffer	FA	—	—	—	16, 57
	—							
2-Deoxy-D-erythro-pentofuranose 5-phosphate (2-deoxy-D-ribose 5-phosphate)	50[f]	100	N HCl	cha	−15.8	—	—	56
				FA	+19	0.47	—	58, 59
				Ba	+10.8, 16.5	0.52	—	60, 61
2-Deoxy-D-erythro-pentofuranose 1,5-diphosphate (2-deoxy-D-ribose)	> 3	100	Water pH 4	FA	—	—	—	62
	< 5[h]	100	N HCl	FA	—	—	—	62
	4	100	N HCl	FA	—	—	—	63
D-Xylose 5-phosphate	1.1	100	6 N H₂SO₄	FA	+8	—	—	64
				FA	+3.2	—	—	63
				Na	+5	—	—	63
L-Fucose 1-phosphate	100	80	Water pH 2	Ba	—	—	—	129
				FA				
α-D-Galactosyl phosphate	5.9	37	0.25 N HCl	FA	+148	0.2 N HCl	—	65
	—	—	—	K	+108	—	—	65
	—	—	—	Ba	+92	—	—	65
β-D-Galactosyl phosphate	—	—	—	dcha	+78.5	—	147–153	44
	5.6	37	0.25 N HCl	Ba	+31.3	—	—	66
	—	—	—	dcha	+21	—	145–151	44

Table 6 (continued)
CARBOHYDRATE PHOSPHATE ESTERS

Substance[a] (synonym) (A)	Hydrolysis Constant[b] $k \times 10^3$ (B)	Hydrolysis Temperature °C (C)	Hydrolysis Medium (D)	Ester group form[c] (E)	Specific rotation[d] (F)	Concentration[e] solvent (G)	Melting point, °C (H)	Reference (I)
D-Galactose 6-phosphate	–	–	–	Ba	+25.2	(16°)	–	67, 68
				CH₃, β-D-glycoside of dcha	−11.9	0.5	138–144d	69
3,6-Dideoxy-D-xylo-hexosyl phosphate (abequose 1-phosphate)	–	–	–	FA	+1.5 (α-anomer)	0.5	–	70
				FA	−3.8 (β-anomer)	0.5	–	70
α-D-Glucopyranosyl phosphate	1.3, 2.99	37	0.25 N HCl	FA	+118	–	–	37, 71, 72
				Ba	+75.5	–	–	37
				dcha	+64	–	163–169	44
				K	+78	–	–	73
β-D-Glucopyranosyl phosphate	5	33	N HCl	dB	+0.5	–	–	74
	15	33	N HCl	dB	−20	–	–	74
				dcha	+7.3	(26°)	–	44
D-Glucose 6-phosphate	0.23	100	N HCl	FA	+35.7	(26°)	137–143	31, 76
				Ba	+18	–	–	31, 76, 77
				K	+21.2	–	157d	77, 78
				CH₃, α-D-glycoside	+61	–	95–97d	69
α-D-Glucose 1,6-diphosphate	0.78	30	N H₂SO₄	FA	+83 ± 4	0.2	157–159d	79
β-D-Glucose 1,6-diphosphate	3.15	30	N H₂SO₄	FA	−19 ± 2	0.2	–	79
2-Deoxy-D-arabino-hexose 6-phosphate (2-deoxy-D-glucose)	>10[f]	100	N HCl	–	–	–	–	80, 81, 123
D-Mannosyl phosphate	–	–	–	FA	+58	–	–	75
	–	–	–	Ba	+36	–	–	75
				dcha	+28.7	–	–	83
D-Mannose 6-phosphate	0.29	100	N HCl	FA	+15.1 (5461A)	–	–	76
	–	–	–	Ba	+3.5 (5461A)	0.7	–	82
D-Mannose 1,6-diphosphate	No constants	–	–	–	–	–	–	84
Dihydroxyacetone phosphate	33.7	100	N HCl	–	–	–	–	37

Table 6 (continued)
CARBOHYDRATE PHOSPHATE ESTERS

Substance[a] (synonym)	Constant[b] $k \times 10^3$	Hydrolysis Temperature °C	Hydrolysis Medium	Ester group form[c]	Specific rotation[d]	Concentration[e] solvent	Melting point, °C	Reference
(A)	(B)	(C)	(D)	(E)	(F)	(G)	(H)	(I)
L-*glycero*-Tetrulose phosphate (L-erythrulose phosphate)	10^f	100	N HCl	—	—	—	—	85, 100
D-*erythro*-Pentulosyl 5-phosphate (D-ribulose phosphate)	5	100	N H_2SO_4	FA	−29.6	0.2 N HCl	—	86, 87
L-*erythro*-Pentulosyl 5-phosphate (L-ribulose phosphate)	5–12	90	N H_2SO_4	FA	+28	0.26, 0.2 N HBr	—	88
D-*erythro*-Pentulose 1,5-diphosphate (D-ribulose diptiosphate)	15^i	100	N H_2SO_4		—	—	—	89
D-*threo*-Pentulose phosphate (D-xylulose phosphate)	86	100	N HCl		—	—	—	90, 91
D-Fructose 1-phosphate	70	100	N HCl	FA	−64.2 (5461 A)	11.3	—	92
	—	—	—	Ba	−39 (5461 A)	6.1	—	92
	—	—	—	B	−52.1 (5461 A)	—	—	92
	—	—	—	Ba	−30.4	(26°)	—	93
D-Fructose 6-phosphate	4.4	100	N HCl	Ba	+3.6	10	—	76, 94
D-Fructose 1,6-diphosphate	52	100	N HCl	FA	+4.1	13.6	—	94, 95
D-*threo*-2,5-Hexodiulose phosphate (5-keto-D-fructose phosphate)	70	98	N HCl	trcha	—	—	163–166d	96
	—	—	—	FA	—	—	—	130
L-Fuculosyl phosphate	60	100	N HCl	Ba	−2.3	—	—	97
α-D-*ribo*-Hexos-3-ulose 1-phosphate (3-keto-D-glucose 1-phosphate)	100	100	N H_2SO_4	FA	+68 (15°)	0.7	—	131
6-Deoxy-L-*arabino*-hexosyl phosphate (L-rhamnulose phosphate)	46^f	100	N HCl	Ba	+8.9	(30°) 5.2, pH 4 Acetic acid	—	98
L-Sorbose 1-phosphate	60^f	—	N HCl	dcha	−16.5	—	171–173d	99
	—	—	—	mono K	−7.2	—	—	101
	0.28^f	100	N H_2SO_4	Ba	—	0.1 N HCl	—	102
Sedoheptulose 7-phosphate (D-*altro*-2-heptulose 7-phosphate)	20	100	N H_2SO_4	FA	—	—	—	103
Sedoheptulose 1,7-diphosphate	0.28^h	100	N H_2SO_4	FA	—	—	—	103
	—	100	N H_2SO_4	FA	—	—	—	103
D-*arabino*-3-Heptulose phosphate	No constants	—	—		—	—	—	104
D-*manno*-Heptulose phosphate	No constants	—	—		—	—	—	105

Table 6 (continued)
CARBOHYDRATE PHOSPHATE ESTERS

Substance[a] (synonym)	Hydrolysis			Ester group form[c]	Specific rotation[d]	Concentration[e] solvent	Melting point, °C	Reference
(A)	Constant[b] $k \times 10^3$ (B)	Temperature °C (C)	Medium (D)	(E)	(F)	(G)	(H)	(I)
A heptulose monophosphate	4	100	N HCl	Ba	+8 (5461 A)	—	—	106
D-glycero-D-altro-Octulose 1-phosphate	20[f]	100	N HCl	FA	—	—	—	132
D-glycero-D-altro-Octulose 8-phosphate	< 2[f]	100	N HCl	FA	—	—	—	132
D-glycero-D-altro-Octulose 1,8-diphosphate	ca 10	100	N HCl	FA	—	—	—	132
2-Amino-2-deoxy-D-galactosyl phosphate (glucosamine-1-phosphate)	—	—	—	FA N-acetyl der	+178	—	—	107
				K N-acetyl der	+112.4	—	—	108
				FA	+142.6	—	—	108
2-Amino-2-deoxy-D-galactose 6-phosphate	0.8[f]	110	6 N HCl	FA	+57.8	0.1	—	109, 11
				N-acetyl der	+48.4	0.05 M Na acetate	—	110
2-Amino-2-deoxy-α-D-glucosyl phosphate (glucosamine-1-phosphate)	60[f]	100	N HClO$_4$	FA	+100	—	—	111
	230[f]	100	N HCl	FA	+79	—	—	112
2-Amino-2-deoxy-β-D-glucosyl phosphate	3.7[f]	37	N H$_2$SO$_4$	K N-acetyl der	—43 (calcd)	—	—	112
				FA	—40 (calcd)	—	—	112
2-Amino-2-deoxy-D-glucose 6-phosphate	86[f]	26	N H$_2$SO$_4$	K N-acetyl der	—	—	—	112
				dNA N-acetyl der	—1.7	0.5	170—171d	113, 114
	0.06[f]	100	N HCl	FA	+54	(18°)0.3, pH 2.5	170—180d	111, 115
				Ba	+53	8, 0.5 M Na acetate	—	115
				FA N-acetyl der	+29.5	—	—	110
2-Amino-2-deoxy-D-gluconic acid 6-phosphate	1.24	100	N H$_2$SO$_4$	FA	—6.8	—	—	116
2-Amino-3-O-(2-carboxyethyl)-2-deoxy-D-glucose phosphate (muramic acid phosphate)	0.8[f]; No constants	100	6 N HCl	—	—	—	—	109
α-Lactosyl phosphate	2[f]	37	N HCl	Ba	+73.3	—	—	117, 118
β-Lactosyl phosphate	6[f]	37	N HCl	Ba	+24.8	—	—	117, 118
2-O-α-D-Mannosyl-L-myo-inositol 1-phosphate	—	—	—	—	—	—	—	83
Sucrose 1-phosphate	5.9[f]	100	N H$_2$SO$_4$	—	+147	—	—	119
Maltose-1-phosphate	—	—	—	—	+185	—	—	124
Trehalose phosphate	0.16	—	—	F A	—	0.1 N HCl	—	120
Trehalose 6,6'-diphosphate	—	—	—	Ba	+132 (5461 A)	—	—	121
	1.6[f]	100	3 N HCl	FA	+99.3	0.7	—	122

Compiled by George G. Maher.

Table 6 (continued)
CARBOHYDRATE PHOSPHATE ESTERS

REFERENCES

1. Grollman and Osborn, *Biochemistry*, 3, 1571 (1964).
2. Baer and Kates, *J. Am. Chem. Soc.*, 70, 1394 (1948).
3. Kiessling and Schuster, *Ber. Dtsch. Chem. Ges.*, 71, 123 (1938).
4. Weil-Malherbe and Green, *Biochem. J.*, 49, 286 (1951).
5. Shetter, *J. Am. Chem. Soc.*, 78. 3722 (1956).
6. MacDonald, Fischer, and Ballou, *J. Am. Chem. Soc.*, 78, 3720 (1956).
7. Baddiley, Buchanan, Carss, and Mathias, *J. Chem. Soc.* (Lond.) p. 4583 (1956).
8. Ballou and Pizer, *J. Am. Chem. Soc.*, 81, 4745 (1959).
9. Posternak, *Helv. Chim. Acta*, 41, 1891 (1958); 42, 390 (1959).
10. Eisenberg, Jr. and Bolden, *Biochem. Biophys. Res. Commun.*, 21, 100 (1965).
11. Woolley, *J. Biol. Chem.*, 147, 581 (1943).
12. Pizer and Ballou, *J. Am. Chem. Soc.*, 81, 915 (1959).
13. Brown and Hall, *J. Chem. Soc.* (Lond.), p. 357 (1959).
14. Angyal and Tate, *J. Chem. Soc.* (Lond.), p. 4122 (1961).
15. Wolff and Kaplan, *J. Biol. Chem.*, 218, 849 (1957).
16. Weiss and Mingioli, *J. Am. Chem. Soc.*, 78, 2894 (1956).
17. Maruo and Benson, *J. Am. Chem. Soc.*, 79, 4564 (1957).
18. Lepage, Mumma, and Bensen, *J. Am. Chem. Soc.*, 82, 3713 (1960).
19. Ballou and Fischer, *J. Am. Chem. Soc.*, 76. 3188 (1954).
20. Kiessling, *Ber. Dtsch. Chem. Ges.*, 68, 243 (1935).
21. Meyerhof and Oesper, *J. Biol. Chem.*, 179, 1371, 1381 (1949).
22. Wright and Khorana, *J. Am. Chem. Soc.*, 80, 1994 (1958).
23. Negelein and Bromel, *Biochem. Z.*, 303, 132 (1939).
24. Baer, *J. Biol. Chem.*, 185, 763 (1950).
25. Greenwald, *J. Biol. Chem.*, 63, 339 (1925).
26. Sutherland, Posternak, and Cori, *J. Biol. Chem.*, 181, 153 (1949).
27. Ballou and Hesse, *J. Am. Chem. Soc.*, 78, 3718 (1956).
28. Barker and Wold, *J. Org. Chem.*, 28, 1847 (1963).
29. Ishii, Hashimoto, Tachibana, and Yoshikawa, *Biochem. Biophys. Res. Commun.*, 10, 19 (1963).
30. Patwardhan, *Biochem. J.*, 28, 1854 (1934).
31. Robison and King, *Biochem. J.*, 25, 323 (1931).
32. Ciferri, Blakley, and Simpson, *Can. J. Microbiol.*, 5, 277 (1959).
33. MacGee and Doudoroff, *J. Biol. Chem.*, 210, 617 (1954).
34. Barker, Bourne, Fleetwood, and Stacey, *J. Chem. Soc.*, (Lond.), p. 4128 (1958).
35. Moses, Ferrier, and Calvin, *Proc. Natl. Acad. Sci.* (U.S.A.), 48, 1644 (1962).
36. Fischer and Baer, *Ber. Dtsch. Chem. Ges.*, 65, 337, 1040 (1932).
37. Kiessling, *Ber. Dtsch. Chem. Ges.*, 67, 869 (1934).
38. Meyerhof and Junowicz-Kocholaty, *J. Biol. Chem.*, 71, 149 (1943).
39. Ballou and Fischer, *J. Am. Chem. Soc.*, 77, 3329 (1955).
40. Ballou, Fischer, and MacDonald, *J. Am. Chem. Soc.*, 77.5967 (1955).
41. Volk, *J. Biol. Chem.*, 234, 1931 (1959).
42. Volk, *Biochim. Biophys. Acta*, 37, 365 (1960).
43. Wright and Khorana, *J. Am. Chem. Soc.*, 78, 811 (1956).
44. Putman and Hassid, *J. Am. Chem. Soc.*, 79, 5057 (1957).
45. Tener, Wright, and Khorana, *J. Am. Chem. Soc.*, 79, 441 (1957).
46. Khym, Doherty, and Cohn, *J. Am. Chem. Soc.*, 76, 5523 (1954).
47. Loring, Moss, Levy, and Hain, *Arch. Biochem. Biophys.*, 65, 578 (1956).
48. Albaum and Umbreit, *J. Biol. Chem.*, 167, 369 (1947).
49. Levene and Harris, *J. Biol. Chem.*, 101, 419 (1933).
50. Horecker and Smyrniotis, *Arch. Biochem. Biophys.*, 29, 232 (1950).
51. Michelson and Todd, *J. Chem. Soc.* (Lond.), p. 2476 (1949).
52. Levene and Stiller, *J. Biol. Chem.*, 104, 299 (1934).
53. Tener and Khorana, *J. Am. Chem. Soc.*, 80, 1999 (1958).
54. Klenow, *Arch. Biochem. Biophys.*, 46, 186 (1953).
55. Kornberg, Lieberman, and Simms, *J. Biol. Chem.*, 215, 389 (1955).
56. MacDonald and Fletcher, Jr., *J. Am. Chem. Soc.*, 84, 1262 (1962).
57. Friedkin, *J. Biol. Chem.*, 184, 449 (1950).

Table 6 (continued)
CARBOHYDRATE PHOSPHATE ESTERS

58. Racker, *J. Biol. Chem.*, 196, 347 (1952).
59. MacDonald and Fletcher, Jr., *J. Am. Chem. Soc.*, 81, 3719 (1959).
60. Szabó and Szabó, *J. Chem. Soc.*, (Lond.), p. 5139 (1964).
61. Ukita and Nagasawa, *Chem. Pharm. Bull.* (Tokyo), 7, 655 (1959).
62. Tarr, *Chem. Ind.*, 562 (1957).
63. Levene and Raymond, *J. Biol. Chem.*, 102, 347 (1933).
64. Gorin, Hough, and Jones, *J. Chem. Soc.* (Lond.), p. 582 (1955).
65. Kosterlitz, *Biochem. J.*, 33, 1087 (1939); 37, 318 (1943).
66. Reithel, *J. Am. Chem. Soc.*, 67, 1056 (1945).
67. Inouye, Tannenbaum, and Hsia, *Nature*, 193, 67 (1962).
68. Tanaka, *Yakugaku Zasshi*, 81, 797 (1961); *Chem. Abstr.*, 55, 27064 (1961).
69. Szabó and Szabó, *J. Chem. Soc.* (Lond.), p. 3762 (1960).
70. Antonakis, *Bull. Soc. Chim. Fr.*, p. 2112 (1965).
71. Cori, Colowick, and Cori, *J. Biol. Chem.*, 121, 465 (1937).
72. Meagher and Hassid, *J. Am. Chem. Soc.*, 68, 2135 (1946).
73. Wolfrom and Pletcher, *J. Am. Chem. Soc.*, 63, 1050 (1941).
74. Wolfrom, Smith, Pletcher, and Brown, *J. Am. Chem. Soc.*, 64, 23 (1942).
75. Colowick, *J. Biol. Chem.*, 124, 557 (1938).
76 Robison, *Biochem. J.*, 26, 2191 (1932).
77. Saito and Noguchi, *Nippon Kagaku Zasshi*, 82, 469 (1961); *Chem. Abstr.*, 56, 11678 (1962).
78. Lardy and Fischer, *J. Biol. Chem.*, 164, 513 (1946).
79. Posternak, *J. Biol. Chem.*, 180, 1269 (1949).
80. Crane and Sols, *J. Biol. Chem.*, 210, 597 (1954).
81. DeMoss and Happel, *J. Bacteriol.*, 70, 104 (1955).
82. Leloir, *Fortschr. Chem. Org. Naturst.*, 8, 47 (1951).
83. Hill and Ballou, *J. Biol. Chem.*, 241, 895 (1966).
84. Leloir, in *Phosphorus Metabolism*, Vol. 1, McElroy and Glass, Eds., Johns Hopkins Press, Baltimore, 1951, 67.
85. Charalampous and Mueller, *J. Biol. Chem.*, 201, 161 (1953).
86. Horecker, Smyrniotis, and Seegmiller, *J. Biol. Chem.*, 193, 383 (1951).
87. Hurwitz, Weissbach, Horecker, and Smyrniotis, *J. Biol. Chem.*, 218, 769 (1956).
88. Simpson and Wood, *J. Am. Chem. Soc.*, 78, 5452 (1956); *J. Biol. Chem.*, 230, 473 (1958).
89. Horecker, Hurwitz, and Weissbach, *J. Biol. Chem.*, 218, 785 (1956).
90. Glock, *Biochem. J.*, 52, 575 (1952).
91. Stumpf and Horecker, *J. Biol. Chem.*, 218, 753 (1956).
92. Tanko and Robison, *Biochem. J.*, 29, 961 (1935).
93. Pogell, *J. Biol. Chem.*, 201, 645 (1953).
94. Neuberg, Lustig, and Rothenberg, *Arch. Biochem. Biophys.*, 3, 33, (1944).
95. MacLeod and Robison, *Biochem. J.*, 27, 286 (1933).
96. McGilvery, *J. Biol. Chem.*, 200, 835 (1953).
97. Heath and Ghalambar, *J. Biol. Chem.*, 237, 2423 (1962).
98. Chiu and Feingold, *Biochem. Biophys. Acta*, 92, 489 (1964).
99. Chiu, Otto, Power, and Feingold, *Biochim. Biophys. Acta*, 127, 249 (1966).
100. Gillett and Ballou, *Biochemistry*, 2, 547 (1963).
101. Hers, *Biochim. Biophys. Acta*, 8, 416 (1952).
102. Mann and Lardy, *J. Biol. Chem.*, 187, 339 (1950).
103. Horecker, Smyrniotis, Hiatt, and Marks, *J. Biol. Chem.*, 212, 827 (1955).
104. Sie, Nigam, and Fishman, *J. Am. Chem. Soc.*, 81, 6083 (1959); 82, 1007 (1960).
105. Nordahl and Benson, *J. Am. Chem. Soc.*, 76, 5054 (1954).
106. Robison, Macfarlane, and Tazelaar, *Nature*, 142, 114 (1938).
107. Cardini and Leloir, *J. Biol. Chem.*, 225, 318 (1957).
108. Carlson, Swanson, and Roseman, *Biochemistry*, 3, 402 (1964).
109. Liu and Gotschlich, *J. Biol. Chem.*, 238, 1928 (1963).
110. Distler, Merrick, and Roseman, *J. Biol. Chem.*, 230, 497 (1958).
111. Brown, *J. Biol. Chem.*, 204, 877 (1953).
112. Maley, Maley, and Lardy, *J. Am. Chem. Soc.*, 78, 5303 (1956).
113. O'Brien, *Biochim. Biophys. Acta*, 86, 628 (1964).
114. Baluja, Chase, Kenner, and Todd, *J. Chem. Soc.* (Lond.), p. 4678 (1960).
115. Anderson and Percival, *J. Chem. Soc.* (Lond.), p. 814 (1956).
116. Grieling and Kisters, *Hoppe-Seyler's Z. Physiol. Chem.*, 346, 77 (1966).

Table 6 (continued)
CARBOHYDRATE PHOSPHATE ESTERS

117. Gander, Petersen, and Boyer, *Arch. Biochem. Biophys.*, 69, 85 (1957).
118. Sasaki and Taniguchi, *Nippon Nogeikagaku Kasihi*, 33, 183 (1959); *Chem. Abstr.*, 54, 308 (1960).
119. Leloir and Cardini, *J. Biol. Chem.*, 214, 157 (1955).
120. Cabib and Leloir, *J. Biol. Chem.*, 231, 259 (1958).
121. Robison and Morgan, *Biochem. J.*, 22, 1277 (1928).
122. Narumi and Tsumita, *J. Biol. Chem.*, 240, 2271 (1965).
123. Brooks, Lawrence, and Ricketts, *Biochem. J.*, 73, 566 (1959); *Nature*, 187, 1028 (1960).
124. Narumi and Tsumita, *J. Biol. Chem.*, 242, 2233 (1967).
125. Angval and Russell, *Aust. J. Chem.*, 22, 383 (1969).
126. Seamark, Tate, and Smeaton, *J. Biol. Chem.*, 243, 2424 (1968).
127. Volk, *J. Bacteriol.*, 95, 782 (1968).
128. Pippen and McCready, *J. Org. Chem.*, 16, 262 (1951).
129. Ishihara, Massaro, and Heath, *J. Biol. Chem.*, 243, 1103 (1968).
130. Avigad and England, *J. Biol. Chem.*, 243, 1511 (1968).
131. Fukui, *J. Bacteriol.*, 97, 793 (1969).
132. Bartlett and Bucolo, *Biochem. Biophys. Res. Commun.*, 3, 474 (1960).

CARBOHYDRATE PHOSPHATE ESTERS

Substance[a] (synonym)	Hydrolysis Constant[b] $k \times 10^3$	Hydrolysis Temp. °C	Hydrolysis Medium	Ester group form[c]	Specific rotation	Concentration[e] solvent	Melting point, °C	Reference
Trioses								
D-Glycerol 1-phosphate (α-L-glycerophosphate, L-glycerol 3-phosphate)	0.15	80	Water pH 6.3	Ag FA	+1.0 −1.45	6.5 10	—	1–3
Bis (2,3-dihydroxypropyl) hydrogen phosphate (α,α-diglycerophosphate)	350[f]	100	*N* HNO₃	FA	—	—	—	4
D-Glyceraldehyde 3-phosphate	86	100	*N* HCl	FA	+14	*N* HCl	—	5–8
Dihydroxyacetone phosphate	77	100	*N* HCl	—	—	—	—	6
D-Glyceric acid 2-phosphate	0.40[f]	125	*N* HCl	FA —	+13 +5	*N* HCl (NH₄)₂MoO₄	— —	9, 10 9
D-Glyceric acid 3-phosphate	0.40[f]	125	*N* HCl —	Ba Ba	−14.5 −745	*N* HCl (NH₄)₂MoO₄	— —	9, 10, 11 9
D-Glyceric acid 1,3-diphosphate	26	38	Water	FA	−2.3	—	—	12
D-Glyceric acid 2,3-diphosphate	— —	— —	— —	Ba Na	−2, −4 −4, +4.6	6–17, *N* HNO₃ 6–28	— —	13, 14 13–15
3-Hydroxypropionic acid phosphate (2-deoxyglyceric acid phosphate)	35[f]	90	*N* HCl	—	—	—	—	16
Tetroses								
D-Erythritol 4-phosphate	—	—	—	FA	+2.6	—	183–186	17
L-Erythritol 4-phosphate	— —	— —	— —	dcha dcha	−2.3, −2.6 +2.3	— —	186–190 —	17, 18 17
D-Erythrose 4-phosphate	86	100	*N* H₂SO₄	FA	0	—	—	19

[a] Compounds are grouped in order of increasing chain length. Within each group, they are arranged in the order alcohols, aldoses, ketoses, and acids.

[b] For the ester group at the lowest numbered carbon atom. The k values are in min^{-1} (natural logarithms).

[c] FA = free acid, Ag = silver salt, B = brucine salt, Ba = barium salt, cha = cyclohexylammonium salt, K = potassium salt, Na = sodium salt, d = di, tr = tri, t = tetra.

[d] $[\alpha]$, at the sodium D line, 5890A, unless otherwise indicated in parenthesis.

[e] Concentrations are 1–5 g/100 ml of solution at 20–25°; solvents other than water are indicated, and other temperatures are given in parentheses.

[f] Calculated by the contributor from the data of the reference cited; k = 0.69/time in minutes for 50% hydrolysis of the ester linkage.

[g] For the pyrophosphate group.

[h] For the second ester group.

[i] Both ester groups hydrolyze with equal ease.

CARBOHYDRATE PHOSPHATE ESTERS (continued)

Substance[a] (synonym)	Hydrolysis			Ester group form[c]	Specific rotation	Concentration[e] solvent	Melting point, °C	Reference
	Constant[b] $k \times 10^3$	Temp. °C	Medium					
Tetroses (continued)								
D-glycero-Tetrulose 1-phosphate	100	100	1 N HCl	—	—	—	—	20
D-glycero-Tetrulose 4-phosphate (D-erythrulose phosphate)	46	100	1 N HCl	—	—	—	—	20
D-glycero-Tetrulose 1,4-diphosphate	23[f]	100	N HCl	—	—	—	—	21, 22
D-Erythronic acid 4-phosphate	—	—	—	FA	-1.4	—	—	23
	—	—	—	FA	-11.7 (4000)	—	—	23
D-Erythronolactone 2-phosphate	—	—	—	trcha	-20	—	—	24, 25
4-Deoxy-D-erythronic acid 2-phosphate	—	—	—	cha	-55.0	N HCl	—	24
	—	—	—	FA	+15	N HCl	—	26
4-Deoxy-D-erythronic acid 3-phosphate	—	—	—	FA	-14.5	N HCl	—	26
	—	—	—	FA	-737	(NH$_4$)$_2$MoO$_4$	—	26
Pentoses								
L-Ribitol 1-phosphate (D-ribitol 5-phosphate)		100	N HCl	FA	—	—	—	27?
Ribitol 1,5-diphosphate	No constants	—	—	—	—	—	—	28
D-Xylitol 5-phosphate	—	—	—	Ba	+1.27	—	—	29
2-Deoxy-D-erythro-pentitol 5-phosphate	—	—	—	Ba	-16.8	—	—	30
α-D-Apio-D-furanosyl phosphate	35	26	0.25 N H$_2$SO$_4$	cha	-10.0	—	—	31
α-D-Apio-L-furanosyl phosphate	83	26	0.25 N H$_2$SO$_4$	FA	+16.9	—	—	32
L-Arabinofuranosyl phosphate	—	—	—	Ba	+48.2	—	—	33
L-Arabinopyranosyl phosphate	—	—	—	dcha(α-Anomer)	+30.8	(26°)	144—150	34
	—	—	—	dcha(β-Anomer)	+91	(26°)	155—161	34
α-D-Arabinofuranosyl phosphate	—	—	—	Ba	+6.4	—	—	33
α-D-Arabinopyranosyl phosphate	—	—	—	cha	-39.1	—	—	33
D-Arabinose 5-phosphate	3[f]	100	N H$_2$SO$_4$	FA	—	—	—	35, 36
	—	—	—	Ba	-18.8	—	—	37
	—	—	—	B	-48.6	50% Pyridine	—	37
α-D-Ribofuranosyl phosphate	2.9	20	0.01 N HCl	FA	+40.3	—	—	38
	—	—	—	dcha	—	—	—	39

CARBOHYDRATE PHOSPHATE ESTERS (continued)

Substance[a] (synonym)	Hydrolysis			Ester group form[c]	Specific rotation	Concentration[e] solvent	Melting point, °C	Reference
	Constant[b] $k \times 10^3$	Temp. °C	Medium					
Pentoses (continued)								
β-D-Ribofuranosyl phosphate	275	25	0.5 N HCl	—	—	—	—	40
	6[f]	25	0.01 N HCl	—	—	—	—	41
	5	25	0.01 N HCl	—	—	—	—	41
	1.5[f]	20	0.01 N HCl	Ba	-9.3	—	—	38
	—	—	—	dcha	-13.6	Ethanol	—	39
β-D-Ribopyranosyl phosphate	0.4	25	0.01 N HCl	Ba	-47.1	5% Acetic acid	—	41
D-Ribopyranosyl phosphate	2.9[f]	20	0.01 N HCl	Ba	-6.8	—	—	38
D-Ribose 2-phosphate	—	—	—	dB	-27.5	$H_2O{:}C_5H_5N$, 1:1	112–114d	42
	—	—	—	Ba	-6.8	—	—	42
D-Ribose 3-phosphate	—	—	—	dB	-35; -28	$H_2O{:}C_5H_5N$, 1:1	114–117d	42, 43
	—	—	—	Na	-97	Half-saturated boric acid	—	44, 45
D-Ribose 5-phosphate	13	100	0.25 N H₂SO₄	Na	+38	—	—	45
	0.5	100	0.25 N HCl	FA	18 ± 2	0.2, 1 N HCl	—	46, 47
	—	—	—	Ba	+6	—	—	44, 48
α-D-Ribofuranose 1,5-diphosphate	1.66	70	0.01 N HCl	FA	+20.8	0.43	—	49, 50
	—	—	—	tcha	+33.5	—	—	49
	—	—	—	FA	—	—	—	51
D-Ribofuranose 5-phosphate 1-pyrophosphate	69[g]	65	Acetate pH 4 buffer	—	—	—	—	52
α-D-Xylopyranosyl phosphate	6.2	36	0.38 N HCl	Ba	+65	—	—	53
	—	—	—	Ba	+70.9	5% Acetic	—	53
	—	—	—	K	+76	—	—	53, 54
	—	—	—	cha	+58	—	—	34
β-D-Xylopyranosyl phosphate	—	—	—	cha	+0.8	—	—	34
	—	—	—	Ba	-13.3	5% acetic	—	54
D-Xylose 3-phosphate	—	—	—	FA	-1.27	—	—	29
D-Xylose 5-phosphate	9	100	N HCl	FA	+8	—	—	55
	1.1	100	6 N H₂SO₄	Na	+3.2	—	—	56
	—	—	—	Ba	+5	$H_2O{:}C_5H_5N$, 1:1	—	55
2-Deoxy-α-D-*erythro*-pentofuranosyl phosphate (2-deoxy-α-D-ribosyl phosphate)	57[f]	21	Acetate pH 4.5 buffer	cha	+34.5, +38.8	—	—	57–59

CARBOHYDRATE PHOSPHATE ESTERS (continued)

Substance[a] (synonym)	Hydrolysis — Constant[b] $k \times 10^3$	Hydrolysis — Temp. °C	Hydrolysis — Medium	Ester group form[c]	Specific rotation	Concentration[e] solvent	Melting point, °C	Reference
Pentoses (continued)								
2-Deoxy-β-D-*erythro*-pentofuranosyl phosphate (2-deoxy-β-D-ribosyl phosphate)	—	—	—	cha	−15.8	—	—	58
2-Deoxy-D-*erythro*-pentofuranose 5-phosphate (2-deoxy-D-ribose 5-phosphate)	110[f]	100	N HCl	FA	+19	0.47	—	60, 61
	—	—	—	Ba	+10.8, 16.5	0.52	—	30,31
2-Deoxy-D-*erythro*-pentofuranose 1,5-diphosphate (2-deoxy-D-ribose 1,5-diphosphate)	33	20	Water pH 4	FA	—	—	—	62
	65[h]	100	N HCl	FA	—	—	—	62
2-Deoxy-D-*threo*-pentose 5-phosphate	—	—	—	Ba	−35	—	—	63
3-Deoxy-D-*erythro*-pentose 5-phosphate	—	—	—	Ba	−10.6	—	—	64
D-*erythro*-Pentulose 1-phosphate	No constants	—	—	—		—	—	65
D-*erythro*-Pentulose 5-phosphate (D-ribulose phosphate)	11[f]	100	N H_2SO_4	FA	−29.6	0.2N HCl	—	66, 67
	—	—	—	Ba	−40	0.02N HCl	—	68
D-*erythro*-Pentulose 1,5-diphosphate (D-ribulose diphosphate)	20[i]	100	N H_2SO_4	—	—	—	—	69
	57[i]	100	0.1 N HCl	—	—	—	—	70
L-*erythro*-Pentulose 5-phosphate (L-ribulose phosphate)	30[f]	90	N H_2SO_4	FA	+28	0.26, 0.2 N HBr	—	71
D-*threo*-Pentulose 5-phosphate (D-Xylulose phosphate)	200[f]	100	N HCl	B	−37.8	—	—	72, 73
	—	—	—	Ba	+1.95	—	—	29, 74
2-Deoxy-D-*erythro*-pentonic acid 5-phosphate	—	—	—	Ba	—	—	—	30
Hexoses								
D-Mannitol 1-phosphate	—	100	N HCl	FA	—	—	—	75
2-Amino-2-deoxy-D-glucitol 3-phosphate	—	—	—	FA	−20.5	—	—	76
β-D-Galactofuranosyl phosphate	—	—	—	Ba	+16.7	—	—	77
α-D-Galactopyranosyl phosphate	14	37	0.25 N HCl	FA	+148	0.2 N HCl	—	78
	—	—	—	K	+98	—	—	78
	—	—	—	Ba	+92	—	—	78
β-D-Galactopyranosyl phosphate	—	—	—	dcha	+78.5	—	147−153	34
	12	37	0.25 N HCl	Ba	+31.3	—	—	79
	—	—	—	dcha	+21	—	145−151	34

CARBOHYDRATE PHOSPHATE ESTERS (continued)

Substance[a] (synonym)	Hydrolysis			Ester group form[c]	Specific rotation	Concentration[e] solvent	Melting point, °C	Reference
	Constant[b] $k \times 10^3$	Temp. °C	Medium					
Hexoses (continued)								
D-Galactose 3-phosphate	–	–	–	K	+25.2	–	–	80
D-Galactose 6-phosphate	–	–	–	FA	+36.5	–	–	80
α-D-Galactopyranose 1,6-diphosphate	–	–	–	Ba	+25.2	(16°)	–	81, 82
	–	–	–	FA	+111	–	–	51
α-D-Glucopyranosyl phosphate	3.0	37	0.25 N HCl	FA	+118	–	–	83, 53
	–	–	–	Ba	+75.5	–	–	83
	–	–	–	dcha	+64	(26°)	163–169	34
	–	–	–	K	+78	–	–	84
β-D-Glucopyranosyl phosphate	11.5	33	N HCl	dB	+0.5	–	–	85
	35	33	N HCl	dB	–20	–	–	85
	–	–	–	dcha	+7.3	(26°)	137–143	34
α-L-Glucopyranosyl phosphate	–	–	–	Ba	–73.2	–	–	86
	–	–	–	K	–78.2	–	–	86
D-Glucose 2-phosphate	5	100	0.1 N HCl	K	+15	–	–	87
	–	–	–	FA	+35	–	–	87
D-Glucose 3-phosphate	–	–	–	FA	+39 (5461)	–	–	88
	–	–	–	Ba	+26.5	–	–	89
D-Glucose 4-phosphate	–	–	–	B	–14.5	50% Pyridine	–	90
D-Glucose 5-phosphate	–	–	–	B	–45.3	Pyridine	–	91
	–	–	–	Ba	+15	–	–	92
D-Glucose 6-phosphate	0.5	100	N HCl	FA	+35.7	–	157d	93, 94
	–	–	–	Ba	+18	–	95–97d	93–95
	–	–	–	K	+21.2	–	–	95, 96
3-O-Methyl-D-glucose 6-phosphate	–	–	–	cha	+22	–	–	97
α-D-Glucose 1,6-diphosphate	0.78	30	N H$_2$SO$_4$	FA	+83 ± 4	0.2	–	98
	–	–	–	dcha	+31.0	0.5	–	99
β-D-Glucose 1,6-diphosphate	3.15	30	N H$_2$SO$_4$	FA	–19 ±2	0.2	–	98
	–	–	–	Li	–27.5	–	–	100
α-L-Idopyranosyl phosphate	–	–	–	cha	–32	–	–	100
α-D-Mannopyranosyl phosphate	1.9	30	0.95 N H$_2$SO$_4$	FA	+58	0.4	–	101, 102
	–	–	–	Ba	+36	–	–	101
	–	–	–	dcha	+28.7	–	–	103
	–	–	–	Li	+46.3	–	–	100

CARBOHYDRATE PHOSPHATE ESTERS (continued)

Substance[a] (synonym)	Hydrolysis Constant[b] $k \times 10^3$	Hydrolysis Temp. °C	Hydrolysis Medium	Ester group form[c]	Specific rotation	Concentration[e] solvent	Melting point, °C	Reference
Hexoses (continued)								
β-D-Mannopyranosyl phosphate	—	—	—	cha	-6.5	—	180	104
D-Mannose 6-phosphate	0.67	100	N HCl	FA	+15.1 (5461)	—	—	94
α-D-Mannopyranose 1,6-diphosphate	—	—	—	Ba	+3.5 (5461)	0.7	—	70
	0.48	30	0.95 N HCl	K	+29.9	—	—	102
2-Acetamido-2-deoxy-α-D-galactopyranosyl phosphate	22	37	1 N HCl	FA	28.5	—	—	51
	—	—	—	—	—	—	—	105
	—	—	—	Li	+189 (5780)	—	—	106
	—	—	—	Li	+197 (5780)	—	—	107
	—	—	—	K	+112	—	—	108
	—	—	—	FA	+178	—	—	109
	—	—	—	Ba	+71.5	—	—	110
2-Acetamido-2-deoxy-α-D-galactopyranosyl phosphate 6-sulfate	—	—	—	FA	—	—	—	111
2-Amino-2-deoxy-α-D-galactopyranosyl phosphate (galactosamine 1-phosphate)	170	100	1 N HCl	FA	+143	—	—	108
2-Amino-2-deoxy-D-galactose 6-phosphate	0.8[f]	110	6 N HCl	FA	+57.8	0.1	—	112, 113
	—	—	—	N-Acetyl der	+48.4	0.5 M Na acetate	—	113
6-Deoxy-6-fluoro-α-D-galactopyranosyl phosphate	3.1	37	0.25 N HCl	K	+81	0.2(18°)	—	114
	69	60	0.25 N HCl	—	—	—	—	114
2-Acetamido-2-deoxy-α-D-glucopyranosyl phosphate	3.7	37	1 N HCl	K	+79	—	—	115
	4.1	37	1 N HCl	Ca	+107	—	—	116
	1.2	26	1.33 N HCl	K	+76	—	—	117
	—	—	—	Li	+144	—	—	107
2-Acetamido-2-deoxy-β-D-glucopyranosyl phosphate	86	26	1.33 N HCl	Na	-1.7	-40 (Calcd)	170–171d	117, 118
2-Amino-2-deoxy-α-D-glucopyranosyl phosphate (glucosamine-1-phosphate)	—	—	—	K	+100	—	—	115
	230	100	1 N HCl	K	—	—	—	115
	140[f]	100	N HClO₄	FA	-20 (Calcd)	—	—	119
2-Amino-2-deoxy-β-D-glucopyranosyl phosphate	—	—	—	FA	+70	—	178–179d	115, 118
	—	—	—	FA	+79	—	—	120
2-Acetamido-2-deoxy-D-glucose 6-phosphate	—	—	—	FA	+29.5	8, 0.5 M Na acetate	—	76
2-Amino-2-deoxy-D-glucose 6-phosphate	0.16	100	N HCl	FA	+54	0.5	—	113
	—	—	—	Ba	+53	(18°)	170–180d	119, 121
	—	—	—	—	0.3, pH 2.5	—	—	121

CARBOHYDRATE PHOSPHATE ESTERS (continued)

Substance[a] (synonym)	Hydrolysis — Constant[b] $k \times 10^3$	Temp. °C	Medium	Ester group form[c]	Specific rotation	Concentration[e] solvent	Melting point, °C	Reference
Hexoses (continued)								
2-Acetamido-2-deoxy-D-glucose 1,6-diphosphate	—	—	—	FA	+73	—	—	51
2-Amino-2-deoxy-D-glucose 1,6-diphosphate	—	—	—	FA	+84	—	—	51
2-Amino-3-O-(2-carboxyethyl)-2-deoxy-D-glucose 6-phosphate (muramic acid phosphate)	0.8[f]	100	6 N HCl	—	—	—	—	112
	—	—	—	FA	+79	—	—	122
N-Acetylmuramic acid 1-phosphate	No constants	—	—	—	—	—	—	123
3-Deoxy-3-fluoro-α-D-glucopyranosyl phosphate	—	—	—	cha	+60.5	—	158–162	124
3-Deoxy-3-fluoro-D-glucose-6-phosphate	No constants	—	—	FA	+60.5	—	—	124
4-Thio-α-D-glucopyranosyl phosphate	—	—	—	cha	+136.6	0.29	—	125
5-Thio-α-D-glucopyranosyl phosphate	—	—	—	cha	+21.3	—	—	126
2-Acetamido-2-deoxy-α-D-mannopyranosyl phosphate	—	—	—	cha	—	—	159–163	127
2-Deoxy-α-D-arabino-hexopyranosyl phosphate (2-deoxy-α-D-glucose 1-phosphate)	—	—	—	cha	+45	0.5	136–141	128
2-Deoxy-D-arabino-hexose 6-phosphate (2-deoxy-D-glucose 6-phosphate)	>10[f]	100	—	—	—	—	—	129 131
2-Deoxy-D-lyxo-hexose 3-phosphate (2-deoxy-D-galactose 3-phosphate)	—	—	—	FA	+25	—	—	80
2-Deoxy-D-lyxo-hexose 6-phosphate (2-deoxy-D-galactose 6-phosphate)	—	—	—	FA	+41	—	—	80
3-Deoxy-α-D-ribo-hexopyranosyl phosphate (3-deoxy-α-D-glucose 1-phosphate)	—	—	—	Et₃, N	+61.2	0.47	—	132
3-Deoxy-β-ribo-hexopyranosyl phosphate (3-deoxy-β-D-glucose 1-phosphate)	—	—	—	Et₃, N	+0.7	0.42	—	132
3-Deoxy-D-ribo-hexose 6-phosphate (3-deoxy-D-glucose 6-phosphate)	—	—	—	Ba	+6.6	—	—	30
	—	—	—	Ba	+3.8	—	—	133
	—	—	—	B	−24.2	—	—	133

CARBOHYDRATE PHOSPHATE ESTERS (continued)

Substance[a] (synonym)	Hydrolysis			Ester group form[c]	Specific rotation	Concentration[e] solvent	Melting point, °C	Reference
	Constant[b] $k \times 10^3$	Temp. °C	Medium					
Hexoses (continued)								
3-Deoxy-α-D-xylo-hexopyranosyl phosphate (3-deoxy-α-D-galactose 1-phosphate)	—	—	—	Ba	+4	—	—	134
3-Deoxy-β-D-xylo-hexopyranosyl phosphate (3-deoxy-β-D-galactose 1-phosphate)	—	—	—	Ba	-96	—	—	134
4-Deoxy-α-D-xylo-hexopyranosyl phosphate (4-deoxy-α-D-glucose 1-phosphate)	—	—	—	Et₃N	+72.5	0.43	—	132
4-Deoxy-β-D-xylo-hexopyranosyl phosphate (4-deoxy-β-D-glucose 1-phosphate)	—	—	—	Et₃N	+3.3	0.21	—	132
3,6-Dideoxy-D-xylo hexosyl phosphate	—	—	—	FA	1.5 (α-Anomer)	0.5		135
(abequose 1-phosphate)	—	—	—	FA	-3.8 (β-Anomer)	0.5		135
6-Deoxy-α-D-glucopyranosyl phosphate	—	—	—	Et₃N	+80.1	—	—	132
6-Deoxy-β-D-glucopyranosyl phosphate	—	—	—	Et₃N	+1.8	—	—	132
α-L-Fucopyranosyl phosphate	—	—	—	cha	-77.8	0.11	—	136
β-L-Fucopyranosyl phosphate	230	80	Water pH 2	FA	—	—	—	137
α-L-Rhamnopyranosyl phosphate	—	—	—	cha	-20.5	—	—	138
β-L-Rhamnopyranosyl phosphate	—	—	—	cha	-21.5	—	—	139
β-L-Rhamnopyranosyl phosphate	—	—	—	cha	+11.9	—	—	138
β-D-Fructopyranosyl phosphate	25	37	pH 4	Ba	-83.3	—	—	140
β-D-Fructopyranosyl phosphate	34	37	pH 4	cha	-77.9	—	—	141
β-D-Fructopyranosyl phosphate	86	37	pH 4	Na	-53.6	—	—	140
β-D-Fructofuranosyl phosphate	21	100	0.1 N HCl	FA	-64.2 (5461)	11.3	—	142
D-Fructose 1-phosphate	160	100	N HCl	Ba	-39 (5461)	6.1	—	142
	—	—	—	B	-52.1 (5461)	(26°)	—	142
	—	—	—	Ba	-30.4	—	—	143
D-Fructose 6-phosphate	10	100	N HCl	Ba	+3.6	10	—	94, 144

CARBOHYDRATE PHOSPHATE ESTERS (continued)

Substance[a] (synonym)	Hydrolysis — Constant[b] $k \times 10^3$	Temp. °C	Medium	Ester group form[c]	Specific rotation	Concentration[e] solvent	Melting point, °C	Reference
Hexoses (continued)								
D-Fructose 1,6-diphosphate	112	100	N HCl	FA	+4.0	13.6	—	144, 145
L-Fuculose 1-phosphate	140	—	—	trcha	-2.3	—	163–166d	146
	—	100	N HCl	Ba	—	—	—	147
L-Rhamnulose 1-phosphate	106f	100	N HCl	Ba	+8.9 (30°)	5.2 pH 4 Acetic acid	—	148
L-Sorbose 1-phosphate	90	99	1 N HCl	dcha	-16.5	—	171–173d	149
	—	—	—	K	-7.2	0.1 N HCl	—	150
L-Sorbose 6-phosphate	11	99	1 N HCl	Ba	-12.0	—	—	150
D-Tagatose 6-phosphate	—	—	—	Ba	+5.6	—	—	150
α-D-*ribo*-Hexopyranosyl-3-ulose phosphate (3-keto-D-glucose 1-phosphate)	—	100	N H$_2$SO$_4$	Ba / FA	+68 (15°)	0.7	—	151 / 152
D-*xylo*-Hexos-5-ulose-6-phosphate (5-ketoglucose 6-phosphate)	No constants	—	—	—	—	—	—	153
D-*threo*-2,5-Hexodiulose phosphate (5-keto-D-fructose phosphate)	125	98	N HCl	FA	—	—	—	154
D-Gluconic acid 6-phosphate	0.48	100	N HCl	FA	+0.2 (5461)	—	—	93, 155
	—	—	—	FA lactone	+21 (5461)	—	—	93
D-Mannono-1,4-lactone 6-phosphate	0.117	100	N HCl	—	+54.1 (5461)	—	—	155
D-Mannono-1,5-lactone 6-phosphate	0.117	100	N HCl	—	+60.6 (5461)	—	—	155
2-Amino-2-deoxy-D-gluconic acid 6-phosphate	1.24	100	N H$_2$SO$_4$	FA	-6.8	—	—	156
2-Deoxy-D-*arabino*-hexonic acid 6-phosphate	—	—	—	cha	+6	Ethanol	—	157
3-Deoxy-D-*ribo*-hexonic acid 6-phosphate	—	—	—	B	-20.2	—	—	133
D-Glucosaccharinic acid 6-phosphate	—	—	—	—	+62	—	—	158
α,β-D-Glucometasaccharinic acid 6-phosphate	—	—	—	Ba	-5.5	—	—	97
α,β-D-Glucometasaccharinic acid 5-phosphate	—	—	—	Ba	-6.7	—	—	97
β-D-Galactopyranosyluronic acid phosphate (β-D-galacturonic acid 1-phosphate)	—	—	—	Benzylamine	-14	—	—	159

CARBOHYDRATE PHOSPHATE ESTERS (continued)

Substance[a] (synonym)	Hydrolysis Constant[b] $k \times 10^3$	Hydrolysis Temp. °C	Hydrolysis Medium	Ester group form[c]	Specific rotation	Concentration[e] solvent	Melting point, °C	Reference
Hexoses (continued)								
α-D-Glucopyranosyluronic acid phosphate (α-D-glucuronic acid 1-phosphate)	0.23	61	0.01 N HCl	K	+53.6	–	–	160
	–	–	–	K	+51	–	–	161
α-L-Idopyranosyluronic acid phosphate (α-L-Iduronic acid phosphate)	–	–	–	cha	–15.8	–	135–138	100
α-D-Mannopyranosyluronic acid phosphate (α-D-mannuronic acid 1-phosphate)	–	–	–	Li	+19.1	–	–	100
D-arabino-Hexulosonic acid 6-phosphate (2-keto-D-gluconic acid 6-phosphate)	3[f]	94	N H₂SO₄	K	+3.3	–	–	162
3-Deoxy-D-erythro-hexulosonic acid 6-phosphate (3-deoxy-2-keto-D-gluconic acid 6-phosphate)	16	100	N HCl	FA	–	–	–	163
L-xylo-Hexulosonic acid diphosphate (2-keto-L-gluonic acid diphosphate)	No constants	–	–	–	–	–	–	164
α-D-xylo-Hexopyranos-4-ulosyluronic acid phosphate (4-keto-α-D-glucuronic acid 1-phosphate)	–	–	–	–	+30	–	–	165
Heptoses, Octoses								
D-glycero-D-gala-Heptose phosphate	–	–	–	Ba	+26.8	–	–	166
L-glycero-α-D-manno-Heptopyranosyl phosphate	–	–	–	cha	+32	–	–	167
Sedoheptulose 7-phosphate (D-altro-2-heptulose 7-phosphate)	9	100	N H₂SO₄	FA	+8 (5461)	–	–	168
	9	100	1 N HCl	Ba	–	–	–	169, 170
Sedoheptulose 1,7-diphosphate	17[f]	100	N H₂SO₄	FA	–	–	–	168
	9	100	N H₂SO₄	FA	–	–	–	168
D-gluco-3-Heptulose phosphate	No constants	–	–	–	–	–	–	171
D-manno-Heptulose phosphate	No constants	–	–	–	–	–	–	172
A heptulose monophosphate	9–2	100	N HCl	Ba	+8 (5461)	–	–	170

CARBOHYDRATE PHOSPHATE ESTERS (continued)

Substance[a] (synonym)	Hydrolysis			Ester group form[c]	Specific rotation	Concentration[e] solvent	Melting point, °C	Reference
	Constant[b] $k \times 10^3$	Temp. °C	Medium					
Heptoses, Octoses (continued)								
3-Deoxy-D-*gluco*-heptonic acid 7-phosphate	–	–	–	cha	+9.2	–	–	173
3-Deoxy-D-*arabino*-Heptulosonic acid 7-phosphate	–	–	–	FA	+42	–	–	173
	–	–	–	K	+15.7	–	–	173
D-*glycero*-D-*altro*-Octulose 1-phosphate	46[f]	100	N HCl	FA	–	–	–	174
D-*glycero*-D-*altro*-Octulose 8-phosphate	<2[f]	100	N HCl	FA	–	–	–	174
D-*glycero*-D-*altro*-Octulose 1,8-diphosphate	ca. 23	100	N HCl	FA	–	–	–	174
Cyclitols								
D-*myo*-Inositol 1-phosphate (*myo*-inositol 3-phosphate)	–	–	–	dcha	+9.3	pH 2.0	210–215d	175–177
	–	–	–	dcha	–3.2	pH 9.0	–	175
				B	–	–	238	178
L-*myo*-Inositol 1-phosphate (*myo*-inositol 3-phosphate)	2[f]	100	Water pH 2.0	dcha	–9.8	pH 2.0	–	179
				–	+3.4	pH 9.0	–	179
myo-Inositol 2-phosphate				FA	0 (meso.)	–	196–198	180
				B	–	–	244–247	180
				cha	–	–	203–205	180
				dcha	–	–	210–212	180
myo-Inositol 1,4-diphosphate	–	–	–	trcha	–	–	186–197d	181
myo-Inositol 4,5-diphosphate	–	–	–	trcha	–	–	182–183d	181
myo-Inositol hexaphosphate (phytic acid)	–	–	–	d CH$_3$ ester	–	–	247–249	182
(-)-Inositol 3-phosphate	–	–	–	FA	–25.6	–	>250	183
3-O-Methyl-(+)-inositol 4-phosphate (pinitol 4-phosphate)	–	–	–	FA	+20.5	–	>250	183
2,3-Dihydroxypropyl *myoinositol* hydrogen phosphate (1-O-glycerophosphoryl-*myoinositol*)	35[f]	100	N HCl	FA	–	–	–	184
		–	–	cha	–14	6, pH 3.5	115–117d	184–185
2-O-α-D-Mannosyl-L-*myo*-inositol 1-phosphate	No constants	–	–	–	–	–	–	103
Shikimic acid 5-phosphate	–	–	–	K H$_2$O	–107.6	(29°)	–	186

CARBOHYDRATE PHOSPHATE ESTERS (continued)

Substance[a] (synonym)	Hydrolysis			Ester group form[c]	Specific rotation	Concentration[e] solvent	Melting point, °C	Reference
	Constant[b] $k \times 10^3$	Temp. °C	Medium					
Disaccharides								
α-Cellobiosyl phosphate	—	—	—	cha	—	—	—	187
N-Acetyl α-chondrosinyl phosphate	—	—	—	Bu_3N	+66.4	—	—	188
α-Lactosyl phosphate	4[f]	37	N HCl	Ba	+73.3	—	—	189, 190
				FA	+99.5	—	—	191
β-Lactosyl phosphate	13[f]	37	N HCl	Ba	+24.8	—	—	189, 190
				FA	+31.5	—	—	191
α-Maltosyl phosphate	3.2	36	0.38 N HCl	Ba	+107	—	—	53
	140	100	N HCl	—	+147	—	—	192
Sucrose 6-phosphate	—	—	—	Ba	+35.4	—	—	193
	13[f]	100	$N\ H_2SO_4$	K	+34	—	—	193
				—	—	—	—	194
Trehalose 6-phosphate	—	—	—	B	+31 (5461)	—	—	195
				Ba	+99	—	—	196
	0.6	—	—	FA	+185	0.1 N HCl	—	197
Trehalose 6,6'-diphosphate	—	—	—	Ba	+132 (5461)	—	—	195
				cha	+62	—	—	196
	3.8[f]	100	3 N HCl	FA	+99.3	0.7	—	198

Compiled by Donald L. MacDonald, with acknowledgments to George C. Maher and the late Melville L. Wolfrom, compilers of the corresponding tables in earlier editions.

CARBOHYDRATE PHOSPHATE ESTERS (continued)

REFERENCES

1. Kiessling and Schuster, *Ber. Dtsch. Chem. Ges.*, 71, 123 (1938).
2. Weil-Malherbe and Green, *Biochem. J.*, 49, 286 (1951).
3. Baer and Fischer, *J. Biol. Chem.*, 128, 491 (1939).
4. Maruo and Benson, *J. Am. Chem. Soc.*, 79, 4564 (1957).
5. Fischer and Baer, *Ber. Dtsch. Chem. Ges.*, 65, 337, 1040 (1932).
6. Kiessling, *Ber. Dtsch. Chem. Ges.*, 67, 869 (1934).
7. Meyerhof and Junowicz-Kocholaty, *J. Biol. Chem.*, 71, 149 (1943).
8. Ballou and Fischer, *J. Am. Chem. Soc.*, 77, 3329 (1955).
9. Ballou and Fischer, *J. Am. Chem. Soc.*, 76, 3188 (1954).
10. Kiessling, *Ber. Dtsch. Chem. Ges.*, 68, 243 (1935).
11. Meyerhof and Schultz, *Biochem. Z.*, 297, 60 (1938).
12. Negelein and Brömel, *Biochem. Z.*, 303, 132 (1939).
13. Baer, *J. Biol. Chem.*, 185, 763 (1950).
14. Greenwald, *J. Biol. Chem.*, 63, 339 (1925).
15. Sutherland, Posternak, and Cori, *J. Biol. Chem.*, 181, 153 (1949).
16. Ballou and Hesse, *J. Am. Chem. Soc.*, 78, 3718 (1956).
17. MacDonald, Fischer, and Ballou, *J. Am. Chem. Soc.*, 78, 3720 (1956).
18. Shetter, *J. Am. Chem. Soc.*, 78, 3722 (1956).
19. Ballou, Fischer, and MacDonald, *J. Am. Chem. Soc.*, 77, 5967 (1955).
20. Chu and Ballou, *J. Am. Chem. Soc.*, 83, 1711 (1961).
21. Charalampous and Mueller, *J. Biol. Chem.*, 201, 161 (1953).
22. Gillett and Ballou, *Biochemistry*, 2, 547 (1963).
23. Taylor and Ballou, *Biochemistry*, 2, 553 (1963).
24. Barker and Wold, *J. Org. Chem.*, 28, 1847 (1963).
25. Ishii, Hashimoto, Tachibana, and Yoshikawa, *Biochem. Biophys. Res. Commun.*, 10, 19 (1963).
26. Ballou, *J. Am. Chem. Soc.*, 79, 984 (1957).
27. Baddiley, Buchanan, Carss, and Mathias, *J. Chem. Soc.* (Lond.), p. 4583 (1956).
28. Applegarth, Buchanan, and Baddiley, *J. Chem. Soc.* (Lond.), p. 1213 (1965).
29. Moffatt and Khorana, *J. Am. Chem. Soc.*, 79, 1194 (1957).
30. Szabó and Szabó, *J. Chem. Soc.* (Lond.), p. 5139 (1964).
31. Ukita and Nagasawa, *Chem. Pharm. Bull.* (Tokyo), 7, 655 (1959).
32. Mendicino and Hanna, *J. Biol. Chem.*, 245, 6113 (1970).
33. Wright and Khorana, *J. Am. Chem. Soc.*, 80, 1994 (1958).
34. Putman and Hassid, *J. Am. Chem. Soc.*, 79, 5057 (1957).
35. Volk, *J. Biol. Chem.*, 234, 1931 (1959).
36. Volk, *Biochim. Biophys. Acta*, 37, 365 (1960).
37. Levene and Christman, *J. Biol. Chem.*, 123, 607 (1938).
38. Wright and Khorana, *J. Am. Chem. Soc.*, 78, 811 (1956).
39. Tener, Wright, and Khorana, *J. Am. Chem. Soc.*, 79, 441 (1957).
40. Kalckar, *J. Biol. Chem.*, 167, 477 (1947); Plesner and Klenow, *Methods Enzymol.*, 3, 181 (1957).
41. Halmann, Sanchez, and Orgel, *J. Org. Chem.*, 34, 3702 (1969).
42. Khym, Doherty, and Cohn, *J. Am. Chem. Soc.*, 76, 5523 (1954).
43. Loring, Moss, Levy, and Hain, *Arch. Biochem. Biophys.*, 65, 578 (1956).
44. Albaum and Umbreit, *J. Biol. Chem.*, 167, 369 (1947).
45. Levene and Harris, *J. Biol. Chem.*, 101, 419 (1933).
46. Horecker and Smyrniotis, *Arch. Biochem. Biophys.*, 29, 232 (1950).
47. Michelson and Todd, *J. Chem. Soc.* (Lond.), p. 2476 (1949).
48. Levene and Stiller, *J. Biol. Chem.*, 104, 299 (1934).
49. Tener and Khorana, *J. Am. Chem. Soc.*, 80, 1999 (1958).
50. Klenow, *Arch. Biochem. Biophys.*, 46, 186 (1953).
51. Hanna and Mendicino, *J. Biol. Chem.*, 245, 4031 (1970).
52. Kornberg, Lieberman, and Simms, *J. Biol. Chem.*, 215, 389 (1955).
53. Meagher and Hassid, *J. Am. Chem. Soc.*, 68, 2135 (1946).
54. Antia and Watson, *J. Am. Chem. Soc.*, 80, 6134 (1958).
55. Levene and Raymond, *J. Biol. Chem.*, 102, 347 (1933).
56. Gorin, Hough, and Jones, *J. Chem. Soc.* (Lond.), p. 582 (1955).
57. Friedkin, *J. Biol. Chem.*, 184, 499 (1950).
58. MacDonald and Fletcher, Jr., *J. Am. Chem. Soc.*, 84, 1262 (1962).

59. Tarr, *Can. J. Biochem. Physiol.*, 36, 517 (1958).
60. Racker, *J. Biol. Chem.*, 196, 347 (1952).
61. MacDonald and Fletcher, Jr., *J. Am. Chem. Soc.*, 81, 3719 (1959).
62. Tarr, *Chem. Ind.* (Lond.), p. 562 (1957).
63. Antonakis, Dowgiallo, and Szabo, *Bull. Soc. Chim. Fr.*, 1355 (1962).
64. Szabó and Szabó, *J. Chem. Soc.* (Lond.), p. 2944 (1965).
65. Stewart and Ballou, *J. Org. Chem.*, 32, 1065 (1967).
66. Horecker, Smyrniotis, and Seegmiller, *J. Biol. Chem.*, 193, 383 (1951).
67. Hurwitz, Weissbach, Horecker, and Smyrniotis, *J. Biol. Chem.*, 218, 769 (1956).
68. Kornberg, quoted in Horecker, *Methods Enzymol.*, 3, 190 (1957).
69. Horecker, Hurwitz, and Weissbach, *J. Biol. Chem.*, 218, 785 (1956).
70. Leloir, *Fortschr. Chem. Org. Naturst.*, 8, 47 (1951).
71. Simpson and Wood, *J. Am. Chem. Soc.*, 78, 5452 (1956); *J. Biol. Chem.*, 230, 473 (1958).
72. Glock, *Biochem. J.*, 52, 575 (1952).
73. Stumpf and Horecker, *J. Biol. Chem.*, 218, 753 (1956).
74. Barnwell, Saunders, and Watson, *Can. J. Chem.*, 33, 711 (1955).
75. Wolff and Kaplan, *J. Biol. Chem.*, 218, 849 (1957).
76. Lambert and Zilliken, *Chem. Ber.*, 96, 2350 (1963).
77. Chittenden, *Carbohydr. Res.*, 25, 35 (1972).
78. Kosterlitz, *Biochem. J.*, 33, 1087 (1939); 37, 318 (1943).
79. Reithel, *J. Am. Chem. Soc.*, 67, 1056 (1945).
80. Foster, Overend, and Stacey, *J. Chem. Soc.* (Lond.), p. 980 (1951).
81. Inouye, Tannenbaum, and Hsia, *Nature*, 193, 67 (1962).
82. Tanaka, *Yakugaku Zasshi*, 81, 797 (1961); *Chem. Abstr.*, 55, 27064 (1961).
83. Cori, Colowick, and Cori, *J. Biol. Chem.*, 121, 465 (1937).
84. Wolfrom and Pletcher, *J. Am. Chem. Soc.*, 63, 1050 (1941).
85. Wolfrom, Smith, Pletcher, and Brown, *J. Am. Chem. Soc.*, 64, 23 (1942).
86. Potter, Sowden, Hassid, and Doudoroff, *J. Am. Chem. Soc.*, 70, 1751 (1948).
87. Farrar, *J. Chem. Soc.* (Lond.), p. 3131 (1949).
88. Josephson and Proffe, *Ann.*, 481, 91 (1930).
89. Levene and Raymond, *J. Biol. Chem.*, 89, 479 (1930).
90. Levene and Raymond, *J. Biol. Chem.*, 91, 751 (1931).
91. Raymond, *J. Biol. Chem.*, 113, 375 (1936).
92. Josephson and Proffe, *Biochem. Z.*, 258, 147 (1933).
93. Robison and King, *Biochem. J.*, 25, 323 (1931).
94 Robison, *Biochem. J.*, 26, 2191 (1932).
95. Saito and Noguchi, *Nippon Kagaku Zasshi*, 82, 469 (1961); *Chem. Abstr.*, 56, 11678 (1962).
96. Lardy and Fischer, *J. Biol. Chem.*, 164, 513 (1946).
97. Lewak and Szabó, *J. Chem. Soc.* (Lond.), p. 3975 (1963).
98. Posternak, *J. Biol. Chem.*, 180, 1269 (1949).
99. Buck, *Carbohydr. Res.*, 6, 247 (1968).
100. Perchimlides, Osawa, Davidson, and Jeanloz, *Carbohydr. Res.*, 3, 463 (1967).
101. Colowick, *J. Biol. Chem.*, 124, 557 (1938).
102. Posternak and Rosselet, *Helv. Chim. Acta*, 36, 1614 (1953).
103. Hill and Ballou, *J. Biol. Chem.*, 241, 895 (1966).
104. Pridhar and Behrman, *Carbohydr. Res.*, 23, 456 (1972).
105. Leloir, Cardini, and Olavarria, *Arch. Biochem. Biophys.*, 74, 84 (1958).
106. Davidson and Wheat, *Biochim. Biophys. Acta*, 72, 112 (1963).
107. Kim and Davidson, *J. Org. Chem.*, 28, 2475 (1963).
108. Carlson, Swanson, and Roseman, *Biochemistry*, 3, 402 (1964).
109. Cardini and Leloir, *J. Biol. Chem.*, 225, 317 (1958).
110. Olavesen and Davidson, *Biochim. Biophys. Acta*, 101, 245 (1965).
111. Cardini and Leloir, *Arch. Biochem. Biophys.*, 45, 55 (1953).
112. Liu and Gotschlich, *J. Biol. Chem.*, 238, 1928 (1963).
113. Distler, Merrick, and Roseman, *J. Biol. Chem.*, 230, 497 (1958).
114. Kent and Wright, *Carbohydr. Res.*, 22, 193 (1972).
115. Maley, Maley, and Lardy, *J. Am. Chem. Soc.*, 78, 5503 (1956).
116. Leloir and Cardini, *Biochim. Biophys. Acta*, 20, 33 (1956).
117. O'Brien, *Biochim. Biophys. Acta*, 86, 628 (1964).
118. Baluja, Chase, Kenner, and Todd, *J. Chem. Soc.* (Lond.), p. 4678 (1960).

CARBOHYDRATE PHOSPHATE ESTERS (continued)

119. Brown, *J. Biol. Chem.*, 204, 877 (1953).
120. Westphal and Stadler, *Angew. Chem.*, 75, 452 (1963).
121. Anderson and Percival, *J. Chem. Soc.* (Lond.), 814 (1956).
122. Jeanloz, Konami, and Osawa, *Biochemistry*, 10, 192 (1971).
123. Heymann, Turdiu, Lee, and Barkulis, *Biochemistry*, 7, 1393 (1968).
124. Wright, Taylor, Brunt, and Brownsley, *J. Chem. Soc. Chem. Commun.*, 691 (1972); Wright and Taylor, *Carbohydr. Res.*, 32, 366 (1974).
125. Kochetkov, Shibaev, Kusov, and Troitskii, *Izv. Akad. Nauk SSSR, Ser. Khim.*, 425 (1973); *Bull. Acad. Sci. USSR, Div. Chem. Sci.*, 22, 408 (1973).
126. Whistler and Stark, *Carbohydr. Res.*, 13, 15 (1970).
127. Salo and Fletcher, Jr., *Biochemistry*, 9, 878 (1970).
128. Shibaev, Kusov, Kuchar, and Kochetkov, *Izv. Akad. Nauk SSSR, Ser. Khim.*, 992 (1973); *Bull. Acad. Sci. USSR, Div. Chem. Sci.*, 22, 886 (1973).
129. Crane and Sols, *J. Biol. Chem.*, 210, 597 (1954).
130. DeMoss and Happel, *J. Bacteriol.*, 70, 104 (1955).
131. Brooks, Lawrence, and Ricketts, *Biochem. J.*, 73, 566 (1959); *Nature*, 187, 1028 (1960).
132. Shibaev, Kusov, Kuchar, and Kochetkov, *Izv. Akad. Naud SSSR, Ser. Khim.*, 430 (1973); *Bull. Acad. Sci. USSR, Div. Chem. Sci.*, 22, 408 (1973).
133. Dahlgard and Kaufmann, *J. Org. Chem.*, 25, 781 (1960).
134. Antonakis, *Compt. Rend.*, 258, 3511 (1964).
135. Antonakis, *Bull. Soc. Chim. Fr.*, 2112 (1965).
136. Schanbacher and Wilken, *Biochim. Biophys. Acta*, 141, 646 (1967); Leaback, Heath, and Roseman, *Biochemistry*, 8, 1351 (1969).
137. Ishihara, Massaro, and Heath, *J. Biol. Chem.*, 243, 1103 (1968).
138. Pridhar and Behrman, *Biochemistry*, 12, 997 (1973).
139. Barber, *Biochim. Biophys. Acta*, 141, 174 (1967); Chatterjee and MacDonald, *Carbohydr. Res.*, 6, 253 (1968).
140. Pontis and Fischer, *Biochem. J.*, 89, 452 (1963).
141. MacDonald, *J. Org. Chem.*, 31, 513 (1966).
142. Tako and Robison, *Biochem. J.*, 29, 961 (1935).
143. Pogell, *J. Biol. Chem.*, 201, 645 (1953).
144. Neuberg, Lustig, and Rothenberg, *Arch. Biochem. Biophys.*, 3, 33 (1944).
145. MacLeod and Robison, *Biochem. J.*, 27, 286 (1933).
146. McGilvery, *J. Biol. Chem.*, 200, 835 (1953).
147. Heath and Ghalambar, *J. Biol. Chem.*, 237, 2423 (1962).
148. Chiu and Feingold, *Biochim. Biophys. Acta*, 92, 489 (1964).
149. Chiu, Otto, Power, and Feingold, *Biochim. Biophys. Acta*, 127, 249 (1966).
150. Mann and Lardy, *J. Biol. Chem.*, 187, 339 (1950).
151. Totton and Lardy, *J. Biol. Chem.*, 181, 701 (1949).
152. Fukui, *J. Bacteriol.*, 97, 793 (1969).
153. Kiely and Fletcher, Jr., *J. Org. Chem.*, 33, 3723 (1968).
154. Avigad and England, *J. Biol. Chem.*, 243, 1511 (1968).
155. Patwardhan, *Biochem. J.*, 28, 1854 (1934).
156. Greiling and Kisters, *Hoppe-Seyler's Z. Physiol. Chem.*, 346, 77 (1966).
157. Wolfrom and Franks, *J. Org. Chem.*, 29, 3645 (1964).
158. Lee, *J. Org. Chem.*, 28, 2473 (1963).
159. Touster and Reynolds, *J. Biol. Chem.*, 197, 863 (1952).
160. Barker, Bourne, Fleetwood, and Stacey, *J. Chem. Soc.* (Lond.), 4128 (1958).
161. Marsh, *J. Chem. Soc.* (Lond.), 1578 (1952).
162. Ciferri, Blakley, and Simpson, *Can. J. Microbiol.*, 5, 277 (1959).
163. MacGee and Doudoroff, *J. Biol. Chem.*, 210, 617 (1954).
164. Moses, Ferrier, and Calvin, *Proc. Natl. Acad. Sci. U.S.A.*, 48, 1644 (1962).
165. Stroud and Hassid, *Biochem. Biophys. Res. Commun.*, 15, 65 (1964).
166. Strobach and Szabó, *J. Chem. Soc.* (Lond.), 3970 (1963).
167. Teuber, Bevill, and Osborn, *Biochemistry*, 7, 3303 (1968).
168. Horecker, Smyrniotis, Hiatt, and Marks, *J. Biol. Chem.*, 212, 827 (1955).
169. Benson, in *Modern Methods of Plant Analysis*, Vol. II, Paech and Tracy, Eds., Springer-Verlag, Berlin, 1955, 113.
170. Robison, Macfarlane, and Tazelaar, *Nature*, 142, 114 (1938).
171. Sie, Nigam, and Fishman, *J. Am. Chem. Soc.*, 81, 6083 (1959); 82, 1007 (1960).
172. Nordahl and Benson, *J. Am. Chem. Soc.*, 76, 5054 (1954).
173. Sprinson, Rothschild, and Sprecher, *J. Biol. Chem.*, 238, 3170 (1963).

CARBOHYDRATE PHOSPHATE ESTERS (continued)

174. Bartlett and Bucolo, *Biochem. Biophys. Res. Commun.*, 3, 474 (1960).
175. Ballou and Pizer, *J. Am. Chem. Soc.*, 81, 4745 (1959); 82, 3333 (1960).
176. Posternak, *Helv. Chim. Acta,* 41, 1891 (1958); 42, 390 (1959).
177. Eisenberg, Jr. and Bolden, *Biochem. Biophys. Res. Commun.*, 21, 100 (1965).
178. Woolley, *J. Biol. Chem.*, 147, 581 (1943).
179. Pizer and Ballou, *J. Am. Chem. Soc.*, 81, 915 (1959).
180. Brown and Hall, *J. Chem. Soc.* (Lond.), p. 357 (1959).
181. Angyal and Tate, *J. Chem. Soc.* (Lond.), p. 4122 (1961).
182. Angyal and Russell, *Aust. J. Chem.*, 22, 383 (1969).
183. Kilgour and Ballou, *J. Am. Chem. Soc.*, 80, 3956 (1958).
184. Lepage, Mumma, and Bensen, *J. Am. Chem. Soc.*, 82, 3713 (1960).
185. Seamark, Tate, and Smeaton, *J. Biol. Chem.*, 243, 2424 (1968).
186. Weiss and Mingioli, *J. Am. Chem. Soc.*, 78, 2894 (1956).
187. Shibaev, Kusov, Troitskii, and Kochetkov, *Izv. Akad. Nauk SSSR, Ser. Khim.*, 182 (1974); *Bull. Acad. Sci. USSR, Div. Chem. Sci.*, 23, 171 (1974).
188. Olavesen and Davidson, *J. Biol. Chem.*, 240, 992 (1965).
189. Gander, Petersen, and Boyer, *Arch. Biochem. Biophys.*, 69, 85 (1957).
190. Sasaki and Taniguchi, *Nippon Nogeikagaku Kasihi*, 33, 183 (1959); *Chem. Abstr.*, 54, 308 (1960).
191. Reithel and Young, *J. Am. Chem. Soc.*, 74, 4210 (1952).
192. Narumi and Tsumita, *J. Biol. Chem.*, 242, 2233 (1967).
193. Buchanan, Cummerson, and Turner, *Carbohydr. Res.*, 21, 283 (1972).
194. Leloir and Cardini, *J. Biol. Chem.*, 214, 157 (1955).
195. Robison and Morgan, *Biochem. J.*, 22, 1277 (1928).
196. MacDonald and Wong, *Biochim. Biophys. Acta*, 86, 390 (1964).
197. Cabib and Leloir, *J. Biol. Chem.*, 231, 259 (1958).
198. Narumi and Tsumita, *J. Biol. Chem.*, 240, 2271 (1965).

Table 1
STRUCTURE OF DISACCHARIDE UNITS ISOLATED FROM COMPLEX CARBOHYDRATES OF MAMMALIAN ORIGIN

Linkage[a]	Source
Fucose	
Fuc(α, 1 → 3)GlcNAc	Le[a], Le[b] type 2 blood group chains (1) (reports of presence in IgG (2) and IgA (3) myeloma globulins were tentative; linkage probably involves C-6 of GlcNAc)
Fuc(α, 1 → 4)GlcNAc	Le[a], Le[b] Type 1 chains (1)
Fuc(α, 1 → 6)GlcNAc	IgA (3) and IgE (4) myeloma globulins; storage material in fucosidosis (5), probably ubiquitous in glycoproteins
Fuc(α, 1 → 2)Gal	A, B, H, Le[b] Type 1 and Type 2 blood group chains (1) (glycolipids (6), glycoproteins (1, 7), and oligosaccharides), fucosyllactose etc; storage material in fucosidosis (8)
Fuc(α, 1 → 3)Glc	Lactodifucotetraose (1), lacto-N-difucohexaose II (1)
Fuc(α, 1 → 4)Man	Existence suggested in IgG and ribonuclease B but not verified
Galactose	
Gal(β, 1 → 3)GlcNAc	Le[a] glycoprotein (9) orosomucoid (10) IgA-myeloma globulin (3), transferrin (11)
Gal(β, 1 → 4)GlcNAc	Orosomucoid- (10), IgA-, IgG- (2), and IgE-(4) myeloma globulins, transferrin (11), blood group substances (1), storage material in G_{M1}-gangliosidosis liver (12, 13)
Gal(β, 1 → 6)GlcNAc	IgG-myeloma globulin (2), ribonuclease (14)
Gal(β, 1 → 3)GalNAc	Pig submaxillary gland (15), gangliosides (G_{M1}, G_{D1a}, etc.) (16)
Gal(β, 1 → 6)GalNAc	IgA-myeloma globulin (3)
Gal(α, 1 → 4)Gal	Human digalactosylceramide (17) human trihexosylceramide (18), globoside (cytolipin K) (18), digalactosyldiglycerides (19)
Gal(α, 1 → 3)Gal	Rat trihexosylceramide (20), cytolipin R (21), rabbit erythrocyte pentaglycosyl-ceramide (22), blood group B (1)
Gal(β, 1 → 3)Gal	Mucopolysaccharide linkage region (23)
Gal(β, 1 → 4)Glc	Many glycosphingolipids (15), lactose
Gal(β, 1 → 4)Xyl	Mucopolysaccharide linkage region (23)
Glucose	
Glc(α, 1 → 4)Glc	Glycogen (24)
Glc(α, 1 → 6)Glc	Glycogen (24)
Glc(α, 1 → 2)Gal	Collagen (glomerular basement membrane) (25)
N-Acetylglucosamine (2-acetamido-2-deoxy-D-glucose)	
GlcNAc(β, 1 → 3)Gal	Blood group substances (1, 6), keratan-sulfate (26), G_{M1}-gangliosidosis liver (13)
GlcNAc(β, 1 → 4)Gal	Some bovine spleen gangliosides (27)
GlcNAc(β, 1 → 6)Gal	Le[a] glycoprotein (1, 9)

[a]Abbreviations: Fuc, L-fucose (6-deoxy-L-galactose); Gal, D-galactose; Glc, D-glucose; Man, D-mannose; Xyl, D-xylose; GlcNAc, N-acetyl-D-glucosamine; GalNAc, N-acetyl-D-galactosamine; NeuNAc, N-acetyl-neuraminic acid; NeuNGly, N-glycolylneuraminic acid; GlcUA, D-glucuronic acid; IdUA, L-iduronic acid; Ig, immunoglobulin; G_{M1}- etc., ganglioside nomenclature according to Svennerholm (15); Le, Lewis antigen.

Table 1 (continued)

STRUCTURE OF DISACCHARIDE UNITS ISOLATED FROM COMPLEX CARBOHYDRATES OF MAMMALIAN ORIGIN

Linkage[a]	Source
GlcNAc(β, 1 → 2)Man	IgG-myeloma globulin (2), IgE myeloma globulin (4), oligosaccharide stored in G_{M1}-gangliosidosis liver (12); believed related to erythrocyte MN glycoprotein
GlcNAc(β, 1 → 3)Man	Transferrin (11), orosomucoid (10), ribonuclease (14)
GlcNAc(β, 1 → 4)Man	Ovalbumin (28), orosomucoid (10), ribonuclease (14), IgG-myeloma globulin (2)
GlcNAc(β, 1 → 4)GlcNAc	IgG- and IgE-myeloma globulin linkage region (asparagine) (2, 4) (also found as the repeating disaccharide in chitin)
GlcNAc(α, 1 → 4)GlcUA	Heparin (29)
GlcNAc(β, 1 → 4)GlcUA	Hyaluronic acid (29)
GlcNAc(β, 1 → 6)Gal	Group specific H and Le[a] glycoproteins from ovarian cysts (1, 7, 9)
GlcNAc(β, 1 → 6)GalNAc	Le[a] glycoprotein (13) glycopeptide stored in G_{M1}-gangliosidosis liver (13)
GlcNAc(α, 1 → 3)Man	IgE-myeloma globulin (30)
GlcNAc(α, 1 → 3)IdUA	Heparin, heparan sulfates (29)

N-Acetylgalactosamine (2-acetamido-2-deoxy-D-galactose)

GalNAc(α 1 → 3)Gal	Blood group A (1) Le[a] (9) rabbit pentaglycosyl-ceramide (22) porcine submaxillary gland mucin Type A (15)
GalNAc(α, 1 → 3)GalNAc	Forssman hapten (31)
GalNAc(β, 1 → 3)Gal	Cytolipin K (18) (human erythrocyte globoside) and R (21)
GalNAc(β, 1 → 4)Gal	Gangliosides (16), IgA-myeloma globulin (3)
GalNAc(β, 1 → 4)GalNAc	IgA-myeloma globulin (3)
GalNAc(β, 1 → 4)GlcUA	Chondroitin 4/6 sulfates (29)
GalNAc(β, 1 → 4)IdUA	Dermatan sulfate (29)

Mannose

Man α(1 → 6)Man	Ribonuclease (14), IgG-myeloma globulin (2) IgE-myeloma globulin (4)
Man α(1 → 4)Man	Ovalbumin (28, 32)
Man α(1 → 3)Man	IgG- and IgE-myeloma globulins (3, 30) ovalbumin (28, 32), G_{M1}-gangliosidosis liver (12), IgE-myeloma globulin (4)
Man α(1 → 2)Man	IgA-myeloma globulin (3), storage material in mannosidosis (33—35)
Man α(1 → 4)GlcNAc	Ribonuclease (14), orosomucoid (10), IgA-myeloma globulin (2)
Man α(1 → 3)GlcNAc	Ovalbumin (27), orosomucoid (10), IgA- and gG-myeloma globulins (2, 3)
Man β(1 → 3)GlcNAc	Ovalbumin (28, 32), ribonuclease (14)
Man β(1 → 4)GlcNAc	IgE-myeloma globulin (4), oligosaccharide stored in G_{M1}-gangliosidosis (12) and mannosidosis liver (33—35)

Sialic Acid

NeuNAc(α, 2 → 2/4)Gal	IgG-heavy chain glycoprotein (36)
NeuNAc (α, 2 → 3)Gal	Gangliosides (G_{M3}, G_{M2}, G_{M1}, etc.) (15)
NeuNGly	sialolactose, IgA-myeloma globulin (2)

Table 1 (continued)
STRUCTURE OF DISACCHARIDE UNITS ISOLATED FROM COMPLEX CARBOHYDRATES OF MAMMALIAN ORIGIN

Linkage[a]	Source
NeuNAc(α, 2 → 6)Gal	Fetuin (37), orosomucoid (10), thyro-globulin (38)
NeuNAc (α, 2 → 6)GalNAc NeuNGly	Submaxillary gland glycoproteins (15)
NeuNAc (α, 2 → 8)NANA NeuNGly	Gangliosides (G$_{D1b}$, G$_{T1a}$, G$_{T1b}$, G$_{D3}$, G$_{D2}$ (16)
Uronic Acids	
IdUA(α, 1 → 3)GalNAc	Dermatan sulfate, heparan sulfate (29)
GlcUA(β, 1 → 3)GlcNAc	Hyaluronic acid (29)
GlcUA(β, 1 → 3)GalNAc	Chondroitin 4/6 sulfates, heparin (29)
GlcUA(β, 1 → 3)Gal	Mucopolysaccharide linkage region (29)

Compiled by Glyn Dawson.

REFERENCES

1. Marcus, *N. Engl. J. Med.*, 280, 944 (1969).
2. Kornfeld, Keller, Baenziger, and Kornfeld, *J. Biol. Chem.*, 246, 3259 (1971).
3. Dawson and Clamp, *Biochem. J.*, 107, 341 (1968).
4. Baenziger, Kochwa, and Kornfeld, *J. Biol. Chem.*, 249, 1897 (1974).
5. Tsay and Dawson, *Biochem. Biophys. Res. Commun.*, 63, 807 (1975).
6. Hakomori, *Chem. Phys. Lipids*, 5, 96 (1970).
7. Watkins, *Science*, 152, 172 (1966).
8. Dawson, in *Sphingolipids, Sphingolipidoses and Allied Disorders*, Aronson and Volk, Eds., Academic Press, New York, 1972, 395.
9. Lloyd, Kabat, and Licerio, *Biochemistry*, 7, 2976 (1968).
10. Wagh, Bornstein, and Winzler, *J. Biol. Chem.*, 244, 658 (1969).
11. Jamieson, Jett, and DeBernado, *J. Biol. Chem.*, 246, 3686 (1971).
12. Wolfe, Senior, and Ng Ying Kin, *J. Biol. Chem.*, 249, 1828 (1974).
13. Tsay and Dawson, *Biochem. Biophys. Res. Commun.*, 52, 759 (1973).
14. Kabasawa and Hirs, *J. Biol. Chem.*, 245, 1610 (1972).
15. Carlson, *J. Biol. Chem.*, 243, 616 (1968).
16. Svennerholm, *J. Lipid Res.*, 5, 145 (1964).
17. Li, Li, and Dawson, *Biochim. Biophys. Acta*, 260, 1163 (1971).
18. Hakomori, Siddiqui, Li, Li, and Hellerquist, *J. Biol. Chem.*, 246, 2271 (1971).
19. Wenger, SubbaRao, and Pieringer, *J. Biol. Chem.*, 245, 2513 (1970).
20. Stoffyn, Stoffyn, and Hauser, *Biochim. Biophys. Acta*, 360, 174 (1974).
21. Laine, Sweeley, Li, Kisic, and Rapport, *J. Lipid Res.*, 13, 519 (1972).
22. Eto, Ichikawa, Ando, and Yamakawa, *J. Biochem.* (Tokyo), 64, 205 (1968).
23. Rodén, in *Chemical and Molecular Basis of the Intracellular Matrix*, Balasz, Ed., Academic Press, London, 1970.
24. Northcote, *Annu. Rev. Biochem.*, 33, 51 (1964).
25. Spiro, *J. Biol. Chem.*, 242, 4813 (1967).
26. Bray, Lieberman, and Meyer, *J. Biol. Chem.*, 242, 3373 (1967).
27. Wiegandt, *Chem. Phys. Lipids*, 5, 198 (1970).
28. Makino and Yamashina, *J. Biochem.* (Tokyo), 60, 262 (1966).
29. Dorfman and Matalon, in *The Metabolic Basis of Inherited Disease*, Stanbury, Wyngaarden, and Fredrickson, Eds., McGraw-Hill, New York, 1972, 1218.
30. Baenziger, Kornfeld, and Kochwa, *J. Biol. Chem.*, 249, 1889 (1974).
31. Siddiqui and Hakomori, *J. Biol. Chem.*, 246, 5766 (1971).
32. Sukeno, Tarentino, Plummer, and Maley, *Biochem. Biophys. Res. Commun.*, 45, 219 (1971).

Table 1 (continued)
STRUCTURE OF DISACCHARIDE UNITS ISOLATED FROM COMPLEX CARBOHYDRATES OF MAMMALIAN ORIGIN

33. Nordén, Lundblad, Svensson, Öckerman, and Autio, *J. Biol. Chem.*, 248, 6210 (1973).
34. Nordén, Lundblad, Svensson, and Autio, *Biochemistry*, 13, 871 (1974).
35. Tsay, Dawson, and Matalon, *J. Pediatr.*, 84, 865 (1974).
36. Clamp, Dawson, and Franklin, *Biochem. J.*, 110, 385 (1968).
37. Spiro, *N. Engl. J. Med.*, 281, 991 (1969).
38. Fukuda and Egami, *Biochem. J.*, 123, 415 (1971).

Table 2
CARBOHYDRATE-AMINO ACID LINKAGES FOUND IN MAMMALIAN GLYCOPROTEINS AND RELATED GLYCOCONJUGATES

Linkage[a]	Source
GlcNAc-Asn	Many glycoproteins (1–15)
GalNAc-Ser/Thr	Typical of mucins (16, 17), blood group substances (18, 4, 5) but also found in IgA myeloma globulin (2) and renal glomerular basement membrane glycoprotein (13)
Gal Ser(sphingosine) Glc	Glycosphingolipids (19–27)
Gal-HyLys	Collagen (28)
Xyl-Ser	Mucopolysaccharides (29)
Gal-Cys	Human urine glycopeptide (30), origin unknown

Compiled by Glyn Dawson.

[a]Abbreviations: GlcNAc, N-acetyl-D-glucosamine; GalNAc, N-acetyl-D-galactos-amine; Gal, D-galactose; Glc, D-glucose; Xyl, D-yxlose.

REFERENCES

1. Kornfeld, Keller, Baenziger, and Kornfeld, *J. Biol. Chem.*, 246, 3256 (1971).
2. Dawson and Clamp, *Biochem. J.*, 107, 341 (1968).
3. Baenziger, Kochwa, and Kornfeld, *J. Biol. Chem.*, 249, 1897 (1974).
4. Watkins, *Science*, 152, 172 (1966).
5. Lloyd, Kabat, and Licerio, *Biochemistry*, 7, 2976 (1968).
6. Wagh, Bornstein, and Winzler, *J. Biol. Chem.*, 244, 658 (1969).
7. Jamieson, Jett, and DeBernado, *J. Biol. Chem.*, 246, 3686 (1971).
8. Kabasawa and Hirs, *J. Biol. Chem.*, 245, 1610 (1972).
9. Makino and Yamashina, *J. Biochem.* (Tokyo), 60, 262 (1966).
10. Baenziger, Kornfeld, and Kochwa, *J. Biol. Chem.*, 249, 1889 (1974).
11. Sukeno, Tarentino, Plummer, and Maley, *Biochem. Biophys. Res. Commun.*, 45, 219 (1971).
12. Clamp, Dawson, and Franklin, *Biochem. J.*, 110, 385 (1968).
13. Spiro, *N. Engl. J. Med.*, 281, 991 (1969).
14. Fukuda and Egami, *Biochem. J.*, 123, 415 (1971).
15. Marshall and Neuberger, *Biochemistry*, 3, 1596 (1964).
16. Carlson, *J. Biol. Chem.*, 243, 616 (1968).
17. Carubelli, Bhavanandan, and Gottschalk, *Biochim. Biophys. Acta*, 101, 67 (1965).

Table 2 (continued)
CARBOHYDRATE-AMINO ACID LINKAGES FOUND IN MAMMALIAN GLYCOPROTEINS AND RELATED GLYCOCONJUGATES

18. Marcus, *N. Engl. J. Med.*, 280, 944 (1969).
19. Hakomori, *Chem. Phys. Lipids*, 5, 96 (1970).
20. Svennerholm, *J. Lipid Res.*, 5, 145 (1964).
21. Li, Li, and Dawson, *Biochim. Biophys. Acta*, 260, 1163 (1971).
22. Hakomori, Siddiqui, Li, Li, and Hellerquist, *J. Biol. Chem.*, 246, 2271 (1971).
23. Wenger, SubbaRao, and Pieringer, *J. Biol. Chem.*, 245, 2513 (1970).
24. Stoffyn, Stoffyn, and Hauser, *Biochim. Biophys. Acta*, 360, 174 (1974).
25. Laine, Sweeley, Li, Kisic, and Rapport, *J. Lipid Res.*, 13, 519 (1972).
26. Eto, Ichikawa, Ando, and Yamakawa, *J. Biochem.* (Tokyo), 64, 205 (1968).
27. Wiegandt, *Chem. Phys. Lipids*, 5, 198 (1970).
28. Spiro, *J. Biol. Chem.*, 242, 4813 (1967).
29. Rodén, in *Chemical and Molecular Basis of the Intracellular Matrix*, Balasz, Ed., Academic Press, London, 1970.
30. Lotte and Weiss, *FEBS Lett.*, 16, 81 (1971).

OLIGOSACCHARIDES (INCLUDING DISACCHARIDES)

Substance[a] (synonym)	Derivative	Chemical formula	Melting point °C	Specific rotation[b] $[\alpha]_D$	Reference
(A)	(B)	(C)	(D)	(E)	(F)
		Disaccharides			
O-6-Deoxy-3-O-methyl-β-D-Allp-(1 → 4)-D-digitoxose (Drebyssobiose)					
	Drebyssobionic acid lactone	$C_{13}H_{24}O_8$	108–110	+25.8	324
		$C_{13}H_{22}O_8$	125–131	+29.6 (c 0.7, CHCl$_3$)	324
O-(4-O-Benzoyl)-D-apiosyl-(1 → 2)-D-glucopyranosyl benzoate					
	Pentaacetate	$C_{25}H_{36}O_{12}$	148–150	−106 (CH$_3$OH)	1,2
		$C_{35}H_{36}O_{17}$	203–204	−35 (CHCl$_3$)	1
O-D-Fruf-(2 → 2)-D-Fruf-anhydride (Alliuminoside)					
	Hexaacetate	$C_{12}H_{20}O_{10}$	92–93	−23.8	3
		$C_{24}H_{32}O_{16}$	98–99	−29.3	3
O-β-D-Fruf-(2 → 1)-D-Fru (Inulobiose)					
	Octaacetate	$C_{12}H_{22}O_{11}$	—	−32.5, −72.4	4, 5
		$C_{28}H_{38}O_{19}$	—	−6.5, −14.2 (CHCl$_3$)	4. 5
O-β-D-Fruf-(2 → 1)-D-Fru		$C_{12}H_{22}O_{11}$	—	−26.3	6

[a] In alphabetical order by the sequence (starting at the nonreducing end) of the component monosaccharide glycosyl units constituting the oligosaccharide arranged within the groups — disaccharides, trisaccharides, etc. The oligosaccharides entered are only those which have been isolated as a naturally existing entity or have been found to derive from the known reaction of a known natural enzyme on a known natural carbohydrate substrate under conditions not foreign to natural biological systems.

[b] $[\alpha]_D$ for 1–5 g solute, c per 100 ml aqueous solution at 20–25°C unless otherwise given.

[c] Crystallizes in one of two forms, depending on solvent used.

OLIGOSACCHARIDES (INCLUDING DISACCHARIDES)

Substance[a] (synonym) (A)	Derivative (B)	Chemical formula (C)	Melting point °C (D)	Specific rotation[b] $[\alpha]_D$ (E)	Reference (F)
Disaccharides (continued)					
O-D-Fruf-(2→6)-D-Fruf (Levanbiose)	Octaacetate	$C_{28}H_{38}O_{19}$	—	+14.2 (CHCl₃)	6
O-D-Fruf-(2→?)-D-Fru (Sogdianose)		$C_{12}H_{22}O_{11}$	—	−20.8 (17°)	322, 323
O-β-D-Fruf-(2→1)-α-D-Glcp (Sucrose)	Octaacetate	$C_{12}H_{22}O_{11}$; $C_{28}H_{38}O_{19}$	156–158 ; 94–95	−16.4 ; −28.7 (CHCl₃)	3 ; 3
O-β-D-Fruf-(2→?)-D-Glc (Ceratose)	Octaacetate	$C_{12}H_{22}O_{11}$; $C_{28}H_{38}O_{19}$	188, 170[c] ; 69, 75[c]	+66.5 ; +59.6 (CHCl₃)	7 ; 8, 9
O-β-D-Fruf-(2→6)-D-Glc		$C_{12}H_{22}O_{11}$	—	+21	10
O-β-Fruf-(2→6)-D-2dGlc		$C_{12}H_{22}O_{11}$	—	+5	11
O-β-D-Galp-(1→4)-D-Allp		$C_{12}H_{22}O_{10}$	s 56, 85	+62 → +26.8	12
O-β-D-Galf-(1→2)-D-arabinitol (Umbilicin)	Octaacetate	$C_{12}H_{22}O_{10}$; $C_{27}H_{38}O_{18}$	112–113 ; 138–139, 84–85	+29 ; −81, −20 (CHCl₃)	13 ; 14, 14
O-β-D-Galp-(1→4)-D-arabinitol		$C_{11}H_{22}O_{10}$	178–181	—	13
O-α-D-Galp-(1→3)-L-Ara	Heptamethyl ether	$C_{11}H_{20}O_{9}$; $C_{18}H_{34}O_{10}$	192–194 ; 89	+80 → +65 ; +164	15, 16 ; 17, 18
O-β-D-Galp-(1→3)-L-Ara		$C_{11}H_{20}O_{10}$	177–178	+30 → +45	13
O-β-D-Galp-(1→4)-L-Arap	Methyl β-glycoside	$C_{11}H_{20}O_{10}$; $C_{11}H_{22}O_{10}$	No constants known ; 216–218	— ; +163	13 ; 13
O-β-D-Galp-(1→5)-L-Araf	Heptamethyl ether	$C_{11}H_{20}O_{10}$; $C_{18}H_{34}O_{10}$	— ; —	−13, −18, +85 ; −36, −45 (CH₃OH)	13, 19, 20 ; 19, 20

OLIGOSACCHARIDES (INCLUDING DISACCHARIDES)

Substance[a] (synonym)	Derivative	Chemical formula	Melting point °C	Specific rotation[b] $[\alpha]_D$	Reference
(A)	(B)	(C)	(D)	(E)	(F)
		Disaccharides (continued)			
O-β-D-Galp-(1 → 2)-D-erythritol		$C_{10}H_{20}O_9$	182–184	+7	13, 21
	Heptaacetate	$C_{24}H_{34}O_{16}$	114	+109 (c 0.6, acetone)	22
O-α-D-Galp-(1 → 2)-D-Fruf		$C_{12}H_{22}O_{11}$	s 170, 179	+81.5	23
O-β-D-Galp-(1 → 2)-D-Fruf		$C_{12}H_{22}O_{11}$	169–170	−33	24
	Octaacetate	$C_{28}H_{38}O_{19}$	—	+41.3 (CHCl$_3$)	25
O-β-D-Galp-(1 → 3)-D-Fucp		$C_{12}H_{22}H_{10}$	245–246	+78	13
O-α-D-Galp-(1 → 3)-D-Galp		$C_{12}H_{22}O_{11}$	157.5–158.5	+161	317
	Octaacetate	$C_{28}H_{38}O_{19}$	151–152,	+110.2 (c 0.5, CHCl$_3$)	318
O-β-D-Galp-(1 → 3)-D-Galp		$C_{12}H_{22}O_{11}$	163–170,	+69 → +55	16
			204–206	+75 → +60	26
				+56	13
O-α-D-Galp-(1 → 4)-D-Galp	O-α-D-Galp-(1 → 4)-D-galactitol	$C_{12}H_{22}O_{11}$	210–211	+172	209, 317
		$C_{12}H_{24}O_{11}$	—	+119	317
O-β-D-Galp-(1 → 4)-D-Galp		$C_{12}H_{22}O_{11}$	195–198	+85 → +67	13
	Octaacetate	$C_{28}H_{38}O_{19}$	172–173	+57.3 (CHCl$_3$)	27
O-α-D-Galp-(1 → 5)-D-Galf		$C_{12}H_{22}O_{11}$	—	+133	317
	O-α-D-Galp-(1 → 5)-D-galactitol	$C_{12}H_{24}O_{11}$	—	+122	317
O-α-D-Galp-(1 → 6)-D-Galp (Swietenose)		$C_{12}H_{22}O_{11}$	—	+149	28, 29
	Octaacetate	$C_{28}H_{38}O_{19}$	223–227	+186 (c 0.5, CHCl$_3$)	29

OLIGOSACCHARIDES (INCLUDING DISACCHARIDES)

Disaccharides (continued)

Substance[a] (synonym) (A)	Derivative (B)	Chemical formula (C)	Melting point °C (D)	Specific rotation[b] $[\alpha]_D$ (E)	Reference (F)
O-β-D-Galp-(1 → 6)-D-Galp		$C_{12}H_{22}O_{11}$	97–100 (·CH$_3$OH)	+26	24, 30
	Octamethyl ether	$C_{20}H_{38}O_{11}$	168–170	+28	31
			68–70	-5.7 (CH$_3$OH)	31
O-β-D-Galp-(1 → 4)-3,6-anhydro-L-Gal (Agarobiose)		$C_{12}H_{20}O_{10}$	—	-21.5 → -16.4	32
	Dimethyl acetal	—	—	+19	33
		$C_{14}H_{24}O_{10}$	163–166	-36 (MeOH)	34
O-D-Galp-(1 → 6)-D-GalNAcp		$C_{14}H_{25}NO_{11}$	—	+142	35
O-α-D-Galp-(1 → 2)-D-Glc		$C_{12}H_{22}O_{11}$	118–120	+145	36
			155d	+161 → +153	37
	Octaacetate	$C_{28}H_{38}O_{19}$	176–178	+153 (CHCl$_3$)	37
O-β-D-Galp-(1 → 2)-D-Glc		$C_{12}H_{22}O_{11} \cdot H_2O$	175d	+48 → +39	38
O-β-D-Galp-(1 → 3)-D-Glc		$C_{12}H_{22}O_{11}$	167–169	+37 (c 0.8)	13
	Monohydrate	$C_{12}H_{22}O_{11} \cdot H_2O$	202–204	+77 → +41	39
	Phenylosazone	$C_{24}H_{34}N_4O_9$	184–185	—	39
	Methyl α-glycoside	$C_{13}H_{24}O_{11}$	148.5–150	+18.3 (c 0.5)	325
O-β-D-Galp-(1 → 4)-α-D-Glcp		$C_{12}H_{22}O_{11} \cdot H_2O$	202	+83.5 → +52.6	40 41
	Octaacetate	$C_{28}H_{38}O_{19}$	152	+53.6 (c 10, CHCl$_3$)	42
O-β-D-Galp-(1 → 4)-β-D-Glcp (Lactose)		$C_{12}H_{22}O_{11}$	252	+34.2 → 53.6	43
	Octaacetate	$C_{28}H_{38}O_{19}$	90	-4.7 (c 10, CHCl$_3$)	42
O-α-D-Galp-(1 → 6)-α-D-Glc		$C_{12}H_{22}O_{11}$	183–184	+166 → 142	44
O-α-D-Galp-(1 → 6)-β-D-Glcp (Melibiose)	Melibiitol	$C_{12}H_{22}O_{11} \cdot 2H_2O$	85–86	+123 → +143	7 44
		$C_{12}H_{24}O_{11}$	173–175	+111	45
	Octaacetate	$C_{28}H_{38}O_{19}$	177	+102.5	46

OLIGOSACCHARIDES (INCLUDING DISACCHARIDES)

Substance[a] (synonym) (A)	Derivative (B)	Chemical formula (C)	Melting point °C (D)	Specific rotation[b] $[\alpha]_D$ (E)	Reference (F)
		Disaccharides (continued)			
O-β-D-Galp-(1 → 6)-D-Glcp (Allolactose, Lactobiose)		$C_{12}H_{22}O_{11}$	165, 174–176	+25 → +37.5	27, 47–49
	Octaacetate	$C_{28}H_{38}O_{19}$	165	-0.5 (CHCl$_3$)	50
O-D-Gal-(? → ?)-D-Glc		$C_{12}H_{22}O_{11}$	205	-27	49
O-β-D-Galp-(1 → 3)-D-6d-Glcp		$C_{12}H_{22}O_{10}$	246–248	+25	13
O-β-D-Galp-(1 → 3)-D-GlcNAc (Lacto-N-biose I)		$C_{14}H_{25}NO_{11}$	166–167	+32 → +14	51, 52
O-β-D-Galp-(1 → 4)-D-GlcNAcp (Lactosamine, N-acetyl)		$C_{14}H_{25}NO_{11}$	No constants known	+51.2 → +27.8	53
	Monomethanolate	$C_{14}H_{25}NO_{11} \cdot CH_3OH$	172	—	53
	Heptaacetate	$C_{28}H_{39}NO_{18}$	222–223	+61.5 (30°) (CHCl$_3$)	53
	Methyl β-glycoside	$C_{15}H_{27}NO_{11}$	243–245d	-23.1	54
O-α-D-Galp-(1 → 6)-D-GlcNAcp		$C_{14}H_{25}NO_{11}$	138d	+118	35, 317
	Heptaacetate	$C_{28}H_{39}NO_{18}$	141–142	+50.2 (CHCl$_3$)	317
O-β-D-Galp-(1 → 6)-D-GlcNAcp		$C_{14}H_{25}NO_{11}$	157–159	+32.1 → +27.3	51, 53
O-α-D-Galp-(1 → 1)-glycerol		$C_9H_{18}O_8$	150–152	+155	55
O-β-D-Galp-(1 → 1)-glycerol		$C_9H_{18}O_8$	139–140	+3.8, -7, -73	55–57
	Hexabenzoate	$C_{51}H_{42}O_{14}$	133–134	-6 (CHCl$_3$)	57
O-α-D-Galp-(1 → 2)-glycerol (Floridoside)		$C_9H_{18}O_8$	86–87, 129–130	+151, +163	22, 58, 59
	Hexaacetate	$C_{21}H_{30}O_{14}$	101	+114 (acetone)	60
O-α-D-Galp-(1 → 1)-myo-inositol (Galactinol)		$C_{12}H_{22}O_{11} \cdot 2H_2O$	220–222	+135.6	61
	Nonamethyl ether	$C_{21}H_{40}O_{11}$	96.5–98	+119	62

OLIGOSACCHARIDES (INCLUDING DISACCHARIDES)

Substance[a] (synonym) (A)	Derivative (B)	Chemical formula (C)	Melting point °C (D)	Specific rotation[b] $[\alpha]_D$ (E)	Reference (F)
		Disaccharides (continued)			
O-β-D-Galp-(1 → 5)-myo-Inositol		$C_{12}H_{22}O_{11}$	248–252	0	63
O-β-D-Galp-(1 → 3)-D-mannitol (Peltigeroside)		$C_{12}H_{24}O_{11}$	161–163	−55.5 .–61	64. 65
O-D-Galp-(1 → ?)-D-Man	Methyl glycoside	$C_{12}H_{22}O_{11}$ $C_{13}H_{24}O_{11}$	No constants given 168–170	+51 (c 0.7) —	13 13
O-β-D-Galp-(1 → 3)-α-L-Rha		$C_{12}H_{22}O_{10}$	200–202	+2 → +15	15
O-β-D-Galp-(1 → 3)-D-Rib		$C_{11}H_{20}O_{10}$	No constants given	—	13
O-β-D-Galp-(1 → 5)-D-Rib		$C_{11}H_{20}O_{10}$	No constants given	—	13
O β-D-Galp (1 → 2)-D-Xyl		$C_{11}H_{20}O_{10}$ $C_{18}H_{34}O_{10}$	159–160 —	+25 −5.9 (CH₃OH)	13 66
O-β-D-Galp-(1 → 3)-D-Xyl	Heptamethyl ether	$C_{11}H_{20}O_{10}$	196–200	+27 → +10	13
O-3,6-anhydro-α-D-Galp-(1 → 3)-D-Galp 4-sulfate		$C_{12}H_{20}O_{13}S$	No constants known	—	326
O-3,6-anhydro-L-Galp-(1 → 3)-D-Gal (Neoagarobiose)	Hexaacetate	$C_{12}H_{20}O_{10}$ $C_{24}H_{32}O_{16}$	207–208 112	+34.4 → +20.3 +1.6 (27°) (CHCl₃)	67 67
O-α-D-GalUAp-(1 → 4)-D-GalUA (Digalacturonic acid)	Methyl α-glycoside dimethyl ester	$C_{12}H_{18}O_{13}$ $C_{15}H_{24}O_{13}$	125–135d 120–122	+154 +162.6	68, 69 70
O-4,5-anhydro-α-D-GalUAp-(1 → 4)-D-GalUA		$C_{12}H_{16}O_{12}$	—	+177.8	71

OLIGOSACCHARIDES (INCLUDING DISACCHARIDES)

Substance[a] (synonym) (A)	Derivative (B)	Chemical formula (C)	Melting point °C (D)	Specific rotation[b] $[\alpha]_D$ (E)	Reference (F)
O-β-D-Glcp-(1 → 3)-L-Ara		$C_{11}H_{20}O_{10}$	199–201	+70	13
O-β-D-Glcp-(1 → 4)-D-Ara		$C_{11}H_{20}O_{10}$	135	-104	327
	Heptaacetate	$C_{25}H_{34}O_{17}$	214	-62 (CHCl₃)	327
O-α-D-Glcp-(1 → 1)-D-Fruf		$C_{12}H_{22}O_{11}$	—	+49	72
O-α-D-Glcp-(1 → 3)-D-Fru (Turanose)		$C_{12}H_{22}O_{11}$	157	+22 → +75.3	45, 73
	Octaacetate I	$C_{28}H_{38}O_{19}$	216–217	+20.5 (CHCl₃)	74
	Octaacetate II	$C_{28}H_{38}O_{19}$	158	+107 (CHCl₃)	74
O-α-D-Glcp-(1 → 4)-D-Fru (Maltulose)		$C_{12}H_{22}O_{11}$	113–115d	+58 → +64	75
O-α-D-Glcp-(1 → 5)-D-Fru (Leucrose)		$C_{12}H_{22}O_{11}$	161–163	-8.8 → -6.8	76
	Heptaacetate	$C_{24}H_{36}O_{18}$	150–151	—	76
O-α-D-Glcp-(1 → 6)-D-	Phenylosazone	$C_{24}H_{34}N_4O_9$	186–188	—	77
Fruf (Palatinose, Isomaltulose)		$C_{12}H_{22}O_{11}$	173–175	+97.2	72, 78
	Phenylosazone	$C_{24}H_{34}N_4O_9$	—	—	72, 77
O-α-D-Glcp-(1 → 3)-D-Fuc		$C_{12}H_{22}O_{10}$	250–252	+45	13
O-α-D-Glcp-(1→1)-D-Galf		$C_{12}H_{22}O_{11}$	No constants given	—	79
O-β-D-Glcp-(1 → 6)-D-Gal	Octaacetate	$C_{12}H_{22}O_{11}$ / $C_{28}H_{38}O_{19}$	128–130 / —	+15 ±1 / +1 (CHCl₃)	80, 328 / 81
O-α-Glcp-(1 → 1)-α-D-Glcp (α,α-Trehalose)		$C_{12}H_{22}O_{11}$	214–216	+199	7, 82
	Dihydrate	$C_{12}H_{22}O_{11}$·2H₂O	94–100	+180	82
	Octaacetate	$C_{28}H_{38}O_{19}$	98	+162.3 (c 10) (CHCl₃)	8
O-β-D-Glcp-(1 → 1)-β-D-Glcp (β,β-Trehalose)		$C_{12}H_{22}O_{11}$	130–135	-41.5	83, 84
	Octaacetate	$C_{28}H_{38}O_{19}$	181	-19 (CHCl₃)	85

OLIGOSACCHARIDES (INCLUDING DISACCHARIDES)

Substance[a] (synonym) (A)	Derivative (B)	Chemical formula (C)	Melting point °C (D)	Specific rotation[b] $[\alpha]_D$ (E)	Reference (F)
		Disaccharides (continued)			
O-α-D-Glcp-(1 → 1)-β-D-Glcp		$C_{12}H_{22}O_{11}$	80d, 150–153	+70 (c 0.2)	84, 86
	Octaacetate	$C_{28}H_{38}O_{19}$	120, 140	+67, +82 (CHCl$_3$)	84–86
O-α-D-Glcp-(1 → 2)-D-Glc (Kojibiose)		$C_{12}H_{22}O_{11}$	175	+135	87,88
	α-Octaacetate	$C_{28}H_{38}O_{19}$	166	+153 (CHCl$_3$)	89
	β-Octaacetate	$C_{28}H_{38}O_{19}$	118	+112 (CHCl$_3$)	90
O-β-D-Glcp-(1 → 2)-D-Glc (Sophorose)		$C_{12}H_{22}O_{11}$	195–196	+20	83, 91, 92
	β-Octaacetate	$C_{28}H_{38}O_{19}$	191–192	–8 (CHCl$_3$)	91–93
	α-Octaacetate	$C_{28}H_{38}O_{19}$	111	+45 (CHCl$_3$)	94
O-α-D-Glcp-(1 → 3)-D-Glc (Nigerose, Sakebiose)		$C_{12}H_{22}O_{11}$	151–153	+135, +145	89, 95, 96
	Octaacetate	$C_{28}H_{38}O_{19}$	—	+80 (CHCl$_3$)	97
O-β-D-Glcp-(1 → 3)-α-D-Glc (α-Laminaribiose)		$C_{12}H_{22}O_{11}$	202–205	+25.5 → +17.5	98
	α-Octaacetate ethanolate	$C_{28}H_{38}O_{19}\cdot C_2H_5OH$	77–78	+20 (CHCl$_3$)	99
O-β-D-Glcp-(1 → 3)-β-D-Glc (β-Laminaribiose)		$C_{12}H_{22}O_{11}$	188–192	+7.5 → +20.8	100
	β-Octaacetate	$C_{28}H_{38}O_{19}$	160–161	–28.6 (17°) (CHCl$_3$)	101
O-β-D-Glcp-(1 → 4)-β-D-Glcp (β-Cellobiose)		$C_{12}H_{22}O_{11}$	225	+14.2 → +34.6 (c 8)	83, 102
	β-Octaacetate	$C_{28}H_{38}O_{19}$	202	–14.7 (CHCl$_3$)	42
	α-Octaacetate	$C_{28}H_{38}O_{19}$	229	+41.0 (CHCl$_3$)	42
O-α-D-Glcp-(1 → 4)-α-D-Glcp (α-Maltose)		$C_{12}H_{22}O_{11}$	108	+173	103, 104
	α-Octaacetate	$C_{28}H_{38}O_{19}$	125	+123 (CHCl$_3$)	42
O-α-D-Glcp-(1 → 4)-β-D-Glcp (β-Maltose)	Monohydrate	$C_{12}H_{22}O_{11}\cdot H_2O$	102–103	+112 → +130	103, 104
	β-Octaacetate	$C_{28}H_{38}O_{19}$	159–160	+62.6 (CHCl$_3$)	42

OLIGOSACCHARIDES (INCLUDING DISACCHARIDES)

Substance[a] (synonym) (A)	Derivative (B)	Chemical formula (C)	Melting point °C (D)	Specific rotation[b] $[\alpha]_D$ (E)	Reference (F)
		Disaccharides (continued)			
O-α-D-Glcp-(1 → 6)-Glcp (Isomaltose)	β-Octaacetate α-Octaacetate	$C_{12}H_{22}O_{11}$ $C_{28}H_{38}O_{19}$	Amorph 144–145	+103.2, +122 +96.9 (CHCl$_3$)	105, 106 105
O-β-D-Glcp-(1 → 6)-α-D-Glcp (α-Gentiobiose)	Dimethanolate	$C_{12}H_{22}O_{11}\cdot2CH_3OH$ $C_{28}H_{38}O_{19}$	85–86 189	+31 → +9.6 +52.4 (CHCl$_3$)	7 107, 108
O-β-D-Glcp-(1 → 6)-β-D-Glcp (β-Gentiobiose)	β-Octaacetate	$C_{12}H_{22}O_{11}$ $C_{28}H_{38}O_{19}$	190 193	–3 → +10.5 –5.4 (c 6, CHCl$_3$)	83, 109 107, 108
O-D-Glcp-(1 → 4)-D-2d-Glcp		$C_{12}H_{22}O_{10}$	204–205	+23, +123	110, 327
O-D-Glcp-(1 → ?)-3-O-methyl-D-6d-Glcp (Kondurangobiose)	Hexaacetate	$C_{13}H_{24}O_{10}$ $C_{25}H_{36}O_{16}$	202–204d 188	+20	111 112
O-D-Glcp-(1 → ?)-3-O-methyl-D-6d-Glcp (Thevetobioside)	Hexaacetate	$C_{13}H_{24}O_{10}$ $C_{25}H_{36}O_{16}$	233 168–170	–64.4 (CH$_3$OH) –70 (18°) (CHCl$_3$)	113 113
O-α-D-Glcp-(1 → 1)-α-D-GlcNp (Trehalosamine)	Hydrochloride N-Acetyl heptaacetate	$C_{13}H_{25}NO_{10}\cdot HCl$ $C_{28}H_{39}NO_{18}$	197d 100–102	+176 (c 0.02) +152 (CHCl$_3$)	114, 330 114, 330
O-D-Glcp-(1 → 4)-D-GlcNp	N-Acetyl derivative	$C_{12}H_{23}NO_{10}$ $C_{14}H_{25}NO_{11}$	180–185d 144.5–146	+147, +100 → +81 +85 → +39	110, 115 115
O-β-D-Glcp-(1 → 4)-D-GlcNAcp		$C_{14}H_{25}NO_{11}$	160	+23	327
O-D-Glcp(1 → 2)-D-GlcUA		$C_{12}H_{20}O_{12}$		+89	116

OLIGOSACCHARIDES (INCLUDING DISACCHARIDES)

Disaccharides (continued)

Substance[a] (synonym) (A)	Derivative (B)	Chemical formula (C)	Melting point °C (D)	Specific rotation[b] $[\alpha]_D$ (E)	Reference (F)
O-α-D-Glcp-(1 → 1)-glycerol		$C_9H_{18}O_8$	—	+128 (27°) (c 0.7)	117
	Hexaacetate	$C_{21}H_{30}O_{14}$	92	+110 (27°) (acetone)	117
O-β-D-Glcp-(1 → 1)-glycerol		$C_9H_{18}O_8$	—	+12, −32 (c 0.5)	118, 331
	Hexa-p-nitrobenzoate	$C_{21}H_{36}N_6O_{20}$	105–108	−4.4 ± 1 (c 0.4, CHCl$_3$)	119
	Hexaacetate	$C_{21}H_{30}O_{14}$	144	—	331
O-D-Glcp-(1 → 1)-myo-inositol		$C_{12}H_{22}O_{11}$	256–260	−17.5	63
	Nonamethyl ether	$C_{21}H_{40}O_{11}$	95–98	−10 (C$_2$H$_5$OH)	63
O-D-Glcp-(1 → 5)-myo-inositol		$C_{12}H_{22}O_{11}$	158–162	−20	63
O-β-D-Glcp-(1 → 1)-mannitol		$C_{12}H_{24}O_{11}$	140–141	−18	120
	Nonabenzoate	$C_{57}H_{46}O_{20}$	88–94	+39.7 (18°) (CHCl$_3$)	101
O-β-D-Glcp-(1 → 3)-mannitol		$C_{12}H_{24}O_{11}$	97–100	−6	121
O-β-D-Glcp-(1 → 4)-D-Manp		$C_{12}H_{22}O_{11}$	179–182	+6	122
	Monohydrate	$C_{12}H_{22}O_{11}\cdot H_2O$	133–135	+5.5	123
	Octaacetate	$C_{28}H_{38}O_{19}$	201	+34 (CHCl$_3$)	124
O-D-Glc-(1 → 2)-L-Rha (Bryobioside)		$C_{12}H_{22}O_{10}$	175, 188–190	+61.5, +66.1	125, 126
	Heptaacetate	$C_{26}H_{36}O_{17}$	127	+67.2 (CHCl$_3$)	126
O-α-D-Glcp-(1 → 1)-L-Sor		$C_{12}H_{22}O_{11}$	178–180	+33	127
	Octaacetate	$C_{28}H_{38}O_{18}$	—	+38 (CHCl$_3$)	127
O-α-D-Glcp-(1 → 2)-β-D-threo-pentuloside (Gluco-xyluloside)		$C_{11}H_{40}O_{10}$	156–157	+43	128
	Heptaacetate	$C_{23}H_{44}O_{17}$	180–181	+22 (CHCl$_3$)	128

OLIGOSACCHARIDES (INCLUDING DISACCHARIDES)

Disaccharides (continued)

Substance[a] (synonym) (A)	Derivative (B)	Chemical formula (C)	Melting point °C (D)	Specific rotation[b] $[\alpha]_D$ (E)	Reference (F)
O-β-D-Glcp-(1 → 2)-D-Xyl	Phenylosazone	$C_{11}H_{20}O_{10}$ / $C_{23}H_{32}N_4O_8$	202–206 / 213–215	+7 / —	13 / 129
O-α-D-Glcp-(1 → 3)-D-Xyl		$C_{11}H_{20}O_{10}$	—	+87.5	130
O-β-D-Glcp-(1 → 3)-D-Xyl	Phenylosazone	$C_{11}H_{20}O_{10}$ / $C_{23}H_{32}N_4O_8$	120 / 204–206	-6.4	129, 336 / 332
O-α-D-Glcp-(1 → 4)-D-Xyl	Dihydrate	$C_{11}H_{20}O_{10} \cdot 2H_2O$	78, s 58	+97.5	131
O-β-D-Glcp-(1 → 4)-D-Xyl (Securidabiose)	Heptaacetate	$C_{11}H_{20}O_{10}$ / $C_{25}H_{34}O_{17}$	154–157	-7, -27.3 / -18.2 (CHCl₃)	327, 329, 333 / 333
O-3-O-methyl-D-Glcp-(1 → 4)-D-Glc		$C_{13}H_{24}O_{11}$	No constants known	—	334
O-β-D-GlcNAcp-(1 → 3)-D-Gal (Lacto-N-biose II)	Heptaacetate	$C_{14}H_{25}NO_{11}$ / $C_{28}H_{39}NO_{18}$	131–133 / 212–213	+45.5 → +35.7 / +79.5	132 / 335
O-α-D-GlcNAcp-(1 → 6)-D-Galp		$C_{14}H_{25}NO_{11}$	—	+125.6 (c 0.2)	133
O-β-D-GlcNAcp-(1 → 6)-D-Galp	Heptaacetate	$C_{14}H_{25}NO_{11}$ / $C_{28}H_{39}NO_{18}$	197–198	+9.2 / +6.3 (CHCl₃)	132, 133 / 134
O-β-D-GlcNAcp-(1 → 4)-3-O-(D-1-carboxyethyl)-D-GlcNAc	Pentaacetate methyl ester	$C_{19}H_{32}N_2O_{13}$ / $C_{30}H_{44}N_2O_{18}$	235–236	+10 → +4.5 / +40 (c 0.2, CHCl₃)	135 / 135
O-β-D-GlcNAcp-(1 → 4)-6-O-acetyl-3-O-(D-1-carboxyethyl)-D-GlcNAc		$C_{21}H_{34}N_2O_{14}$	—	+23.5	136

OLIGOSACCHARIDES (INCLUDING DISACCHARIDES)

Disaccharides (continued)

Substance[a] (synonym) (A)	Derivative (B)	Chemical formula (C)	Melting point °C (D)	Specific rotation[b] $[\alpha]_D$ (E)	Reference (F)
O-β-D-GlcNAc*p*-(1 → 6)-3-*O*-(D-1-carboxyethyl)-D-GlcNAc	Pentaacetate methyl ester Methyl α-glycoside	$C_{19}H_{33}N_2O_{13}$ $C_{30}H_{44}N_2O_{18}$	240–241 —	+16 → +14 +40 (c 0.4, CHCl$_3$)	135 135
O-β-D-GlcNAc*p*-(1 → 4)-α-D-GlcNAc*p* (*N,N'*-Diacetyl-chitobiose)	methyl ester tetraacetate	$C_{23}H_{44}N_2O_{17}$	288–289	+54 (CHCl$_3$)	137
	Hexaacetate	$C_{16}H_{28}N_2O_{11}$ $C_{28}H_{40}N_2O_{17}$	260–262d 308–309d	+16.6 +55 (18°) (c 0.5, CH$_3$COOH)	138 139
O-D-GlcNAc-(1 → 4)-D-GlcUA		$C_{14}H_{23}NO_{12}$	—	+106	140, 141
O-3-*O*-(D-1-carboxyethyl)-β-D-GlcNAc*p*-(1 → 4)-D-GlcNAc*p* (*N*-acetyl-muramyl-D-glucose)		$C_{19}H_{32}N_2O_{13}$	—	+12.4 (c 0.5)	142
O-6-*O*-acetyl-3-*O*-(D-1-carboxyethyl)-β-D-GlcNAc*p*-(1 → 4)-D-GlcNAc*p*		$C_{21}H_{34}N_2O_{14}$	—	+15.4 (c 0.5)	142
O-β-D-GlcUA*p*-(1 → 3)-D-GalNac (*N*-acetyl-chondrosine)	Heptaacetate Methyl ester hydrochloride	$C_{14}H_{23}NO_{12}$ $C_{28}H_{37}NO_{19}$ $C_{13}H_{23}NO_{11}$ ·HCl	221–222 — 155–156	+35 −2.1 (CHCl$_3$) +39 (CH$_3$OH)	143, 144 144 145
O-β-D-GlcUA*p*-(1 → 3)-D-GalNAc 6-sulfate	Barium salt	$BaC_{14}H_{22}NO_{15}S$	—	−4.4 (c 0.2)	143, 337

OLIGOSACCHARIDES (INCLUDING DISACCHARIDES)

Substance[a] (synonym) (A)	Derivative (B)	Chemical formula (C)	Melting point °C (D)	Specific rotation[b] $[\alpha]_D$ (E)	Reference (F)
		Disaccharides (continued)			
O-β-D-GlcUAp-(1 → 3)-D-GlcNAc (N-acetyl hyalobiuronic acid)	Methyl α-glycoside methyl ester pentaacetate	$C_{14}H_{13}NO_{12}$	—	−32 (28°)	146
O-4,5-dideoxy-β-L-threo-hex-4-enopyrano-syluronic acid-(1 → 3)-D-GlcNAc		$C_{26}H_{37}NO_{17}$	236–238	+30 (c 0.7, CHCl₃)	147
O-2,6-diamino-2,6-dideoxy-D-arabino-hexopyranosyl-(1 → 2)-deoxystreptamine (Neamine, Neomycin A)	Pentaacetate	$C_{14}H_{11}NO_{11}$ $C_{24}H_{31}NO_{16}$	190–192	−20 —	148 148
O-[2-amino-4-[[(1-carboxyformimidoyl)-amino]-2,3,4,6-tetra-deoxy-D-hexopyranosyl]-(1 → 2)-D-(+)-inositol (Kasugamycin)	Hydrochloride N-Salicylidene derivative	$C_{12}H_{26}N_4O_6$ $C_{12}H_{26}N_4O_6\cdot 4HCl$ $C_{40}H_{?1}N_4O_{10}$	256d 233d 198–201	+123 (c 0.5) +82 —	149 150, 338 151
O-α-D-ribo-he:o-pyranosyl-3-ulose-(1 → 2)-β-D-Fruf-(3-Keto-sucrose)		$C_{14}H_5N_5O_{10}$	206–210d	+125	152
O-α-D-ribo-hexo-pyranosyl-3-ulose-(1 → 1)-α-D-Glcp (3-Keto-trehalose)	Trihydrate	$C_{12}H_{20}O_{11}\cdot 3H_2O$ $C_{12}H_{20}O_{11}$	82–83 114	+40 (c 7.5) +151.1	153 154

OLIGOSACCHARIDES (INCLUDING DISACCHARIDES)

Substance[a] (synonym)	Derivative	Chemical formula	Melting point °C	Specific rotation[b] $[\alpha]_D$	Reference
(A)	(B)	(C)	(D)	(E)	(F)
		Disaccharides (continued)			
O-α-D-ribo-hexo-pyranosyl-3-ulose-(1→4)-D-Glcp (3-Keto-maltose)		$C_{12}H_{20}O_{11}$	107	+87.2	154
O-β-D-ribo-hexo-pyranosyl-3-ulose-(1→4)-D-Glcp (3-Keto-cellobiose)		$C_{12}H_{20}O_{11}$	135	+19.9	339
O-β-D-xylo-hexo-pyranosyl-3-ulose-(1→4)-D-Glcp (3-Keto-lactose)		$C_{12}H_{20}O_{11}$	118–120	+39.2	154
O-β-D-Manp-(1→4)-meso-erythritol		$C_{10}H_{20}O_9$	160–162	−38	155, 156
O-D-Manp-(1→1)-D-GlcNp	Hydrochloride N-Acetyl octaacetate	$C_{12}H_{23}NO_{10}$ $C_{12}H_{23}NO_{10} \cdot HCl$ $C_{28}H_{39}NO_{18}$	No constants known b 230 91.5–93	— +91.3 +250 (CHCl$_3$)	340 340 340
O-β-D-Manp-(1→4)-α-D-Glcp	Octaacetate	$C_{12}H_{22}O_{11}$ $C_{28}H_{38}O_{19}$	210–212 162–168	— +12, +18	123, 157 158
O-α-D-Manp-(1→?)-glyceric acid	Sodium salt	$C_9H_{16}O_9$ $C_9H_{15}O_9Na$	88–89 270d	— +105 (15°)	159 159
O-β-D-Manp-(1→4)-α-D-Manp	Octamethyl ether	$C_{12}H_{22}O_{11}$ $C_{20}H_{38}O_{11}$	204 —	−5 → −8 −12 (CHCl$_3$)	160 161
O-β-D-Manp-(1→4)-β-D-Manp	Monohydrate	$C_{12}H_{22}O_{11}$ $C_{12}H_{22}O_{11} \cdot H_2O$	193–194 122–124	— −7.7 → −2.2	162 123
O-4,5-anhydro-β-D-ManUAp-(1→4)-D-ManUA		$C_{12}H_{16}O_{12}$	135–136.5d	−8	163

OLIGOSACCHARIDES (INCLUDING DISACCHARIDES)

Substance[a] (synonym) (A)	Derivative (B)	Chemical formula (C)	Melting point °C (D)	Specific rotation[b] $[\alpha]_D$ (E)	Reference (F)
Disaccharides (continued)					
O-β-L-Rhap-(1 → 6)-D-Galp (Robinobiose)		$C_{12}H_{22}O_{10}$	Amorph	+2.70	164
	Heptaacetate	$C_{26}H_{36}O_{17}$	113	−9.9, −19.2 (CHCl$_3$)	165
O-β-L-Rhap-(1 → 6)-D-Glcp (Rutinose)		$C_{12}H_{22}O_{10}$	189−192d, Amorph	+3.2 → −0.8	166, 167
	Heptaacetate	$C_{26}H_{36}O_{17}$	168−169	−29.7 (CHCl$_3$)	168
O-α-D-Xylp-(1 → 2)-β-D-Fruf		$C_{11}H_{20}O_{10}$	−	+62	169
O-D-Xylp-(1 → 1)-D-Glcp dibenzoate		$C_{25}H_{28}O_{12}$	147−148	−106.7 (CH$_3$OH)	1, 2, 170
	Pentaacetate	$C_{35}H_{36}O_{17}$	203	−	1, 170
O-D-Xylp-(1 → 4)-D-Glcp		$C_{11}H_{20}O_{10}$	−	+70	123, 171
O-α-D-Xylp-(1 → 6)-D-Glc		$C_{11}H_{20}O_{10}$	−	+122	341
O-β-D-Xylp-(1 → 6)-D-Glc (Primeverose)		$C_{11}H_{20}O_{10}$	208	+24.1 → −3.3	10, 66, 172
	Heptaacetate	$C_{25}H_{34}O_{17}$	216	−23.5 (CHCl$_3$)	172
O-β-D-Xylp-(1 → 3)-D-Xyl (Rhodymenabiose)		$C_{10}H_{18}O_9$	192−193	−35 → −22	173, 174
O-β-D-Xylp-(1 → 4)-D-Xylp (Xylobiose)		$C_{10}H_{18}O_9$	195−197	−40 → −27	173, 175
	Hexaacetate	$C_{22}H_{30}O_{15}$	155−156	−75 (c 10, CHCl$_3$)	176
Trisaccharides					
O-L-Araf-(1 → 3)-O-D-Xylp-(1 → 4)-D-Xylp		$C_{16}H_{28}O_{13}$	−	−19.3	177
	Octamethyl ether	$C_{23}H_{42}O_{13}$	−	−13.3 (CH$_3$OH)	177, 178
O-D-Fruf-(2 → 1)-O-D-Fruf-(2 → 1)-D-Fru (Inulotriose)		$C_{18}H_{32}O_{16}$	−	No constants known	179

OLIGOSACCHARIDES (INCLUDING DISACCHARIDES)

Trisaccharides (continued)

Substance[a] (synonym) (A)	Derivative (B)	Chemical formula (C)	Melting point °C (D)	Specific rotation[b] $[\alpha]_D$ (E)	Reference (F)
O-D-Fruf-(2 → ?)-O-D-Fruf-(2 → 2)-D-Fruf-anhydride (Polygontin)	Nonaacetate	$C_{18}H_{30}O_{15}$ $C_{36}H_{48}O_{24}$	207–208 84–85	−52.9 −38.4 (CHCl$_3$)	3 3
O-D-Fruf-(2 → ?)-O-D-Fruf-(2 → 2)-D-Fruf (Trifructan)	Decaacetate	$C_{18}H_{32}O_{16}$ $C_{38}H_{52}O_{26}$	— —	−22.3 +8.5	6 6
O-D-Fruf-(2 → ?)-O-D-Fruf-(2 → 1)-DFru		$C_{18}H_{32}O_{16}$	—	−10.2	180
O-D-Fruf-(2 → ?)-O-D-Fruf-(2 → ?)-D-Gal (Labiose)	Hendecaacetate	$C_{18}H_{32}O_{16}$ $C_{40}H_{54}O_{27}$	s 126–128, 205d 88	+136.7 +122.5 (CHCl$_3$)	181 181
O-D-Fruf-(2 → 1)-O-D-Fruf-(2 → 1)-D-Glcp		$C_{18}H_{32}O_{16}$	193	+28, +33	11, 182–184
O-D-Fruf-(2 → 6)-O-D-Fruf-(2 → 1)-D-Glcp		$C_{18}H_{32}O_{16}$	143	+22	11, 185, 342
O-β-D-Fruf-(2 → 6)-O-α-D-Glcp-(1 → 2)-β-D-Fruf (Neokestose)	Hendecamethyl ether	$C_{18}H_{32}O_{16}$ $C_{29}H_{50}O_{16}$	— —	+15, +22.2 −28 (c 10)	185–187 187
O-α-D-Fucp-(1 → 2)-O-β-D-Galp-(1 → 4)-D-Galp (Fucisido-lactose)	p-Tolylsulfonyl-hydrazone	$C_{18}H_{32}O_{15}$ $C_{25}H_{40}N_2O_{17}S$	230–231d 205–206	−53.5 → −57.5 (c 0.2) −73 (C$_5$H$_5$N:H$_2$O)	51 51
O-α-D-Galp-(1 → 1)-O-β-D-Fruf-(2 → 1)-D-Glcp		$C_{18}H_{32}O_{16}$	—	+131	188
O-α-D-Galp-(1 → 3)-O-β-D-Fruf-(2 → 1)-D-Glcp		$C_{18}H_{32}O_{16}$	—	+98	188

OLIGOSACCHARIDES (INCLUDING DISACCHARIDES)

Substance[a] (synonym) (A)	Derivative (B)	Chemical formula (C)	Melting point °C (D)	Specific rotation[b] $[\alpha]_D$ (E)	Reference (F)
Trisaccharides (continued)					
O-β-D-Galp-(1 → 4)-O-β-D-Fruf-(2 → 1)-D-Glcp		$C_{18}H_{32}O_{16}$	—	+44.1	189
O-α-D-Galp-(1 → 6)-O-β-D-Fruf-(2 → 1)-D-Glcp (Planteose)	Dihydrate Hendecaacetate	$C_{18}H_{32}O_{16} \cdot 2H_2O$ $C_{40}H_{54}O_{27}$	123–124 135	+125.2 +97 (CHCl₃)	190 190
O-β-D-Galp-(1 → 3)-O-[α-L-Fucp-(1 → 4)]-D-GlcNAcp		$C_{20}H_{35}NO_{15}$	—	−44 ± 3 (c 0.3)	191
O-β-D-Galp-(1 → 6)-O-β-D-Galp-(1 → ?)-D-Fru		$C_{18}H_{32}O_{16}$	—	−28	24
O-D-Galp-(1 → ?)-O-D-Galp-(1 → ?)-D-Glc (Lactotriose)	Hendecaacetate	$C_{18}H_{32}O_{16}$ $C_{40}H_{54}O_{27}$	No constants known 120–122	— —	192 192
O-β-D-Galp-(1 → 3)-O-β-D-Galp-(1 → 4)-α-D-Glcp	Trihydrate Hendecaacetate	$C_{18}H_{32}O_{16} \cdot 3H_2O$ $C_{40}H_{54}O_{27}$	197–200 108–110	+56 → +43 +17.2 (c 0.6, CHCl₃)	15, 24 343
O-β-D-Galp-(1 → 4)-O-β-D-Galp-(1 → 4)-D-Glcp		$C_{18}H_{32}O_{16}$	228–231	+68 → +45	13
O-β-D-Galp-(1 → 6)-O-β-D-Gal-(1 → 4)-D-Glcp	Dihydrate	$C_{18}H_{32}O_{16} \cdot 2H_2O$	187, s 167	+34	24, 193
O-α-D-Galp-(1 → 6)-O-α-D-Galp-(1 → 6)-D-Glc (Manninotriose)	Hendecaacetate	$C_{18}H_{32}O_{16}$ $C_{40}H_{54}O_{27}$	Amorph 150 s 105	+167 +135 (C₂H₅OH)	194 194

OLIGOSACCHARIDES (INCLUDING DISACCHARIDES)

Trisaccharides (continued)

Substance[a] (synonym) (A)	Derivative (B)	Chemical formula (C)	Melting point °C (D)	Specific rotation[b] $[\alpha]_D$ (E)	Reference (F)
O-β-D-Galp-(1 → 6)-O-β-D-Galp-(1 → 6)-D-Glc		$C_{18}H_{32}O_{16}$	No constants known	—	195
O-α-D-Galp-(1 → 6)-O-β-D-Galp-(1 → 1)-glycerol		$C_{15}H_{28}O_{13}$	188–189	—	196
		—	196–198	+90	55
	Nonamethyl ether	$C_{24}H_{44}O_{13}$	Oil	+65 ($CHCl_3$)	344
O-D-Galp-(1 → 6)-O-D-Galp-(1 → 1)-*myo*-inositol		$C_{18}H_{32}O_{16}$	—	+145.1	197
O-α-D-Galp-(1 → 2)-O-α-D-Glcp-(1 → 2)-β-D-Fruf (Umbelliferose)		$C_{18}H_{32}O_{16}$	—	+125	198
O-α-Galp-(1 → 3)-O-α-D-Glcp-(1 → 2)-β-D-Fruf		$C_{18}H_{32}O_{16}$	No constants given	—	199
O-β-D-Galp-(1 → 4)-O-α-D-Glcp-(1 → 2)-β-D-Fruf (Lactsucrose)	Pentahydrate	$C_{18}H_{32}O_{16}\cdot 5H_2O$	181, s 150	+59	200
	Hendecaacetate	$C_{40}H_{54}O_{27}$	131	+44 ($CHCl_3$)	201
O-α-D-Galp-(1 → 6)-O-α-D-Glcp-(1 → 2)-β-D-Fruf (Raffinose)	Pentahydrate	$C_{18}H_{32}O_{16}\cdot 5H_2O$	77–78, 118	+101, +123	202
	Hendecaacetate	$C_{40}H_{54}O_{27}$	99–101	+92, +100 (c 8, C_2H_5OH)	203, 204
O-D-Galp-(1 → 4)-O-D-Glcp-(1 → ?)-L-Fuc		$C_{18}H_{32}O_{15}$	No constants known	—	205
O-β-D-Galp-(1 → 4)-O-[α-D-Glcp-(1 → 2)]-β-D-Glcp		$C_{18}H_{32}O_{16}$	—	+103	206, 207
O-α-D-Galp-(1 → 2)-O-α-D-Glcp-(1 → 1)-glycerol		$C_{15}H_{28}O_{13}$	171	+170 ± 3	208
	Nonaacetate	$C_{33}H_{46}O_{22}$	97	+145 ± 3(c 0.5, $CHCl_3$)	208

OLIGOSACCHARIDES (INCLUDING DISACCHARIDES)

Substance[a] (synonym) (A)	Derivative (B)	Chemical formula (C)	Melting point °C (D)	Specific rotation[b] $[\alpha]_D$ (E)	Reference (F)
		Trisaccharides (continued)			
O-α-D-GalUAp-(1 → 4)-O-α-D-GalUAp-(1 → 4)-O-D-GalUAp (Tri-galacturonic acid)		$C_{18}H_{26}O_{19}$	135–142d	+154, +187	69, 209
O-α-D-Glcp-(1 → 2)-O-β-D-Fruf-(1 → 2)-β-D-Fruf (Isokestose, 1-Kestose)		$C_{18}H_{32}O_{16}$	82–88d, 90–92, 105–110; 148; 200–201	+25; +29.3; +28.9; +27.9	184, 210; 211; 212; 211–214
	Hendecamethyl ether	$C_{29}H_{54}O_{16}$	–		
O-α-D-Glcp-(1 → 2)-O-β-D-Fruf-(6 → 2)-β-D-Fruf (Kestose)		$C_{18}H_{32}O_{16}$	145	+28	212, 215
	Hendecamethyl ether	$C_{29}H_{54}O_{16}$	–	+25.8 (18°)	215
O-α-D-Glcp-(1 → 2)-O-β-D-Fruf-(3 → 1)-α-D-Galp		$C_{18}H_{32}O_{16}$	No constants known	–	216
O-α-D-Glcp-(1 → 3)-O-β-D-Fruf-(2 → 1)-α-D-Glcp (Melezitose)	Dihydrate; Hendecaacetate	$C_{18}H_{32}O_{16} \cdot 2H_2O$; $C_{40}H_{54}O_{27}$	153–154; 117	+88.2; +103.6 (CHCl₃)	217, 218; 219
O-α-D-Glcp-(1 → 4)-O-α-D-Glcp-(1 → 2)-β-D-Fruf (Erlose)	Hendecaacetate	$C_{18}H_{32}O_{16}$; $C_{40}H_{54}O_{27}$	68–73; –	+121.8; +92.7 (15°) (CHCl₃)	220, 221; 222
O-α-D-Glcp-(1 → 6)-O-α-D-Glcp-(1 → 2)-β-D-Fruf		$C_{18}H_{32}O_{16}$	118–120	+102.5 (18°)	223, 224
O-β-D-Glcp-(1 → 6)-O-α-D-Glcp-(1 → 2)-β-D-Fruf (Gentianose)		$C_{18}H_{32}O_{16}$	210	+33.4	225, 226

OLIGOSACCHARIDES (INCLUDING DISACCHARIDES)

Trisaccharides (continued)

Substance[a] (synonym) (A)	Derivative (B)	Chemical formula (C)	Melting point °C (D)	Specific rotation[b] $[\alpha]_D$ (E)	Reference (F)
O-α-D-Glcp-(1 → 6)-O-α-D-Glcp-(1 → 5)-D-Fruf (5-O-α-Isomaltosylfructose)		$C_{18}H_{32}O_{16}$	No constants known	—	77
O-α-D-Glcp-(1 → 6)-O-α-D-Glcp-(1 → 6)-D-Fruf (Isomaltotriulose)		$C_{18}H_{32}O_{16}$	—	+118	72
O-α-D-Glcp-(1 → 3)-O-β-D-Glcp-(1 → 1)-α-D-Glcp		$C_{18}H_{32}O_{16}$	183–184	+139	227
	Hendecaacetate	$C_{40}H_{44}O_{27}$	—	+110.5 (CHCl₃)	345
O-β-D-Glcp-(1 → 3)-O-β-D-Glcp-(1 → 3)-β-D-Glcp (Laminaritriose)	Hendecaacetate	$C_{18}O_{32}O_{16}$	120–121	+2.4 (17°)	101, 228
		$C_{40}H_{54}O_{27}$		−40 (CHCl₃)	101
O-α-D-Glcp-(1 → 3)-O-α-D-Glcp-(1 → 4)-D-Glcp		$C_{18}H_{32}O_{16}$	—	+169.5	231, 232
O-β-D-Glcp-(1 → 3)-O-β-D-Glcp-(1 → 4)-α-D-Glcp	Hendecaacetate	$C_{18}H_{32}O_{16}$	229–231	+18.7 → +13	229, 230
		$C_{40}H_{54}O_{27}$	121–123	−22.2 (CHCl₃)	230
O-α-D-Glcp-(1 → 2)-O-[α-D-Glcp-(1 → 4)]-D-Glcp		$C_{18}H_{32}O_{16}$	—	+140 (27°)	346
O-α-D-Glcp-(1 → 2)-O-[β-D-Glcp-(1 → 4)]-D-Glcp		$C_{18}H_{32}O_{16}$	—	+93	88
O-α-D-Glcp-(1 → 4)-O-α-D-Glcp-(1 → 3)-D-Glc		$C_{18}H_{32}O_{16}$	No constants known	—	231, 232

OLIGOSACCHARIDES (INCLUDING DISACCHARIDES)

Trisaccharides (continued)

Substance[a] (synonym) (A)	Derivative (B)	Chemical formula (C)	Melting point °C (D)	Specific rotation[b] $[\alpha]_D$ (E)	Reference (F)
O-β-D-Glcp-(1 → 4)-O-β-D-Glcp-(1 → 3)-D-Glc	Hendecaacetate I Hendecaacetate II	$C_{18}H_{32}O_{16}$ $C_{40}H_{54}O_{27}$ $C_{40}H_{54}O_{27}$	236–239 108–110 186–188	+16.5 → +11.7 −8.3 (CHCl₃) −24 (CHCl₃)	229 230 233
O-α-D-Glcp-(1 → 4)-O-α-D-Glcp-(1 → 4)-D-Glcp (Maltotriose)	Hendecaacetate	$C_{18}H_{32}O_{16}$ $C_{40}H_{54}O_{27}$	150, Amorph 134–136	+160 +86 (CHCl₃)	234, 235 234, 236
O-β-D-Glcp-(1 → 4)-O-β-D-Glcp-(1 → 4)-D-Glcp (Cellotriose)	α-Hendecaacetate β-Hendecaacetate	$C_{18}H_{32}O_{16}$ $C_{40}H_{54}O_{27}$ $C_{40}H_{54}O_{27}$	— 220–222 199.5–200.5	+25 +22.6 (CHCl₃) −10.8 (CHCl₃)	230, 237 238 230
O-α-D-Glcp-(1 → 4)-O-β-D-Glcp-(1 → 6)-D-Glc	Hendecaacetate	$C_{18}H_{32}O_{16}$ $C_{40}H_{54}O_{27}$	139–141 —	+159 +112 (CHCl₃)	239 239
O-α-D-Glcp-(1 → 6)-O-α-D-Glcp-(1 → 4)-D-Glcp (Panose)	O-α-Isomaltopyranosyl-(1 → 4)-D-glucitol dodecaacetate	$C_{18}H_{32}O_{16}$ $C_{42}H_{58}O_{28}$	222–224 147–149	+154 +120 (0.5% C_2H_5OH in CHCl₃)	222, 240 241
O-α-D-Glcp-(1 → 6)-O-α-D-Glcp-(1 → 6)-D-Glc (Isomaltotriose, Dextrantriose)					
O-β-D-Glcp-(1 → 6)-O-β-D-Glcp-(1 → 6)-D-Glc (Gentiotriose,	Hendecabenzoate	$C_{18}H_{32}O_{16}$ $C_{9}H_{7}O_{27}$	226–227 —	+145 +131 (CHCl₃)	106 242

OLIGOSACCHARIDES (INCLUDING DISACCHARIDES)

Trisaccharides (continued)

Substance[a] (synonym) (A)	Derivative (B)	Chemical formula (C)	Melting point °C (D)	Specific rotation[b] $[\alpha]_D$ (E)	Reference (F)
Luteose)					
O-α-D-Glcp-(1 → 6)-O-α-D-Glcp-(1 → 2)-D-GlcUA	Hendecaacetate	$C_{18}H_{32}O_{16}$ $C_{40}H_{54}O_{27}$	214–215 —	−10.3 −9.4 ($CHCl_3$)	243, 244 244
O-α-D-Glcp-(1 → 2)-O-α-D-Glcp-(1 → 1)-glycerol		$C_{18}H_{30}O_{17}$	—	+110 (c 0.07)	116
O-α-D-Glcp-(1 → 6)-O-α-D-Glcp-(1 → 1)-glycerol		$C_{15}H_{28}O_{13}$	·	+172 ± 2	347
O-β-D-Glcp-(1 → 1)-O-[β-D-Glcp-(1 → 6)]-D-mannitol		$C_{15}H_{28}O_{13}$	—	+148	117
	Dodecaacetate	$C_{18}H_{34}O_{16}$ $C_{42}H_{58}O_{28}$	136–138 —	−14 −7.7 ($CHCl_3$)	120 245
O-β-D-Glcp-(1 → 6)-O-β-D-Glcp-(1 → 2)-L-Rha (Bryodulcoside)	Nonaacetate	$C_{18}H_{32}O_{15}$ $C_{36}H_{50}O_{24}$	No constants known 172–173	— 	126 126
O-β-D-Glcp-(1 → 4)-O-β-D-Manp-(1 → 4)-D-Manp		$C_{18}H_{32}O_{16}$	—	+54 ($CHCl_3$)	123, 246
O-3-O-methyl-D-Glcp-(1 → 4)-O-D-Glcp-(1 → 4)-D-Glcp		$C_{18}H_{32}O_{16}$		−9	334
O-(N-methyl-α-L-GlcNp)-(1 → 2)-O-(3-C-formyl-α-L-Sd-Lyxf)-(1 → 1)-2,4-dideoxy-2,4-diguanidino-scyllo-inositol (Streptomycin)	Trihydrochloride	$C_{21}H_{37}N_7O_{12} \cdot 3HCl$	No constants known	— −86.7	247

OLIGOSACCHARIDES (INCLUDING DISACCHARIDES)

Substance[a] (synonym) (A)	Derivative (B)	Chemical formula (C)	Melting point °C (D)	Specific rotation[b] $[\alpha]_D$ (E)	Reference (F)
		Trisaccharides (continued)			
O-(N-methyl-α-L-GlcNp)-(1 → 2)-O-3-C-hydroxymethyl-β-L-5d-Lyxf-(1 → 1)-(2-O-carbamoyl-4-deoxy-4-guanidino-scyllo-inositol) (Bluensomycin)		$C_{21}H_9N_5O_{14}$	No constants known	—	248
O-β-D-GlcNAcp-(1 → 4)-O-β-D-GlcNAcp-(1 → 4)-D-GlcNAcp (Chitotriose)		$C_{24}H_{41}N_3O_{16}$	304—306d	+3.8 → +2.2	139, 140
O-β-D-GlcNAcp-(1 → ?)-O-β-D-GlcUAp-(1 → 3)-D-GlcNAc		$C_{40}H_{17}N_3O_{24}$	315	+33 (c 0.2, CH₃COOH)	249
	Octaacetate	$C_{23}H_{36}N_2O_{17}$	—	−16	250
O-β-D-GlcNAcp-(1 → 4)-O-N-acetylmuramic acid-(1 → 4)-D-GlcNAcp		$C_{27}H_{45}N_3O_{18}$	No constants known	—	348
O-α-3-amino-3-deoxy-D-Glcp-(1 → 6)-O-[6-amino-6-deoxy-α-D-Glcp-type (1 → 4)]-1,3-diamino-1,2,3-trideoxy-scyllo-inositol (Kanamycin A)	Tetra-N-acetyl kanomycin	$C_{18}H_{36}N_4O_{11}$	200	+99, +149 (H₂O)	349, 350
	Tetra-N-2,4-di-nitrophenylheptaacetate	$C_{55}H_{44}N_4O_{15}$	250—255d, 280—282d	+146 (0.1 N H₂SO₄)	252
		$C_{56}H_{58}N_{12}O_{34}$	210—213d	+115	252, 350
O-3-amino-3-deoxy-α-D-Glcp-(1 → 6)-O-[α-D-				+52 (acetone)	349

OLIGOSACCHARIDES (INCLUDING DISACCHARIDES)

Substance[a] (synonym) (A)	Derivative (B)	Chemical formula (C)	Melting point °C (D)	Specific rotation[b] $[\alpha]_D$ (E)	Reference (F)
		Trisaccharides (continued)			
GlcNp-(1 → 4)]-1,3-diamino-1,2,3-trideoxy-scyllo-inositol (Kanamycin C)	Tetra-N-2,4-nitrophenylheptaacetate	$C_{18}H_{36}N_4O_{11}$	270d	+126, +139	351, 352
O-3-amino-3-deoxy-α-D-Glcp-(1 → 6)-O-[2,6-diamino-2,6-dideoxy-α-D-Glcp-(1 → 4)]-1,3-diamino-1,2,3-trideoxy-scyllo-inositol (Kanamycin B)		$C_5H_{58}N_{12}O_{54}$	208–211d	+299 (c 0.8, acetone)	352
	Penta-N-acetyl-kanamycin B	$C_{18}N_3N_5O_{10}$	178–182d	+130 (c 0.5)	353
	Penta-N-2,4-nitrophenylhexaacetate	$C_{28}H_{47}N_5O_{15}$	250d	+110	353
Destomycin A (an aminoheptosidohexosido-scyllo-diamino-dideoxy-inositol)		$C_{60}H_{59}N_{15}O_{36}$	217–218d	+240 (c 0.4, acetone)	354
	Tri-N-acetyl destomycin A	$C_{20}H_{39}N_5O_{14}$	180–190d	+7	253
Destomycin B		$C_{26}H_{45}N_5O_{17}$	240–260d	—	253, 254
		$C_{20}H_{39}N_5O_{14}$	140–200d	+6	253
	Tri-N-acetyl destomycin B	$C_{26}H_{45}N_5O_{17}$	220–240d	—	253
O-N-Acetylmuramic acid-(1 → 4)-O-D-GlcNAcp-(1 → 4)-N-acetylmuramic acid					
O-(N-Acetylneuraminic acid)-(2 → 3)-O-β-D-Galp-(1 → 4)-		$C_{30}H_{49}N_3O_{20}$	No constants known	—	355

OLIGOSACCHARIDES (INCLUDING DISACCHARIDES)

Substance[a] (synonym)	Derivative	Chemical formula	Melting point °C	Specific rotation[b] $[\alpha]_D$	Reference
(A)	(B)	(C)	(D)	(E)	(F)
Trisaccharides (continued)					
β-D-Glcp (Neuraminyl lactose, Lactaminyl lactose, Sialyl lactose)		$C_{23}H_{39}NO_{19}$, / —	— / —	+16.8 / +6 (CH, SOCH₃)	255 / 256
O-(N-Acetylneuraminic acid)-(2 → 3)-O-(β-D-Galp 6-sulfate)-(1 → 4)-β-D-Glcp (Neuraminyl lactose sulfate)		$C_{23}H_{39}NO_{23}S$	No constants known	—	257
O-(N-Acetylneuraminic acid)-(2 → 6)-O-β-D-Galp-(1 → 4)-β-D-Glcp (6-Neuraminyl lactose)		$C_{23}H_{39}NO_{19}$	—	+27.9	255
O-α-D-Manp-(1 → 3)-O-α-D-Galp-(1 → 2)-glycerol (Mannosyl glycerol floridoside)	Nonaacetate	$C_{15}H_{28}O_{13}$ / $C_{33}H_{46}O_{22}$	Amorph / 153–154	— / +103 (CHCl₃)	258 / 258
O-β-D-Manp-(1 → 4)-O-β-D-Glcp-(1 → 4)-D-Glcp		$C_{18}H_{32}O_{16}$		+9.5 (28°)	123
O-β-D-Manp-(1 → 4)-O-β-D-Manp-(1 → 4)-D-Glcp		$C_{18}H_{32}O_{16}$	—	−12 ± 3	123, 259
O-D-Manp-(1 → 6)-O-D-Manp-(1 → 6)-D-Glcp (Laevidulinose)	Hendecaacetate	$C_{18}H_{32}O_{16}$ / $C_9H_{54}O_{27}$	95–100	−11.5, −15 / +18	260, 261 / 260, 261
O-β-D-Manp-(1 → 4)-O-β-D-Manp-(1 → 4)-α-D-Manp	Monohydrate	$C_{18}H_{32}O_{16}\cdot H_2O$ / $C_{18}H_{32}O_{16}\cdot H_2O$	214–216 / 166–167	−23 / —	123 / 123

OLIGOSACCHARIDES (INCLUDING DISACCHARIDES)

Substance[a] (synonym) (A)	Derivative (B)	Chemical formula (C)	Melting point °C (D)	Specific rotation[b] $[\alpha]_D$ (E)	Reference (F)
		Trisaccharides (continued)			
Rhamninose	Mannobiosyl mannitol dodecaacetate	$C_{42}H_{58}O_{29}$ $C_{18}H_{32}O_{14}$	112 135–140d, Amorph	-20 ± 5 (CHCl$_3$) -41	160 319
	Hexaacetate?	$C_{30}H_{44}O_{20}$	95–100	-30.9 (C$_2$H$_5$OH)	319
O-α-D-Xylp-(1 → 6)-O-β-D-Glcp-(1 → 4)-D-Glcp		$C_{17}H_{30}O_{15}$	147–150	$+150$	123
O-D-Xylp-(1 → 3)-O-D-Xylp-(1 → 4)-D-Xylp O-β-D-Xylp-(1 → 4)-O-β-D-Xylp-(1 → 4)-β-D-Xylp (Xylotriose)		$C_{15}H_{26}O_{13}$	225	$-52 \to -47$	173
	Octaacetate	$C_{15}H_{26}O_{13}$ $C_{31}H_{42}O_{21}$	215–216 108–109.5	-48.1 -83 (CHCl$_3$)	262, 263 263
		Tetrasaccharides			
D-Fructose tetraose (Verolnicin) (non-reducing)	Tetradecaacetate	$C_{24}H_{42}O_{21}$ $C_{52}H_{70}O_{35}$	170, 188 92	-29.4 -21.1 (CHCl$_3$)	264 264
D-Fructose tetraose O-D-Fruf-(2 → 1)-O-[D-Fruf-(2 → 2)]-O-[D-Fruf-(2 → 6)]-D-Glcp (Neobifurcose)	Tetradecaacetate	$C_{24}H_{42}O_{21}$	—	-17.3	180
[O-D-Fruf-(2 → 1)-], D-Glcp (Inulotriosyl glucose)	Tridecamethyl ether	$C_{24}H_{42}O_{21}$ $C_{37}H_{68}O_{21}$	— —	$+14.4, +16.7$ -35.4	184, 265 278
O-L-Fucp-(1 → 2)-O-D-Galp-(1 → 4)-O-[L-Fucp-(1 → 3)]-D-		$C_{24}H_{42}O_{21}$	—	-2	266

OLIGOSACCHARIDES (INCLUDING DISACCHARIDES)

Substance[a] (synonym) (A)	Derivative (B)	Chemical formula (C)	Melting point °C (D)	Specific rotation[b] $[\alpha]_D$ (E)	Reference (F)
Tetrasaccharides (continued)					
Glcp (Lactodifuco-tetraose)		$C_{24}H_{42}O_{19}$	—	$-17.1, -106$	205, 267
O-D-Galp-(1 → ?)-O-D-Galp-(1 → ?)-O-D-Fruf-(2 → 1)-D-Glcp (Sesamose)		$C_{24}H_{42}O_{21}$	No constants given	—	268
[O-β-D-Galp-(1 → 4)-]$_3$ D-Glcp		$C_{24}H_{42}O_{21}$	—	$+43$	13
[O-α-D-Galp-(1 → 6)-]$_2$ O-β-D-Galp-(1 → 1)-glycerol		$C_{21}H_{38}O_{18}$	—	$+114$	344
	Dodecamethyl ether	$C_{33}H_{62}O_{18}$	—	$+79.8$ (CHCl$_3$)	344
[O-α-D-Galp-(1 → 6)-]$_2$ α-D-Glcp-(1 → 2)-D-Fruf (Stachyose, Manneotetrose)		$C_{24}H_{42}O_{21}$	140, 170	$+131, +146$	194, 269
	Tetradecaacetate	$C_{52}H_{70}O_{35}$	95—96, Amorph	$+120$ (C$_2$H$_5$OH)	270
	Tetradecamethyl ether	$C_{38}H_{70}O_{21}$	—	$+130$ (CHCl$_3$)	271
O-D-Galp-(1 → 4)-O-D-Galp-(1 → 6)-O-α-D-Glcp-(1 → 2)-D-Fruf		$C_{24}H_{42}O_{21}$	—	$+143$	272
D-Galactose-3,6-anhydro-L-galactose tetrasaccharide (Neoagarotetrose)	Dihydrate	$C_{24}H_{38}O_{19} \cdot 2H_2O$	104—107	-2.8	273
	Decaacetate	$C_{44}H_{58}O_{29} \cdot 2H_2O$	121	-15.8 (CHCl$_3$)	273
O-α-D-Galp-(1 → 6)-O-α-D-Glcp-(1 → 2)-O-β-D-Fruf-(1 → 1)-α-D-Galp (Lychnose)		$C_{24}H_{42}O_{21}$	—	$+155$	272
O-α-D-Galp-(1 → 6)-O-α-D-Glcp-(1 → 2)-O-β-D-Fruf-(3 → 1)-α-D-Galp (Isolychnose)		$C_{24}H_{42}O_{21}$	No constants given	—	274

OLIGOSACCHARIDES (INCLUDING DISACCHARIDES)

Substance[a] (synonym) (A)	Derivative (B)	Chemical formula (C)	Melting point °C (D)	Specific rotation[b] $[\alpha]_D$ (E)	Reference (F)
Tetrasaccharides (continued)					
O-β-D-Galp-(1 → 3)-O-β-D-GlcNAcp-(1 → 3)-O-β-D-Galp-(1 → 4)-D-Glcp (Lacto-N-tetraose)		$C_{26}H_{45}NO_{21}$	205d	+25.2	51
O-α-D-GalUAp-(1 → 4)-O-α-D-GalUAp-(1 → 4)-O-α-D-GalUAp-(1 → 4)-D-GalUAp (Tetragalacturonic acid)	Trihydrate	$C_{24}H_{34}O_{25} \cdot 3H_2O$	160–170d	—	275
O-α-D-Glcp-(1 → 2)-[O-β-D-Fruf-(1 → 2)-]₂ O-β-D-Fruf (Nystose)		$C_{24}H_{42}O_{21}$ / —	131–132 / 110–115	+10.6 / +17.9	276 / 277, 278
O-α-D-Glcp-(1 → 2)-O-[β-D-Fruf-(2 → 6)]-O-β-D-Fruf-(1 → 2)-D-Fruf (Bifurcose)		$C_{24}H_{42}O_{21}$ / $C_{36}H_{60}O_{21}$	156 / —	+8 / +3 (CHCl₃)	211 / 211
O-α-D-Glcp-(1 → 2)-[O-β-D-Fruf-(6 → 2)-]₂ β-D-Fruf	Tetradecamethyl ether	$C_{24}H_{42}O_{21}$	—	−7	279
[O-α-D-Glcp-(1 → 4)-]₂ O-D-Glcp-(1 → 2)-D-Fruf (Maltosylsucrose)		$C_{24}H_{42}O_{21}$	No constants given	—	221
[O-β-D-Glcp-(1 → 3)-]₃ β-D-Glcp (Laminaritetraose)	Tetradecaacetate	$C_{24}H_{42}O_{21}$ / $C_{38}H_{70}O_{35}$	122–123 / —	−5.9 / −46.2 (CHCl₃)	101, 228 / 101
O-α-D-Glcp-(1 → 3)-O-α-D-Glcp-(1 → 4)-O-α-D-Glcp-(1 → 3)-D-Glcp		$C_{24}H_{42}O_{21}$	—	+181 (c 0.7)	356

OLIGOSACCHARIDES (INCLUDING DISACCHARIDES)

Tetrasaccharides (continued)

Substance[a] (synonym) (A)	Derivative (B)	Chemical formula (C)	Melting point °C (D)	Specific rotation[b] $[\alpha]_D$ (E)	Reference (F)
O-β-D-Glcp-(1 → 3)-[O-β-D-Glcp-(1 → 4)-]₂ D-Glcp	α-Anomer β-Anomer·2H₂O	$C_{24}H_{42}O_{21}$ $C_{24}H_{42}O_{21} \cdot 2H_2O$	221–224d 180–181	+12.9 → +10.6 +7 → +10	280 280
O-β-D-Glcp-(1 → 4)-O-β-D-Glcp-(1 → 3)-O-β-D-Glcp-(1 → 4)-D-Glcp		$C_{24}H_{42}O_{21}$	223–226	+19.8 (90% CH₃COOH)	280, 281
[O-β-D-Glcp-(1 → 4)-]₂ O-β-D-Glcp-(1 → 3)-β-D-Glcp	Tetradecaacetate	$C_{24}H_{42}O_{21}$ $C_{52}H_{70}O_{35}$	241–245d 118–121	+11.4 → +8.4 —	280 282
[O-α-D-Glcp-(1 → 4)-]₃-D-Glcp (Maltotetraose)	Methyl glycoside	$C_{24}H_{42}O_{21}$ $C_{25}H_{44}O_{21}$	— —	+166 +213	235, 283 235
[O-β-D-Glcp-(1 → 4)-]₃ D-Glcp (Cellotetraose)	α-Tetradecaacetate β-Tetradecaacetate	$C_{24}H_{42}O_{21}$ $C_{52}H_{70}O_{35}$ $C_{52}H_{70}O_{35}$	251 226–227 223–225	+11.3 → +17 +12.5 (CHCl₃) -18.2 (CHCl₃)	237, 301 284 284
O-α-D-Glcp-(1 → 6)-[O-α-D-Glcp-(1 → 4)-]₂ D-Glcp		$C_{24}H_{42}O_{21}$	—	+177 (15°) (c 0.5)	285
O-α-D-Glcp-(1 → 6)-[O-α-D-Glcp-(1 → 4)-]₂ O-α-D-Glcp-(1 → 4)-D-Glcp	Methyl glycoside monomethanolate	$C_{24}H_{42}O_{21}$ $C_{25}H_{44}O_{21} \cdot CH_3OH$	192–193	+164 +189	240 286
Glucose tetrasaccharide, cyclic?	Dodecaacetate	$C_{24}H_{40}O_{20}$ $C_{48}H_{64}O_{32}$	— —	+168 +157	287 287

OLIGOSACCHARIDES (INCLUDING DISACCHARIDES)

Substance[a] (synonym) (A)	Derivative (B)	Chemical formula (C)	Melting point °C (D)	Specific rotation[b] $[\alpha]_D$ (E)	Reference (F)
		Tetrasaccharides (continued)			
[O-α-D-Glcp-(1 → 6)-], 3-O-methyl-D-Glc		$C_{25}H_{44}O_{21}$	—	+129	357
[O-α-D-Glcp-(1 → 6)-], O-α-D-Glcp-(1 → 1)-glycerol		$C_{21}H_{39}O_{18}$	—	+166 (27°) (c 0.5)	117
O-3-O-methyl-D-Glcp-(1 → 4)-[O-D-Glcp-(1 → 4)-], D-Glc		$C_{25}H_{44}O_{21}$	No constants known	—	334
O-D-GlcNAcp-(1 → 4)-O-N-acetylmuramic acid-(1 → 4)-O-D-GlcNAcp-(1 → 4)-N-acetylmuramic acid		$C_{36}H_{62}N_4O_{33}$	No constants known	—	355
O-β-D-GlcNAcp-(1 → 6)-O-β-N-acetylneuraminic acid-(1 → 4)-O-β-D-GlcNAcp-(1 → 6)-N-acetylneuraminic acid		$C_{36}H_{62}N_4O_{25}$	No constants given	—	288
O-β-D-GlcUAp-(1 → 3)-O-β-D-GlcNAcp(1 → ?)-O-β-D-GlcUAp-(1 → 3)-D-GlcNAc		$C_{28}H_{44}N_2O_{23}$	200d	-41 → -53 (27°)	289
O-4-O-methyl-α-D-GlcUA-(1 → 2)-[O-β-D-Xylp-(1 → 4)-]₃ D-Xylp		$C_{27}H_{36}O_{19}$	—	+23.4	263
O-(2,6-diamino-2,6-dideoxy-α-D-arabino-hexopyranosyl)-(1 → 3)-O-β-D-Ribf-(1 → 5)-[2,6-diamino-2,6-dideoxy-α-D-arabino-hexo-					

OLIGOSACCHARIDES (INCLUDING DISACCHARIDES)

Substance[a] (synonym)	Derivative	Chemical formula	Melting point °C	Specific rotation[b] $[\alpha]_D$	Reference
(A)	(B)	(C)	(D)	(E)	(F)
		Tetrasaccharides (continued)			
pyranosyl-(1 → 4)]-1,3-diamino-1,2,3-tri-deoxy-*scyllo*-inositol (Neomycin C, Streptothricin B II, Framycetin)	Hexa-*N*-acetyl neomycin C	$C_3H_{46}N_6O_{13}$	No constants given	—	290
		$C_{35}H_{58}N_6O_{19}$	—	+94.5 (28°)	291
O-(2,6-diamino-2,6-dideoxy-α-D-*arabino*-hexopyranosyl)-(1 → 3)-*O*-β-D-Rib*f*-(1 → 5)-*O*-[α-D-GlcN*p*-(1 → 4)]-1,3-diamino-1,2,3-tri-deoxy-*scyllo*-inositol (Paromomycin II)	Penta-*N*-acetyl paromomycin II	$C_3H_{45}N_5O_{14}$	No constants given	—	290
		$C_{33}H_{55}N_5O_{19}$	—	+64 (27°)	292
O-(2,6-diamino-2,6-dideoxy-α-L-*xylo*-hexopyranosyl)-(1 → 3)-*O*-β-D-Rib*f*-(1 → 5)-*O*-[2,6-diamino-2,6-dideoxy-α-D-*arabino*-hexo-pyranosyl-(1 → 4)]-1,3-diamino-1,2,3-tri-deoxy-*scyllo*-inositol (Neomycin B, Streptothricin B I)	Hexa-*N*-acetyl neomycin B	$C_3H_{46}N_6O_{13}$	No constants given	—	290
		$C_{35}H_{58}N_6O_{19}$	—	+47.8 (28°)	291

OLIGOSACCHARIDES (INCLUDING DISACCHARIDES)

Tetrasaccharides (continued)

Substance[a] (synonym) (A)	Derivative (B)	Chemical formula (C)	Melting point °C (D)	Specific rotation[b] $[\alpha]_D$ (E)	Reference (F)
O-(2,6-diamino-2,6-dideoxy-α-L-xylo-hexopyranosyl)-(1 → 3)-O-β-D-Ribf-(1 → 5)-O-[α-D-GlcNp-(1 → 4)]-1,3-diamino-1,2,3-trideoxy-scyllo-inositol (Paromomycin I)		$C_{23}H_{45}N_5O_{14}$	No constants given	—	290
O-α-D-Manp-(1 → 4)-O-N-methyl-α-L-GlcNp-(1 → 2)-O-(3-C-formyl-β-L-5d-Lyxf)-(1 → 1)-2,4-dideoxy-2,4-diguanidino-scyllo-inositol (Streptomycin B)	Trihydrochloride	$C_{27}H_{47}N_7O_{17}\cdot 3HCl$	179–182d	-47	293
O-β-D-Xylp-(1 → 4)-O-[α-L-Araf-(1 → 3)]-O-β-D-Xylp-(1 → 4)-D-Xyl	Decaacetate	$C_{20}H_3O_{17}$ $C_{40}H_5O_{27}$	179–180 —	-75 -85 (CHCl₃)	294 294
O-D-Xyl-(1 → 4)-O-D-Xyl-(1 → 3)-O-D-Xyl-(1 → 4)-D-Xylp [O-β-D-Xylp-(1 → 4)]₃, D-Xylp (Xylotetraose)		$C_{20}H_{34}O_{17}$	—	-56.7	173
Scorodose	Decaacetate Acetate	$C_{20}H_3O_{17}$ $C_6H_5O_{27}$ $C_{24}H_{42}O_{21}$ Unknown	224–226 200–201 200, Amorph 85–90	-61.9 -92.4 (CHCl₃) -41.5 -28.5 (CHCl₃)	262, 263 263 295 295

OLIGOSACCHARIDES (INCLUDING DISACCHARIDES)

Substance[a] (synonym) (A)	Derivative (B)	Chemical formula (C)	Melting point °C (D)	Specific rotation[b] $[\alpha]_D$ (E)	Reference (F)
Pentasaccharides					
Fructose pentasaccharide		$C_{30}H_{52}O_{24}$		+8, −23	180, 279
O-Fruf-(2 → ?)-stachyose		$C_{30}H_{52}O_{26}$	No constants given		179
O-α-L-Fucp-(1 → 2)- (Lacto-N-tetraose) (Lacto-N-fucopentaose I)		$C_{32}H_{55}NO_{25}$	216	−11 → −16.3	51
O-β-D-Galp-(1 → 3)O-[α-L-Fucp-(1 → 4)]-O-β-D-GlcNAcp-(1 → 3)-O-β-D-Galp-(1 → 4)-D-Glcp (Lacto-N-fucopentaose II)		$C_{32}H_{55}NO_{25}$	213–215	−28 → +30.4	297
Lacto-pentaose B		$C_{37}H_{42}N_2O_{25}$	—	+15	298
Lacto-pentaose C		$C_{37}H_{42}N_2O_{25}$	—	+13	298
[O-α-D-Galp-(1 → 6)-]₃ O-α-D-Glcp-(1 → 2)-β-D-Fruf (Verbascose)		$C_{30}H_{52}O_{26}$	219–220, 253	+169.9	299, 300
	Heptadecaacetate	$C_{64}H_{86}O_{43}$	132	+130.4	299, 300
O-D-Glcp-(1 → 2)-O-[D-Fruf-(2 → 6)]-O-D-Fruf-(1 → 2)-O-D-Fruf-(1 → 2)-D-Fruf		$C_{30}H_{52}O_{24}$	—	−3.5	211
	Heptadecamethyl ether	$C_{74}H_{62}O_{26}$	—	−10.5 (CHCl₃)	211
O-α-D-Glcp-(1 → 2)- [O-β-D-Fruf- (6 → 2)-]₃ ᷓD-Fruf		$C_{30}H_{52}O_{26}$	—	−11.2	279, 296
[O-α-D-Glcp- (1 → 4)-]₄-D-Glcp (Maltopentaose)		$C_{30}H_{52}O_{26}$	—	+178	302, 320

OLIGOSACCHARIDES (INCLUDING DISACCHARIDES)

Substance[a] (synonym) (A)	Derivative (B)	Chemical formula (C)	Melting point °C (D)	Specific rotation[b] $[\alpha]_D$ (E)	Reference (F)
Pentasaccharides (continued)					
[O-β-D-Glcp-(1 → 4)-]₄-D-Glcp (Cellopentaose)	α-Heptadecaacetate	$C_{50}H_{72}O_{36}$	No constants given	—	237
	β-Heptadecaacetate	$C_{64}H_{66}O_{35}$	246–249	—	303
		$C_{64}H_{66}O_{35}$	238.5–239	−18.5 (CHCl₃)	284
[O-α-D-Glcp-(1 → 6)-], O-α-D-Glcp-(1 → 4)-D-Glcp	Methyl α-glycoside monoethanolate	$C_{30}H_{52}O_{26}$	161–164	+167 (c 0.7)	240
		$C_{31}H_{54}O_{26}·C_2H_5OH$	—	+188.7	286
O-4-O-methyl-α-D-GlcUA-(1 → 2)-[O-β-D-Xylp-(1 → 4)-]₃, D-Xyl		$C_{27}H_{44}O_{23}$	—	+0.6	263
[O-β-D-Xylp-(1 → 4)-]₄, β-D-Xylp (Xylopentaose)	Dodecaacetate	$C_{23}H_{42}O_{21}$	240–242	−72.9	262, 263
		$C_{43}H_{66}O_{33}$	249–250	−98 (CHCl₃)	263
Hexasaccharides					
Fructose hexasaccharides (Arctose) Nonreducing	Eicosaacetate	$C_{36}H_{52}O_{31}$	178	−41	264
		$C_{76}H_{102}O_{51}$	108	−36.5 (15°) (CHCl₃)	264
(Campanulin) (Nonreducing)	Eicosaacetate	$C_{36}H_{52}O_{31}$	170	−23	264
		$C_{76}H_{102}O_{51}$	73	−0.2 (CH₃COCH₃)	264
O-α-L-Fucp-(1 → 4)-O-[β-D-Galp-(1 → 3)-O-β-D-GlcNAcp-(1 → 3)-O-β-D-Galp-(1 → 4)-[O-α-LFucp-(1 → 3)]-					

OLIGOSACCHARIDES (INCLUDING DISACCHARIDES)

Substance[a] (synonym)	Derivative	Chemical formula	Melting point °C	Specific rotation[b] $[\alpha]_D$	Reference
(A)	(B)	(C)	(D)	(E)	(F)
		Hexasaccharides (continued)			
D-Glcp (Lacto-N-difucohexaose II)		$C_5H_6,NO_2,$	218–220d	−68.8	191, 304
(O-D-Galp-)$_4$, O-D-Galp-(1 → 2)-D-Fruf (Lycopose) (Non-reducing)	Eicosaacetate	$C_6H_{12}O_{31}$ $C_7H_{10}O_{51}$	270 150	+187 +174.5 (9°) (CH, COCH$_3$,)	305 305
[O-α-D-Galp-(1 → 6)-]$_5$ O-α-D-Glcp-(1 → 2)-β-D-Fruf (Ajugose)	Hexahydrate	$C_{36}H_{62}O_{31}\cdot6H_2O$	204–205	+163	306
O-α-D-Glup-(1 → 2)-[O-β-D-Fruf (6 → 2)-]$_4$ β-D-Fruf		$C_{36}H_{62}O_{31}$	—	−19	279
O-D-Glcp-(1 → ?)-[O-D-Fruf-(? → 2)-]4D-Fruf	Eicosamethyl ether	$C_6H_{12}O_{31}$ $C_6H_{10}O_{51}$	— —	−5.3 −37	278 278
[O-α-D-Glcp-(1 → 4)-]$_5$ D-Glcp (Maltohexaose)		$C_{36}H_{62}O_{31}$	—	+180	302, 320
[O-β-D-Glcp-(1 → 4)-]$_5$ D-Glcp (Cellohexaose)	α-Eicosaacetate β-Eicosaacetate	$C_6H_{12}O_{31}$ $C_6H_{10}O_{51}$ $C_7H_{10}O_{51}$	229–231 252–255 241–243	+168 (15°) — −18.9 (CHCl$_3$)	237, 307 303 284
[O-α-D-Glcp-(1 → 4)-]$_6$ (Schardinger α-dextrin, cyclohexaamylose)	Octadecaacetate	$C_6H_{60}O_{50}$ $C_7H_6O_{48}$	— —	+151 +107 (CHCl$_3$)	308 309
[O-α,β-D-Glcp-(1 → 5?)-]$_6$	Dodecahydrate Octadecamethyl ether	$C_{36}H_{60}O_{30}\cdot12H_2O$ $C_{54}H_{86}O_{30}$	290–300 98–103	+152 +161	310 310

OLIGOSACCHARIDES (INCLUDING DISACCHARIDES)

Substance[a] (synonym) (A)	Derivative (B)	Chemical formula (C)	Melting point °C (D)	Specific rotation[b] $[\alpha]_D$ (E)	Reference (F)
Hexasaccharides (continued)					
O-4-O-methyl-α-D-GlcUA-(1 → 2)-[*O*-β-D-Xylp-(1 → 4)-]₄ D-Xylp		$C_{31}H_{52}O_{27}$	—	-11.8	263
[*O*-D-Xylp-(1 → 4)-], *O*-D-Xylp-(1 → 3)-[*O*-D-Xylp-(1 → 4)-]₂ D-Xylp		$C_{30}H_{50}O_{25}$	169–173	-154 $[\alpha]_{436}$	311
[*O*-β-D-Xylp-(1 → 4)-], D-Xylp (Xylohexaose)	Dihydrate Tetradecaacetate	$C_{30}H_{50}O_{25} \cdot 2H_2O$ $C_{58}H_{78}O_{39}$	236–237 260–261	+72.8 —	262, 312 312
Heptasaccharides					
Fructose heptasaccharide (Asparagose)		$C_{42}H_{72}O_{36}$	—	-35.7	313
[*O*-α-D-Galp-(1 → 6)-], *O*-α-D-Glcp-(1 → 2)-β-D-Fruf	Tetrahydrate	$C_{42}H_{72}O_{36} \cdot 4H_2O$	246–248	+168	306, 321
[*O*-α-D-Galp-(1 → 6)-]₄ *O*-α-D-Glcp-(1 → 2)-*O*-β-D-Fruf-(3 → 1)-α-D-Galp		$C_{42}H_{72}O_{36}$	No constants given	—	314
[*O*-α-D-Glcp-(1 → 4)-], (Schardinger β dextrin, cycloheptaamylose)	Heneicosaacetate	$C_{42}H_{70}O_{35}$ $C_{84}H_{112}O_{56}$	— —	+162 +121 (CHCl₃)	308 309

OLIGOSACCHARIDES (INCLUDING DISACCHARIDES)

Substance[a] (synonym)	Derivative	Chemical formula	Melting point °C	Specific rotation[b] $[\alpha]_D$	Reference
(A)	(B)	(C)	(D)	(E)	(F)
Heptasaccharides (continued)					
O-4-O-methyl-α-D-GlcUA-(1 → 2)-[O-β-D-Xylp-(1 → 4)-]₃, D-Xylp		$C_{37}H_{60}O_{31}$	—	−20.8	263
[O-β-D-Xylp-(1 → 4)-]₆, D-Xylp		$C_{35}H_{58}O_{29}$	232–234	−74	262, 312
Octasaccharides					
[O-α-D-Galp-(1 → 6)-]₆, O-α-D-Glcp-(1 → 2)-β-D-Fruf	Tetrahydrate	$C_{48}H_{82}O_{41} \cdot 4H_2O$	267–268	+168	306
Di(lacto-N-tetraose)		$C_{32}H_{56}N_2O_{41}$	No constants given		315
[O-α-D-Glcp-(1 → 4)-]₈ (Schardinger γ-dextrin, cyclooctaasmylose)		$C_{48}H_{80}O_{40}$	—	+180	316
	Tetracosaacetate	$C_{96}H_{128}O_{64}$	—	+137 (CHCl₃)	309
O-4-O-methyl-α-D-GlcUA-(1 → 2)-[O-β-D-Xylp-(1 → 4)-]₆, D-Xylp		$C_{42}H_{68}O_{35}$		−25.7	263
[O-β-D-Xylp-(1 → 4)-]₇, D-Xylp (Xylooctaose)		$C_{40}H_{66}O_{33}$	No constants given		262

Compiled by George G. Maher.

OLIGOSACCHARIDES (INCLUDING DISACCHARIDES)

REFERENCES

1. Hansson, Johansson, and Lindberg, *Acta Chem. Scand.*, 20, 2358 (1966).
2. Hemming and Ollis, *Chem. Ind.*, p. 85 (1953).
3. Strepkov, *Zh. Obshch. Khim.*, 28, 3143 (1958).
4. Pazur and Gordon, *J. Am. Chem. Soc.*, 75, 3458 (1953).
5. Schlubach and Scheffler, *Justus Liebigs Ann. Chem.*, 588, 192 (1954).
6. Strepkov, *Dokl. Akad. Nauk SSSR.*, 124, 1344 (1959).
7. Bates, *Polarimetry, Saccharimetry and the Sugars*, Nat. Bur. Stand. Circ. C440, U.S. Gov. Print. Off., Washington, D.C., 1942.
8. Hudson and Johnson, *J. Am. Chem. Soc.*, 37, 2748 (1915).
9. Brigl and Scheyer, *Hoppe-Seyler's Z. Physiol. Chem.*, 160, 214 (1926).
10. Wallenfels and Lehmann, *Ber. Dtsch. Chem. Ges.*, 90, 1000 (1957).
11. Bacon, *Biochem. J.*, 57, 320 (1954).
12. Barber, *J. Am. Chem. Soc.*, 81, 3722 (1959).
13. Gorin, Spencer, and Phaff, *Can. J. Chem.*, 42, 1341, 2307 (1964).
14. Lindberg, Wachmeister, and Wickberg, *Acta Chem. Scand.*, 6, 1052 (1952).
15. Gorin, Haskins, and Westlake, *Can. J. Chem.*, 44, 2083 (1966).
16. Aspinall, Auret, and Hirst, *J. Chem. Soc.* (Lond.), p. 4408 (1958).
17. Charlson, Nunn, and Stephan, *J. Chem. Soc.* (Lond.), p. 269 (1955).
18. Shaw, Stephan, and Fuller, *J. Chem. Soc.* (Lond.), p. 2287 (1965).
19. Goldstein, Smith, and Srivastava, *J. Am. Chem. Soc.*, 79, 3858 (1957).
20. Srivastava and Smith, *J. Am. Chem. Soc.*, 79, 982 (1957).
21. Charlson, Gorin, and Perlin, *Can. J. Chem.*, 34, 1811 (1956).
22. Austin, Hardy, Buchanan, and Baddiley, *J. Chem. Soc.* (Lond.), p. 1419 (1965).
23. Feingold, Avigad, and Hestrin, *J. Biol. Chem.*, 224, 295 (1957).
24. Ballio and Russi, *J. Chromatogr.*, 4, 117 (1960).
25. Helferich and Steinpreis, *Ber. Dtsch. Chem. Ges.*, 91, 1794 (1958).
26. Ball and Jones, *J. Chem. Soc.* (Lond.), p. 905 (1958).
27. Masamune and Kamiyama, *Jap. J. Exp. Med.*, 66, 43 (1957).
28. Ingle and Bhide, *J. Indian Chem. Soc.*, 35, 516 (1958).
29. Turton, Bebbington, Dixon, and Pacsu, *J. Am. Chem. Soc.*, 77, 2565 (1955).
30. Meier, *Acta Chem. Scand.*, 16, 2275 (1962).
31. Haq and Adams, *Can. J. Chem.*, 39, 1563 (1961).
32. Hirase and Araki, *Bull. Chem. Soc. Jap.*, 27, 105 (1953).
33. Yoshikawa and Watanabe, *Hyogo Noka Daigaku Kenkyu Hokoku*, 3, 53 (1957); *Chem. Abstr.*, 52, 19198 (1958).
34. Clingman, Nunn, and Stephan, *J. Chem. Soc.* (Lond.), p. 197 (1957).
35. Watkins, *Nature*, 181, 117 (1958).
36. Wickstrom, *Acta Chem. Scand.*, 11, 1473 (1957).
37. Lehmann and Beck, *Justus Liebigs Ann. Chem.*, 630, 56 (1960).
38. Beck and Wallenfels, *Justus Liebigs Ann. Chem.*, 655, 173 (1962).
39. Kuhn and Baer, *Ber. Dtsch. Chem. Ges.*, 87, 1560 (1954).
40. Trey, *Z. Phys. Chem.*, 46, 620 (1903).
41. Gillis, *Recl. Trav. Chem. Pays-Bas*, 39, 88, 677 (1920).
42. Hudson and Johnson, *J. Am. Chem. Soc.*, 37, 1270, 1276 (1915).
43. Tanret, *Z. Phys. Chem.*, 53, 692 (1905).
44. Fletcher and Diehl, *J. Am. Chem. Soc.*, 74, 5774 (1952).
45. Assarson and Theander, *Acta Chem. Scand.*, 12, 1319 (1958).
46. Hudson and Johnson, *J. Am. Chem. Soc.*, 37, 2752 (1915).
47. Pazur, Tipton, Budovich, and Marsh, *J. Am. Chem. Soc.*, 80, 119 (1958).
48. Helferich and Sparmberg, *Ber. Dtsch. Chem. Ges.*, 66, 806 (1933).
49. Polonovski and Lespangol, *C. R. Acad. Sci.*, 192, 1319 (1931); 195, 465 (1932).
50. Bredereck, Wagner, Geissel, Gross, Hutten, and Ott, *Ber. Dtsch. Chem. Ges.*, 95, 3056 (1962).
51. Kuhn, Gauhe, and Baer, *Ber. Dtsch. Chem. Ges.*, 87, 289, 1553 (1954); 88, 1135, 1713 (1955); 89, 2513, 2514 (1956).
52. Glick, Chen, and Zillikin, *J. Biol. Chem.*, 237, 981 (1962).
53. Zilliken, Smith, Rose, and Gyorgy, *J. Biol. Chem.*, 208, 299 (1954); 217, 79 (1955).
54. Kuhn and Kirschenlohr, *Justus Liebigs Ann. Chem.*, 600, 135 (1956).
55. Wickberg, *Acta Chem. Scand.*, 12, 1183, 1187 (1959).

OLIGOSACCHARIDES (INCLUDING DISACCHARIDES)

56. Carter, McCluer, and Slifer, *J. Am. Chem. Soc.*, 78, 3735 (1956).
57. Reeves, Latour, and Lousteau, *Biochemistry*, 3, 1248 (1964).
58. Colin, *Bull. Soc. Chim. Fr. Ser. 5*, 4, 277 (1937).
59. Su and Hassid, *Biochemistry*, 1, 468 (1962).
60. Putman and Hassid, *J. Am. Chem. Soc.*, 76, 2221 (1954).
61. Brown and Serro, *J. Am. Chem. Soc.*, 75, 1040 (1953).
62. Kabat, MacDonald, Ballou, and Fischer, *J. Am. Chem. Soc.*, 75, 4507 (1953).
63. Gorin, Horitsu and Spencer, *Can. J. Chem.*, 43, 2259 (1965).
64. Pueyo, *C. R. Acad. Sci.*, 248, 2788 (1959).
65. Lindberg, Silvander, and Wachtmeister, *Acta Chem. Scand.*, 18, 213 (1964).
66. Kooiman, *Recl. Trav. Chim. Pays-Bas*, 80, 849 (1961).
67. Araki and Arai, *Bull. Chem. Soc. Jap.*, 29, 339 (1956).
68. McCready, McComb, and Black, *J. Am. Chem. Soc.*, 76, 3035 (1954).
69. Bhattacharjee and Timell, *Can. J. Chem.*, 43, 758 (1965).
70. Gee, Jones, and McCready, *J. Org. Chem.*, 23, 620 (1958).
71. Nagel and Vaughn, *Arch. Biochem. Biophys.*, 94, 328 (1961).
72. Avigad, *Biochem. J.*, 73, 587 (1959).
73. Hudson and Pacsu, *J. Am. Chem. Soc.*, 52, 2519 (1930).
74. Pacsu, *J. Am. Chem. Soc.*, 54, 3649 (1932).
75. Hough, Jones, and Richards, *J. Chem. Soc.* (Lond.), p. 2005 (1953).
76. Stodola, Koepsell, and Sharpe, *J. Am. Chem. Soc.*, 74, 3202 (1952); 78, 2514 (1956).
77. Bourne, Hutson, and Weigel, *Biochem. J.*, 79, 549 (1961).
78. Weidenhagen and Lorenz, *Angew. Chem.*, 69, 641 (1957).
79. Bourne, Hartigan, and Weigel, *J. Chem. Soc.* (Lond.), p. 1088 (1961).
80. Knox, *Biochem. J.*, 94, 534 (1965).
81. Goldstein and Whelan, *J. Chem. Soc.* (Lond.), p. 4264 (1963).
82. Birch, *J. Chem. Soc.* (Lond.), p. 3489 (1965).
83. Peat, Whelan, and Hinson, *Nature*, 170, 1056 (1952).
84. Sharp and Stacey, *J. Chem. Soc.* (Lond.), p. 285 (1951).
85. Micheel and Hagel, *Ber. Dtsch. Chem. Ges.*, 85, 1087 (1952).
86. Matsuda, *J. Agric. Chem. Soc. Jap.*, 30, 119 (1956).
87. Takiura and Koizuma, *Yakugaku Zasshi*, 82, 852 (1962).
88. Bailey, Barker, Bourne, Grant, and Stacey, *J. Chem. Soc.* (Lond.), p. 1895 (1958).
89. Peat, Whelan, and Hinson, *Chem. Ind.*, p. 385 (1955).
90. Sato and Aso, *Nature*, 180, 984 (1957).
91. Freudenberg, Knauber, and Cramer, *Ber. Dtsch. Chem. Ges.*, 84, 114 (1951).
92. Finan and Warren, *J. Chem. Soc.* (Lond.), p. 5229 (1963).
93. Vis and Fletcher, *J. Am. Chem. Soc.*, 78, 4709 (1956).
94. Rabate, *Bull. Soc. Chim. Fr. Ser. 5*, 7, 565 (1940).
95. Haq and Whelan, *J. Chem. Soc.* (Lond.), p. 1342 (1958).
96. Watanabe and Aso, *J. Agr. Res.* (Tokyo), 11, 109 (1960).
97. Wolfrom and Thompson, *J. Am. Chem. Soc.*, 77, 6403 (1955); 78, 4116 (1956).
98. Weismann and Meyer, *J. Am. Chem. Soc.*, 76, 1753 (1954).
99. Freudenberg and Oertzen, *Justus Liebigs Ann. Chem.*, 574, 37 (1951).
100. Connell, Hirst, and Percival, *J. Chem. Soc.* (Lond.), p. 3494 (1950).
101. Peat, Whelan, and Lawley, *J. Chem. Soc.* (Lond.), p. 724, 729 (1958).
102. Peterson and Spencer, *J. Am. Chem. Soc.*, 49, 2822 (1927).
103. Gillis, *Natuurwet. Tijdschr.*, 12, 193 (1930); *Chem. Zentralbl.*, 1, 256 (1931).
104. Hudson and Yanovsky, *J. Am. Chem. Soc.*, 39, 1013 (1917).
105. Wolfrom, Georges, and Miller, *J. Am. Chem. Soc.*, 71, 125 (1949).
106. Jeanes, Wilham, Jones, Tsuchiya, and Rist, *J. Am. Chem. Soc.*, 75, 5911 (1953).
107. Zemplén, *Hoppe-Seyler's Z. Physiol. Chem.*, 85, 399 (1913).
108. Hudson and Johnson, *J. Am. Chem. Soc.*, 39, 1272 (1917).
109. Thompson and Wolfrom, *J. Am. Chem. Soc.*, 75, 3605 (1953).
110. Selinger and Schramm, *J. Biol. Chem.*, 236, 2183 (1961).
111. Baytop, Tanher, Tekman, and Oner, *Folia Pharm.* (Istanbul), 4, 464 (1960).
112. Korte, *Ber. Dtsch. Chem. Ges.*, 88, 1527 (1955).
113. Frérejacque, *C. R. Acad. Sci.*, 246, 459 (1958).

OLIGOSACCHARIDES (INCLUDING DISACCHARIDES)

114. Arcamone and Bizioli, *Gazz. Chim. Ital.*, 87, 896 (1957).
115. Wolfrom, Vercellotti, and Horton, *J. Org. Chem.*, 27, 705 (1962); 28, 278 (1963).
116. Barker, Gomez-Sanchez, and Stacey, *J. Chem. Soc.* (Lond.), p. 3264 (1959).
117. Sawai and Hehre, *J. Biol. Chem.*, 237, 2047 (1962).
118. Jermyn, *Aust. J. Biol. Sci.*, 11, 114 (1958).
119. Dutton and Unrau, *Can. J. Chem.*, 42, 2048 (1964).
120. Lindberg, *Acta Chem. Scand.*, 7, 1119 (1953).
121. Lindberg, Silvander, and Wachtmeister, *Acta Chem. Scand.*, 17, 1348 (1963).
122. Meier, *Acta Chem. Scand.*, 14, 749 (1960).
123. Perila and Bishop, *Can. J. Chem.*, 39, 815 (1961).
124. Gyaw and Timell, *Can. J. Chem.*, 38, 1957 (1960).
125. Palleroni and Doudoroff, *J. Biol. Chem.*, 219, 957 (1956).
126. Tunmann and Schehrer, *Arch. Pharm.*, 292, 745 (1959).
127. Hassid, Doudoroff, Barker, and Dore, *J. Am. Chem. Soc.*, 67, 1394 (1945).
128. Hassid, Doudoroff, Barker, and Dore, *J. Am. Chem. Soc.*, 68, 1465 (1946).
129. Barker, Bourne, Hewitt, and Stacey, *J. Chem. Soc.* (Lond.), p. 3541 (1957).
130. Barker, Stackey, and Stroud, *Nature*, 189, 138 (1961).
131. Putman, Litt, and Hassid, *J. Am. Chem. Soc.*, 77, 4351 (1955).
132. Yosizawa, *Biochim. Biophys. Acta*, 52, 588 (1961).
133. Lloyd and Roberts, *J. Chem. Soc.* (Lond.), p. 6910 (1965).
134. Kuhn and Kirschenlohr, *Ber. Dtsch. Chem. Ges.*, 87, 384 (1954).
135. Sharon, Osawa, Flowers, and Jeanloz, *J. Biol. Chem.*, 241, 223 (1966).
136. Tipper, Ghuysen, and Strominger, *Biochemistry*, 4, 468 (1965).
137. Flowers and Jeanloz, *J. Org. Chem.*, 28, 1564 (1963).
138. Osawa and Nakazawa, *Biochim. Biophys. Acta*, 130, 56 (1966).
139. Barker, Foster, Stacey, and Webber, *Chem. Ind.*, p. 208 (1957); *J. Chem. Soc.* (Lond.), p. 2218 (1958).
140. Barker, Foster, Khmelnitski, and Webber, *Bull. Soc. Chim. Biol.*, 42, 1799 (1960).
141. Danishefsky and Steiner, *Biochim. Biophys. Acta*, 101, 37 (1965).
142. Tipper and Strominger, *Biochem. Biophys. Res. Commun.*, 22, 48 (1966).
143. Martinez, Wolfe, and Nakada, *J. Bacteriol.*, 78, 217 (1959).
144. Olavesen and Davidson, *J. Biol. Chem.*, 240, 992 (1965).
145. Wolfrom, Madison, and Cron, *J. Am. Chem. Soc.*, 74, 1491 (1952).
146. Weissmann and Meyer, *J. Am. Chem. Soc.*, 74, 4729 (1952); 76, 1753 (1954).
147. Jeanloz and Jeanloz, *Biochemistry*, 3, 121 (1964).
148. Linker, Meyer, and Hoffman, *J. Biol. Chem.*, 219, 13 (1956).
149. Leach and Teeters, *J. Am. Chem. Soc.*, 73, 2794 (1951); 74, 3187 (1952).
150. Carter, Dyer, Shaw, Rinehart, and Hichens, *J. Am. Chem. Soc.*, 83, 3723 (1961).
151. Ito, Nishio, and Ogawa, *J. Antibiot. Ser. A*, 17, 189 (1964).
152. Suhara, Maeda, Umezawa, and Ohno, *Tetrahedron Lett.*, 1239 (1966).
153. Fukui, Hochster, Durbin, Grebner, and Feingold, *Bull. Res. Counc. Isr.*, 11A, 262 (1963).
154. Fukui and Hochster, *Can. J. Biochem.*, 41, 2363, (1963).
155. Gorin, Haskins, and Spencer, *Can. J. Biochem. Physiol.*, 38, 165 (1960).
156. Gorin and Perlin, *Can. J. Chem.*, 39, 2474 (1961).
157. Tyminski and Timell, *J. Am. Chem. Soc.*, 82, 2823 (1960).
158. Merler and Wise, *Tappi*, 41, 80 (1958).
159. Colin and Angier, *C. R. Acad. Sci.*, 208, 1450 (1939).
160. Jones and Painter, *J. Chem. Soc.* (Lond.), p. 669 (1959).
161. Jones and Nicholson, *J. Chem. Soc.* (Lond.), p. 27 (1958).
162. Whistler and Stein, *J. Am. Chem. Soc.*, 73, 4187 (1951).
163. Tsujino, *Agric. Biol. Chem.*, 27, 236 (1963).
164. Zemplén and Gerecs, *Ber. Dtsch. Chem. Ges.*, 68, 2054 (1935).
165. Zemplén, Gerecs, and Flesch, *Ber. Dtsch. Chem. Ges.*, 71, 774 (1938).
166. Charaux, *C. R. Acad. Sci.*, 178, 1312 (1924); 180, 1419 (1925).
167. Gorin and Perlin, *Can. J. Chem.*, 37, 1930 (1959).
168. Zemplén and Gerecs, *Ber. Dtsch. Chem. Ges.*, 71, 2520 (1938).
169. Hestrin, Feingold, and Avigad, *J. Am. Chem. Soc.*, 77, 6710 (1955).
170. Power and Salway, *J. Chem. Soc.* (Lond.), p. 1062 (1914).
171. Amanmuradov and Abubakirov, *Chem. Nat. Compd.* (USSR), 1, 292 (1965).
172. Helferich and Rouch, *Justus Liebigs Ann. Chem.*, 455, 168 (1927).

OLIGOSACCHARIDES (INCLUDING DISACCHARIDES)

173. Howard, *Biochem. J.*, 67, 643 (1957).
174. Curtis and Jones, *Can. J. Chem.*, 38, 1305 (1960).
175. Ball and Jones, *J. Chem. Soc.* (Lond.), p. 33 (1958).
176. Whistler, Bachrack, and Tu, *J. Am. Chem. Soc.*, 74, 3059 (1952).
177. Bishop, *J. Am. Chem. Soc.*, 78, 2840 (1956).
178. Banerji and Rao, *Aust. J. Chem.*, 17, 1059 (1964).
179. Pazur, *J. Am. Chem. Soc.*, 75, 6323 (1953).
180. Schlubach and Berndt, *Justus Liebigs Ann. Chem.*, 677, 172 (1964).
181. Strepkov, *Zh. Obshch. Khim.*, 9, 1489 (1939).
182. Bacon, *Nature*, 184, 1957 (1959).
183. Pridham, *Biochem. J.*, 76, 13 (1960).
184. Barker and Carrington, *J. Chem. Soc.* (Lond.), p. 3588 (1953).
185. Haq and Adams, *Can. J. Chem.*, 39, 1165 (1961).
186. Allen and Bacon, *Biochem. J.*, 63, 200 (1956).
187. Gross, Blanchard, and Bell, *J. Chem. Soc.* (Lond.), p. 1727 (1954).
188. Davy and Courtois, *C. R. Acad. Sci.*, 261, 3483 (1965).
189. Suzuki and Hehre, *Arch. Biochem. Biophys,*. 105, 339 (1964).
190. French, Wild, Young, and James, *J. Am. Chem. Soc.*, 75, 709, 3664 (1953).
191. Rege, Painter, Watkins, and Morgan, *Nature*, 204, 740 (1964).
192. Wallenfels, Bernt, and Limberg, *Justus Liebigs Ann. Chem.*, 579, 113 (1952).
193. Ballio and Russi, *Tetrahedron*, 9, 125 (1960).
194. Tanret, *Bull. Soc. Chim. Fr. Ser. 3*, 27, 947 (1902).
195. Pazur, Marsh, and Tipton, *J. Am. Chem. Soc.*, 80, 1433 (1958).
196. Sastry and Kates, *Biochemistry*, 3, 1271 (1964).
197. Petek, Villarroya, and Courtois, *C. R. Acad. Sci.*, 265D, 195 (1966).
198. Wickstrom and Baerheim-Svendsen, *Acta Chem. Scand.*, 10, 1199 (1956).
199. MacLeod and McCorquodale, *Nature*, 182, 815 (1958).
200. Avigad, *J. Biol. Chem.*, 229, 121 (1957).
201. Aso and Yamauchi, *Agric. Biol. Chem.*, 25, 10 (1961).
202. Haworth, Hirst, and Ruell, *J. Chem. Soc.*, p. 3125 (1923).
203. Scheibler and Mittelmeier, *Ber. Dtsch. Chem. Ges.*, 23, 1438 (1890).
204. Tanret, *Bull. Soc. Chim. Fr. Ser. 3*, 13, 261 (1895).
205. Montreuil, *C. R. Acad. Sci.*, 242, 192, 828 (1956).
206. Bailey, Barker, Bourne, and Stacey, *Nature*, 176, 1164 (1955).
207. Yamauchi and Aso, *Nature*, 189, 753 (1961).
208. Brandish, Shaw, and Baddiley, *J. Chem. Soc. Sect. C Org. Chem.*, p. 521 (1966).
209. Jones and Reid, *J. Chem. Soc.* (Lond.), p. 1361 (1954); p. 1890 (1955).
210. Kurasawa, Yamamoto, Igaue and Nakamura, *Nippon Nogei-Kagaku Kaishi*, 30, 624 (1956).
211. Schlubach and Koehn, *Justus Liebigs Ann. Chem.*, 614, 126 (1958).
212. Binkley, *Int. Sugar J.*, 66, 46 (1964).
213. Barker, Bourne, and Carrington, *J. Chem. Soc.* (Lond.), p. 2125 (1954).
214. Bacon and Bell, *J. Chem. Soc.* (Lond.), p. 2528 (1953).
215. Albon, Bell, Blanchard, Gross, and Rundell, *J. Chem. Soc.* (Lond.), p. 24 (1953).
216. Courtois, LeDizet, and Petek, *Bull. Soc. Chim. Biol.*, 41, 1261 (1959).
217. Kuhn and von Grundherr, *Ber. Dtsch. Chem. Ges.*, 59, 1655 (1926).
218. Von Lippmann, *Ber. Dtsch. Chem. Ges.*, 60, 161 (1927).
219. Hudson and Sherwood, *J. Am. Chem. Soc.*, 40, 1456 (1918).
220. White and Maher, *J. Am. Chem. Soc.*, 75, 1259 (1953).
221. Wolf and Ewart, *Arch. Biochem. Biophys.*, 58, 365 (1955).
222. Takiura and Nakagawa, *Yakugaku Zasshi*, 83, 301, 305 (1963).
223. Barker, Bourne, and Theander, *J. Chem. Soc.* (Lond.), p. 2064 (1957).
224. Baron and Guthrie, *Ann. Entomol. Soc. Am.*, 53, 220 (1960).
225. Meyer, *Hoppe-Seyler's Z. Physiol. Chem.*, 6, 135 (1882).
226. Binaghi and Falqui, *Chem. Zentralbl.*, 2, 44 (1926).
227. Krieglstein and Fischer, *Hoppe-Seyler's Z. Physiol. Chem.*, 344, 209 (1966).
228. Feingold, Neufeld, and Hassid, *J. Biol. Chem.*, 233, 783 (1958).
229. Perlin and Suzuki, *Can. J. Chem.*, 40, 50 (1962).
230. Peat, Whelan, and Roberts, *J. Chem. Soc.* (Lond.), p. 3916 (1957).

OLIGOSACCHARIDES (INCLUDING DISACCHARIDES)

231. Barker, Bourne, O'Mant, and Stacey, *J. Chem. Soc.* (Lond.), p. 2448 (1957).
232. Reese and Mandels, *Can. J. Microbiol.*, 10, 103 (1964).
233. Moscatelli, Ham, and Rickes, *J. Biol. Chem.*, 236, 2858 (1961).
234. Wolfrom, Georges, Thompson, and Miller, *J. Am. Chem. Soc.*, 71, 2873 (1949).
235. Peat, Whelan, and Jones, *J. Chem. Soc.* (Lond.), p. 2490 (1957).
236. Sugihara and Wolfrom, *J. Am. Chem. Soc.*, 71, 3357 (1949).
237. Walker and Wright, *Arch. Biochem. Biophys.*, 69, 362 (1957).
238. Wolfrom and Fields, *Tappi*, 41, 204 (1958).
239. French, Taylor, and Whelan, *Biochem. J.*, 90, 616 (1964).
240. Bailey, Barker, Bourne, and Stacey, *J. Chem. Soc.* (Lond.), p. 3536 (1957).
241. Wolfrom, Thompson, and Galkowski, *J. Am. Chem. Soc.*, 73, 4093 (1951).
242. Turvey and Whelan, *Biochem. J.*, 67, 49 (1957).
243. Conchie, Moreno, and Cardini, *Arch. Biochem. Biophys.*, 94, 342 (1961).
244. Haq and Whelan, *J. Chem. Soc.* (Lond.), p. 4543 (1956).
245. Peat, Whelan, and Evans, *J. Chem. Soc.* (Lond.), p. 175 (1960).
246. Schwarz and Timell, *Can. J. Chem.*, 41, 1381 (1963).
247. Kuehl, Peck, Hoffhine, Graber, and Folkers, *J. Am. Chem. Soc.*, 68, 1460 (1946).
248. Bannister and Argoudelis, *J. Am. Chem. Soc.*, 85, 119, 234 (1963).
249. Zechmeister and Toth, *Ber. Dtsch. Chem. Ges.*, 65, 161 (1932).
250. Linker, Meyer, and Weissmann, *J. Biol. Chem.*, 213, 237 (1955).
251. Umezawa, Ueda, Maeda, Yagashita, Kondo, Okami, Utahara, Osato, Nitta, and Takeushi, *J. Antibiot. Ser. A.*, 23, 298 (1957).
252. Cron, Johnson, Palermiti, Perron, Taylor, Whitehead, and Hooper, *J. Am. Chem. Soc.*, 80, 752 (1958).
253. Kondo, Sezaki, Koike, Shimura, Akita, Satoh, and Hara, *J. Antibiot. Ser. A*, 18, 38 (1965).
254. Kondo, Akita, and Koike, *J. Antibiot. Ser. A*, 19, 139 (1966).
255. Schneir and Rafelson, *Biochim. Biophys. Acta*, 130, 1 (1966).
256. Kuhn and Brossmer, *Ber. Dtsch. Chem. Ges.*, 92, 1667 (1959).
257. Ryan, Carubelli, Caputto, and Trucco, *Biochim. Biophys. Acta*, 101, 252 (1965); *J. Biol. Chem.*, 236, 2381 (1961).
258. Lindberg, *Acta Chem. Scand.*, 9, 1093, 1097 (1955).
259. Aspinall, Begbie, and McKay, *J. Chem. Soc.* (Lond.), p. 214 (1962).
260. Mayeda, *J. Biochem.* (Tokyo), 1, 131 (1922).
261. Ohtsuki, *Acta Phytochim.* (Japan), 4, 1 (1928).
262. Whistler and Masak, *J. Am. Chem. Soc.*, 77, 1241 (1955).
263. Marchessault and Timell, *J. Polymer. Sci. C.*, 2, 49 (1963).
264. Murakami, *Acta Phytochim.*, 14, 101 (1944); 15, 105, 109 (1949).
265. Schlubach and Berndt, *Justus Liebigs Ann. Chem.*, 647, 41 (1961).
266. Pazur, *J. Biol. Chem.*, 199, 217 (1952).
267. Kuhn and Gauhe, *Justus Liebigs Ann. Chem.*, 611, 249 (1958).
268. Hatanaka, *Arch. Biochem. Biophys.*, 82, 188 (1959).
269. French, Wild, and James, *J. Am. Chem. Soc.*, 75, 3664 (1953).
270. Onuki, *Sci. Pap. Inst. Phys. Chem. Res.* (Tokyo), 20, 201 (1933).
271. Laidlaw and Wylam, *J. Chem. Soc.* (Lond.), p. 567 (1953).
272. Davy and Courtois, *C. R. Acad. Sci.*, 261, 3483 (1965).
273. Araki and Arai, *Bull. Chem. Soc. Jap.*, 30, 287 (1957).
274. Courtois and Ariyoshi, *Bull. Soc. Chim. Biol.* (Paris), 42, 737 (1960).
275. Demain and Phaff, *Arch. Biochem. Biophys.*, 51, 114 (1954).
276. Binkley and Altenburg, *Int. Sugar J.*, 67, 110 (1965).
277. Kurasawa, Yamamoto, Igaue, and Nakamura, *Nippon Nogei Kagaku Kaishi*, 30, 696 (1956).
278. Strepkov, *Dokl. Akad. Nauk SSSR*, 125, 216 (1959).
279. Schlubach and Koehn, *Justus Liebigs Ann. Chem.*, 606, 130 (1957).
280. Parrish, Perlin, and Reese, *Can. J. Chem.*, 38, 2094 (1960).
281. Perlin and Suzuki, *Can. J. Chem.*, 40, 50 (1962).
282. Igarashi, Igoshi, and Sakurai, *Agric. Biol. Chem.*, 30, 1254 (1966).
283. Whistler and Hickson, *J. Am. Chem. Soc.*, 76, 1671 (1954).
284. Wolfrom and Fields, *Tappi*, 41, 204 (1958); 40, 335 (1957).
285. Duncan and Manners, *Biochem. J.*, 69, 343 (1958).
286. Jones, Jeanes, Stringer, and Tsuchiya, *J. Am. Chem. Soc.*, 78, 2499 (1956).
287. Akiya, *J. Pharm. Soc. Jap.*, 58, 71 (1938).
288. Salton and Ghuysen, *Biochim. Biophys. Acta*, 45, 355 (1960).

OLIGOSACCHARIDES (INCLUDING DISACCHARIDES)

289. Weissman, Meyer, Sampson, and Linker, *J. Biol. Chem.*, 208, 417 (1954).
290. Rinehart, Hichens, Argoudelis, Chilton, Carter, Georgiadis, Schaffner, and Schillings, *J. Am. Chem. Soc.*, 84, 3218 (1962).
291. Rinehart, Argoudelis, Goss, Sohler, and Schaffner, *J. Am. Chem. Soc.*, 82, 3938 (1960).
292. Haskell, French, and Bartz, *J. Am. Chem. Soc.*, 81, 3482 (1959).
293. Fried and Titus, *J. Biol. Chem.*, 168, 391 (1947).
294. Goldschmid and Perlin, *Can. J. Chem.*, 41, 2272 (1963).
295. Kihara, *Proc. Imp. Acad.* (Tokyo), 5, 349 (1929); 11, 552 (1935); *J. Agric. Chem. Soc.* (Japan), 12, 1044 (1936).
296. Schlubach, Berndt, and Chiemprasert, *Justus Liebigs Ann. Chem.*, 665, 191 (1963).
297. Kuhn, Baer, and Gauhe, *Ber. Dtsch. Chem. Ges.*, 91, 364 (1958).
298. Kuhn and Gauhe, *Ber. Dtsch. Chem. Ges.*, 95, 513 (1962).
299. Bourquelot and Bridel, *C. R. Acad. Sci.*, 151, 760 (1910).
300. Murakami, *Proc. Imp. Acad.* (Tokyo), 16, 14 (1940).
301. Zechmeister and Toth, *Ber. Dtsch. Chem. Ges.*, 64, 854 (1931).
302. Hoover, Nelson, Milner, and Wei, *J. Food Sci.*, 30, 253 (1965).
303. Wolfrom, Dacons, and Fields, *Tappi*, 39, 803 (1956).
304. Kuhn and Gauhe, *Ber. Dtsch. Chem. Ges.*, 93, 647 (1960).
305. Murakami, *Acta Phytochim.*, 13, 37 (1942).
306. Herissey, Fleury, Wickstrom, Courtois, and Dizet, *C.R. Acad. Sci.*, 239, 824 (1954); *Bull. Soc. Chim. Biol.* (Paris), 36, 1507 (1954).
307. Akiya and Tomoda, *J. Pharm. Soc. Jap.*, 76, 571 (1956).
308. French and Rundle, *J. Am. Chem. Soc.*, 64, 1651 (1942).
309. Fruedenberg and Jacobi, *Justus Liebigs Ann. Chem.*, 518, 102 (1935).
310. Akiya and Watanabe, *J. Pharm. Soc. Jap.*, 70, 576 (1950).
311. Bjorndel, Eriksson, Garegg, Lindberg, and Swan, *Acta Chem. Scand.*, 19, 2309 (1965).
312. Whistler and Tu, *J. Am. Chem. Soc.*, 74, 3609 (1952); 75, 645 (1954).
313. Murakami, *Acta Phytochim.*, 10, 43 (1937).
314. Courtois, Dizet, and Wickstrom, *Bull. Soc. Chim. Biol.* (Paris), 40, 1059 (1958).
315. Malpress and Hytten, *Biochem. J.*, 68, 708 (1958).
316. French, Knapp, and Pazur, *J. Am. Chem. Soc.*, 72, 5150 (1950).
317. Clancy and Whelan, *Arch. Biochem. Biophys.*, 118, 724, 730 (1967).
318. Morgan and O'Neill, *Can. J. Chem.*, 37, 1201 (1959).
319. Tanret, *Bull. Soc. Chim. Fr. Ser. 3*, 21, 1065 (1899).
320. Maher, unpublished results (1957).
321. Herissey, Fleury, Wickstrom, Courtois, and Dizet, *Bull. Soc. Chim. Biol.* (Paris), 36, 1507 (1964).
322. Aspinall and Telfer, *J. Chem. Soc.* (Lond.), p. 1106 (1955).
323. Anderson, *Acta Chem. Scand.*, 21, 828 (1967).
324. Allgeier, *Helv. Chim. Acta*, 51, 668 (1968).
325. Glaudemans, *Carbohydr. Res.*, 10, 213 (1969).
326. Anderson, Dolan, and Rees, *J. Chem. Soc. Sect. C Org. Chem.*, p. 596 (1968).
327. Alexander, *Arch. Biochem. Biophys.*, 123, 240 (1968).
328. Levene and Tipson, *J. Biol. Chem.*, 125, 355 (1938).
329. Manners and Stark, *Carbohydr. Res.*, 3, 102 (1966).
330. Umezawa, Tatsuta, and Muto, *J. Antibiot. Ser. A*, 20, 388 (1967).
331. Brundish and Baddiley, *Carbohydr. Res.*, 8, 308 (1968).
332. Ferrier and Prasad, *J. Chem. Soc.* (Lond.), p. 7429 (1965).
333. Zatula and Kolesnikov, *Chem. Natur. Compd.* (USSR), 3, 138 (1967).
334. Saier and Ballou, *J. Biol. Chem.*, 243, 992 (1968).
335. Shapiro, Acher, and Rachaman, *J. Org. Chem.*, 32, 3767 (1967).
336. Duncan, Manners, and Thompson, *Biochem. J.*, 73, 295 (1959).
337. Olavesen and Davidson, *Biochim. Biophys. Acta*, 101, 245 (1965).
338. Umezawa, Tatsuta, Tsuchiya, and Kitazawa, *J. Antibiot. Ser. A*, 20, 53 (1967).
339. Hayano and Fukui, *J. Biochem.* (Tokyo), 64, 901 (1968).
340. Uramoto, Otake, and Yonehara, *J. Antibiot. Antibiot. Ser. A*, 20, 236 (1967).
341. Srivastava and Singh, *Carbohydr. Res.*, 4, 326 (1967).
342. Bollman, Hirschmüller, and Schmidt-Berg-Lorenz, *Int. Sugar J.*, 67, 143 (1965).
343. Beith-Halahmi and Flowers, *Carbohydr. Res.*, 81, 340 (1968).
344. Urbas, *Can. J. Chem.*, 46, 49 (1968).

OLIGOSACCHARIDES (INCLUDING DISACCHARIDES)

345. Fischer and Krieglstein, *Hoppe-Seyler's Z. Physiol. Chem.*, 348, 1252 (1967).
346. Siddiqui and Furgala, *Carbohydr. Res.*, 6, 250 (1968).
347. Fischer and Seyferth, *Hoppe-Seyler's Z. Physiol. Chem.*, 349, 1662 (1968).
348. Pollock, Chipman, and Sharon, *Arch. Biochem. Biophys.*, 120, 235 (1967).
349. Umezawa, Tatsuta, and Koto, *J. Antibiot. Ser. A*, 21, 367 (1968); *Bull. Chem. Soc. Jap.*, 42, 533 (1969).
350. Hasegawa, Kurihara, Nishimura, and Nakajima, *Agric. Biol. Chem.*, 32, 1130 (1968).
351. Murase, *J. Antibiot. (Tokyo) Ser. A*, 14, 156, 367 (1961).
352. Umezawa, Koto, Tatsuta, and Tsumura, *Bull. Chem. Soc. Jap.*, 42, 529 (1969).
353. Ito, Nishio, and Ogawa, *J. Antibiot. Ser. A*, 17, 189 (1964).
354. Umezawa, Koto, Tatsuta, Hineno, Nishimura, and Tsumura, *J. Antibiot. Ser. A*, 21, 424 (1968).
355. Leyh-Bouille, Ghuysen, Tipper, and Strominger, *Biochemistry*, 5, 3079 (1966).
356. Tung and Nordin, *Biochim. Biophys. Acta*, 158, 154 (1968).
357. Barker, Bourne, Grant, and Stacey, *J. Chem. Soc.* (Lond.), p. 601 (1958).

OLIGOSACCHARIDES (INCLUDING DISACCHARIDES)

Substance[a] (synonym)	Derivative	Chemical formula	Melting point °C	Specific rotation[b] $[\alpha]_D$	Reference
(A)	(B)	(C)	(D)	(E)	(F)
		Disaccharides			
O-α-L-Ara$f$-(1→3)-L-Ara		$C_{10}H_{18}O_9$	–	0	4
O-β-L-Ara$f$-(1→3)-L-Ara$f$		$C_{10}H_{18}O_9$	–	+89, +94	1, 2
	Phenylosazone	$C_{22}H_{30}N_4O_7$	200	–	1, 2
O-β-L-Ara$p$-(1→3)-L-Ara$f$		$C_{10}H_{18}O_9$		–	3
O-α-L-Ara$f$-(1→5)-L-Ara$f$		$C_{10}H_{18}O_9$	–	-72, -87	2, 4
	Phenylosazone	$C_{22}H_{30}N_4O_7$	177	–	2, 4
O-β-L-Ara$p$-(1→4)-L-Ara		$C_{10}H_{18}O_9$	–	+193	5
	Hexaacetate	$C_{22}H_{30}O_{15}$	167	–	5
O-α-L-Ara$p$-(1→5)-L-Ara		$C_{10}H_{18}O_9$	143	-14→-18	4
O-L-Ara$f$-(1→3)-D-Xyl		$C_{10}H_{18}O_9$	–		6
O-β-L-Ara$p$-(1→2)-D-Glc		$C_{11}H_{20}O_{10}$	210-220	+151	7
O-α-L-Ara$p$-(1→3)-D-Glc		$C_{11}H_{20}O_{10}$	176-178	+54.4	8
O-α-L-Ara$p$-(1→4)-D-Glc		$C_{11}H_{20}O_{10}$	–	+41.9	8
O-α-L-Ara$f$-(1→6)-D-Glc	Heptaacetate	$C_{25}H_{34}O_{17}$	108	-20	9
O-α-L-Ara$p$-(1→6)-D-Glc		$C_{11}H_{20}O_{10}$	210	+37.2, +56	8, 10
O-β-L-Ara$f$-(1→6)-D-Glc		$C_{11}H_{20}O_{10}$	–	+73	9
O-L-Ara$f$-(1→6)-D-Gal		$C_{11}H_{20}O_{10}$			11
O-L-Ara-(1→?)-D-Man	Heptaacetate	$C_{25}H_{34}O_{17}$	147-149	–	12
O-β-D-Xyl$p$-(1→2)-L-Ara		$C_{10}H_{18}O_9$	167-168	+32→+33	13
O-α-D-Xyl$p$-(1→3)-L-Ara		$C_{10}H_{18}O_9$	117-119	+173→+182	14
	Hexaacetate	$C_{22}H_{30}O_{15}$	168-170	+106	14
O-α-Xyl-(1→5)-L-Ara		$C_{10}H_{18}O_9$	–	+74	15
O-β-D-Xyl$p$-(1→5)-L-Ara		$C_{10}H_{18}O_9$	–	-41→-47	16, 17
O-α-D-Xyl$p$-(1→2)-D-Xyl		$C_{10}H_{18}O_9$	–	–	18
O-α-D-Xyl$p$-(1→3)-D-Xyl		$C_{10}H_{18}O_9$	178	+118	19
O-β-D-Xyl$p$-(1→3)-D-Xyl		$C_{10}H_{18}O_9$	192-193	-18.4→-22	20
(Rhodymenabiose)	Phenylosazone	$C_{22}H_{30}N_4O_7$	194-196	+47	20
O-α-D-Xyl$p$-(1→4)-D-Xyl		$C_{10}H_{18}O_9$	–	–	19
O-β-D-Xyl$p$-(1→4)-D-Xyl		$C_{10}H_{18}O_9$	185-190	-20→-30	21, 22
(Xylobiose)	Hexaacetate	$C_{22}H_{30}O_{15}$	155-156	-74→-75	23
O-β-D-Xyl-(1→6)-D-Gal		$C_{11}H_{20}O_{10}$	194-196	-3.6	24
O-β-D-Xyl$p$-(1→3)-D-Glc		$C_{11}H_{20}O_{10}$	–	–	25
O-D-Xyl$p$-(1→4)-D-Glc$p$		$C_{11}H_{20}O_{10}$	–	+70	284
O-α-D-Xyl$p$-(1→6)-D-Glc		$C_{11}H_{20}O_{10}$	205	+121→+127	26
(Isoprimeverose)	Methylglycoside pentaacetate	$C_{21}H_{30}O_{14}$	123-124	+66	26
O-β-D-Xyl$p$-(1→6)-D-Glc		$C_{11}H_{20}O_{10}$	215	-23	27, 28
(Primeverose)	Phenylosazone	$C_{23}H_{32}N_4O_8$	224-226	–	26, 29
O-α-D-Rib$f$-(1→6)-D-Glc		$C_{11}H_{20}O_{10}$	–	+77	30
O-β-D-Rib$f$-(1→6)-D-Glc		$C_{11}H_{20}O_{10}$	–	0	30
	Heptaacetate	$C_{25}H_{34}O_{17}$	108-110	+3	30
O-α-D-Xyl$p$-(1→2)-β-D-Fru$f$		$C_{11}H_{20}O_{10}$	–	+62	283
O-D-Gal$p$-(1→2)-D-Ara		$C_{11}H_{20}O_{10}$	143-144	+34.4	31
	Heptaacetate	$C_{25}H_{34}O_{17}$	139-142	+40.6(CHCl₃)	31
O-β-D-Gal$p$-(1→3)-D-Ara		$C_{11}H_{20}O_{10}$	166-168	-55→-65	32
	Heptaacetate	$C_{25}H_{34}O_{17}$	154	-80.8(CHCl₃)	32
O-α-D-Gal$p$-(1→3)-L-Ara$f$	Heptamethyl ether	$C_{18}H_{34}O_{10}$	–	+102(CHCl₃)	33

[a] In the order of pentose, hexose, methylpentose, hexosamine, hexuronic acid, and sialic acid at the nonreducing end of the oligosaccharide, arranged within the groups–disaccharides, trisaccharides, etc. Oligosaccharides which have other component than sugar are entered at the end of each group.

[b] $[\alpha]_D$ for 1–5 g solute, c, per 100 ml aqueous solution at 20–25°C unless otherwise noted.

OLIGOSACCHARIDES (INCLUDING DISACCHARIDES) (continued)

Substance[a] (synonym)	Derivative	Chemical formula	Melting point °C	Specific rotation[b] $[\alpha]_D$	Reference
(A)	(B)	(C)	(D)	(E)	(F)

Disaccharides (continued)

Substance[a] (synonym)	Derivative	Chemical formula	Melting point °C	Specific rotation[b] $[\alpha]_D$	Reference
O-β-D-Gal*p*-(1→4)-L-Ara*p*		$C_{11}H_{20}O_{10}$	177–178	+30→+45	34
	Methyl β-glycoside	$C_{12}H_{22}O_{10}$	216–218	+163	34
O-β-D-Gal*p*-(1→5)-L-Ara*f*		$C_{11}H_{20}O_{10}$	–	-13, -18	35, 36
O-β-D-Gal*f*-(1→2)-D-Arabinitol (Umbilicin)		$C_{11}H_{22}O_{10}$	138–139	-81	37
	Octaacetate	$C_{27}H_{38}O_{18}$	84–85	-20(CHCl₃)	37
O-β-D-Gal*p*-(1→4)-D-Arabinitol		$C_{11}H_{22}O_{10}$	178–181	–	34
O-β-D-Gal*p*-(1→2)-D-Xyl		$C_{11}H_{20}O_{10}$	159–160	+25, +30	34, 38
O-β-D-Gal*p*-(1→3)-D-Xyl		$C_{11}H_{20}O_{10}$	196–200	+27→+10	34
O-β-D-Gal*p*-(1→4)-D-Xyl		$C_{11}H_{20}O_{10}$	201–211	+15	38
O-β-D-Gal*p*-(1→3)-D-Rib		$C_{11}H_{20}O_{10}$	200–202	+2→+15	39
O-β-D-Gal*p*-(1→5)-D-Rib		$C_{11}H_{20}O_{10}$	–	–	34
O-α-D-Gal*p*-(1→3)-D-Gal		$C_{12}H_{22}O_{11}$	–	+161	40
	Octaacetate	$C_{28}H_{38}O_{19}$	157.5–158.5	+110.2 (*c* 0.5 CHCl₃)	41
O-β-D-Gal*p*-(1→3)-D-Gal		$C_{12}H_{22}O_{11}$	151–152	+69→+55	42
			163–170	+75→+60	43
			204–206	+56	34
O-α-D-Gal*p*-(1→4)-D-Gal		$C_{12}H_{22}O_{11}$	210–211	+172	40, 44
O-β-D-Gal*p*-(1→4)-D-Gal		$C_{12}H_{22}O_{11}$	195–198	+85→+67	34
	Octaacetate	$C_{28}H_{38}O_{19}$	172–173	+57.3(CHCl₃)	45
O-α-D-Gal*f*-(1→5)-D-Gal		$C_{12}H_{22}O_{11}$	–	+133	40
O-β-D-Gal*f*-(1→5)-D-Gal		$C_{12}H_{22}O_{11}$	–	-65	46
O-β-D-Gal*f*-(1→5)-D-Galactitol		$C_{12}H_{24}O_{11}$	149–151	-65	46
O-α-D-Gal*p*-(1→6)-D-Gal (Swietenose)		$C_{12}H_{22}O_{11}$	-	+149	47, 48
	Octaacetate	$C_{28}H_{38}O_{19}$	223–227	+189(*c* 0.5 CHCl₃)	48
O-β-D-Gal*p*-(1→6)-D-Gal		$C_{12}H_{22}O_{11}$	97–100	+26	49, 50
			168–170	+28	51
	Octamethyl ether	$C_{20}H_{38}O_{11}$	68–70	-5.7(CH₃OH)	51
O-α-D-Gal*p*-(1→2)-D-Glc		$C_{12}H_{22}O_{11}$	118–120	+145	52
			155d	+161→+153	53
	Octaacetate	$C_{28}H_{38}O_{19}$	176–178	+153(CHCl₃)	53
O-β-D-Gal*p*-(1→2)-D-Glc		$C_{12}H_{22}O_{11}$	175	+48→+39	54
O-α-D-Gal*p*-(1→3)-D-Glc		$C_{12}H_{22}O_{11}$	169–170	+64.5	55
O-β-D-Gal*p*-(1→3)-D-Glc		$C_{12}H_{22}O_{11}$	167–169	+37(*c* 0.8)	34
	Monohydrate	$C_{12}H_{24}O_{12}$	202–204	+77→+41	56
O-β-D-Gal*p*-(1→4)-α-D-Glc*p* (α-lactose)	Monohydrate	$C_{12}H_{24}O_{12}$	202	+83.5→+52.6	57, 58
	Octaacetate	$C_{28}H_{38}O_{19}$	152	+53.6 (*c* 10, CHCl₃)	59
O-β-D-Gal*p*-(1→4)-β-D-Glc*p* (β-lactose)		$C_{12}H_{22}O_{11}$	252	+34.2→+53.6	60
	Octaacetate	$C_{28}H_{38}O_{19}$	90	-4.7 (*c* 10, CHCl₃)	59
O-α-D-Gal*p*-(1→6)-α-D-Glc (α-Melibiose)		$C_{12}H_{22}O_{11}$	183–184	+166→+142	61
O-α-D-Gal*p*-(1→6)-β-D-Glc (β-Melibiose)		$C_{12}H_{22}O_{11}$	85–86	+123→+143	61
	Octaacetate	$C_{28}H_{38}O_{19}$	177	+102.5	62
O-β-D-Gal*p*-(1→6)-D-Glc (Allolactose)		$C_{12}H_{22}O_{11}$	165,174–176	+25,+37.5	15, 63–65
	Octaacetate	$C_{28}H_{38}O_{19}$	165	-0.5(CHCl₃)	66

OLIGOSACCHARIDES (INCLUDING DISACCHARIDES) (continued)

Substance[a] (synonym) (A)	Derivative (B)	Chemical formula (C)	Melting point °C (D)	Specific rotation[b] $[\alpha]_D$ (E)	Reference (F)

Disaccharides (continued)

Substance[a] (synonym)	Derivative	Chemical formula	Melting point °C	Specific rotation[b] $[\alpha]_D$	Reference
O-β-D-Galp-(1→4)-α-D-Man (α-Epilactose)	Monohydrate	$C_{12}H_{24}O_{12}$	150–160 ⎫		67
			⎬ +30→+38		
O-β-D-Galp-(1→4)-β-D-Man (β-Epilactose)		$C_{12}H_{22}O_{11}$	196–197 ⎭		67
	Octaacetate	$C_{28}H_{38}O_{19}$	96–97		67
O-α-D-Galp-(1→6)-D-Man (Epimelibiose)		$C_{12}H_{22}O_{11}$	201–202	+123→+124	68
O-α-D-Galp-(1→2)-D-Fruf		$C_{12}H_{22}O_{11}$	170	+81.5	85
O-β-D-Galp-(1→2)-D-Fruf		$C_{12}H_{22}O_{11}$	–	–33	49
	Octaacetate	$C_{28}H_{38}O_{19}$	169–170	+41.3(CHCl₃)	69
O-β-D-Galp-(1→3)-D-Fruf		$C_{12}H_{22}O_{11}$	245–246	+78	34
O-β-D-Galp-(1→3)-D-GlcNAc (Lacto-N-biose I)		$C_{14}H_{25}NO_{11}$	166–170	+14	70, 71
O-β-D-Galp-(1→4)-D-GlcNAc (N-Acetyllactosamine)		$C_{14}H_{25}NO_{11}$	168–170	+27→+28	72, 73
	Heptaacetate	$C_{28}H_{39}NO_{18}$	222–223	+61.5	72, 73
O-α-D-Galp-(1→6)-D-GlcNAcp		$C_{14}H_{25}NO_{11}$	138	+118	74
O-β-D-Galp-(1→6)-D-GlcNAcp (N-Acetylallolactosamine)		$C_{14}H_{25}NO_{11}$	157–159	+32.1→+27.3	75, 76
O-α-D-Galp-(1→6)-D-GalNAc		$C_{14}H_{25}NO_{11}$	–	+142	74
O-β-D-Galp-(1→4)-D-ManNAc		$C_{14}H_{25}NO_{11}$	233	+38.5	77
O-β-D-Galp-(1→4)-3,6-anhydro-L-Gal (Agarobiose)		$C_{12}H_{20}O_{10}$	–	–21.5→–16.4	78, 79
	Dimethylacetal	$C_{14}H_{24}O_{10}$	163–166	–36(CH₃OH)	78, 79
O-β-D-Galp-(1→3)-D-6dGlc		$C_{12}H_{22}O_{10}$	246–248	+25	34
O-α-D-Glcp-(1→2)-D-Ara	Heptaacetate	$C_{25}H_{34}O_{17}$	138–140	+46	80
O-β-D-Glcp-(1→2)-D-Ara	Heptaacetate	$C_{25}H_{34}O_{17}$	199–200	–46→–47	81
O-α-D-Glcp-(1→3)-D-Ara	Monohydrate	$C_{11}H_{22}O_{11}$	119–121	+47	82
O-β-D-Glcp-(1→3)-D-Ara		$C_{11}H_{20}O_{10}$	161	–90→–94	83, 84
O-α-D-Glcp-(1→3)-L-Ara	Dihydrate	$C_{11}H_{24}O_{12}$	–	+156	86
O-β-D-Glcp-(1→3)-L-Ara		$C_{11}H_{20}O_{10}$	199–201	+70	34
O-α-D-Glcp-(1→4)-L-Ara		$C_{11}H_{20}O_{10}$	–	–	87
O-α-D-Glcp-(1→2)-D-Xyl	Heptamethyl ether	$C_{18}H_{34}O_6$	–	+109→+112	88, 89
O-β-D-Glcp-(1→2)-D-Xyl		$C_{11}H_{20}O_{10}$	202–206	+7	34
	Phenylosazone	$C_{23}H_{32}N_4O_8$	213–215	–	90
O-α-D-Glcp-(1→3)-D-Xyl		$C_{11}H_{20}O_{10}$	–	+87.5	91
O-β-D-Glcp-(1→3)-D-Xyl		$C_{11}H_{20}O_{10}$	–	–0.6(c 0.4)	90
O-α-D-Glcp-(1→4)-D-Xyl	Dihydrate	$C_{11}H_{24}O_{12}$	78	+97.5	92
O-c-D-Glcp-(1→1)-D-Galf		$C_{12}H_{22}O_{11}$	–	–	72
O-β-D-Glcp-(1→2)-D-Gal		$C_{12}H_{22}O_{11}$	171–172	+42.6	93
O-α-D-Glcp-(1→3)-D-Gal		$C_{12}H_{22}O_{11}$	–	+138	94
O-β-D-Glcp-(1→3)-D-Gal (Solabiose)		$C_{12}H_{22}O_{11}$	200	+35→+40	95
	Octaacetate	$C_{28}H_{38}O_{19}$	75	+27	95
O-α-D-Glcp-(1→4)-D-Gal		$C_{12}H_{22}O_{11}$	–	+140	96
O-β-D-Glcp-(1→4)-D-Gal		$C_{12}H_{22}O_{11}$	246–247	+41.5	97
	Octaacetate	$C_{28}H_{38}O_{19}$	165–166	+26.8	97
O-α-D-Glcp-(1→6)-D-Gal		$C_{12}H_{22}O_{11}$	–	–	98
O-β-D-Glcp-(1→6)-D-Gal		$C_{12}H_{22}O_{11}$	–	+10→+20	98, 99
	Octaacetate	$C_{28}H_{38}O_{19}$	149–150	–	98, 99
O-α-D-Glcp-(1→1)-α-D-Glcp (αα'-Trehalose)		$C_{12}H_{22}O_{11}$	214–216	+199	103
	Octaacetate	$C_{28}H_{38}O_{19}$	98	+162.3(c 10, CHCl₃)	104
O-β-D-Glcp-(1→1)-β-D-Glcp (ββ'-Trehalose)		$C_{12}H_{22}O_{11}$	130–135	–41.5	105, 106
	Octaacetate	$C_{28}H_{38}O_{19}$	181	–19(CHCl₃)	107

OLIGOSACCHARIDES (INCLUDING DISACCHARIDES) (continued)

Substance[a] (synonym) (A)	Derivative (B)	Chemical formula (C)	Melting point °C (D)	Specific rotation[b] $[\alpha]_D$ (E)	Reference (F)
		Disaccharides (continued)			
O-α-D-Glc$p$-(1→1)-β-D-Glc$p$		$C_{12}H_{22}O_{11}$	150–153	+70(c 0.2)	106, 108
(αβ-Trehalose)	Octaacetate	$C_{28}H_{38}O_{19}$	120,140	+67,+82(CHCl₃)	106, 108
O-α-D-Glc$p$-(1→2)-D-Glc		$C_{12}H_{22}O_{11}$	188	+137	100, 101
(Kojibiose)	α-Octaacetate	$C_{28}H_{38}O_{19}$	166	+152(CHCl₃)	113
	β-Octaacetate	$C_{28}H_{38}O_{19}$	118	+112(CHCl₃)	114
O-β-D-Glc$p$-(1→2)-D-Glc		$C_{12}H_{22}O_{11}$	195–196	+20	105, 109, 110
(Sophorose)	α-Octaacetate	$C_{28}H_{38}O_{19}$	111	+45(CHCl₃)	109, 110, 112
	β-Octaacetate	$C_{28}H_{38}O_{19}$	191–192	-8(CHCl₃)	111
O-α-D-Glc$p$-(1→3)-D-Glc		$C_{12}H_{22}O_{11}$	–	+135,+145	113, 115, 116
(Nigerose)	Octaacetate	$C_{28}H_{38}O_{19}$	151–153	+80(CHCl₃)	117
O-β-D-Glc$p$-(1→3)-α-D-Glc		$C_{12}H_{22}O_{11}$	202–205	+25.5→+17.5	118
(α-Laminaribiose)	α-Octaacetate	$C_{28}H_{38}O_{19}$	77–78	+20(CHCl₃)	119
O-β-D-Glc$p$-(1→3)-β-D-Glc		$C_{12}H_{22}O_{11}$	188–192	+7.5→+20.8	120
(β-Laminaribiose)	β-Octaacetate	$C_{28}H_{38}O_{19}$	160–161	-28.6(17°)(CHCl₃)	121
O-α-D-Glc$p$-(1→4)-α-D-Glc$p$		$C_{12}H_{22}O_{11}$	108	+173	122, 123
(α-Maltose)	α-Octaacetate	$C_{28}H_{38}O_{19}$	125	+123(CHCl₃)	59
O-α-D-Glc$p$-(1→4)-β-D-Glc$p$	Monohydrate	$C_{12}H_{24}O_{12}$	102–103	+112→+130	122, 123
(β-Maltose)	β-Octaacetate	$C_{28}H_{38}O_{19}$	159–160	+62.6(CHCl₃)	59
O-β-D-Glc$p$-(1→4)-β-D-Glc$p$		$C_{12}H_{22}O_{11}$	225	+14.2→+34.6(c 8)	105, 124
(β-Cellobiose)	α-Octaacetate	$C_{28}H_{38}O_{19}$	229	+41.0(CHCl₃)	59
	β-Octaacetate	$C_{28}H_{38}O_{19}$	202	-14.7(CHCl₃)	59
O-α-D-Glc$p$-(1→6)-D-Glc$p$		$C_{12}H_{22}O_{11}$	–	+103.2,+122	125, 126
(Isomaltose)	β-Octaacetate	$C_{28}H_{38}O_{19}$	144–145	+96.9(CHCl₃)	125
O-β-D-Glc$p$-(1→6)-α-D-Glc$p$	Dimethanolate	$C_{14}H_{30}O_{13}$	85–86	+31→+9.6	127
(α-Gentiobiose)	α-Octaacetate	$C_{28}H_{38}O_{19}$	189	+52.4(CHCl₃)	128, 129
O-β-D-Glc$p$-(1→6)-β-D-Glc$p$		$C_{12}H_{22}O_{11}$	190	-3→+10.5	105, 130
(β-Gentiobiose)	β-Octaacetate	$C_{28}H_{38}O_{19}$	193	-5.4(c 6,CHCl₃)	128, 129
O-β-D-Glc$p$-(1→1)-Mannitol		$C_{12}H_{24}O_{11}$	140–141	-18	161
O-D-Glc-(1→3)-D-Man		$C_{12}H_{22}O_{11}$	165	+27.9	131
	Octaacetate	$C_{28}H_{38}O_{19}$	142–143	+35.6(CHCl₃)	131
O-β-D-Glc$p$-(1→3)-Mannitol		$C_{12}H_{24}O_{11}$	97–100	-6	162
O-α-D-Glc$p$-(1→4)-D-Man		$C_{12}H_{22}O_{11}$	213–215	+115	132, 133
(Epimaltose)	Octaacetate	$C_{28}H_{38}O_{19}$	157	+117(CHCl₃)	132, 133
O-β-D-Glc$p$-(1→4)-α-D-Man		$C_{12}H_{22}O_{11}$	135–137	+5.8,+12.5	134, 135
(α-Epicellobiose)	α-Octaacetate	$C_{28}H_{38}O_{19}$	202–204	+36(CHCl₃)	135, 136
O-β-D-Glc$p$-(1→4)-β-D-Man		$C_{12}H_{22}O_{11}$	–	-6.5→+5.8(CHCl₃)	135, 136
(β-Epicellobiose)	β-Octaacetate	$C_{28}H_{38}O_{19}$	165	-13	135, 136
O-β-D-Glc$p$-(1→6)-D-Man	Monohydrate	$C_{12}H_{22}O_{11}$	137–138	-11	137, 138, 139
(Epigentiobiose)	α-Octaacetate	$C_{28}H_{38}O_{19}$	110–112	+26→+29(CHCl₃)	137, 138, 139
	β-Octaacetate	$C_{28}H_{38}O_{19}$	132–140	-20.6	137, 138, 139
O-α-D-Glc$p$-(1→1)-D-Fru		$C_{12}H_{22}O_{11}$	–	+49	140
O-β-D-Glc$p$-(1→1)-D-Fru	Dihydrate	$C_{12}H_{26}O_{13}$	132–135	-59.2	141, 142
	Octaacetate	$C_{28}H_{38}O_{19}$	128–129	-14	143
O-α-D-Glc$p$-(1→3)-D-Fru		$C_{12}H_{22}O_{11}$	157	+22→+75.3	144
(Turanose)	Octaacetate I	$C_{28}H_{38}O_{19}$	216–217	+20.5(CHCl₃)	145
	Octaacetate II	$C_{28}H_{38}O_{19}$	158	+107(CHCl₃)	145

OLIGOSACCHARIDES (INCLUDING DISACCHARIDES) (continued)

Substance[a] (synonym)	Derivative	Chemical formula	Melting point °C	Specific rotation[b] $[\alpha]_D$	Reference
(A)	(B)	(C)	(D)	(E)	(F)

Disaccharides (continued)

Substance[a] (synonym)	Derivative	Chemical formula	Melting point °C	Specific rotation[b] $[\alpha]_D$	Reference
O-α-D-Glc$p$-(1→4)-D-Fru (Maltulose)		$C_{12}H_{22}O_{11}$	113–115	+58→+64	146
O-β-D-Glc$p$-(1→4)-D-Fru (Cellobiulose)		$C_{12}H_{22}O_{11}$	–	-60.1	149
O-α-D-Glc$p$-(1→5)-D-Fru (Leucrose)		$C_{12}H_{22}O_{11}$	161–163	-8.8→-6.8	147
	Heptaacetate	$C_{26}H_{36}O_{18}$	150–151	–	147
	Phenylosazone	$C_{24}H_{34}N_4O_9$	186–188	–	148
O-α-D-Glc$p$-(1→6)-D-Fru (Palatinose, Isomaltulose)		$C_{12}H_{22}O_{11}$	–	+97.2	140, 150
	Phenylosazone	$C_{24}H_{34}N_4O_9$	173–175	–	140, 148
O-α-D-Glc$p$-(1→1)-α-D-GlcNp (Trehalosamine)	Hydrochloride	$C_{12}H_{24}NO_{10}Cl$	–	+176(c 0.02)	151
	N-Acetylhepta- acetate	$C_{28}H_9NO_{18}$	100–102	–	151
O-α-D-Glc$p$-(1→4)-D-GlcN	Hydrochloride	$C_{12}H_{24}NO_{10}Cl$	180–185	+81	153
O-α-D-Glc$p$-(1→4)-D-GlcNAc		$C_{14}H_{25}NO_{11}$	144–146	+39	153
O-β-D-Glc$p$-(1→4)-D-GlcNAc		$C_{14}H_{25}NO_{11}$	–	–	154
O-β-D-Glc$p$-(1→3)-D-GalNAc	Dihydrate	$C_{14}H_{29}NO_{13}$	155–157	+19	152
O-β-D-Glc$p$-(1→4)-L-Fuc		$C_{12}H_{22}O_{10}$	–	-71	155
	Heptaacetate	$C_{26}H_{36}O_{17}$	228–230	-59	155
O-β-D-Glc$p$-(1→4)-L-Rha (Scillabiose)		$C_{12}H_{22}O_{10}$	–	-24.8	156, 157
	Heptaacetate	$C_{26}H_{36}O_{17}$	96–97	-50.4	156, 157
O-D-Glc-(1→2)-L-Rha (Bryobioside)		$C_{12}H_{22}O_{10}$	175,188–190	+61.5,+66.1	159, 160
	Heptaacetate	$C_{26}H_{36}O_{17}$	127	+67.2(CHCl$_3$)	160
O-α-D-Glc$p$-(1→2)-D-GlcUA		$C_{12}H_{20}O_{12}$	–	+89	158
O-D-Glc$p$-(1→4)-D-2d-Glc$p$		$C_{12}H_{22}O_{10}$	–	+123	163
O-D-Glc$p$-(1→?)-3-O-Methyl- 6d-D-Glc$p$ (Kondurangobiose)		$C_{13}H_{24}O_{10}$	202–204	+20	164
	Hexaacetate	$C_{25}H_{36}O_{16}$	188	–	165
O-D-Glc$p$-(1→?)-3-O-Methyl- 6d-D-Glc (Thevetobioside)		$C_{13}H_{24}O_{10}$	233	-66.4(CH$_3$OH)	166
	Hexaacetate	$C_{25}H_{36}O_{16}$	168–170	-70(18°)(CHCl$_3$)	166
O-α-D-Man$p$-(1→3)-D-Gal		$C_{12}H_{22}O_{11}$	–	–	167
O-D-Man$p$-(1→6)-D-Gal		$C_{12}H_{22}O_{11}$	–	+134	168
O-β-D-Man$p$-(1→4)-α-D-Glc		$C_{12}H_{22}O_{11}$	210–212	+12,+18	169, 170
	Octaacetate	$C_{28}H_{38}O_{19}$	162–168	–	171
O-α-D-Man$p$-(1→6)-D-Glc		$C_{12}H_{22}O_{11}$	–	+73	172
	Octaacetate	$C_{28}H_{38}O_{19}$	83–87	+33	172
O-β-D-Man$p$-(1→6)-D-Glc		$C_{12}H_{22}O_{11}$	209–210	-5	173
O-α-D-Man$p$-(1→2)-D-Man		$C_{12}H_{22}O_{11}$	–	+42	480
O-α-D-Man$p$-(1→3)-D-Man		$C_{12}H_{22}O_{11}$	–	+50	174
O-α-D-Man$p$-(1→4)-D-Man		$C_{12}H_{22}O_{11}$	–	+49	175
O-β-D-Man$p$-(1→4)-α-D-Man$p$		$C_{12}H_{22}O_{11}$	204	-5→-8	176
	Octamethyl ether	$C_{20}H_{38}O_{11}$	–	-12	177
O-β-D-Man$p$-(1→4)-β-D-Man$p$		$C_{12}H_{22}O_{11}$	193–194	-7.7→-2.2	178
O-α-D-Man$p$-(1→6)-D-Man$p$		$C_{12}H_{22}O_{11}$	196–197	+52,+62	177, 179
	Octaacetate	$C_{28}H_{38}O_{19}$	152–153	+19.6	180
O-β-D-Man$p$-(1→6)-D-Man$p$		$C_{12}H_{22}O_{11}$	–	-12.4	177
O-α-D-Man$p$-(1→3)-D-GlcNAc		$C_{14}H_{25}NO_{11}$	129–130	+61→+58	181
O-α-D-Man$p$-(1→4)-D-GlcNAc		$C_{14}H_{25}NO_{11}$	154–156	+77→+66(50% CH$_3$OH)	182
	Heptaacetate	$C_{28}H_{39}NO_{18}$	113–114	+1.5(CHCl$_3$)	182
O-α-D-Man$p$-(1→6)-D-GlcNAc		$C_{14}H_{25}NO_{11}$	142–144	+38→+35	183
	Heptaacetate	$C_{28}H_{39}NO_{18}$	75–77	+68(CHCl$_3$)	183
O-β-D-Man$p$-(1→6)-D-GlcN	Hydrochloride	$C_{12}H_{24}NO_{10}$	–	+55	184

OLIGOSACCHARIDES (INCLUDING DISACCHARIDES) (continued)

Substance[a] (synonym)	Derivative	Chemical formula	Melting point °C	Specific rotation[b] $[\alpha]_D$	Reference
(A)	(B)	(C)	(D)	(E)	(F)

Disaccharides (continued)

Substance[a] (synonym)	Derivative	Chemical formula	Melting point °C	Specific rotation[b] $[\alpha]_D$	Reference
O-β-D-Fruf-(2→1)-α-D-Glc*p*		$C_{12}H_{22}O_{11}$	188,170	+66.5	127
(Sucrose)	Octaacetate	$C_{28}H_{38}O_{19}$	69, 75	+59.6(CHCl₃)	104
O-β-D-Fruf-(2→?)-D-Glc		$C_{12}H_{22}O_{11}$	...	+21	191
(Ceratose)					
O-β-D-Fruf-(2→6)-D-Glc		$C_{12}H_{22}O_{11}$	–	+5	192
O-D-Fruf-(2→2)-D-Fruf-anhydride		$C_{12}H_{20}O_{10}$	92–93	–23.8	185
(Alliuminoside)	Hexaacetate	$C_{24}H_{32}O_{16}$	98–99	–29.3	185
O-β-D-Fruf-(2→1)-D-Fru		$C_{12}H_{22}O_{11}$	–	–32.5,72.4	186, 187
(Inulobiose)	Octaacetate	$C_{28}H_{38}O_{19}$	–	–6.5,–14.2 (CHCl₃)	186, 187
O-D-Fruf-(2→6)-D-Fru		$C_{12}H_{22}O_{11}$	–	–20.8(17°)	188,189
(Levanbiose)					
O-D-Fruf-(2→?)-D-Fru		$C_{12}H_{22}O_{11}$	156–158	–16.4	185
(Sogdianose)	Octaacetate	$C_{28}H_{38}O_{19}$	94–95	–28.7(CHCl₃)	185
O-β-D-Fruf-(2→6)-D-2dGlc		$C_{12}H_{22}O_{10}$	56, 85	+62→+26.8	193
O-α-L-Fuc*p*-(1→2)-D-Gal		$C_{12}H_{22}O_{10}$	–	–56.7	194, 195
	Benzylglycoside	$C_{19}H_{29}O_{11}$	205–207	–97.8(*c* 0.92)	194
O-L-Fuc-(1→?)-D-Glc		$C_{12}H_{22}O_{10}$	–	–	196
O-α-D-Fuc*p*-(1→6)-D-Glc		$C_{12}H_{22}O_{10}$	–	+125	197
O-α-L-Fuc*p*-(1→2)-L-Fuc		$C_{12}H_{22}O_{9}$	185–190	–169	198, 199
O-α-L-Fuc*p*-(1→3)-L-Fuc		$C_{12}H_{22}O_{9}$	198–200	–191	198
O-α-L-Fuc*p*-(1→4)-L-Fuc		$C_{12}H_{22}O_{9}$	–	–170	198
O-α-L-Fuc*p*-(1→4)-D-GlcNAc		$C_{14}H_{25}NO_{10}$	128–129	–24→–25	200
	Hexaacetate	$C_{26}H_{37}NO_{16}$	94–96	(*c* 0.8,50%CH₃OH) –10°(CHCl₃)	200
O-α-L-Fuc*p*-(1→6)-D-GlcNAc		$C_{14}H_{25}NO_{10}$	–	–51	201
O-α-L-Fuc*p*-(1→2)-D-Tal		$C_{12}H_{22}O_{10}$	–	–120	195
O-α-L-Rha*p*-(1→2)-D-Gal		$C_{12}H_{22}O_{10}$	75–80	–3.5	202
O-α-L-Rha*p*-(1→6)-D-Gal		$C_{12}H_{22}O_{10}$	–	0→+2.7	203, 204
(Robinobiose)	Heptaacetate	$C_{26}H_{36}O_{17}$	113	–19	203
O-β-L-Rha*p*-(1→2 or 4)-D-Glc		$C_{12}H_{22}O_{10}$			205
(Neohesperidose)					
O-α-L-Rha*p*-(1→6)-D-Glc		$C_{12}H_{22}O_{10}$	189–192	+0.8→+3.2	206, 204
(Rutinose)	β-Heptaacetate	$C_{26}H_{36}O_{17}$	167	–28	206
O-α-D-GalNAc*p*-(1→3)-D-Gal		$C_{14}H_{25}NO_{11}$	179–181	+150,+200.7	212, 213
O-α-D-GalNAc*p*-(1→4)-D-Gal		$C_{14}H_{25}NO_{11}$	186–187	+203	214
O-β-D-GlcNAc*p*-(1→3)-D-Gal		$C_{14}H_{25}NO_{11}$	131–133	+45.5→+35.7	207
(Lacto-*N*-biose II)					
O-β-D-GlcNAc*p*-(1→6)-α-D-Gal*p*		$C_{14}H_{25}NO_{11}$	–	+125.6(*c* 0.2)	208
O-β-D-GlcNAc*p*-(1→6)-β-D-Glc		$C_{14}H_{25}NO_{11}$	–	+3.7	209
	Heptaacetate	$C_{28}H_{39}NO_{18}$	218–219	–9.5	209
O-β-D-GlcNAc*p*-(1→4)-D-GlcNAc*p*		$C_{14}H_{25}N_2O_{11}$	260–262	+16.6	268
(*N,N'*-Diacetyl-chitobiose)	Hexaacetate	$C_{28}H_{40}N_2O_{17}$	308–309	+55(18°) (*c* 0.5,CH₃COOH)	269
O-α-D-GlcNAc*p*-(1→6)-D-GlcNAc		$C_{14}H_{25}N_2O_{11}$	215	+125	210
O-β-D-GlcNAc*p*-(1→6)-D-GlcNAc		$C_{14}H_{25}N_2O_{11}$	200	+6	211
O-D-GlcNAc-(1→4)-D-GlcUA		$C_{14}H_{23}NO_{12}$	–	+106	270, 271
O-D-GalUA-(1→?)-L-Ara		$C_{11}H_{18}O_{11}$	–	+58.2	215

OLIGOSACCHARIDES (INCLUDING DISACCHARIDES) (continued)

Substance[a] (synonym) (A)	Derivative (B)	Chemical formula (C)	Melting point °C (D)	Specific rotation[b] $[\alpha]_D$ (E)	Reference (F)
Disaccharides (continued)					
O-α-D-GalUA*p*-(1→4)-D-Xyl*p*		$C_{11}H_{18}O_{11}$	–	+67	216
O-D-GalUA*p*-(1→3)-D-Gal		$C_{12}H_{20}O_{12}$	–	–	217
O-D-GalUA*p*-(1→4)-D-Gal		$C_{12}H_{20}O_{12}$	–	–	218
O-β-D-GalUA*p*-(1→6)-D-Gal		$C_{12}H_{20}O_{12}$	–	–	219
O-GalUA-(1→?)-Fuc		$C_{12}H_{20}O_{11}$	–	–	220
O-α-GalUA*p*-(1→2)-L-Rha		$C_{12}H_{20}O_{11}$	–	+65→+69	221, 222
O-α-D-GalUA*p*-(1→4)-D-GalUA		$C_{12}H_{18}O_{13}$	125–135	+154	223, 224
	Methyl α-glycoside dimethyl ester	$C_{15}H_{24}O_{13}$	120–122	+162.6	225
O-α-D-GlcUA*p*-(1→2)-D-Xyl		$C_{11}H_{18}O_{11}$	–	+88→+98	233
O-β-D-GlcUA*p*-(1→2)-D-Xyl		$C_{11}H_{18}O_{11}$	–	+5.7	234
O-α-D-GlcUA*p*-(1→3)-D-Xyl*p*		$C_{11}H_{18}O_{11}$	–	+18→+57	235
O-β-D-GlcUA*p*-(1→3)-D-Xyl		$C_{11}H_{18}O_{11}$	–	+3.7	236
O-α-D-GlcUA*p*-(1→4)-D-Xyl		$C_{11}H_{18}O_{11}$	–	–	237
O-β-GlcUA-(1→2)-Lyx		$C_{11}H_{18}O_{11}$	–	–	238
O-α-D-GlcUA*p*-(1→3)-D-Gal		$C_{12}H_{20}O_{12}$	–	–	226
O-α-D-GlcUA-(1→4)-D-Gal	Ba-salt	$C_{12}H_{19}O_{12}Ba$	–	+67	227
O-β-D-GlcUA*p*-(1→4)-D-Gal		$C_{12}H_{20}O_{12}$	–	+15	228
O-β-D-GlcUA*p*-(1→6)-D-Gal		$C_{12}H_{20}O_{12}$	116–120	–3	229
O-β-D-GlcUA*p*-(1→4)-D-Glc (Cellobiouronic acid)		$C_{12}H_{20}O_{12}$	189	+7.6	230, 231
	Heptaacetate	$C_{26}H_{34}O_{19}$	239	+32.9	230
O-β-D-GlcUA*p*-(1→6)-D-Glc	α-Heptaacetate methyl ester	$C_{27}H_{36}O_{19}$	201–202	+48.4	232
O-β-D-GlcUA*p*-(1→2)-D-Man*p*		$C_{12}H_{20}O_{12}$	–	–32→–33	239, 240
O-α-D-GlcUA*p*-(1→4)-D-Man*p*		$C_{12}H_{20}O_{12}$	–	–	241
O-α-D-GlcUA*p*-(1→2)-L-Rha		$C_{12}H_{20}O_{11}$	–	+63	242
O-β-D-GlcUA*p*-(1→4)-L-Rha		$C_{12}H_{20}O_{11}$	–	–6 to –22	243,244
O-β-D-GlcUA*p*-(1→3)-D-GalNAc (*N*-Acetylchondrosine)		$C_{14}H_{23}NO_{12}$	–	+35	276, 277
O-β-D-GlcUA*p*-(1→3)-D-GlcNAc (*N*-Acetylhyalobiuronic acid)		$C_{14}H_{23}NO_{12}$	–	–32(28°)	278
O-GlcUA*p*-(1→6)-D-GlcN		$C_{12}H_{21}NO_{11}$	–	–	245
O-β-D-GlcUA*p*-(1→2)-D-GlcUA	Ba-salt	$C_{12}H_{16}O_{13}Ba_2$	–	–5.2	246
O-α-NANA-(2→6)-D-GalNAc		$C_{19}H_{32}N_2O_{14}$	–	–	247
O-α-NANA-(2→6)-D-GlcNAc		$C_{19}H_{32}N_2O_{14}$	–	–	248
O-α-D-Gal*p*-(1→1)-glycerol		$C_9H_{18}O_8$	150–152	+155	249
O-β-D-Gal*p*-(1→1)-glycerol		$C_9H_{18}O_8$	139–140	+3.8,–7,–73	249–251
	Hexabenzoate	$C_{51}H_{42}O_{14}$	133–134	–6(CHCl₃)	251
O-α-D-Gal*p*-(1→2)-glycerol		$C_9H_{18}O_8$	86–87 129–130	+151,+163	252, 253
(Floridoside)	Hexaacetate	$C_{21}H_{30}O_{14}$	101	+114(acetone)	255
O-β-D-Gal*p*-(1→2)-D-erythritol		$C_{10}H_{20}O_9$	182–184	+7	275
	Heptaacetate	$C_{24}H_{34}O_{11}$	114	+109(*c* 0.6 acetone)	252
O-α-D-Gal*p*-(1→1)-myo-inositol (Galactinol)	Dihydrate	$C_{12}H_{26}O_{13}$	220–222	+135.6	256
	Nonamethyl ether	$C_{21}H_{40}O_{11}$	96.5–98	+119	257
O-β-D-Gal*p*-(1→5)-myo-inositol		$C_{12}H_{22}O_{11}$	248–252	0	258

OLIGOSACCHARIDES (INCLUDING DISACCHARIDES) (continued)

Substance[a] (synonym)	Derivative	Chemical formula	Melting point °C	Specific rotation[b] $[\alpha]_D$	Reference
(A)	(B)	(C)	(D)	(E)	(F)

Disaccharides (continued)

Substance[a] (synonym)	Derivative	Chemical formula	Melting point °C	Specific rotation[b] $[\alpha]_D$	Reference
O-β-D-Gal$p$-(1→3)-D-mannitol (Peltigeroside)		$C_{12}H_{24}O_{11}$	161–163	−55.5,−61	259, 260
O-3,6-anhydro-L-Gal$p$-(1→3)-D-Gal (Neoagarobiose)		$C_{12}H_{20}O_{10}$	207–208	+34.4→+203	261
	Hexaacetate	$C_{24}H_{32}O_{16}$	112	+1.6(27°) (CHCl$_3$)	261
O-(4,5-anhydro-α-D-GalUAp)-(1→4)-D-GalUA		$C_{12}H_{16}O_{12}$	–	+177.8	262
O-α-D-Glc$p$-(1→1)-glycerol		$C_9H_{18}O_8$	–	+128(27°) (c 0.7)	263
	Hexaacetate	$C_{21}H_{30}O_{14}$	92	+110(27°) (acetone)	263
O-β-D-Glc$p$-(1→1)-glycerol		$C_9H_{18}O_8$	–	+12	264, 265
	Hexa-P-nitro-benzoate	$C_{51}H_{36}N_6O_{26}$	105–108	–	265
O-D-Glc$p$-(1→1)-myoinositol		$C_{12}H_{22}O_{11}$	256–260	−17.5	258
	Nonamethylether	$C_{21}H_{40}O_{11}$	95–98	−10(C$_2$H$_5$OH)	258
O-D-Glc$p$-(1→5)-myoinositol		$C_{12}H_{22}O_{11}$	158–162	−20	258
O-α-D-Glc$p$-(1→1)-L-Sor		$C_{12}H_{22}O_{11}$	178–180	+33	266
	Octaacetate	$C_{28}H_{38}O_{19}$	–	+38(CHCl$_3$)	266
O-α-D-Glc$p$-(1→2)-β-D-threo-pentuloside (Gluco-xyluloside)		$C_{11}H_{20}O_{10}$	156–157	+43	267
	Heptaacetate	$C_{25}H_{34}O_{17}$	180–181	+22(CHCl$_3$)	267
O-β-D-Man$p$-(1→4)-meso-erythritol		$C_{10}H_{20}O_9$	160–162	−38	272, 273
O-α-D-Man$p$-(1→?)-glyceric acid		$C_9H_{16}O_9$	88–89	+105(15°)	274
O-(4,5-dideoxy-α-L-threo-hex-4-enopyranosyluronic acid)-(1→3)-D-GlcNAc		$C_{14}H_{21}NO_{11}$	–	−20	279
	Pentaacetate	$C_{24}H_{31}NO_{16}$	190–192	–	279
O-α-D-ribo-hexopyranosyl-3-ulose-(1→2)-β-D-Fru$f$ (3-Keto-sucrose)	Trihydrate	$C_{12}H_{26}O_{14}$	82–83	+40(c 7.5)	280
O-α-D-ribo-hexopyranosyl-3-ulose-(1→1)-α-D-Glc$p$ (3-Keto-trehalose)		$C_{12}H_{20}O_{11}$	114	+151.1	281
O-α-D-ribo-hexopyranosyl-3-ulose-(1→4)-D-Glc$p$ (3-Keto-maltose)		$C_{12}H_{20}O_{11}$	107	+87.2	281
O-β-D-xylo-hexopyranosyl-3-ulose-(1→4)-D-Glc$p$ (Keto-lactose)		$C_{12}H_{20}O_{11}$	118–120	+39.2	281
O-4,5-anhydro-β-D-ManUAp-(1→4)-D-ManUA		$C_{12}H_{16}O_{12}$	135–136.5	−8	282

Trisaccharides

Substance[a] (synonym)	Derivative	Chemical formula	Melting point °C	Specific rotation[b] $[\alpha]_D$	Reference
O-α-L-Ara$p$-(1→5)-O-α-L-Ara$p$-(1→5)-L-Ara		$C_{15}H_{26}O_{13}$	–	−35	285
O-α-L-Ara$f$-(1→3)-O-D-Xyl$p$-(1→4)-D-Xyl$p$		$C_{15}H_{26}O_{13}$	–	−19.3	286
	Octamethyl ether	$C_{23}H_{42}O_{13}$	–	−13.3(CH$_3$OH)	286, 287

OLIGOSACCHARIDES (INCLUDING DISACCHARIDES) (continued)

Substance[a] (synonym)	Derivative	Chemical formula	Melting point °C	Specific rotation[b] $[\alpha]_D$	Reference
(A)	(B)	(C)	(D)	(E)	(F)

Trisaccharides (continued)

Substance[a] (synonym)	Derivative	Chemical formula	Melting point °C	Specific rotation[b] $[\alpha]_D$	Reference
O-D-Xyl$p$-(1→3)-O-D-Xyl$p$-(1→4)-D-Xyl$p$		$C_{15}H_{26}O_{13}$	225	−52→−47	288
O-β-D-Xyl$p$-(1→4)-O-β-D-Xyl$p$-(1→4)-β-D-Xyl$p$		$C_{15}H_{26}O_{13}$	215−216	−48.1	289, 290
	Octaacetate	$C_{31}H_{42}O_{21}$	108−109.5	−83(CHCl$_3$)	290
(Xylotriose)					
O-α-D-Xyl$p$-(1→6)-O-β-D-Glc$p$-(1→4)-D-Glc$p$		$C_{17}H_{30}O_{15}$	147−150	+150	169
O-L-Gal-(1→4)-Xyl-(1→2)-L-Ara		$C_{16}H_{28}O_{14}$	217−219	−61	291
O-α-D-Gal$p$-(1→3)-O-α-D-Gal$p$-(1→3)-D-Gal		$C_{18}H_{32}O_{16}$	237−239	+146	292
O-β-D-Gal$p$-(1→3)-O-β-D-Gal$p$-(1→3)-D-Gal		$C_{18}H_{32}O_{16}$	240−245	+51	293
O-D-Gal-(1→6)-O-D-Gal-(1→3)-D-Gal		$C_{18}H_{32}O_{16}$	−	+20.5,+36	294, 295
O-α-D-Gal-(1→6)-O-α-D-Gal-(1→6)-D-Gal		$C_{18}H_{32}O_{16}$	−	−	296
O-β-D-Gal$p$-(1→3)-O-β-D-Gal$p$-(1→4)-D-Glc	Trihydrate	$C_{18}H_{38}O_{19}$	197−200	+56→+43	49
	Undecaacetate	$C_{40}H_{54}O_{27}$	108−110	+17.2(c 0.61 CHCl$_3$)	297
O-β-D-Gal$p$-(1→4)-O-β-D-Gal$p$-(1→4)-D-Glc$p$		$C_{18}H_{32}O_{16}$	228−231	+68→+45	34
O-β-D-Gal$p$-(1→6)-O-β-D-Gal$p$-(1→4)-D-Glc		$C_{18}H_{32}O_{16}$	187, 167	+34	49, 298, 299
O-α-D-Gal$p$-(1→6)-O-α-D-Gal$p$-(1→6)-D-Glc		$C_{18}H_{32}O_{16}$	150	+167	300
	Undecaacetate	$C_{40}H_{54}O_{27}$	105	+135(C$_2$H$_5$OH)	300
O-β-D-Gal$p$-(1→6)-O-β-D-Gal$p$-(1→6)-D-Glc		$C_{18}H_{32}O_{16}$	−	−	301
O-D-Gal$p$-(1→?)-O-D-Gal$p$-(1→?)-D-Glc		$C_{18}H_{32}O_{16}$	−	−	302
(Lactotriose)	Undecaacetate	$C_{40}H_{54}O_{27}$	120−122	−	302
O-β-D-Gal$p$-(1→6)-O-β-D-Gal$p$-(1→?)-D-Fru		$C_{18}H_{32}O_{16}$	−	−28	49
O-α-D-Gal$p$-(1→6)-O-α-D-Gal$p$-(1→6)-D-Man$p$		$C_{18}H_{32}O_{16}$	−	+131	303
O-β-D-Gal$p$-(1→4)-O-β-D-Glc$p$-(1→4)-D-Gal		$C_{18}H_{32}O_{16}$	−	+22.2	304
	Phenylosazone	$C_{30}H_{44}N_4O_{14}$	211	−	304
O-β-D-Glc$p$-(1→4)-O-β-D-Glc$p$-(1→6)-D-Glc$p$		$C_{18}H_{32}O_{16}$	257	+22	305
	Phenylosazone	$C_{30}H_{44}N_4O_{14}$	233	−50.5	305
O-α-D-Gal$p$-(1→2)-O-α-D-Glc$p$-(1→2)-β-D-Fru$f$		$C_{18}H_{32}O_{16}$	−	+125	306
(Umbelliferose)					
O-α-D-Gal$p$-(1→3)-O-α-D-Glc$p$-(1→2)-β-D-Fru$f$		$C_{18}H_{32}O_{16}$	−	+90.5	307
O-β-D-Gal$p$-(1→4)-O-α-D-Glc$p$-(1→2)-β-D-Fru$f$	Pentahydrate	$C_{18}H_{42}O_{21}$	181	+59	308
	Undecaacetate	$C_{40}H_{54}O_{27}$	131	+44(CHCl$_3$)	309
(Lactosylsucrose)					

OLIGOSACCHARIDES (INCLUDING DISACCHARIDES) (continued)

Substance[a] (synonym)	Derivative	Chemical formula	Melting point °C	Specific rotation[b] $[\alpha]_D$	Reference
(A)	(B)	(C)	(D)	(E)	(F)

Trisaccharides (continued)

Substance[a] (synonym)	Derivative	Chemical formula	Melting point °C	Specific rotation $[\alpha]_D$	Reference
O-α-D-Gal$p$-(1→6)-O-α-D-Glc$p$-(1→2)-β-D-Fru$f$	Pentahydrate	$C_{18}H_{42}O_{21}$	77–78,118	+101,+123	310
(Raffinose)	Undecaacetate	$C_{40}H_{54}O_{27}$	99–101	+92,+100(c 8, C_2H_5OH)	311, 312
O-α-D-Gal$p$-(1→6)-O-β-D-Man$p$-(1→4)-D-Man		$C_{18}H_{32}O_{16}$	228–229	+98.4	313
O-α-D-Gal$p$-(1→1)-O-β-D-Fru$f$-(2→1)-D-Glc		$C_{18}H_{32}O_{16}$	–	+131	314
O-α-D-Gal$p$-(1→3)-O-β-D-Fru$f$-(2→1)-D-Glc$p$		$C_{18}H_{32}O_{16}$	–	+98	314
O-β-D-Gal$p$-(1→4)-O-β-D-Fru$f$-(2→1)-D-Glc$p$		$C_{18}H_{32}O_{16}$	–	+44.1	315
O-α-D-Gal$p$-(1→6)-O-β-D-Fru$f$-(2→1)-D-Glc$p$	Dihydrate	$C_{18}H_{36}O_{18}$	123–124	+125.2	316
(Planteose)	Undecaacetate	$C_{40}H_{54}O_{27}$	135	+97(CHCl$_3$)	316
O-β-D-Gal$p$-(1→6)-O-β-D-Fru$f$-(2→1)-α-D-Glc$p$		$C_{18}H_{32}O_{16}$	–	–	317
O-D-Gal$p$-(1→3)-O-[β-D-Glc$p$-(1→4)]-L-Fuc		$C_{18}H_{32}O_{15}$	–	+23	318
O-β-D-Gal$p$-(1→4)-O-[α-L-Fuc$p$-(1→3)]-D-Glc (3-Fucosyllactose)		$C_{18}H_{32}O_{15}$	–	–	319
O-β-D-Gal$p$-(1→4)-O-[α-D-Glc$p$-(1→2)]-D-Glc$p$		$C_{18}H_{32}O_{16}$	–	+103	320, 321
O-β-D-Gal$p$-(1→3)-O-β-D-GlcNAcp-(1→3)-D-Gal	Dihydrate	$C_{20}H_{39}NO_{16}$	202	+40.7	322, 323
(Lacto-N-triose I)	Phenylosazone	$C_{32}H_{47}N_5O_{14}$	230	–	324, 325
O-β-D-Gal$p$-(1→4)-O-β-D-GlcNAp-(1→3)-D-Gal		$C_{20}H_{35}NO_{16}$	–	–	326
O-D-Gal-(1→?)-GalUA-(1→?)-L-Rha		$C_{18}H_{30}O_{17}$	–	+5.2	327
O-β-D-Glc$p$-(1→2)-O-β-D-Glc$p$-(1→4)-D-Gal$p$		$C_{18}H_{32}O_{16}$	250–260	+13.1	328, 329
O-β-D-Glc$p$-(1→4)-O-β-D-Glc$p$-(1→6)-D-Gal		$C_{18}H_{32}O_{16}$	–	+9.5	330
	Phenylosazone		207	–	330
O-α-D-Glc$p$-(1→2)-O-[β-D-Gal$p$-(1→4)]-D-Glc$p$		$C_{18}H_{32}O_{16}$	–	+103	331
O-α-D-Glc$p$-(1→2)-O-α-D-Glc$p$-(1→2)-D-Glc (Kojitriose)		$C_{18}H_{32}O_{16}$	–	–	358
O-α-D-Glc$p$-(1→3)-O-β-D-Glc$p$-(1→1)-α-D-Glc$p$		$C_{18}H_{32}O_{16}$	–	+139	367
O-α-D-Glc$p$-(1→3)-O-α-D-Glc$p$-(1→3)-D-Glc		$C_{18}H_{32}O_{16}$	–	–	365
O-β-D-Glc$p$-(1→3)-O-β-D-Glc$p$-(1→3)-β-D-Glc$p$ (Laminaritriose)		$C_{18}H_{32}O_{16}$	–	+2.4(17°)	368
O-α-D-Glc$p$-(1→3)-O-α-D-Glc$p$-(1→4)-D-Glc$p$		$C_{18}H_{32}O_{16}$	–	+169.5	337, 338
O-β-D-Glc$p$-(1→3)-O-β-D-Glc$p$-(1→4)-D-Glc$p$		$C_{18}H_{32}O_{16}$	229–231	+11.6+13.6	332, 333
	Undecaacetate	$C_{40}H_{54}O_{27}$	120–122	−20	332, 333

OLIGOSACCHARIDES (INCLUDING DISACCHARIDES) (continued)

Substance[a] (synonym) (A)	Derivative (B)	Chemical formula (C)	Melting point °C (D)	Specific rotation[b] $[\alpha]_D$ (E)	Reference (F)
Trisaccharides (continued)					
O-β-D-Glcp-(1→3)-O-β-D-Glcp-(1→6)-D-Glc		$C_{18}H_{32}O_{16}$	–	-3.5→-6	353
O-α-D-Glcp-(1→4)-O-α-D-Glcp-(1→3)-D-Glc		$C_{18}H_{32}O_{16}$	–	–	337, 338
O-β-D-Glcp-(1→4)-O-β-D-Glcp-(1→3)-D-Glc		$C_{18}H_{32}O_{16}$	236–239	+16.5→+11.7	339
	Undecaacetate I	$C_{40}H_{54}O_{27}$	108–110	-8.3(CHCl₃)	340
	Undecaacetate II	$C_{40}H_{54}O_{27}$	186–188	-24(CHCl₃)	341
O-α-D-Glcp-(1→4)-O-α-D-Glcp-(1→4)-D-Glcp		$C_{18}H_{32}O_{16}$	150	+160	342, 343
(Maltotriose)	Undecaacetate	$C_{40}H_{54}O_{27}$	134–136	+86(CHCl₃)	342, 344
O-β-D-Glcp-(1→4)-O-β-D-Glcp-(1→4)-D-Glcp		$C_{18}H_{32}O_{16}$	–	+25	340, 345
(Cellotriose)	α-Undecaacetate	$C_{40}H_{54}O_{27}$	220–222	+226(CHCl₃)	346
	β-Undecaacetate	$C_{40}H_{54}O_{27}$	199.5–200.5	-10.8(CHCl₃)	340
O-α-D-Glcp-(1→4)-O-α-D-Glcp-(1→6)-D-Glc		$C_{18}H_{32}O_{16}$	–	+159	347
	Undecaacetate	$C_{40}H_{54}O_{27}$	139–141	+112(CHCl₃)	347
O-α-D-Glcp-(1→4)-O-β-D-Glcp-(1→6)-D-Glc	α-Undecaacetate	$C_{40}H_{54}O_{27}$	174–176	+80	354
	β-Undecaacetate	$C_{40}H_{54}O_{27}$	233	+42	355
O-β-D-Glcp-(1→4)-O-α-D-Glcp-(1→6)-D-Glc		$C_{18}H_{32}O_{16}$	–	–	357
O-β-D-Glcp-(1→4)-O-β-D-Glcp-(1→6)-D-Glc		$C_{18}H_{32}O_{16}$	247–252	+8.4	356
O-α-D-Glcp-(1→6)-O-α-D-Glcp-(1→3)-D-Glc		$C_{18}H_{32}O_{16}$	–	+150	366
	Undecaacetate	$C_{40}H_{54}O_{27}$	117–119	+117→+121	366
O-α-D-Glcp-(1→6)-O-β-D-Glcp-(1→3)-D-Glc		$C_{18}H_{32}O_{16}$	–	+67	359
O-β-D-Glcp-(1→6)-O-[β-D-Glcp-(1→3)]-D-Glc		$C_{18}H_{32}O_{16}$	–	+14.4	360
O-β-D-Glcp-(1→6)-O-β-D-Glcp-(1→3)-D-Glc		$C_{18}H_{32}O_{16}$	–	-3.2→-4.2	360, 361
O-α-D-Glcp-(1→6)-O-[α-D-Glcp-(1→4)]-D-Glcp		$C_{18}H_{32}O_{16}$	–	–	362
O-β-D-Glcp-(1→6)-O-[α-D-Glcp-(1→4)]-D-Glcp		$C_{18}H_{32}O_{16}$	–	+84	363, 364
O-β-D-Glcp-(1→6)-O-β-D-Glcp-(1→4)-D-Glcp		$C_{18}H_{32}O_{16}$	–	+9.2→+10.2	335, 336
	Undecaacetate	$C_{40}H_{54}O_{27}$	205	-13	335
O-α-D-Glcp-(1→6)-O-α-D-Glcp-(1→4)-D-Glcp (Panose)		$C_{18}H_{32}O_{16}$	222–224	+154	348, 349
O-β-D-Glcp-(1→6)-O-[β-D-Glcp-(1→4)]-D-Glcp		$C_{18}H_{32}O_{16}$	–	–	334
O-α-D-Glcp-(1→6)-O-α-D-Glcp-(1→6)-D-Glc		$C_{18}H_{32}O_{16}$	–	+145	126
(Isomaltotriose)	Undecabenzoate	$C_{99}H_{87}O_{27}$	226–227	+131(CHCl₃)	350
O-β-D-Glcp-(1→6)-O-β-D-Glcp-(1→6)-D-Glc		$C_{18}H_{32}O_{16}$	–	-10.3	351, 352
(Gentiotriose)	Undecaacetate	$C_{40}H_{54}O_{27}$	214–215	-9.4(CHCl₃)	352

OLIGOSACCHARIDES (INCLUDING DISACCHARIDES) (continued)

Substance[a] (synonym)	Derivative	Chemical formula	Melting point °C	Specific rotation[b] $[\alpha]_D$	Refere:
(A)	(B)	(C)	(D)	(E)	(F)

Trisaccharides (continued)

Substance[a] (synonym)	Derivative	Chemical formula	Melting point °C	Specific rotation[b] $[\alpha]_D$	Refere:
O-α-D-Glcp-(1→4)-O-α-D-Glcp-(1→2)-β-D-Fruf		$C_{18}H_{32}O_{16}$	–	+121.8	369,
(Erlose)	Undecaacetate	$C_{40}H_{54}O_{27}$	68–73	+92.7(15°)	348
O-α-D-Glcp-(1→6)-O-α-D-Glcp-(1→2)-β-D-Fruf		$C_{18}H_{32}O_{16}$	118–120	+102.5(18°)	371,
O-β-D-Glcp-(1→6)-O-α-D-Glcp-(1→2)-β-D-Fruf (Gentianose)		$C_{18}H_{32}O_{16}$	210	+33.4	373,
O-α-D-Glcp-(1→6)-O-α-D-Glcp-(1→5)-D-Fruf		$C_{18}H_{32}O_{16}$	–	–	148
O-α-D-Glcp-(1→6)-O-α-D-Glcp-(1→6)-D-Fruf (Isomaltotriulose)		$C_{18}H_{32}O_{16}$	–	+118	140
O-α-D-Glcp-(1→6)-O-α-D-Glcp-(1→2)-D-GlcUA		$C_{18}H_{30}O_{17}$	–	+110(c 0.07)	389
O-β-D-Glcp-(1→6)-O-β-D-Glcp-(1→2)-L-Rha		$C_{18}H_{32}O_{15}$	–	–	160
	Nonaacetate	$C_{36}H_{50}O_{24}$	172–173	+54(CHCl₃)	160
O-β-D-Glcp-(1→4)-O-β-D-Manp-(1→4)-D-Manp		$C_{18}H_{32}O_{16}$	–	-9	388
O-α-D-Glcp-(1→2)-O-β-D-Fruf-(1→2)-β-D-Fruf (Isokestose)		$C_{18}H_{32}O_{16}$	200–201	+28.9	375, :
	Undecamethyl ether	$C_{29}H_{54}O_{16}$	–	+27.9	376–
O-α-D-Glcp-(1→2)-O-β-D-Fruf-(6→2)-β-D-Fruf (Kestose)		$C_{18}H_{32}O_{16}$	145	+28	{ 375, : 391, :
	Undecamethyl ether	$C_{29}H_{54}O_{16}$	–	+25.8(18°)	379
O-α-D-Glcp-(1→3)-O-β-D-Fruf-(2→1)-α-D-Glcp	Dihydrate	$C_{18}H_{36}O_{18}$	153–154	+88.2	380, :
(Melezitose)	Undecaacetate	$C_{40}H_{54}O_{27}$	117	+103.6(CHCl₃)	382
O-β-D-Manp-(1→4)-O-α-D-Glcp-(1→4)-D-Glcp		$C_{18}H_{32}O_{16}$	–	+9.5(28°)	169
O-β-D-Manp-(1→4)-O-β-D-Manp-(1→4)-D-Glcp		$C_{18}H_{32}O_{16}$	–	-12±3	169, :
O-D-Manp-(1→6)-O-D-Manp-(1→6)-D-Glcp (Laevidulinose)		$C_{18}H_{32}O_{16}$	–	-11.5,-15	384, :
	Undecaacetate	$C_{40}H_{54}O_{27}$	95–100	+18	384, :
O-α-D-Manp-(1→2)-O-α-D-Manp-(1→2)-D-Man		$C_{18}H_{32}O_{16}$	–	+63.0	480
O-β-D-Manp-(1→4)-O-β-D-Manp-(1→4)-α-D-Manp		$C_{18}H_{32}O_{16}$	214–216	-23	176
O-α-D-Manp-(1→6)-O-α-D-Manp-(1→6)-D-Man		$C_{18}H_{32}O_{16}$	–	+71.4	480
O-α-D-Manp-(1→6)-O-β-D-Glcp-(1→6)-D-Glc	Undecaacetate	$C_{40}H_{54}O_{27}$	118–119	+20.2(CHCl₃)	386
O-α-D-Manp-(1→6)-O-β-D-GlcNAcp-(1→4)-D-GlcNAc		$C_{22}H_{38}N_2O_{16}$	186–188	+36→+34	387
	Nonaacetate	$C_{40}H_{54}N_2O_{25}$	134–135	+37°(CHCl₃)	387
O-β-D-Fruf-(2→6)-O-α-D-Glcp-(1→2)-β-D-Fruf (Neokestose)		$C_{18}H_{32}O_{16}$	–	+21→+22	390

OLIGOSACCHARIDES (INCLUDING DISACCHARIDES) (continued)

Substance[a] (synonym)	Derivative	Chemical formula	Melting point °C	Specific rotation[b] $[\alpha]_D$	Reference
(A)	(B)	(C)	(D)	(E)	(F)

Trisaccharides (continued)

Substance[a] (synonym)	Derivative	Chemical formula	Melting point °C	Specific rotation[b] $[\alpha]_D$	Reference
O-D-Fru-(2→?)-O-D-Gal-(1→?)-D-Fru	Trihydrate	$C_{18}H_{38}O_{19}$	126–128	+136	394
(Labiose)	Undecaacetate	$C_{40}H_{54}O_{27}$	88	+122.5(CHCl₃)	394
O-D-Fruf-(2→1)-O-D-Fruf-(2→1)-D-Fru		$C_{18}H_{32}O_{16}$	–	–	401
(Inulotriose)					
O-D-Fruf-(2→?)-O-D-Fruf-(2→2)-D-Frufanhydride		$C_{18}H_{30}O_{15}$	207–208	–52.9	185
(Polygontin)	Nonaacetate	$C_{36}H_{48}O_{24}$	84–85	–38.4(CHCl₃)	185
O-D-Fruf-(2→?)-O-D-Fruf-(2→2)-D-Fruf		$C_{18}H_{32}O_{16}$	–	–22.3	402
(Trifructan)	Decaacetate	$C_{36}H_{52}O_{26}$	–	+8.5	402
O-α-L-Fucp-(1→2)-O-β-D-Galp-(1→4)-D-Glc		$C_{18}H_{32}O_{15}$	230–231	–53.5→–57.5 (c 0.2)	395
(2'-Fucosyllactose)	p-Tolylsulfonyl hydrazone	$C_{25}H_{40}N_2O_{17}S$	205–206	–73(C₅H₅N:H₂O)	395
O-L-Fucp-(1→4)-O-D-Glcp-(1→4)-D-Glc		$C_{18}H_{32}O_{15}$	–	–	396
O-α-D-GalNAcp-(1→3)-O-β-D-Galp-(1→3)-D-GlcNAc		$C_{22}H_{38}N_2O_{16}$	–	+110,+136	397, 398
O-α-D-GalNAcp-(1→3)-O-β-D-Galp-(1→4)-D-GlcNAc		$C_{22}H_{38}N_2O_{16}$	–	+147	398
O-α-D-GalNAcp-(1→4)-O-β-D-Galp-(1→4)-D-GlcNAc		$C_{22}H_{38}N_2O_{16}$	273–275	+140	400
O-β-D-GlcNAcp-(1→3)-O-β-D-Galp-(1→3)-D-GlcNAcp		$C_{22}H_{38}N_2O_{16}$	–	+19.5	403
O-β-D-GlcNAcp-(1→6)-O-β-D-Galp-(1→3)-D-GlcNAcp		$C_{22}H_{38}N_2O_{16}$	–	+51.6	403
O-β-D-GlcNAcp-(1→3)-O-[β-D-GlcNAcp-(1→6)]-D-Galp		$C_{22}H_{38}N_2O_{16}$	–	+6.5	404
O-β-D-GlcNAcp-(1→3)-O-β-D-Galp-(1→4)-D-Glc		$C_{20}H_{35}NO_{16}$	201–202	+40.7	405–407
(Lacto-N-triose II)	Phenylosazone	$C_{32}H_{47}N_5O_{14}$	230	–	405–407
O-β-D-GlcNAcp-(1→4)-O-β-D-GlcNAcp-(1→4)-D-GlcNAcp		$C_{24}H_{41}N_3O_{16}$	304–306	+3.8→+2.2	269, 270
	Octaacetate	$C_{40}H_{57}N_3O_{24}$	315	+33(c 0.2, CH₃COOH)	408
(Chitotriose)					
O-β-D-GlcNAcp-(1→?)-O-β-D-GlcUAp-(1→3)-D-GlcNAc		$C_{22}H_{36}N_2O_{17}$	–	–16	409
O-D-GalUA-(1→?)-O-L-Ara-(1→?)-Xyl		$C_{16}H_{26}O_{15}$	–	–	410
O-α-D-GalUA-(1→2)-O-L-Rha-(1→4)-D-Gal		$C_{17}H_{28}O_{15}$	–	–	411
O-GlcUA-(1→?)-O-Xyl-(1→?)-Gal		$C_{17}H_{28}O_{16}$	–	+40	412
O-β-D-GlcUAp-(1→2)-O-D-Man-(1→?)-D-Glc		$C_{18}H_{30}O_{17}$	–	–	413
O-α-D-GlcUAp-(1→4)-O-β-D-Xylp-(1→4)-D-Xylp		$C_{16}H_{26}O_{15}$	–	+38	414
O-α-D-GalNAcp-(1→3)-[O-α-L-Fucp-(1→2)]-D-Gal		$C_{20}H_{35}NO_{15}$	–	–	484

OLIGOSACCHARIDES (INCLUDING DISACCHARIDES) (continued)

Substance[a] (synonym)	Derivative	Chemical formula	Melting point °C	Specific rotation[b] $[\alpha]_D$	Reference
(A)	(B)	(C)	(D)	(E)	(F)

Trisaccharides (continued)

Substance[a] (synonym)	Derivative	Chemical formula	Melting point °C	Specific rotation[b] $[\alpha]_D$	Reference
O-α-D-Gal$p$-(1→3)-[O-α-L-Fuc$p$-(1→2)]-D-Gal		$C_{18}H_{32}O_{15}$	–	–	484
O-α-NANA-(2→3)-O-β-D-Gal$p$-(1→3)-D-GalNAc		$C_{25}H_{42}N_2O_{19}$	–	–	485
O-α-NANA-(2→3)-O-β-D-Gal$p$-(1→4)-D-Glc		$C_{23}H_9NO_{19}$	–	+16.8	415
(3'-Sialyllactose)		$C_{23}H_9NO_{19}$	–	+6(DMSO)	416
O-α-NGNA-(2→3)-O-β-D-Gal$p$-(1→4)-D-Glc		$C_{23}H_9NO_{20}$	–	–	462
O-α-NANA-(2→3)-O-β-D-Gal$p$-6-Sulfate-(1→4)-D-Glc		$C_{23}H_9NO_{22}S$	–	–	417
O-α-NANA-(2→6)-O-β-D-Gal$p$-(1→4)-D-Glc		$C_{23}H_9NO_{19}$	–	+27.9	415
(6'-Sialyllactose)					
O-α-D-Gal$p$-(1→2)-O-α-D-Glc$p$-(1→1)-glycerol		$C_{15}H_{28}O_{13}$	171	+170±3	418
	Nonaacetate	$C_{33}H_{46}O_{22}$	97	+145±3(c 0.5, CHCl$_3$)	418
O-α-D-Glc$p$-(1→6)-O-α-D-Glc$p$-(1→1)-glycerol		$C_{15}H_{28}O_{13}$	–	+148	263
O-β-D-Glc$p$-(1→1)-O-[β-D-Glc$p$-(1→6)]-D-Mannitol		$C_{18}H_{34}O_{16}$	–	–14	161
	Dodecaacetate	$C_{42}H_{58}O_{28}$	136–138	–7.7(CHCl$_3$)	419
O-α-D-Man$p$-(1→3)-O-α-D-Gal$p$-(1→2)-glycerol		$C_{15}H_{28}O_{13}$	–	–	420
	Nonaacetate	$C_{33}H_{46}O_{22}$	153–154	+103(CHCl$_3$)	420
O-α-D-GalUAp-(1→4)-O-α-D-GalUAp-(1→4)-D-GalUAp (Trigalacturonic acid)		$C_{18}H_{26}O_{19}$	135–142	+154,+187	224, 421

Tetrasaccharides

Substance[a] (synonym)	Derivative	Chemical formula	Melting point °C	Specific rotation[b] $[\alpha]_D$	Reference
O-β-D-Xyl$p$-(1→4)-O-[α-L-Ara$f$-(1→3)]-O-β-D-Xyl$p$-(1→4)-D-Xyl		$C_{20}H_{34}O_{17}$	–	–75	422
	Decaacetate	$C_{40}H_{54}O_{27}$	179–180	–85(CHCl$_3$)	422
O-D-Xyl-(1→4)-O-D-Xyl-(1→3)-O-D-Xyl-(1→4)-D-Xyl$p$		$C_{20}H_{34}O_{17}$	–	–56.7	288
O-β-D-Xyl$p$-(1→4)-O-β-D-Xyl$p$-(1→4)-O-β-D-Xyl$p$-(1→4)-D-Xyl$p$		$C_{20}H_{34}O_{17}$	224–226	–61.9	289, 290
(Xylotetraose)	Decaacetate	$C_{40}H_{54}O_{27}$	200–201	–92.4(CHCl$_3$)	290
O-D-Gal$p$-(1→?)-O-D-Gal$p$-(1→?)-O-D-Fru$f$-(2→1)-D-Glc$p$ (Sesamose)		$C_{24}H_{42}O_{21}$	–	–	423
O-β-D-Gal$p$-(1→4)-O-β-D-Gal$p$-(1→4)-O-β-D-Gal$p$-(1→4)-D-Glc$p$		$C_{24}H_{42}O_{21}$	–	+43	34
O-D-Gal$p$-(1→4)-O-D-Gal$p$-(1→6)-O-α-D-Glc$p$-(1→2)-D-Fru$f$		$C_{24}H_{42}O_{21}$	–	+143	424

OLIGOSACCHARIDES (INCLUDING DISACCHARIDES) (continued)

Substance[a] (synonym)	Derivative	Chemical formula	Melting point °C	Specific rotation[b] $[\alpha]_D$	Reference
(A)	(B)	(C)	(D)	(E)	(F)

Tetrasaccharides (continued)

Substance[a] (synonym)	Derivative	Chemical formula	Melting point °C	Specific rotation[b]	Reference
O-α-D-Gal$p$-(1→6)-O-α-D-Gal$p$-(1→6)-O-α-D-Glc$p$-(1→2)-D-Fru$f$		$C_{24}H_{42}O_{21}$	140,170	+131,+146	300, 425
(Stachyose)	Tetradecaacetate	$C_{52}H_{70}O_{35}$	95–96	+120(C_2H_5OH)	426
O-α-D-Gal$p$-(1→6)-O-α-D-Glc$p$-(1→2)-O-β-D-Fru$f$-(1→1)-α-D-Gal$p$ (Lychnose)		$C_{24}H_{42}O_{21}$	–	+155	424
O-α-D-Gal$p$-(1→6)-O-α-D-Glc$p$-(1→2)-O-β-D-Fru$f$-(3→1)-α-D-Gal (Isolychnose)		$C_{24}H_{42}O_{21}$	–	–	427
O-D-Gal$p$-(1→6)-O-D-Gal$p$-(1→3)-O-D-Gal$p$-(1→3)-D-Gal		$C_{24}H_{42}O_{21}$	–	–	428
O-D-Gal$p$-(1→6)-O-D-Gal$p$-(1→6)-O-D-Gal$p$-(1→3)-D-Gal		$C_{24}H_{42}O_{21}$	–	–	428
O-β-D-Gal$p$-(1→3)-O-β-D-GlcNAcp-(1→3)-O-β-D-Gal$p$-(1→4)-D-Glc (Lacto-N-tetraose)		$C_{26}H_{45}NO_{21}$	205	+25.2	70
O-β-D-Gal$p$-(1→4)-O-β-D-GlcNAcp-(1→3)-O-β-D-Gal$p$-(1→4)-D-Glc (Lacto-N-neotetraose)	Trihydrate	$C_{26}H_{51}NO_{24}$	214–218	+27	429
O-β-D-Glc$p$(1→2)-O-[β-D-Xyl$p$-(1→3)]-O-β-D-Glc$p$-(1→4)-D-Gal$p$		$C_{23}H_{40}O_{20}$	188	+2	430
O-β-D-Glc$p$-(1→4)-O-β-D-Glc$p$-(1→4)-O-β-D-Gal$p$-(1→4)-D-GlcUA			–	–	431
O-β-D-Glc$p$-(1→3)-O-β-D-Glc$p$-(1→4)-O-β-D-Glc$p$-(1→4)-D-Glc$p$	α-Anomer	$C_{24}H_{42}O_{21}$	221–224	+12.9→+10.6	432
	β-Anomer dihydrate	$C_{24}H_{46}O_{23}$	180–181	+7→+10	432
O-β-D-Glc$p$-(1→4)-O-β-D-Glc$p$-(1→3)-O-β-D-Glc$p$-(1→4)-D-Glc$p$		$C_{24}H_{42}O_{21}$	223–226	+19.8(90% CH_3COOH)	432, 433
O-β-D-Glc$p$-(1→4)-O-β-D-Glc$p$-(1→4)-O-β-D-Glc$p$-(1→3)-β-D-Glc$p$		$C_{24}H_{42}O_{21}$	241–245	+11.4→+8.4	432
	Tetradecaacetate	$C_{52}H_{70}O_{35}$	118–121	–	434
O-α-D-Glc$p$-(1→4)-O-α-D-Glc$p$-(1→4)-O-α-D-Glc$p$-(1→4)-D-Glc$p$ (Maltotetraose)		$C_{24}H_{42}O_{21}$	–	+166	435
	Methyl glycoside	$C_{25}H_{44}O_{21}$	–	+213	435
O-β-D-Glc$p$-(1→4)-O-β-D-Glc$p$-(1→4)-O-β-D-Glc$p$-(1→4)-D-Glc$p$		$C_{24}H_{42}O_{21}$	251	+11.3→+17	436
	α-Tetradecaacetate	$C_{52}H_{70}O_{35}$	226–227	+12.5(CHCl₃)	437
	β-Tetradecaacetate	$C_{52}H_{70}O_{35}$	223–225	-18.2(CHCl₃)	437

OLIGOSACCHARIDES (INCLUDING DISACCHARIDES) (continued)

Substance[a] (synonym)	Derivative	Chemical formula	Melting point °C	Specific rotation[b] $[\alpha]_D$	Reference
(A)	(B)	(C)	(D)	(E)	(F)

Tetrasaccharides (continued)

Substance[a] (synonym)	Derivative	Chemical formula	Melting point °C	Specific rotation $[\alpha]_D$	Reference
O-α-D-Glc$p$-(1→6)-O-α-D-Glc$p$-(1→4)-O-α-D-Glc$p$-(1→4)-D-Glc$p$		$C_{24}H_{42}O_{21}$	–	+177(15°)(c 0.5)	438
O-α-D-Glc$p$-(1→6)-O-α-D-Glc$p$-(1→6)-O-α-D-Glc$p$-(1→4)-D-Glc$p$		$C_{24}H_{42}O_{21}$	–	+164	439
	Methyl glycoside monomethanolate	$C_{26}H_{48}O_{22}$	192–193	+189	439
O-α-D-Glc$p$-(1→4)-O-α-D-Glc$p$-(1→6)-O-α-D-Glc$p$-(1→4)-D-Glc$p$		$C_{24}H_{42}O_{21}$	–	–	440
O-β-D-Glc$p$-(1→4)-O-β-D-Glc$p$-(1→6)-O-β-D-Glc$p$-(1→6)-D-Glc$p$	Tetradecaacetate	$C_{52}H_{70}O_{35}$	239–240	-19.6	441
O-α-D-Glc$p$-(1→6)-O-[α-D-Glc$p$-(1→3)]-O-α-D-Glc$p$-(1→6)-D-Glc$p$		$C_{24}H_{42}O_{21}$	–	–	442
O-α-D-Glc$p$-(1→2)-O-β-D-Fru$f$-(1→2)-O-β-D-Fru$f$-(1→2)-β-D-Fru$f$ (Nystose)		$C_{24}H_{42}O_{21}$	131–132 110–115	+10.6 +17.9	443 444, 445
O-α-D-Glc$p$-(1→4)-O-α-D-Glc$p$-(1→4)-O-α-D-Glc$p$-(1→2)-D-Fru$f$		$C_{24}H_{42}O_{21}$	–	–	370
O-β-D-Glc$p$-(1→3)-O-β-D-Glc$p$-(1→3)-O-β-D-Glc$p$-(1→3)-β-D-Glc$p$		$C_{24}H_{42}O_{21}$	–	-5.9	119, 368
	Tetradecaacetate	$C_{52}H_{70}O_{35}$	122–123	-46.2(CHCl₃)	119
O-α-D-Man$p$-(1→3)-O-α-D-Man$p$-(1→2)-O-α-D-Man$p$-(1→2)-D-Man		$C_{24}H_{42}O_{21}$	–	+65.7	481
O-α-D-Man$p$-(1→6)-O-α-D-Man$p$-(1→6)-O-α-D-Man$p$-(1→6)-D-Man		$C_{24}H_{42}O_{21}$	–	+60.8	481
O-α-D-Man$p$-(1→2)-O-α-D-Man$p$-(1→3)-O-α-D-Man$p$-(1→2)-D-Man		$C_{24}H_{42}O_{21}$	–	–	482
D-Fructose tetraose (Veronicin)(nonreducing)		$C_{24}H_{42}O_{21}$	170,188	-29.4	446
	Tetradecaacetate	$C_{52}H_{70}O_{35}$	92	-21.1(CHCl₃)	446
O-D-Fru$f$-(2→1)-O-[D-Fru$f$-(2→2)]-O-[D-Fru$f$-(2→6)]-D-Glc (Neobifurcose)		$C_{24}H_{42}O_{21}$	–	+14.4,+16.7	447, 448
	Tridecamethyl ether	$C_{37}H_{68}O_{21}$	–	-35.4	445
O-D-Fru$f$-(2→1)-O-D-Fru$f$-(2→1)-O-D-Fru$f$-(2→1)-D-Glc$p$ (Inulotriosylglucose)		$C_{24}H_{42}O_{21}$	–	-2	449
O-α-L-Fuc$p$-(1→2)-O-β-D-Gal$p$-(1→4)-O-[α-L-Fuc$p$-(1→3)]-D-Glc (Lactodifucotetraose)		$C_{24}H_{42}O_{19}$	–	-17.1,-106	450

OLIGOSACCHARIDES (INCLUDING DISACCHARIDES) (continued)

Substance[a] (synonym)	Derivative	Chemical formula	Melting point °C	Specific rotation[b] $[\alpha]_D$	Reference
(A)	(B)	(C)	(D)	(E)	(F)

Tetrasaccharides (continued)

Substance[a] (synonym)	Derivative	Chemical formula	Melting point °C	Specific rotation[b] $[\alpha]_D$	Reference
O-α-D-GalUAp-(1→4)-O-α-D-GalUAp-(1→4)-O-α-D-GalUAp-(1→4)-D-GalUAp	Trihydrate	$C_{24}H_{40}O_{28}$	160–170	–	451
O-α-D-GalNAcp-(1→3)-[O-α-L-Fucp-(1→2)]-O-β-D-Galp-(1→4)-D-Glc		$C_{26}H_{45}NO_{20}$	–	–	486
O-α-NANA-(2→8)-O-α-NANA-(2→3)-O-β-D-Galp-(1→3)-D-GalNAc		$C_{36}H_{59}N_3O_{27}$	–	–	485
O-β-D-GlcUAp-(1→3)-O-D-GlcNAcp-(1→?)-O-β-D-GlcUAp-(1→3)-D-GlcNAc		$C_{28}H_{44}N_2O_{23}$	200	–41→–53(27°)	452
O-α-NANA-(2→8)-O-α-NANA-(2→3)-O-β-D-Galp-(1→4)-D-Glc		$C_{34}H_{56}N_2O_{27}$	–	–	462
O-α-D-Glcp-(1→6)-O-α-D-Glcp-(1→6)-O-α-D-Glcp-(1→1)-glycerol		$C_{21}H_{38}O_{18}$	–	+166(27°)(c 0.5)	263

Pentasaccharides

Substance[a] (synonym)	Derivative	Chemical formula	Melting point °C	Specific rotation[b] $[\alpha]_D$	Reference
[O-β-D-Xylp-(1→4)-]₄-β-D-Xylp (Xylopentaose)		$C_{25}H_{42}O_{21}$	240–242	–72.9	289, 290
	Dodecaacetate	$C_{49}H_{76}O_{33}$	249–250	–98(CHCl₃)	290
[O-α-D-Galp-(1→6)-]₃-O-α-D-Glcp-(1→2)-β-D-Fruf (Verbascose)		$C_{30}H_{52}O_{26}$	219–220,253	+169.9	453, 454
	Heptadecaacetate	$C_{64}H_{86}O_{43}$	132	+130.4	453, 454
O-β-D-Galp-(1→3)-O-[α-L-Fucp-(1→4)]-O-β-D-GlcNAcp-(1→3)-O-β-D-Galp-(1→4)-D-Glcp (Lacto-N-fucopentaose II)		$C_{32}H_{55}NO_{25}$	213–215	–28→+30.4	455
O-D-Glcp-(1→2)-O-[D-Fruf-(2→6)]-O-D-Fruf-(1→2)-O-D-Fruf-(1→2)-D-Fruf		$C_{30}H_{52}O_{26}$	–	–3.5	456
	Heptadeca methylether	$C_{47}H_{86}O_{26}$	–	–10.5(CHCl₃)	456
[O-α-D-Glcp-(1→6)-]₃-O-α-D-Glcp-(1→4)-D-Glcp		$C_{30}H_{52}O_{26}$	–	+167(c 0.7)	349
	Methyl-α-glycoside mono-ethanolate	$C_{33}H_{60}O_{27}$	161–164	+188.7	437
[O-β-D-Glcp-(1→4)-]₄-D-Glcp (Cellopentaose)		$C_{30}H_{52}O_{26}$	–	–	345
	α-Heptaacetate	$C_{64}H_{86}O_{43}$	246–249	–	457
	β-Heptaacetate	$C_{64}H_{86}O_{43}$	238.5–239	–18.5(CHCl₃)	437
[O-α-D-Glcp-(1→4)-]₄-D-Glcp (Maltopentaose)		$C_{30}H_{52}O_{26}$	–	+178	458
O-α-D-Glcp-(1→2)-[O-β-D-Fruf-(6→2)-]₃-β-D-Fruf		$C_{30}H_{52}O_{26}$	–	–11.2	459, 460
O-β-D-Galp-(1→4)-O-[α-L-Fucp-(1→3)]-O-β-D-GlcNAcp-(1→3)-O-β-D-Galp-(1→4)-D-Glcp (Lacto-N-fucopentaose III)		$C_{32}H_{55}NO_{25}$	275–277	+7.35	461

OLIGOSACCHARIDES (INCLUDING DISACCHARIDES) (continued)

Substance[a] (synonym)	Derivative	Chemical formula	Melting point °C	Specific rotation[b] $[\alpha]_D$	Reference
(A)	(B)	(C)	(D)	(E)	(F)

Pentasaccharides (continued)

Substance[a] (synonym)	Derivative	Chemical formula	Melting point °C	Specific rotation $[\alpha]_D$	Reference
[O-α-D-Manp-(1→2)-]₄-D-Man		$C_{30}H_{52}O_{26}$	–	–	483
O-α-L-Fucp-(1→2)-O-β-D-Galp-(1→3)-O-β-D-GlcNAcp-(1→3)-O-β-D-Galp-(1→4)-D-Glcp (Lacto-N-fucopentaose I)		$C_{32}H_{55}NO_{25}$	216	-11→-16.3	70
O-α-D-GalNAcp-(1→3)-[O-α-L-Fucp-(1→2)]-O-β-D-Galp-(1→4)-[O-α-L-Fucp-(1→3)]-D-Glc		$C_{32}H_{55}NO_{24}$	–	–	484
O-α-D-Galp-(1→3)-[O-α-L-Fucp-(1→2)]-O-β-D-Galp-(1→4)-[O-α-L-Fucp-(1→3)]-D-Glc		$C_{30}H_{52}O_{24}$	–	–	484
O-α-NANA-(2→3)-O-β-D-Galp-(1→3)-O-β-D-GlcNAcp-(1→3)-O-β-D-Galp-(1→4)-D-Glc (LST-a)		$C_{37}H_{62}N_2O_{29}$	–	–	462
O-β-D-Galp-(1→3)-[O-α-NANA-(2→6)-]-O-β-D-GlcNAcp-(1→3)-O-β-D-Galp-(1→4)-D-Glc (LST-b)		$C_{37}H_{62}N_2O_{29}$	–	+14.5→+15.0	462
O-α-NANA-(2→6)-O-β-D-Galp-(1→4)-O-β-D-GlcNAcp-(1→3)-O-β-D-Galp-(1→4)-D-Glc (LST-c)		$C_{37}H_{62}N_2O_{29}$	–	+13	462
O-α-NGNA-(2→3)-O-β-D-Galp-(1→4)-O-β-D-GlcNAcp-(1→3)-O-β-D-Galp-(1→4)-D-Glc (G_{LNnT} I NGNA)		$C_{37}H_{62}N_2O_{30}$	–	–	463

Hexasaccharides

Substance[a] (synonym)	Derivative	Chemical formula	Melting point °C	Specific rotation $[\alpha]_D$	Reference
[O-β-D-Xylp-(1→4)-]₅-D-Xylp (Xylohexaose)	Dihydrate	$C_{30}H_{54}O_{27}$	236–237	+72.8	289, 464
	Tetradecaacetate	$C_{58}H_{78}O_{39}$	260–261	–	464
[O-D-Xylp-(1→4)-]₂-O-D-Xylp-(1→3)-[O-D-Xylp-(1→4)-]₂-D-Xylp		$C_{30}H_{50}O_{25}$	169–173	$-154[\alpha]_{436}$	465
(O-D-Galp-)₄-O-D-Galp-n-(1→2)-D-Fruf (Lycopose)		$C_{36}H_{62}O_{31}$	270	+187	466
	Eicosa acetate	$C_{76}H_{102}O_{51}$	150	+174.5(9°) (CH_3COCH_3)	466
[O-α-D-Galp-(1→6)-]₄-O-α-D-Glcp-(1→2)-β-D-Fruf (Ajugose)	Hexahydrate	$C_{36}H_{74}O_{37}$	204–205	+163	467
O-α-D-Glcp-(1→2)-[O-β-D-Fruf-(6→2)-]₄-β-D-Fruf		$C_{36}H_{62}O_{31}$	–	-19	479
O-D-Glcp-(1→?)-[O-D-Fruf-(?→2)-]₄-O-Fruf		$C_{36}H_{62}O_{31}$	–	-5.3	445
	Eicosa methylether	$C_{56}H_{102}O_{31}$	–	-37	445
[O-α-D-Glcp-(1→4)-]₅-D-Glc (Maltohexaose)		$C_{36}H_{62}O_{31}$	–	+180	458

OLIGOSACCHARIDES (INCLUDING DISACCHARIDES) (continued)

Substance[a] (synonym)	Derivative	Chemical formula	Melting point °C	Specific rotation[b] $[\alpha]_D$	Reference
(A)	(B)	(C)	(D)	(E)	(F)

Hexasaccharides (continued)

Substance[a] (synonym)	Derivative	Chemical formula	Melting point °C	Specific rotation[b] $[\alpha]_D$	Reference
[O-β-D-Glcp-(1→4)-]$_5$-D-Glc (Cellohexaose)		$C_{36}H_{62}O_{31}$	229–231	+168(15°)	345, 468
	α-Eicosa-acetate	$C_{76}H_{102}O_{51}$	252–255	–	457
	β-Eicosa-acetate	$C_{76}H_{102}O_{51}$	241–243	-18.9(CHCl$_3$)	437
[O-α-D-Glcp-(1→4)-]$_6$ (Cyclohexaamylose)		$C_{36}H_{60}O_{30}$	–	+151	469
	Octaacetate	$C_{72}H_{96}O_{48}$	–	+107(CHCl$_3$)	470
[O-α-D-Manp-(1→2)-]$_5$-D-Man		$C_{36}H_{62}O_{31}$	–	–	483
O-β-D-Galp-(1→3)-O-β-D-GlcNAcp-(1→3)-[O-β-D-Galp-(1→4)-O-β-D-GlcNAcp-(1→6)]-O-β-D-Galp-(1→4)-D-Glc (Lacto-N-hexaose)		$C_{40}H_{68}N_2O_{31}$	–	–	471
O-β-D-Galp-(1→4)-O-β-D-GlcNAcp-(1→3)-[O-β-D-Galp-(1→4)-O-β-D-GlcNAcp-(1→6)]-O-β-D-Galp-(1→4)-D-Glc (Lacto-N-neohexaose)		$C_{40}H_{68}N_2O_{31}$	–	–	472
O-α-L-Fucp-(1→2)-O-β-D-Galp-(1→3)-[O-α-L-Fucp-(1→4)]-O-β-D-GlcNAcp-(1→3)-O-β-D-Galp-(1→4)-D-Glc (Lacto-N-difucohexaose I)		$C_{38}H_{65}NO_{29}$	–	–	473
O-β-D-Galp-(1→3)-[O-α-L-Fucp-(1→4)]-O-β-D-GlcNAcp-(1→3)-O-β-D-Galp-(1→4)-[O-α-L-Fucp-(1→3)]-D-Glc (Lacto-N-difucohexaose II)		$C_{38}H_{65}NO_{29}$	218–220	-68.8	474
O-α-NANA-(2→3)-O-β-D-Galp-(1→3)-[O-α-NANA-(2→6)]-O-β-D-GlcNAcp-(1→3)-O-β-D-Galp-(1→4)-D-Glc (Disialyl-lacto-N-tetraose)		$C_{48}H_{79}N_3O_{37}$	–	–	475
O-α-D-GalNAcp-(1→3)-[O-α-L-Fucp-(1→2)]-O-β-D-Galp-(1→3)-O-β-D-GlcNAcp-(1→3)-O-β-D-Galp-(1→4)-D-Glc		$C_{40}H_{68}N_2O_{30}$	–	–	486
O-α-D-4-O-methyl-GlcUA-(1→2)-[O-β-D-Xylp-(1→4)-]$_4$-D-Xylp		$C_{32}H_{52}O_{27}$	–	-11.8	290

Heptasaccharides

Substance[a] (synonym)	Derivative	Chemical formula	Melting point °C	Specific rotation[b] $[\alpha]_D$	Reference
Fructose heptasaccharide (Asparagose)		$C_{42}H_{72}O_{36}$	–	-35.7	476
[O-β-D-Xylp-(1→4)-]$_6$-D-Xylp (Xyloheptaose)		$C_{35}H_{58}O_{29}$	232–234	-74	289, 464
[O-α-D-Galp-(1→6)-]$_5$-O-α-D-Glcp-(1→2)-β-D-Fru$f$	Tetrahydrate	$C_{42}H_{80}O_{40}$	246–248	+168	467
[O-α-D-Galp-(1→6)-]$_4$-O-α-D-Glcp-(1→2)-O-β-D-Fru$f$-(3→1)-α-D-Galp		$C_{42}H_{72}O_{36}$	–	–	477

OLIGOSACCHARIDES (INCLUDING DISACCHARIDES) (continued)

Substance[a] (synonym)	Derivative	Chemical formula	Melting point °C	Specific rotation[b] $[\alpha]_D$	Reference
(A)	(B)	(C)	(D)	(E)	(F)

Heptasaccharides (continued)

Substance[a] (synonym)	Derivative	Chemical formula	Melting point °C	Specific rotation[b] $[\alpha]_D$	Reference
[O-α-D-Glcp-(1→4)-]₇, (Cycloheptaamylose)		$C_{42}H_{70}O_{35}$	–	+162	469
	Heneicosa acetate	$C_{84}H_{112}O_{56}$	–	+121(CHCl₃)	470
[O-α-D-Manp-(1→2)-]₆-D-Man		$C_{42}H_{72}O_{36}$	–	–	483
Fucosyllacto-N-hexaose		$C_{46}H_{78}N_2O_{35}$	–	–	472
Fucosyllacto-N-neohexaose		$C_{46}H_{78}N_2O_{35}$	–	–	472
O-α-NANA-(2→6)-O-β-D-Galp-(1→4)-O-β-D-GlcNAcp-(1→6)-[O-β-D-Galp-(1→3)-O-β-D-GlcNAcp-(1→3)-]-O-β-D-Galp-(1→4)-D-Glc		$C_{51}H_{85}N_3O_{39}$	–	–	472
O-α-NANA-(2→6)-O-β-D-Galp-(1→4)-O-β-D-GlcNAcp-(1→6)-[O-β-D-Galp-(1→4)-O-β-D-GlcNAcp-(1→3)-]-O-β-D-Galp-(1→4)-D-Glc		$C_{51}H_{85}N_3O_{39}$	–	–	472
O-α-D-4-O-methyl-GlcUA-(1→2)-[O-β-D-Xylp-(1→4)-]₅-D-Xylp		$C_{37}H_{60}O_{31}$	–	-20.8	290

Octasaccharides

Substance[a] (synonym)	Derivative	Chemical formula	Melting point °C	Specific rotation[b] $[\alpha]_D$	Reference
[O-β-D-Xylp-(1→4)-]₇-D-Xylp (Xylooctaose)		$C_{40}H_{66}O_{33}$	–	–	289
[O-α-D-Galp-(1→6)-]₄-O-α-D-Glcp-(1→2)-β-D-Fruf	Tetrahydrate	$C_{48}H_{90}O_{41}$	267–268	+168	467
[O-α-D-Glcp-(1→4)-]₈ (Cyclooctaamylose)		$C_{48}H_{80}O_{40}$	–	+180	478
	Tetracosa-acetate	$C_{96}H_{128}O_{64}$	–	+137(CHCl₃)	470
Difucosyl-lacto-N-hexaose			–	–	472
Difucosyl-lacto-N-neohexaose			–	–	472
Sialyl-fucosyl-lacto-N-neo hexaose		$C_{57}H_{95}N_3O_{43}$	–	–	472
O-α-D-4-O-methyl-GlcUA-(1→2)-[O-β-D-Xylp-(1→4)-]₆-D-Xylp		$C_{42}H_{68}O_{35}$	–	-25.7	290
O-β-Galp-(1→4)-O-β-GlcNAcp-(1→2)-O-α-Manp-(1→3)-[O-β-Galp-(1→4)-O-β-GlcNAcp-(1→2)-O-α-Manp-(1→6)]-O-β-Manp-(1→4)-GlcNAc		$C_{54}H_{91}N_3O_{41}$	–	–	393

Compiled by Akira Kobata.

OLIGOSACCHARIDES (INCLUDING DISACCHARIDES) (continued)

REFERENCES

1. Aspinall, Hirst, and Nicolson, *J. Chem. Soc.* (Lond.), p. 1697 (1959).
2. Andrews, Hough, and Powell, *Chem. Ind.*, p. 658 (1956).
3. Haq and Adams, *Can. J. Chem.*, 39, 1563 (1961).
4. Smith and Stephen, *J. Chem. Soc.* (Lond.), p. 4892 (1961).
5. Jones and Nicholson, *J. Chem. Soc.* (Lond.), p. 27 (1958).
6. Aspinall and Cairncross, *J. Chem. Soc.* (Lond.), p. 3998 (1960).
7. Lehmann and Beck, *Justus Liebigs Ann. Chem.*, 630, 56 (1960).
8. Wallenfels and Beck, *Justus Liebigs Ann. Chem.*, 630, 46 (1960).
9. Gorin, *Can. J. Chem.*, 40, 275 (1962).
10. Helferich and Bredreck, *Justus Liebigs Ann. Chem.*, 465, 166 (1928).
11. Aspinall and Nicholson, *J. Chem. Soc.* (Lond.), p. 2503 (1960).
12. Gakhokidze and Kutidze, *J. Gen. Chem. U.S.S.R.*, 22, 247 (1952).
13. Aspinall and Ferrier, *J. Chem. Soc.* (Lond.), p. 4188 (1957).
14. Montgomery, Smith, and Srivastava, *J. Am. Chem. Soc.*, 79, 698 (1957).
15. Erskine and Jones, *Can. J. Chem.*, 35, 1174 (1957).
16. Ball and Jones, *J. Chem. Soc.* (Lond.), p. 4871 (1957).
17. Andrews, Ball, and Jones, *J. Chem. Soc.* (Lond.), p. 4090 (1953).
18. Rosenberg and Zamenhof, *J. Biol. Chem.*, 237, 1040 (1962).
19. Ball and Jones, *J. Chem. Soc.* (Lond.), p. 33 (1958).
20. Curtis and Jones, *Can. J. Chem.*, 38, 1305 (1960).
21. Myhre and Smith, *J. Org. Chem.*, 26, 4609 (1961).
22. Aspinall and Ross, *J. Chem. Soc.* (Lond.), p. 3674 (1961).
23. Whistler, Bacchrach, and Tu, *J. Am. Chem. Soc.*, 74, 3059 (1952).
24. Ball and Jones, *J. Chem. Soc.* (Lond.), p. 4871 (1957).
25. Kuhn, Low, and Trischmann, *Angew. Chem.*, 68, 212 (1956).
26. Zemplén and Bognár, *Chem. Ber.*, 72, 1160 (1939).
27. Wallenfels and Lehmann, *Chem. Ber.*, 90, 1000 (1957).
28. Bridel and Charaux, *C.R. Acad. Sci.*, 180, 1219 (1925).
29. Helferich and Steinpreis, *Chem. Ber.*, 91, 1794 (1958).
30. Gorin, *Can. J. Chem.*, 40, 275 (1962).
31. Gakhokide and Kobiashvili, *J. Gen. Chem. U.S.S.R.*, 22, 244, 247 (1952).
32. Whistler and Yagi, *J. Org. Chem.*, 26, 1050 (1961).
33. Smith, *J. Chem. Soc.* (Lond.), p. 744 (1939).
34. Gorin, Spencer, and Phaff, *Can. J. Chem.*, 42, 1341, 2307 (1964).
35. Goldstein, Smith, and Srivastava, *J. Am. Chem. Soc.*, 79, 3858 (1957).
36. Srivastava and Smith, *J. Am. Chem. Soc.*, 79, 982 (1957).
37. Lindberg, Wachmeister, and Wickberg, *Acta Chem. Scand.*, 6, 1052 (1952).
38. Montgomery, Smith, and Srivastava, *J. Am. Chem. Soc.*, 79, 698 (1957).
39. Gorin, Haskins, and Westlake, *Can. J. Chem.*, 44, 2083 (1966).
40. Clancy and Whelan, *Arch. Biochem. Biophys.*, 118, 724 (1967).
41. Morgan and O'Neil, *Can. J. Chem.*, 37, 1201 (1959).
42. Aspinall, Auret, and Hirst, *J. Chem. Soc.* (Lond.), p. 4408 (1958).
43. Ball and Jones, *J. Chem. Soc.* (Lond.), p. 905 (1958).
44. Jones and Reid, *J. Chem. Soc.* (Lond.), p. 1361 (1954); p. 1890 (1955).
45. Masamune and Kamiyama, *J. Exp. Med.* (Tokyo), 66, 43 (1957).
46. Gorin and Spencer, *Can. J. Chem.*, 37, 499 (1959).
47. Ingle and Bhide, *J. Indian Chem. Soc.*, 35, 516 (1958).
48. Turton, Bebbington, Dixon, and Pacsu, *J. Am. Chem. Soc.*, 77, 2565 (1955).
49. Ballio and Russi, *J. Chromatogr.*, 4, 117 (1960).
50. Meier, *Acta Chem. Scand.*, 16, 2275 (1962).
51. Haq and Adams, *Can. J. Chem.*, 39, 1563 (1961).
52. Wickstrom, *Acta Chem. Scand.*, 11, 1473 (1957).
53. Lehmann and Beck, *Justus Liebigs Ann. Chem.*, 630, 56 (1960).
54. Beck and Wallenfels, *Justus Liebigs Ann. Chem.*, 655, 173 (1962).
55. Gakhokide, *Chem. Abstr.*, 47, 6875 (1953).
56. Kuhn and Baer, *Chem. Ber.*, 87, 1560 (1954).
57. Trey, *Z. Phys. Chem.*, 46, 620 (1903).

OLIGOSACCHARIDES (INCLUDING DISACCHARIDES) (continued)

58. Gillis, *Rec. Trav. Chim. Pay-Bas*, 39, 88 677 (1920).
59. Hudson and Johnson, *J. Am. Chem. Soc.*, 37,1270, 1276 (1915).
60. Tanret, *Hoppe-Seyler's Z. Physiol. Chem.*, 53, 692 (1905).
61. Fletcher and Diehl, *J. Am. Chem. Soc.*, 74, 5774 (1952).
62   Hudson and Johnson, *J. Am. Chem. Soc.*, 37, 2752 (1915).
63. Pazur, Tipton, Budovich, and Marsh, *J. Am. Chem. Soc.*, 80, 119 (1958).
64. Helferich and Sparmberg, *Chem. Ber.*, 66, 806 (1933).
65. Polonovski and Lespagnol, *C.R. Acad. Sci.*, 192, 1319 (1931).
66. Bredereck, Wagner, Geissel, Gross, Hutten, and Ott, *Chem. Ber.*, 95, 3056 (1962).
67. Haskins, Hann, and Hudson, *J. Am. Chem. Soc.*, 64, 1852 (1942).
68. Jones, Hough, and Richards, *J. Chem. Soc.* (Lond.), p. 295 (1954).
69. Helfrich and Steinpreis, *Chem. Ber.*, 91, 1794 (1958).
70. Kuhn and Gauhe, *Chem. Ber.*, 93, 647 (1960).
71. Alessandrini, Schmidt, Zilliken, and György, *J. Biol. Chem.*, 220, 71 (1956).
72. Kuhn and Kirschenlohr, *Justus Liebigs Ann. Chem.*, 600, 135 (1956).
73. Okuyama, *Tohoku J. Exp. Med.*, 68, 313 (1958).
74. Watkins, *Nature*, 181, 117 (1958).
75. Kuhn, Baer, and Gauhe, *Chem. Ber.*, 88, 1713 (1955).
76. Zilliken, Smith, Rose, and György, *J. Biol. Chem.*, 208, 299 (1954).
77. Kuhn and Gauhe, *Chem. Ber.*, 94, 842, (1961).
78. Hirase and Araki, *Bull. Chem. Soc. Jap.*, 27, 105 (1953).
79. Clingman, Nunn, and Stephan, *J. Chem. Soc.* (Lond.), p. 197 (1957).
80. Gakhokidze, *J. Gen. Chem. U.S.S.R.*, 16, 1923 (1946).
81. Weissmann and Meyer, *J. Am. Chem. Soc,* 76, 1753 (1954).
82. Lindberg and Wickberg, *Acta Chem. Scand.*, 8, 821 (1954).
83. Zemplén, *Chem. Ber.*, 59, 1254 (1926).
84. Gakhokidze, *J. Gen. Chem. U.S.S.R.*, 16, 1914 (1946).
85. Feingold, Avigad, and Hestrin, *J. Biol. Chem.*, 224, 295 (1957).
86. Hassid, Doudoroff, Potter, and Barker, *J. Am. Chem. Soc.*, 70, 306 (1948).
87. Andrews and Jones, *J. Chem. Soc.* (Lond.), p. 1724 (1954).
88. Gupta, *J. Chem. Soc.*, (Lond.), p. 5262 (1961).
89. Gorrod and Jones, *J. Chem. Soc.* (Lond.), p. 2522 (1954).
90. Barker, Bourne, Hewitt, and Stacey, *J. Chem. Soc.* (Lond.), p. 3541 (1957).
91. Barker, Stacey, and Stroud, *Nature*, 189, 138 (1961).
92. Putman, Litt, and Hassid, *J. Am. Chem. Soc.*, 77, 4351 (1955).
93. Gakhokidze and Kutidze, *J. Gen. Chem. U.S.S.R.*, 22, 139 (1952).
94. Flowers, *Carbohydr. Res.*, 18, 211 (1971).
95. Kuhn, Löw, and Trischmann, *Chem. Ber.*, 88, 1492 (1955).
96. Jones and Perry, *J. Am. Chem. Soc.* 79, 2787 (1957).
97. Kuhn and Löw, *Chem. Ber.*, 86, 1027 (1953).
98. Lloyd and Roberts, *Proc. Chem. Soc.*, p. 250 (1960).
99. Freudenberg, Noe, and Knopf, *Chem. Ber.*, 60, 238, (1927).
100. Matsuda, *Nature*, 180, 985 (1957).
101. Haq and Whelan, *Nature*, 178, 1225 (1956).
102. Bourne, Hartigan, and Weigel, *J. Chem. Soc.* (Lond.), p. 1088 (1961).
103. Birch, *J. Chem. Soc.* (Lond.), p. 3489 (1965).
104. Hudson and Johnson, *J. Am. Chem. Soc.*, 37, 2748 (1915).
105. Peat, Whelan, and Hinson, *Nature*, 170, 1056 (1952).
106. Sharp and Stacey, *J. Chem. Soc.* (Lond.), p. 285 (1951).
107. Micheel and Hagel, *Chem. Ber.*, 85, 1087 (1952).
108. Matsuda, *J. Agric. Chem. Soc. Jap.*, 30, 119 (1956).
109. Freudenberg, Knauber, and Cramer, *Chem. Ber.*, 84, 144 (1951).
110. Finan and Warren, *J. Chem. Soc.* (Lond.), p. 5229 (1963).
111. Rabat, *Bull. Soc. Chim. Fr. Ser. 5*, 7, 565 (1940).
112. Vis and Fletcher, *J. Am. Chem. Soc.*, 78, 4709 (1956).
113. Peat, Whelan, and Hinson, *Chem. Ind.*, p. 385 (1955).
114. Sato and Aso, *Nature*, 180, 984 (1957).
115. Haq and Whelan, *J. Chem. Soc.* (Lond.), p. 1342 (1958).
116. Watanabe and Aso, *J. Agric. Res.* (Tokyo), 11, 109 (1960).

OLIGOSACCHARIDES (INCLUDING DISACCHARIDES) (continued)

117. Wolfrom and Thompson, *J. Am. Chem. Soc.*, 77, 6403 (1955).
118. Weismann and Meyer, *J. Am. Chem. Soc.*, 76, 1753 (1954).
119. Freudenberg and Oertzen, *Justus Liebigs Ann. Chem.*, 574, 37 (1951).
120. Connel. Hirst, and Percival, *J. Chem. Soc.* (Lond.), p. 3494 (1950).
121. Peat, Whelan, and Lawley, *J. Chem. Soc.* (Lond.), pp. 724, 729 (1958).
122. Gillis, *Natuurwet. Tijdschr.* (Ghent), 12, 193 (1930); *Chem. Zentralbl.*, 1, 256 (1931).
123. Hudson and Yanovski, *J. Am. Chem. Soc.*, 39, 1013 (1917).
124. Peterson and Spencer, *J. Am. Chem. Soc.*, 49, 2822 (1927).
125. Wolfrom, Georges, and Miller, *J. Am. Chem. Soc.*, 71, 125 (1949).
126. Jeanes, Wilham, Jonones, Tsuchiya, and Rist, *J. Am. Chem. Soc.*, 75, 5911 (1953).
127. Bates, *Polarimetry, Saccharimetry and the Sugars*, National Bureau of Standards Circ. C440, U. S. Gov. Print. Off., Washington, D. C, 1942.
128. Zemplèn, *Hoppe-Seyler's Z. Physiol. Chem.*, 85, 399 (1913).
129. Hudson and Johnson, *J. Am. Chem. Soc.*, 39, 1272 (1917).
130. Thompson and Wolfrom, *J. Am. Chem. Soc.* 75, 3605 (1953).
131. Gakhokidze and Gvelukashvli, *J. Gen. Chem. U.S.S.R.*, 22, 143 (1952).
132. Hudson, *J. Org. Chem.*, 9, 470 (1944).
133. Haworth, Hirst, and Reynolds, *J. Chem. Soc.* (Lond.), p. 302 (1934).
134. Brauns, *J. Am. Chem. Soc.*, 48, 2776 (1926).
135. Haworth, Hirst, Streight, Thomas, and Welb, *J. Chem. Soc.* (Lond.), p. 2636 (1930).
136. Haskins, Hann, and Hudson, *J. Am. Chem. Soc.*, 63, 1724 (1941).
137. Lindberg, *Acta Chem. Scand.*, 7, 1218 (1953).
138. Bredereck, Wagner, Kuhn, and Ott, *Chem. Ber.*, 93, 1201 (1960).
139. Peat, Whelan, and Evans, *J. Chem. Soc.* (Lond.), p. 175 (1960).
140. Avigad, *Biochem. J.*, 73, 587 (1959).
141. Gakhokidze and Gvelukashvli, *J. Gen. Chem. U.S.S.R.*, 22, 143 (1952).
142. Haworth, Hirst, and Reynolds, *J. Chem. Soc.* (Lond.), p. 302 (1934).
143. Brauns, *J. Am. Chem. Soc.*, 48, 2776 (1926).
144. Hudson and Pacsu, *J. Am. Chem. Soc.*, 52, 2519 (1930).
145. Pacsu, *J. Am. Chem. Soc.*, 54, 3649 (1932).
146. Hough, Jones, and Richards, *J. Chem. Soc.* (Lond.), p. 2005 (1953).
147. Stodola, Koepsell, and Sharpe, *J. Am. Chem. Soc.*, 74, 3202 (1952); 78, 2514 (1956).
148. Bourne, Hutson, and Weigel, *Biochem. J.*, 79, 549 (1961).
149. Corbett and Kenner, *J. Chem. Soc.* (Lond.), p. 1431 (1955).
150. Weidenhagen and Lorenz, *Angew. Chem.*, 69, 641 (1957).
151. Arcamone and Bizioli, *Gazz. Chim. Ital.*, 87, 896 (1957).
152. Wolfrom and Juliano, *J. Am. Chem. Soc.*, 82, 1673 (1960).
153. Selinger and Schramm, *J. Biol. Chem.*, 236, 2183 (1961).
154. Barker, Heidelberger, Stacey, and Tipper, *J. Chem. Soc.* (Lond.), p. 3468 (1958).
155. Gorin and Spencer, *Can. J. Chem.*, 39, 2275 (1961).
156. Zemplén, *Chem. Abstr.*, 33, 4202 (1939).
157. Stoll, Keis, and von Wartburg, *Helv. Chim. Acta*, 35, 2495 (1952).
158. Barker, Gómez-Sánchez, and Stacey, *J. Chem. Soc.* (Lond.), p. 3264 (1959).
159. Palleroni and Doudoroff, *J. Biol. Chem.*, 219, 957 (1956).
160. Tunmann and Schehrer, *Arch. Pharm.*, 292, 745 (1959).
161. Lindberg, *Acta Chem. Scand.*, 7, 1119 (1953).
162. Lindberg, Silvander, and Wachtmeister, *Acta Chem. Scand.*, 17, 1348 (1963).
163. Selinger and Schramm, *J. Biol. Chem.*, 236, 2183 (1961).
164. Baytop, Tanher, Tekman, and Oner, *Folia Pharm.* (Istanbul), 4, 464 (1960).
165. Korte, *Chem. Ber.*, 88, 1527 (1955).
166. Frérejacque, *C. R. Acad. Sci.*, 246, 459 (1958).
167. Lindberg, *Acta Chem. Scand.*, 8, 869 (1954); 9, 1093, 1097 (1954).
168. Freudenberg, Wolf, Knopf, and Zaheer, *Chem. Ber.*, 61, 1743 (1928).
169. Perila and Bishop, *Can. J. Chem.*, 39, 815 (1961).
170. Tyminski and Timell, *J. Am. Chem. Soc.*, 82, 2823 (1960).
171. Merler and Wise, *Tappi (Tech. Assoc. Pulp Pap. Ind.)*, 41, 80 (1958).
172. Gorin and Perlin, *Can. J. Chem.*, 37, 1930 (1959).
173. Gorin and Perlin, *Can. J. Chem.*, 39, 2474 (1961).

OLIGOSACCHARIDES (INCLUDING DISACCHARIDES) (continued)

174. Jones and Nicholson, *J. Chem. Soc.* (Lond.), p. 27 (1958).
175. Aspinall, Rashbrook, and Kessler, *J. Chem. Soc.*, (Lond.) 215 (1958).
176. Jones and Painter, *J. Chem. Soc.* (Lond.), p. 669 (1959).
177. Jones and Nicholson, *J. Chem. Soc.* (Lond.), p. 27 (1958).
178. Wistler and Stein, *J. Am. Chem. Soc.*, 73, 4187, (1951).
179. Peat, Turvey, and Doyle, *J. Chem. Soc.* (Lond.), p. 3918 (1961).
180. Talley, Reynolds, and Evans, *J. Am. Chem. Soc.*, 65, 575 (1943).
181. Shaban and Jeanloz, *Carbohydr. Res.*, 17, 193 (1971).
182. Shaban and Jeanloz, *Carbohydr. Res.*, 20, 17 (1971).
183. Shaban and Jeanloz, *Carbohydr. Res.*, 17, 411, (1971).
184. Barker, Murray, Stacey, and Stroud, *Nature*, 191, 143 (1961).
185. Strepkov, *Zh. Obshch. Khim.*, 28, 3143 (1958).
186. Pazur and Gordon, *J. Am. Chem. Soc.*, 75, 3458 (1953).
187. Schlubach and Scheffler, *Justus Liebigs Ann. Chem.*, 588, 192 (1954).
188. Aspinall and Telfer, *J. Chem. Soc.* (Lond.), p. 1106 (1955).
189. Anderson, *Acta Chem. Scand.*, 21, 828 (1967).
190. Brigl and Scheyer, *Hoppe-Seyler's Z. Physiol. Chem.*, 160, 214 (1926).
191. Wallenfels and Lehmann, *Chem. Ber.*, 90, 1000 (1957).
192. Bacon, *Biochem. J.*, 57, 320 (1954).
193. Barber, *J. Am. Chem. Soc.*, 81, 3722 (1959).
194. Levy, Flowers, and Sharon, *Carbohydr. Res.*, 4, 305 (1967).
195. Kuhn, Baer, and Gauhe, *Justus Liebigs Ann. Chem.*, 611, 242 (1958).
196. Eagon and Dedonder, *C. R. Acad. Sci.*, 241, 579 (1955).
197. Gorin and Perlin, *Can. J. Chem.*, 37, 1930 (1959).
198. Coté, *J. Chem. Soc.* (Lond.), p. 2248 (1959).
199. O'Neill, *J. Am. Chem. Soc.*, 76, 5074 (1954).
200. Shaban and Jeanloz, *Carbohydr. Res.*, 20, 399 (1971).
201. Dejter-Juszynski and Flowers, *Carbohydr. Res.*, 23, 41 (1972).
202. Kuhn, Low, and Trischmann, *Chem. Ber.*, 88, 1492 (1955).
203. Zemplén, Gerecs, and Flesch, *Chem. Ber.*, 71, 2511 (1938).
204. Gorin and Perlin, *Can. J. Chem.*, 37, 1930 (1959).
205. Zemplén, Tettamanti, and Farago, *Chem. Ber.*, 71, 2511 (1938).
206. Zemplén and Gerecs, *Chem. Ber.*, 67, 2049 (1934).
207. Yoshizawa, *Biochim. Biophys. Acta*, 52, 588 (1961).
208. Lloyd and Roberts, *J. Chem. Soc.* (Lond.), p. 6910 (1965).
209. Kuhn and Kirschenlohr, *Chem. Ber.*, 87, 384 (1954).
210. Foster and Horton, *J. Chem. Soc.* (Lond.), p. 1890 (1958).
211. Wang and Tai, *Acta Chem. Sinicia*, 25, 50 (1959).
212. Schiffman, Kabat, and Leskowitz, *J. Am. Chem. Soc.*, 84, 73 (1962).
213. Yoshizawa, *J. Biochem.* (Tokyo), 51, 1 (1962).
214. Shinohara, *Tohoku J. Exp. Med.*, 67, 141 (1958).
215. Anderson and Fireman, *J. Biol. Chem.*, 109, 437 (1935).
216. Roudier and Eberhard, *Bull. Soc. Chim. Fr.*, 28, 2074 (1958).
217. Dhar and Mukherjee, *J. Sci. Ind. Res.* (India), 18B, 219 (1959).
218. Hirst and Dunstan, *J. Chem. Soc.* (Lond.), p. 2332 (1953).
219. Aspinall and Nicholson, *J. Chem. Soc.* (Lond.), p. 2503 (1960).
220. Aspinall and Fanshawe, *J. Chem. Soc.* (Lond.), p. 4215 (1961).
221. Anderson and Crowder, *J. Am. Chem. Soc.*, 52, 3711 (1930).
222. Tipson, Christman, and Levene, *J. Biol. Chem.*, 128, 609 (1939).
223. McCready, McComb, and Black, *J. Am. Chem. Soc.*, 76, 3035 (1954).
224. Bhattacharjee and Timell, *Can. J. Chem.*, 43, 758 (1965).
225. Gee, Jones, and McCready, *J. Org. Chem.*, 23, 620, (1958).
226. Mathur and Mukherjee, *J. Sci. Ind. Res.* (India), 13B 452 (1954).
227. Mukherjee and Stivastava, *J. Am. Chem. Soc.*, 77, 422 (1955).
228. Gorin and Spencer, *Can. J. Chem.*, 39, 2282 (1961).
229. Hotchkiss and Goebel, *J. Biol. Chem.*, 115, 285 (1936).
230. Jayne and Demmig, *Chem. Ber.*, 95, 356 (1960).
231. Jones and Perry, *J. Am. Chem. Soc.*, 79, 2787 (1957).
232. Helferich and Berger, *Chem. Ber.*, 90, 2492 (1957).
233. Hamilton, Spriesterbach, and Smith, *J. Chem. Soc.*, 79, 443 (1957).

OLIGOSACCHARIDES (INCLUDING DISACCHARIDES) (continued)

234. Bowering and Timell, *J. Am. Chem. Soc.*, 82, 2827 (1960).
235. Bishop, *Can. J. Chem.*, 33, 1521 (1955).
236. Bishop, *Can. J. Chem.*, 31, 134 (1953).
237. Whistler and Hough, *J. Am. Chem. Soc.*, 75, 4919 (1953).
238. Davidson and Meyer, *J. Am. Chem. Soc.*, 77, 4796 (1955).
239. Drummond and Percival, *J. Chem. Soc.*, (Lond.), p. 3908 (1961).
240. Smith and Stephen, *J. Chem. Soc.* (Lond.), p. 4892 (1961).
241. Barker, Foster, Siddiqui, and Stacey, *J. Chem. Soc.* (Lond.), p. 2358 (1958).
242. Hirst, Percival, and Williams, *J. Chem. Soc.* (Lond.), p. 1942 (1958).
243. O'Donnell and Percival, *J. Chem. Soc.* (Lond.), p. 2168 (1959).
244. McKinnell and Percival, *J. Chem. Soc.* (Lond.), p. 2082 (1962).
245. Danishefsky, Eiber, and Langholtz, *Biochem. Biophys. Res. Commun.*, 3, 571, (1960).
246. Voss and Pfirschke, *Chem. Ber.*, 70, 132 (1937).
247. Graham and Gottschalk, *Biochim. Biophys. Acta*, 38, 513 (1960).
248. Gottschalk and Graham, *Biochim. Biophys. Acta*, 34, 380, (1959).
249. Wickberg, *Acta Chem. Scand.*, 12, 1183, 1187 (1959).
250. Carter, McCluer, and Slifer, *J. Am. Chem. Soc.*, 78, 3735 (1956).
251. Reeves, Latour, and Lousteau, *Biochemistry*, 3, 1248 (1964).
252. Austin, Hardy, Buchanan, and Baddiley, *J. Chem. Soc.* (Lond.), 1419 (1965).
253. Colin, *Bull. Soc. Chim. Fr. Ser. 5*, 4, 277 (1937).
254. Su and Hassid, *Biochemistry*, 1, 468 (1962).
255. Putman and Hassid, *J. Am. Chem. Soc.*, 76, 2221 (1954).
256. Brown and Serro, *J. Am. Chem. Soc.*, 75, 1040 (1953).
257. Kabat, MacDonald, Ballou, and Fischer, *J. Am. Chem. Soc.*, 75, 4507 (1953).
258. Gorin, Horitsu, and Spencer, *Can. J. Chem.*, 43, 2259 (1965).
259. Pueyo, *C. R. Acad. Sci.*, 248, 2788 (1959).
260. Lindberg, Silvander, and Wachtmeister, *Acta Chem. Scand.*, 18, 213 (1964).
261. Araki and Arai, *Bull. Chem. Soc. Jap.*, 29, 339 (1956).
262. Nagel and Vaughn, *Arch. Biochem. Biophys.*, 94, 328 (1961).
263. Sawai and Hehre, *J. Biol. Chem.*, 237, 2047 (1962).
264. Jermyn, *Aust. J. Biol. Sci.*, 11, 114 (1958).
265. Dutton and Unrau, *Can. J. Chem.*, 42, 2048 (1964).
266. Hassid, Doudoroff, Barker, and Dore, *J. Am. Chem. Soc.*, 67, 1394 (1945).
267. Hassid, Doudoroff, Barker, and Dore, *J. Am. Chem. Soc.*, 68, 1465 (1946).
268. Osawa and Nakazawa, *Biochim. Biophys. Acta*, 130, 56 (1966).
269. Barker, Foster, Stacey, and Webber, *Chem. Ind.*, p. 208 (1957).
270. Barker, Foster, Khmelnitski, and Webber, *Bull. Soc. Chim. Biol.*, 42, 1799 (1960).
271. Danishefski and Steiner, *Biochim. Biophys. Acta*, 101, 37 (1965).
272. Gorin, Haskins, and Spencer, *Can. J. Biochem. Physiol.*, 38, 165 (1960).
273. Gorin and Perlin, *Can. J. Chem.*, 39, 2474 (1941).
274. Colin and Angier, *C. R. Acad. Sci.*, 208, 1450 (1939).
275. Charlson, Gorin, and Perlin, *Can. J. Chem.*, 34, 1811 (1956).
276. Martinez, Wolfe, and Nakada, *J. Bacteriol.*, 78, 217 (1959).
277. Olavesen and Davidson, *J. Biol. Chem.*, 240, 992 (1965).
278. Weissmann and Meyer, *J. Am. Chem. Soc.*, 74, 4729 (1952); 76, 1753 (1954).
279. Linker, Meyer, and Hoffman, *J. Biol. Chem.*, 219, 13 (1956).
280. Fukui, Hochster, Durbin, Grebner, and Feingold, *Bull. Res. Counc. Isr.*, 11A, 262 (1963).
281. Fukui and Hochster, *Can. J. Biochem.*, 41, 2363 (1963).
282. Tsujino, *Agric. Biol. Chem.*, 27, 236 (1963).
283. Hestrin, Feingold, and Avigad, *J. Am. Chem. Soc.*, 77, 6710 (1955).
284. Amanmuradov and Abubakirov, *Chem. Nat. Compd.* (USSR), 1, 292 (1965).
285. Smith and Stephen, *J. Chem. Soc.* (Lond.), p. 4892 (1961).
286. Bishop, *J. Am. Chem. Soc.*, 78, 2840 (1956).
287. Banerji and Rao, *Aust. J. Chem.*, 17, 1059 (1964).
288. Howard, *Biochem. J.*, 67, 643 (1957).
289. Whistler and Masak, *J. Am. Chem. Soc.*, 77, 1241 (1955).
290. Marchessault and Timell, *J. Polym. Sci.*, C2, 49 (1963).
291. Whistler and Corbett, *J. Am. Chem. Soc.*, 77, 6328 (1955).
292. Morgan and O'Neil, *Can. J. Chem.*, 37, 1201 (1959).
293. Aspinall, Hirst, and Ramstad, *J. Chem. Soc.* (Lond.), p. 593 (1958).

OLIGOSACCHARIDES (INCLUDING DISACCHARIDES) (continued)

294. Haq and Adams, *Can. J. Chem.*, 39, 1563 (1961).
295. Smith and Stephen, *J. Chem. Soc.* (Lond.), p. 4892 (1961).
296. Courtois, *Carbohydrate Chemistry of Substances of Biological Interest, 4th Int. Congr. Biochem.*, Vol. 1, Wolfrom, Ed., Pergamon Press, London, 1959, 146.
297. Halahmi, Flowers, and Shapiro, *Carbohydr. Res.*, 5, 25 (1967).
298. Ballio and Russi, *Tetrahedron*, 9, 125 (1960).
299. Yamashita and Kobata, *Arch. Biochem. Biophys.*, 161, 164 (1974).
300. Tanret, *Bull. Soc. Chim. Ser. 3*, 27, 947 (1902).
301. Pazur, Marsh, and Timpton, *J. Am. Chem. Soc.*, 80, 1433 (1958).
302. Wallenfels, Bernt, and Limberg, *Justus Liebigs Ann. Chem.*, 579, 113 (1952).
303. Chaudun, Courtois, and Dizet, *Bull. Soc. Chim. Biol.*, 42, 227 (1960).
304. Freudenberg, Wolf, Knopf, and Zaheer, *Chem. Ber.*, 61, 1743 (1928).
305. Helferich and Schafer, *Justus Liebigs Ann. Chem.*, 450, 229 (1926).
306. Wickstrom and Svendsen, *Acta Chem. Scand.*, 10, 1199 (1956).
307. Macleod and McCorquodale, *Nature*, 182, 815 (1958).
308. Avigad, *J. Biol. Chem.*, 229, 121 (1957).
309. Aso and Yamauchi, *Agric. Biol. Chem.*, 25, 10 (1961).
310. Haworth, Hirst, and Ruell, *J. Chem. Soc.* (Lond.), p. 3125 (1923).
311. Scheibler and Mittelmeier, *Chem. Ber.*, 23, 1438 (1890).
312. Tanret, *Bull. Soc. Chim. Fr. Ser. 3*, 13, 261 (1895).
313. Whistler and Durso, *J. Am. Chem. Soc.*, 74, 5140 (1952).
314. Davy and Courtois, *C.R. Acad. Sci.*, 261, 3483 (1965).
315. Suzuki and Hehre, *Arch. Biochem. Biophys.*, 105, 339 (1964).
316. French, Wild, Young, and James, *J. Am. Chem. Soc.*, 75, 709 (1953).
317. Pazur, Marsh, and Tipton, *J. Biol. Chem.*, 233, 277 (1958).
318. Gorin and Spencer, *Can. J. Chem.*, 39, 2275 (1961).
319. Montreuil, *C.R. Acad. Sci.*, 242, 192 (1956).
320. Bailey, Barker, Bourne, and Stacey, *Nature*, 176, 1164 (1955).
321. Yamauchi and Aso, *Nature*, 189, 753 (1961).
322. Kuhn, Baer, and Gauhe, *Chem. Ber.*, 89, 2514 (1956).
323. Kuhn, Baer, and Gauhe, *Justus Liebigs Ann. Chem.*, 611, 242 (1958).
324. Kuhn, Baer, and Gauhe, *Chem. Ber.*, 91, 364 (1958).
325. Kuhn and Gauhe, *Chem. Ber.*, 93, 647 (1960).
326. Kobata and Ginsburg, *J. Biol. Chem.*, 244, 5496 (1969).
327. Whistler and Conrad, *J. Am. Chem. Soc.*, 76, 3544 (1954).
328. Kuhn and Löw, *Chem. Ber.*, 86, 1027 (1953).
329. Kuhn, Löw, and Trischmann, *Chem. Ber.*, 90, 203 (1957); *Angew. Chem.*, 68, 212 (1958).
330. Freudenberg, Wolf, Knopf, and Zaheer, *Chem. Ber.*, 61, 1743 (1928).
331. Bailey, Barker, Bourne, Grant, and Stacey, *J. Chem. Soc.* (Lond.), p. 1895 (1958).
332. Peat, Whelan, and Roberts, *J. Chem. Soc.* (Lond.), p. 3916 (1957).
333. Parrish, Perlin, and Reese, *Can. J. Chem.*, 38, 2094 (1960).
334. Klemer, *Chem. Ber.*, 89, 2583 (1956).
335. Crook and Stone, *Biochem. J.*, 65, 1 (1957).
336. Berger and Eberhart, *Biochem. Biophys. Res. Comm.*, 6, 62 (1961).
337. Barker, Bourne, O'mant, and Stacey, *J. Chem. Soc.* (Lond.), p. 2448 (1957).
338. Reese and Mandels, *Can. J. Microbiol.*, 10, 103 (1964).
339. Perlin and Suzuki, *Can. J. Chem.*, 40, 50 (1962).
340. Peat, Whelan, and Roberts, *J. Chem. Soc.* (Lond.), p. 3916 (1957).
341. Moscatelli, Ham, and Rickes, *J. Biol. Chem.*, 236, 2858 (1961).
342. Wolfrom, Georges, Thompson, and Miller, *J. Am. Chem. Soc.*, 71, 2873 (1949).
343. Peat, Whelan, and Jones, *J. Chem. Soc.* (Lond.), p. 2490 (1957).
344. Sugihara and Wolfrom, *J. Am. Chem. Soc.*, 71, 3357 (1949).
345. Walker and Wright, *Arch. Biochem. Biophys.*, 69, 362 (1957).
346. Wolfrom and Fields, *Tappi (Tech. Assoc. Pulp Pap. Ind.)*, 41, 204 (1958).
347. French, Taylor, and Whelan, *Biochem. J.*, 90, 616 (1964).
348. Takiura and Nakagawa, *Yakugaku Zasshi*, 83, 301, 305 (1963).
349. Bailey, Barker, Bourne, and Atacey, *J. Chem. Soc.* (Lond.), p. 3536 (1957).
350. Turvey and Whelan, *Biochem. J.*, 67, 49 (1957).
351. Conchie, Moreno, and Cardini, *Arch. Biochem. Biophys.*, 94, 342 (1961).
352. Haq and Whelan, *J. Chem. Soc.* (Lond.), p. 4543 (1956).

OLIGOSACCHARIDES (INCLUDING DISACCHARIDES) (continued)

353. Peat, Whelan, and Evans, *J. Chem. Soc.* (Lond.), p. 175 (1960).
354. Thompson and Wolfrom, *J. Am. Chem. Soc.*, 77, 3567 (1955).
355. Asp and Lindberg, *Acta Chem. Scand.*, 5, 665 (1951).
356. Zemplén and Gerecs, *Chem. Ber.*, 64, 1545 (1931).
357. Zemplén, Bruckner, and Gerecs, *Chem. Ber.*, 64, 744 (1931).
358. Shibasaki, *Tohoku J. Agric. Res.*, 6, 171 (1955).
359. Peat, Whelan, and Lawley, *J. Chem. Soc.* (Lond.), p. 729 (1958).
360. Turvey and Evans, *J. Chem. Soc.* (Lond.), p. 2366 (1960).
361. Handa and Nishizawa, *Nature*, 192, 1078 (1961).
362. Peat, Turvey, and Evans, *J. Chem. Soc.* (Lond.), p. 3223 (1959).
363. Klemer, *Chem. Ber.*, 92, 218 (1959).
364. Goldstein and Lindberg, *Acta Chem. Scand.*, 16, 383 (1962).
365. Peat, Whelan, Turvey, and Morgan, *J. Chem. Soc.* (Lond.), p. 623 (1961).
366. Abdullah, Goldstein, and Whelan, *J. Chem. Soc.* (Lond.), p. 176 (1962).
367. Krieglstein and Fischer, *Hoppe-Seyler's Z. Physiol. Chem.*, 344, 209 (1966).
368. Feingold, Neufeld, and Hassid, *J. Biol. Chem.*, 233, 783 (1958).
369. White and Maher, *J. Am. Chem. Soc.*, 75, 1259 (1953).
370. Wolf and Ewart, *Arch. Biochem. Biophys.*, 58, 365 (1955).
371. Barker, Bourne, and Theander, *J. Chem. Soc.* (Lond.), p. 2064 (1957).
372. Baron and Guthrie, *Ann. Entomol. Soc. Am.*, 53, 220 (1960).
373. Meyer, *Hoppe-Seyler's Z. Physiol. Chem.*, 6, 135 (1882).
374. Binaghi and Falqui, *Chem. Zentralbl.*, 2, 44 (1926).
375. Binkley, *Int. Sugar J.*, 66, 46 (1964).
376. Schlubach and Koehm, *Justus Liebigs Ann. Chem.*, 614, 126 (1958).
377. Barker, Bourne, and Carrington, *J. Chem. Soc.* (Lond.), p. 2125 (1954).
378. Bacon and Bell, *J. Chem. Soc.* (Lond.), 2528 (1953).
379. Albon, Bell, Blanchard, Gross, and Rundell, *J. Chem. Soc.* (Lond.), p. 24 (1953).
380. Kuhn and von Grundherr, *Chem. Ber.*, 59, 1655 (1926).
381. Von Lippmann, *Chem. Ber.*, 60, 161 (1927).
382. Hudson and Sherwood, *J. Am. Chem. Soc.*, 40, 1456 (1918).
383. Aspinall, Begbie, and Mckay, *J. Chem. Soc.* (Lond.), p. 214 (1962).
384. Mayeda, *J. Biochem.* (Tokyo), 1, 131 (1922).
385. Ohtsuki, *Acta Phytochim.*, 4, 1 (1928).
386. Talley and Evans, *J. Am. Chem. Soc.*, 65, 573, 575 (1943).
387. Shaban and Jeanloz, *Carbohydr. Res.*, 19, 311 (1971).
388. Schwarz and Timell, *Can. J. Chem.*, 41, 1381 (1963).
389. Barker, Gomez-Sanchez, and Stacey, *J. Chem. Soc.* (Lond.), p. 3264 (1959).
390. Allen and Bacon, *Biochem. J.*, 63, 200 (1956).
391. Bacon and Bell, *J. Chem. Soc.* (Lond.), p. 2528 (1953).
392. Bacon, *Biochem. J.*, 57, 320 (1954).
393. Wolfe, Senior, and Kin, *J. Biol. Chem.*, 249, 1828 (1974).
394. Strepkov, *J. Gen. Chem. U.S.S.R.*, 9, 1489 (1939).
395. Kuhn, Gauhe, and Baer, *Chem. Ber.*, 87, 289, 1553 (1954); 89, 2513, 2514 (1956).
396. Nakazawa, *J. Biochem.* (Tokyo), 46, 1579 (1959).
397. Schiffman, Kabat, and Leskowitz, *J. Am. Chem. Soc.*, 84, 73 (1962).
398. Lister-Cheese and Morgan, *Nature*, 191, 149 (1961).
399. Masamune, Yoshizawa, and Haga, *Tohoku J. Exp. Med.*, 64, 257 (1956).
400. Masamune and Shinohara, *Tohoku J. Exp. Med.*, 69, 65 (1958).
401. Pazur, *J. Am. Chem. Soc.*, 75, 6323 (1953).
402. Strepkov, *Dokl. Akad. Nauk SSSR*, 124, 1344 (1959).
403. Okuyama, *Seikagaku*, 33, 134, 821 (1961).
404. Yoshizawa, *J. Biochem.* (Tokyo), 51, 145 (1962).
405. Kuhn, Baer, and Gauhe, *Justus Liebigs Ann. Chem.*, 611, 242 (1958).
406. Kuhn and Gauhe, *Chem. Ber.*, 93, 647 (1960).
407. Kuhn, Baer, and Gauhe, *Chem. Ber.*, 91, 364 (1958).
408. Zechmeister and Toth, *Chem. Ber.*, 65, 161 (1932).
409. Linker, Meyer, and Weissmann, *J. Biol. Chem.*, 213, 237 (1955).
410. Anderson, Gillette, and Seely, *J. Biol. Chem.*, 140, 569 (1941).
411. Buchi and Deuel, *Helv. Chim. Acta*, 37, 1392 (1954).
412. Falconer and Adams, *Can. J. Chem.*, 34, 338 (1956).

OLIGOSACCHARIDES (INCLUDING DISACCHARIDES) (continued)

413. Sloneker and Jeanes, *Can. J. Chem.*, 40, 2066 (1962).
414. Whistter and McGilvray, *J. Am. Chem. Soc.*, 77, 2212 (1955).
415. Schneir and Rafelson, *Biochem. Biophys. Acta*, 130, 1 (1966).
416. Kuhn and Brossmer, *Chem. Ber.*, 92, 1667 (1959).
417. Ryan, Carubelli, Caputto, and Trucco, *Biochim. Biophys. Acta*, 101, 252 (1965).
418. Brandish, Shaw, and Baddiley, *J. Chem. Soc.*i (Lond.), p. C521 (1966).
419. Peat, Whelan, and Evans, *J. Chem. Soc.* (Lond.), p. 175 (1960).
420. Lindberg, *Acta Chem. Scand.*, 9, 1093, 1097 (1955).
421. Jones and Reid, *J. Chem. Soc.* (Lond.), p. 1361 (1954); p. 1890 (1955).
422. Goldschmid and Perlin, *Can. J. Chem.*, 41, 2272 (1963).
423. Hatanaka, *Arch. Biochem. Biophys.*, 82, 188 (1959).
424. Davy and Courtois, *C. R. Acad. Sci.*, 261, 3483 (1965).
425. French, Wild, and James, *J. Am. Chem. Soc.*, 75, 3664 (1953).
426. Onuki, *Sci. Pap. Inst. Phys. Chem. Res.* (Japan), 20, 201 (1933).
427. Courtois and Ariyoshi, *Bull. Soc. Chim. Biol.*, 42, 737 (1960).
428. Haq and Adams, *Can. J. Chem.*, 39, 1563 (1961).
429. Kuhn, Gauhe, and Baer, *Chem. Ber.*, 95, 513, 518 (1962).
430. Kuhn, Löw, and Trischmann, *Chem. Ber.*, 90, 203 (1957).
431. Torriani and Pappenheimer, *J. Biol. Chem.*, 237, 1 (1962).
432. Parrish, Perlin, and Reese, *Can. J. Chem.*, 38, 2094 (1960).
433. Perlin and Suzuki, *Can. J. Chem.*, 40, 50 (1962).
434. Igarashi, Igoshi, and Sakurai, *Agric. Biol. Chem.*, 30, 1254 (1966).
435. Whistler and Hickson, *J. Am. Chem. Soc.*, 76, 1671 (1954).
436. Zechmeister and Toth, *Chem. Ber.*, 64, 854 (1931).
437. Wolfrom and Fields, *Tappi (Tech. Assoc. Pulp Pap. Ind.)*, 41, 204 (1958); 40, 335 (1957).
438. Duncan and Manners, *Biochem. J.*, 69, 343 (1958).
439. Jones, Jeanes, Stringer, and Tsuchiya, *J. Am. Chem. Soc.*, 78, 2499 (1956).
440. Pazur and Ando, *J. Biol. Chem.*, 235, 297 (1960).
441. Helferich, Schafer, and Bauerlein, *Justus Liebigs Ann. Chem.*, 465, 166 (1928).
442. Bailey, Hutson, and Weigel, *Biochem. J.*, 80, 514 (1961).
443. Binkley and Altenburg, *Int. Sugar J.*, 67, 110 (1965).
444. Kurosawa, Yamamoto, Igaue, and Nakamura, *Nippon Nogei Kagaku Kaishi*, 30, 696 (1956).
445. Strepkov, *Dokl. Akad. Nauk SSSR*, 125, 216 (1959).
446. Murakami, *Acta Phytochim.*, 14, 101 (1944); 15, 105, 109 (1949).
447. Barker and Carrington, *J. Chem. Soc.* (Lond.), p. 3588 (1953).
448. Schlubach and Berndt, *Justus Liebigs Ann. Chem.*, 647, 41 (1961).
449. Pazur, *J. Biol. Chem.*, 199, 217 (1952).
450. Kuhn and Gauhe, *Justus Liebigs Ann. Chem.*, 611, 249 (1958).
451. Demain and Phaff, *Arch. Biochem. Biophys.*, 51, 114 (1954).
452. Wiessman, Meyer, Sampson, and Linker, *J. Biol. Chem.*, 208, 417 (1954).
453. Bourquelot and Bridel, *C. R. Acad. Sci.*, 151, 760 (1910).
454. Murakami, *Proc. Imp. Acad.* (Tokyo), 16, 14 (1940).
455. Kuhn, Baer, and Gauhe, *Chem. Ber.*, 91, 364 (1958).
456. Schlubach and Koehn, *Justus Liebigs Ann. Chem.*, 614, 126 (1958).
457. Wolfrom, Dacons, and Fields, *Tappi (Tech. Assoc. Pulp Pap. Ind.)*, 39, 803 (1956).
458. Hoover, Nelson, Milner, and Wei, *J. Food Sci.*, 30, 253 (1965).
459. Schlubach and Koehn, *Justus Liebigs Ann. Chem.*, 606, 130 (1957).
460. Schlubach, Berndt, and Chiemprasert, *Justus Liebigs Ann. Chem.*, 665, 191 (1963).
461. Kobata and Ginsburg, *J. Biol. Chem.*, 244, 5496 (1969).
462. Kuhn, Gauhe, and Baer, *Chem. Ber.*, 86, 827 (1953).
463. Wiegandt and Schulze, *Z. Naturforsch.*, 24b, 945 (1969).
464. Whistler and Tu, *J. Am. Chem. Soc.*, 74, 3609 (1952); 75, 645 (1954).
465. Bjorndel, Eriksson, Garegg, Lindberg, and Swan, *Acta Chem. Scand.*, 19, 2309 (1965).
466. Murakami, *Acta Phytochim.*, 13, 37 (1942).
467. Herissey, Fleury, Wickstrom, Courtois, and Dizet, *Compt. Rend.*, 239, 824 (1954).
468. Akiya and Tomoda, *J. Pharm. Soc. Jap.*, 76, 571 (1956).
469. French and Rundle, *J. Am. Chem. Soc.*, 64, 1651 (1942).
470. Freudenberg and Jacobi, *Justus Liebigs Ann. Chem.*, 518, 102 (1935).
471. Kobata and Ginsburg, *J. Biol. Chem.*, 247, 1525 (1972).
472. Kobata and Ginsburg, *Arch. Biochem. Biophys.*, 150, 273 (1972).

OLIGOSACCHARIDES (INCLUDING DISACCHARIDES) (continued)

473. Kuhn, Baer, and Gauhe, *Justus Liebigs Ann. Chem.*, 611, 242 (1958).
474. Kuhn and Gauhe, *Chem. Ber.*, 93, 647 (1960).
475. Grimmonprez and Montreuil, *Bull. Soc. Chim. Biol.*, 50, 843 (1968).
476. Murakami, *Acta Phytochim.*, 10, 43 (1937).
477. Courtois, Dizet, and Wickstrom, *Bull. Soc. Chim. Biol.*, 40, 1059 (1958).
478. French, Knapp, and Pazur, *J. Am. Chem. Soc.*, 72, 5150 (1950).
479. Schlubach and Koehn, *Justus Liebigs Ann. Chem.*, 606, 130 (1957).
480. Suzuki and Sunayama, *Jap. J. Microbiol.*, 13, 95 (1969).
481. Suzuki, Sunayama, and Saito, *Jap. J. Microbiol.*, 12, 19 (1968).
482. Suzuki and Sunayama, *Jap. J. Microbiol.*, 12, 413 (1968).
483. Sunayama, *Jap. J. Microbiol.*, 14, 27 (1970).
484. Lundblad, Hallgren, Rudmark, and Svensson, *Biochemistry*, 12, 3341 (1973).
485. Huttunen and Miettinen, *Acta Chem. Scand.*, 19, 1486 (1965).
486. Kobata and Ginsburg, *J. Biol. Chem.*, 245, 1484 (1970).

MUCOPOLYSACCHARIDES (GLYCOSAMINOGLYCANS)

Name[a]	Repeating unit[b]	[α]$_D$, degrees[c]	Infrared, Cm^{-1},[d]	Intrinsic viscosity (21)	Molecular weight	Occurrence
Chitin	(1 → 4)-O-2-Acetamido-2-deoxy-β-D-glucopyranose (1)	-14 to +56[i] (1)	884–890 (1)	-	-	Skeletal substance of arthropods, molluscs, and annelids, cell wall of many fungi, green algae
Chondroitin	(1 → 4)-O-β-D-Glucopyranosyluronic acid-(1 → 3)-2-acetamido-2-deoxy-β-D-galactopyranose (2, 3)	-21 (3)	-	-	-	Bovine cornea
Chondroitin 4-sulfate (Chondroitin sulfate A)	(1 → 4)-O-β-D-glucopyranosyluronic acid-(1 → 3)-2-acetamido-2-deoxy-4-O-sulfo-β-D-galactopyranose (4)	-26 to -30 (4)	724, 851, 930 (17, 18)	0.2–1.0	5 × 10⁴ (22)	Bone cornea, cartilage, notochord, skin
Chondroitin 6-sulfate (Chondroitin sulfate C)	(1 → 4)-O-Glucopyranosyluronic acid-(1 → 3)-2-acetamido-2-deoxy-6-O-sulfo-β-D-galactopyranose (5)	-12 to -22 (5)	775, 820, 1,000 (17, 18)	0.2–1.3	5 × 10³– 50 × 10³ (21)	Cartilage, aorta, skin, umbilical cord
Dermatan sulfate (Chondroitin sulfate B, β-heparin)	(1 → 4)-O-α-L-Idopyranosyluronic acid-(1 → 3)-2-acetamido-2-deoxy-4-O-sulfo-β-D-galactopyranose (6)[e]	-55 to -63 (13)	724, 851, 930 (18)	0.5–1.0	1.5 × 10⁴– 4 × 10⁴ (21)	Aorta, skin, umbilical cord, tendon
Heparan sulfate (Heparitin sulfate)	Glucopyranosyluronic acid-(1 → 4)-2-amino-2-deoxy-O-sulfo-D-glucopyranose (7)[f]	+39 to +69 (14)	920, 1,050 (19)	-	-	Aorta, lung

[a]Certain mucopolysaccharides have been given different names by various investigators. In such cases, alternative names are given in parentheses.

[b]The repeating unit, which is indicated, is the one that is most prevalent. In many mucopolysaccharides there may be some variations in parts of the chain (microheterogeneity), especially with regard to sulfation. The units involved in the linkage to the proteins are not given here.

[c]Many of the values for specific rotation and intrinsic viscosity are given as ranges because these depend on the method of isolation and the original tissue source. In these cases, the references cited are review articles which include the original research papers.

[d]Fingerprint region.

[e]Also contains small but significant amounts of glucuronic acid.[25,26]

[f]Some amino groups are acetylated and others are sulfated. There are also variations in the position of O-sulfate. Part of the uronic acid is iduronic acid.

[g]There are O-sulfates in about one third of the uronic acid residues. Although both iduronate and glucuronate are present their relative proportion is not completely defined.[27]

[h]Some of the galactose is sulfated on position-6.

[i]In HCl; change in rotation occurs as a result of hydrolysis.

MUCOPOLYSACCHARIDES (GLYCOSAMINOGLYCANS) (continued)

Name[a]	Repeating unit[b]	$[\alpha]_D$, degrees[c]	Infrared, Cm^{-1}, [d]	Intrinsic viscosity (21)	Molecular weight	Occurrence
Heparin	(1 → 4)-O-α-D-Glucopyranosyluronic acid-(1 → 4)-2-deoxy-6-O-sulfo-α-D-glucopyranose and (1 → 4)-O-α-L-idopyranosyluronic acid-2-sulfate-(1 → 4)-2-sulfoamino-2-deoxy-6-O-sulfo-α-D-glucopyranose (8, 9)[g]	+48 (15)	890, 940 (14)	0.1–0.2	8×10^3 – 20×10^3 (23)	Liver, lung, skin, mast cells
Hyaluronic acid	(1 → 4)-O-β-D-Glucopyranosyluronic acid-(1 → 3)-2-acetamido-2-deoxy-β-D-glucopyranose (10)	−68 (16)	900, 950 (16)	2.0–48	2×10^5 – 10×10^5 (24)	Synovial fluid, vitreous humor, umbilical cord, skin
Keratan sulfate (Keratosulfate)	(1 → 3)-O-β-D-Galactopyranose-(1 → 4)-2-acetamido-2-deoxy-6-O-sulfo-β-D-glucopyranose (7, 11)[h]	+4.5	775, 820, 998 (20)	0.2–0.5	8×10^3 – 12×10^3 (21)	Aorta, cornea, cartilage, nucleus pulposus

Compiled by I. Danishefsky.

MUCOPOLYSACCHARIDES (GLYCOSAMINOGLYCANS) (continued)

REFERENCES

1. Foster and Webber, *Adv. Carbohydr. Chem.*, 15, 371 (1960).
2. Meyer, Linker, Davidson, and Weissmann, *J. Biol. Chem.*, 205, 611 (1953).
3. Davidson and Meyer, *J. Biol. Chem.*, 211, 605 (1954).
4. Jeanloz, *Methods Carbohydr. Chem.*, 5, 110 (1965).
5. Jeanloz, *Methods Carbohydr. Chem.*, 5, 113 (1965).
6. Jeanloz, *Methods Carbohydr. Chem.*, 5, 114 (1965).
7. Cifonelli, *Carbohydr. Res.*, 8, 233 (1968).
8. Danishefsky, Steiner, Bella, and Friedlander, *J. Biol. Chem.*, 244, 1741 (1969).
9. Wolfrom, Honda, and Wang, *Carbohydr. Res.*, 10, 259 (1969).
10. Brimacombe and Webber, *Mucopolysaccharides*, Elsevier, Amsterdam, 1964, 43.
11. Bhavanandam and Meyer, *Science*, 151, 1404 (1966).
12. Irvine, *J. Chem. Soc.*, 95, 564 (1909).
13. Brimacombe and Webber, *Mucopolysaccharides*, Elsevier, Amsterdam, 1964, 82.
14. Linker, Hoffman, Sampon, and Meyer, *Biochim. Biophys. Acta*, 29, 443 (1958).
15. Danishefsky, Eiber, and Carr, *Arch. Biochem. Biophys.*, 90, 114 (1960).
16. Danishefsky and Bella, *J. Biol. Chem.*, 241, 143 (1966).
17. Orr, *Biochim. Biophys. Acta*, 14, 173 (1954).
18. Mathews, *Nature*, 181, 421 (1958).
19. Schiller, *Biochim. Biophys. Acta*, 32, 315 (1959).
20. Brimacombe and Webber, *Mucopolysaccharides*, Elsevier, Amsterdam, 1964, 138.
21. Mathews, *Clin. Orthop.*, 48, 267 (1966).
22. Mathews, *Arch. Biochem. Biophys.*, 61, 367 (1956).
23. Barlow, Sanderson, and McNeil, *Arch. Biochem. Biophys.*, 94, 518 (1961).
24. Silpananta, Dunston, and Ogston, *Biochem. J.*, 109, 43 (1968).
25. Hoffman, Linker, and Meyer, *Arch. Biochem. Biophys.*, 69, 435 (1957).
26. Framsson and Roden, *J. Biol. Chem.*, 242, 4161 (1967).
27. Helting and Lindahl, *J. Biol. Chem.*, 246, 5442 (1972).

THE NATURALLY OCCURRING AMINO SUGARS

Compound and formula	Source	Physical constants[a]		R_{GlcN} values on paper solvent systems[b]					R_{GlcN} on ion exchange system[c]		References
		MP	$[\alpha]_D$	A	B	C	D	E	I	II	

I. 2-AMINO SUGARS

Compound and formula	Source	MP	$[\alpha]_D$	A	B	C	D	E	I	II	References
Glucosamine (chitosamine): 2-amino-2-deoxy-D-glucose	Polysaccharides of bacteria, fungi, invertebrates, chitin, antibiotics, higher plants, vertebrates, UDP-complexes	88 / 190–210 / 110–111	(α) FB +100 → +47.5; (α) HCl +100 → +72; (β) FB +28 → +47.5; (β) HCl +25 → +72.6	1.00	1.00	1.00	1.00	1.00	1.00	1.00	1–4
Galactosamine (chondrosamine): 2-amino-2-deoxy-D-galactose	Polysaccharides of bacteria, fungi, invertebrates, antibiotics, vertebrates, UDP-complexes	185	(α) HCl: W–HCl +121 → +80; (β) HCl: W–HCl +44 → +80	0.90 / 0.80^A	0.90	1.04	1.05	0.94	1.17 / 1.20	1.03	1–4

[a] MP. melting point; $[\alpha]_D$. – Rotation solvent; water, unless otherwise indicated in which case W-E = water:ethanol (1:1); W-HCl = water-HCl; E = ethanol; M = methanol. The abbreviations (α) or (β) indicate the anomer; HCl indicates the hydrochloride: Ac the acetate.

[b] Solvent system:

A. n-butanol-pyridine-water (6:4:3)
A^A. solvent system A on paper treated with 0.1 M $BaCl_2$ or $BaAc_2$
B. n-butanol glacial acetic acid-water (5:1:2)
C. phenol-water (70:30)
D. phenol-water (80:20), ammonia atmosphere
E. ethylacetate-pyridine-water-acetic acid (5:5:3:1)
F. pyridine-ethyl acetate-water (10:36:11.5)
G. phenol-water (80:20)
H. n-butanol-acetic acid-water (5:1:2.5)
I. ethylacetate-pyridine-n-butanol-butyric acid water (10:10:5:1:5)

J. isobutyric acid-N ammonia (10:0.6)
K. pyridine-ethyl acetate-water (10:3.0:1.5 upper layer)
L. n-butanol-ethanol-water (13:8:4)
M. n-butanol-acetic acid-water (3:1:1)
N. n-butanol-ethanol-water (4:1:1)
O. n-butanol-pyridine-0.1 N HCl (5:3:2)
P. n-butanol-acetic acid-water (25:6:25)
Q. ethylacetate-pyridine-water (2:1:2)
R. n-butanol-ethanol-water (5:1:4)
S. n-propanol-1 per cent ammonia (7:3)

[c] System I: Dowex 50 H+ column 1 x 50 cm packed according to Gardell and eluted with 0.33 N HCl.[4,4]
System II: Technicon amino acid analyzer modified by Brendel et al.[4] and eluted with 0.133 M pyridine-acetic acid (0.82 M) buffer pH 3.85.

THE NATURALLY OCCURRING AMINO SUGARS (continued)

Compound and formula	Source	Physical constants[a]		R_{GlcN} values on paper solvent systems[b]					R_{GlcN} on ion exchange system[c]		References
		MP	$[\alpha]_D$	A	B	C	D	E	I	II	

I. 2-Amino Sugars—(continued)

Compound and formula	Source	MP	$[\alpha]_D$	A	B	C	D	E	I	II	References
Mannosamine: 2-amino-2-deoxymannose 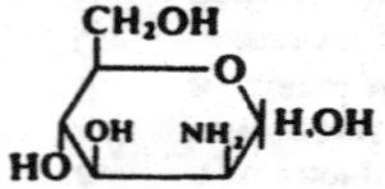 (N-acetyl-D-isomer)	Pneumococcus type XIX polysaccharide E. coli, Salmonella, animal metabolite	178–180	HCl −3	1.05 1.13[A] 1.17[A]	—	1.19	1.05	—	1.06	1.12	1—4, 6[e], 7[e], 8
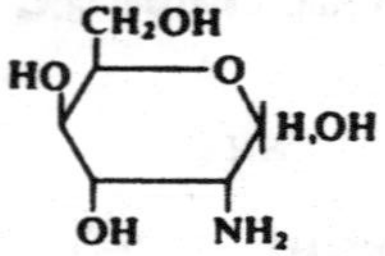 D-Galosamine: 2-amino-2-deoxy-D-galose	Antibiotics: streptolin B, streptothricin	150–170	(α) HCl +6.1 → −17.9	1.00 1.01	—	—	1.05	—	1.21	1.20	1—4
2-Amino heptose: D-glycero-2-deoxy-2-amino-galo-(or ido-) heptose j	Anacystis nidulans cell wall	—	—	—	—	—	—	—	2.19	—	46
6-0-Methyl-D-Glucosamine: 6-0-methyl-2-amino-2-deoxy-D-glucose 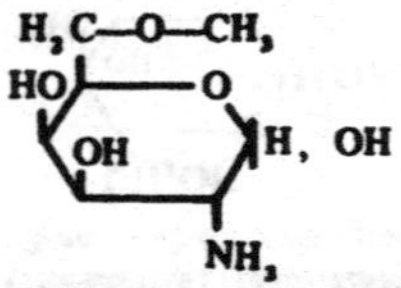	Lipopolysaccharide of Rhodopseudomonas palustris	—	—	—	—	—	—	—	—	—	54
D-Quinovosamine: 2-amino-2,6-dideoxy-D-glucose 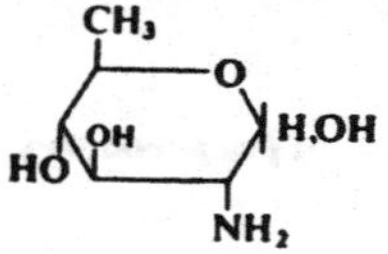	Achromobacter georgio politanum Salmonella, Proteus vulgaris Arizona, Neurospora crassa Vibrio cholera, Brucella species	165–170	HCl +55.5	1.85	2.23	2.5	—	1.40	1.43	1.26	3, 4, 9[d], 10, 45, 47, 55, 56

[d]Denotes the reference describing the characterization of the compound in question.
[e]Denotes chromatographic identification.
[j]The C-2 carbon configuration is in doubt

THE NATURALLY OCCURRING AMINO SUGARS (continued)

Compound and formula	Source	Physical constants[a]		R_{GlcN} values on paper solvent systems[b]					R_{GlcN} on ion exchange system[c]		References
		MP	$[\alpha]_D$	A	B	C	D	E	I	II	
1. 2-Amino Sugars—(continued)											
L-Quinovosamine: 2-amino-2,6-dideoxy-L-glucose	Lipopolysaccharide of *Shigella boydii*	—	—	—	—	—	—	—	—	—	57
D-Fucosamine: 2-amino-2,6-dideoxy-D-galactose 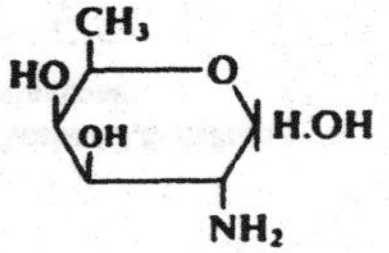	*C. violaceum* *B. licheniformis* *B. cereus* *Erysipelothrix insidiosa* *Pseudomonas aeruginosa*	155 chars 170–175 decomp.	HCl +91 ± 2	1.32	1.94	2.4	1.31	1.20	1.73 1.75 1.95	1.24	1, 2, 4 10, 11, 12 13d 14d 48d, 49d, 53d
L-Fucosamine: 2-amino-2,6-dideoxy-L-galactose 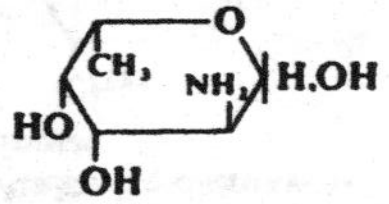	Polysaccharide of pneumococcus type V *Citrobacter freundii* 05: H30 muco-polysaccharide	155 chars	HCl −93.4 ± 2	—	—	—	—	—	—	—	2, 15d, 16d
Pneumosamine: 2-amino-2,6-dideoxy-L-talose 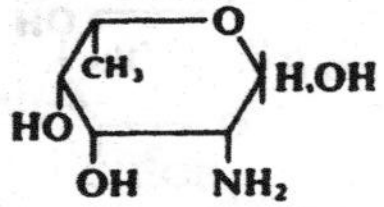	Pneumococcus type V	162–163	HCl +6.9 → +10.4	—	—	—	—	—	—	1.35	2, 4, 16d
L-Rhamnosamine: 2-amino-2,6-dideoxy-L-rhamnose 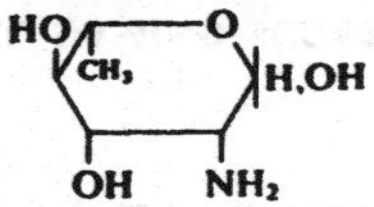	*E. coli* 03:K2ab(L):H2	—	HCl +22.5	—	—	—	—	—	—	1.48	50d

THE NATURALLY OCCURRING AMINO SUGARS (continued)

Compound and formula	Source	Physical constants[a]		R_{GlcN} values on paper solvent systems[b]					R_{GlcN} on ion exchange system[c]		References
		MP	$[\alpha]_D$	A	B	C	D	E	I	II	
II. 3-AMINO SUGARS											
Kanosamine: 3-amino-3-deoxy-D-glucose 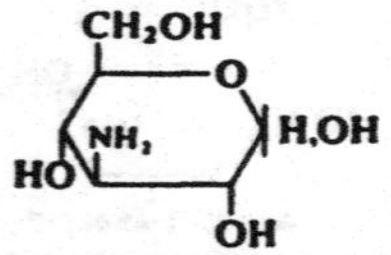	Antibiotics: kanamycin group	—	—	—	—	—	—	—	—	—	2[e], 17[d] 18, 21
3-Amino-3,6-dideoxy-D-glucose 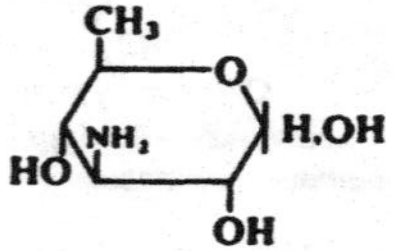	Lipopolysaccharides, *Citrobacter freundii, Salmonella, E. coli*	Syrup	—	1.6	2.0 2.2	—	—	1.36	1.34 1.37	129	10[e], 19[d] 20[e], 21[e]
3-Amino-3,6-dideoxy-D-galactose 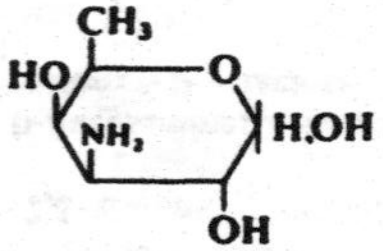	Lipopolysaccharides, *Xanthomonas campestris, Salmonella, E. coli Arizona*	—	—	1.2	1.6 1.8	—	—	—	1.54	120	20[e], 21[e] 22[d]
Mycosamine: 3-amino-3,6-dideoxy-D-mannose 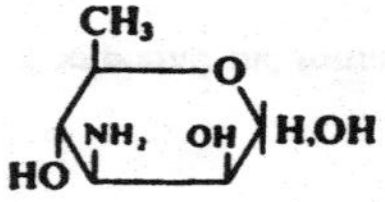	Antibiotics: amphotericin B, nystatin pimaricin	—	—	1.4 1.8	1.8 2.2	—	—	—	1.28	1.26	2, 17[d] 20, 21

THE NATURALLY OCCURRING AMINO SUGARS (continued)

Compound and formula	Source	Physical constants[a] MP	Physical constants[a] [α]$_D$	R$_{GlcN}$ values on paper solvent systems[b] A	B	C	D	E	R$_{GlcN}$ on ion exchange system[c] I	II	References

II. 3-Amino Sugars—(continued)

3-Aminoribose: 3-amino-3-deoxy-D-ribose

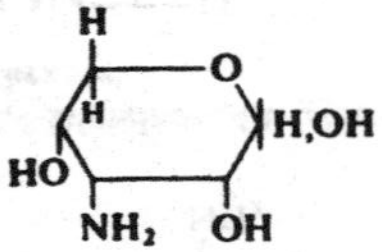

Source: 3'-amino-3'-deoxy-adenosine from *Helminthosporium* sp. and *Cordyceps militaris*, antibiotic: puromycin
MP: 154–155, 157–158, 161
[α]$_D$: HCl −37 → −24.0; Ac −25
References: 2, 17, 23, 24

III. 4-AMINO SUGARS

Viosamine: 4-amino-4,6-dideoxy-D-glucose

Source: Lipopolysaccharide *Chromobacterium violaceum*, *E. coli*, TDP-nucleotides in *Echerichia* and *Salmonella*
MP: 132–138
[α]$_D$: HCl −9 → +21
A: 1.47   B: 1.45   C: 1.3   I: 1.43
References: 2, 3, 11[d], 12, 25[d], 51

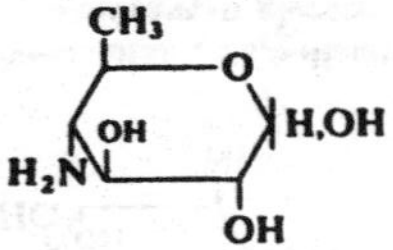

4-Amino-4,6-dideoxy-D-galactose

Source: TDP-nucleotide in *Escherichia*, *Salmonella* and *Pasteurella*, Lipopolysaccharide of *E. coli.*

	R$_{rhamnose}$				
	J	K	L	M	N
(4-amino-4,6-dideoxy-D-glucose)	1.38	0.42	0.94	0.5 / 0.7	1.0 / 1.5	References 26[d]
(4-amino-4,6-dideoxy-D-galactose) 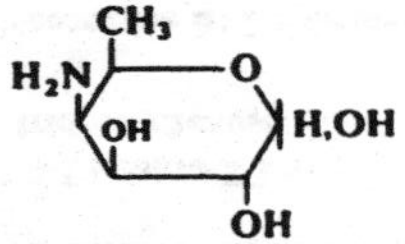	1.25	0.88	1.16	0.5 / 0.7	1.0 / 1.5	References 26[d], 51

IV. 6-AMINO SUGARS

6-Amino-6-deoxy-D-glucose

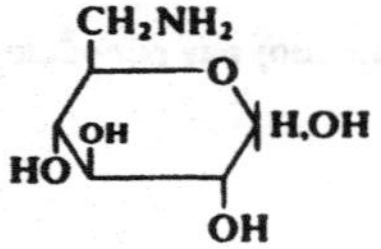

Source: Antibiotics: kanamycin A
MP: 161–162
[α]$_D$: HCl +23.0 → +50.1
References: 2, 17[d], 18[d]

THE NATURALLY OCCURRING AMINO SUGARS (continued)

Compound and formula	Source	Physical constants[a]		R_{GlcN} values on paper solvent systems[b]					R_{GlcN} on ion exchange system[c]		References
		MP	$[\alpha]_D$	A	B	C	D	E	I	II	
V. DIAMINO-SUGARS											
2,3-Diamino-2,3,6-trideoxyhexose:	Lipopolysaccharides of *Rhodospirillaceae*	—	—	—	—	—	—	—	—	—	58
Neosamine B: 2,6-diamino-2,6-dideoxy-L-idose 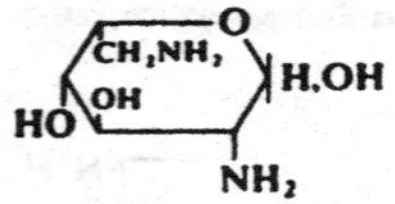	Antibiotics: neomycin, paronomycin, zygomycin	—	HCl +17	—	—	—	—	—	—	—	2, 27, 28
Neosamine C: 2,6-diamino-2,6-dideoxy-D-glucose 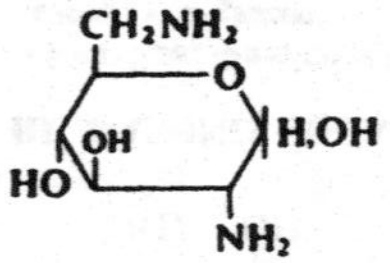	Antibiotics: neomycin B, neomycin A, zygomycin A	—	HCl +67	N —	R_{GlcN} S —	—	—	—	—	4.7g	2, 27, 28
2,4-Diamino-2,4,6-trideoxy-hexose 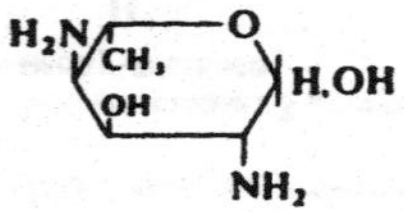	Polysaccharide from *Bacillus lichenformis*	—	—	0.92	1.09	—	—	—	—	—	2, 29d, 30
2,4-Diamino-2,4,6-trideoxy hexose	UDP-nucleotide synthesized by *D. pneumoniae* Type XIV	—	—	—	—	—	—	—	—	—	31

gBrendel et al. system using 3.1 *M* pyridine-acetic buffer at pH 4.5.[a]

THE NATURALLY OCCURRING AMINO SUGARS (continued)

VI. N-ACETYLATED[i] AND N-METHYLATED AMINO SUGARS

Compound and formula	Source	MP	$[\alpha]_D$	A	B	C	D	E	F	G	H	I	ion I	ion II	References
				R_{GlcN}					R_{fucose}						
2-Acetamido-D-glucose	—	205 / 182–184	(α) +64 → +40.9 / (β) −21.5 → +40.9	1.71, 1.84[i], 0.96[Δ]	—	—	1.10	—	—	—	—	—	—	—	1, 3
2-Acetamido-D-galactose	—	172–173	(α) +115 → +86	1.59, 1.70[i], 0.75[Δ]	—	—	1.19	—	—	—	—	—	—	—	1, 3
2-Acetamido-D-mannose	—	105–108	(β) −21 → +10	1.79, 1.84[i], 1.05[Δ]	—	—	1.12	—	—	—	—	—	—	—	1, 2, 3
2-Acetamido-D-gulose	—	—	−55 → −59	1.87	—	—	1.18	—	—	—	—	—	—	—	1[e], 3
2-Acetamido-2,6-dideoxy-D-glucose	—	—	—	—	—	—	—	—	—	—	—	—	—	—	
2-Acetamido-2,6-dideoxy-D-galactose	—	—	—	2.12	—	—	1.35	—	—	—	—	—	—	—	3
2-Acetamido-2,6-dideoxy-L-galactose	—	195–198	−79	—	—	—	—	—	—	—	—	—	—	—	16[d]
2-Acetamido-2,6-dideoxy-L-talose	—	—	—	—	—	—	—	—	—	—	—	—	—	—	
3-Acetamido-3-deoxy-D-glucose	—	199–202	−43	—	—	—	—	—	0.71	1.13	0.90	0.92	—	—	18, 32
3-Acetamido-3,6-dideoxy-D-glucose	—	—	—	1.2 / 1.3	1.3 / 1.5	—	—	—	—	—	—	—	—	—	20, 21
3-Acetamido-3,6-dideoxy-D-galactose	—	174–176	+114	1.1 / 1.2	1.4	—	—	—	1.20	1.31	1.24	1.18	—	—	20, 21 / 22[d], 32
3-Acetamido-3,6-dideoxy-D-mannose	—	191–192	−46E	1.4	1.6	—	—	—	1.88	1.31	1.37	1.37	—	—	20, 21, 32, 33
3-Acetamido-3-deoxy-D-ribose	—	—	—	—	—	—	—	—	1.71	1.33	1.28	1.29	—	—	32

[b] Not all of the N-acetamido compounds have necessarily been found in nature, but are listed here for convenience.

[i] N-acetylmannosamine and N-acetylgalactosamine have an $R_{N\text{-acetylglucosamine}}$ of 0.4—0.5 when run on Borate-treated paper with solvent A.

THE NATURALLY OCCURRING AMINO SUGARS (continued)

VI. N-Acetylated[h] and N-Methylated Amino Sugars—(continued)

Compound and formula	Source	Physical constants[a]		R_GlcN values on paper solvent systems[b]						R_GlcN on ion exchange system[c]		References
		MP	[α]_D	A	B	C	D	E	M	I	II	
				A	J	G	K	L	M			
						R_rhamnose						
4-Acetamido-4,6-dideoxy-D-glucose	—	—	—	0.97	1.20	1.27	0.61	1.02	1.09	—	—	26[d]
4-Acetamido-4,6-dideoxy-D-galactose	—	—	—	0.94	1.30	1.39	0.56	0.99	1.07	—	—	26[d]
				A	N	Q	R	S				
						R_GlcN						
6-Acetamido-6-deoxy-D-glucose	—	196–198	+44.0 → +34.9	1.70					—	—	—	18[d]
2-Amino-4-acetamido-2,4,6-trideoxy-L-altrose-HCl	—	216–219	+115 → +94		2.33	1.38	1.8	1.38	—	—	—	23, 30
2,4-Diacetamido-2,4,6-trideoxy-hexose	—	262–264	+67 W-E		7.50	—	—	—	—	—	—	29, 30
N-methyl-L-glucosamine: 2-deoxy-2-methylamino-L-glucose	Antibiotics: Streptomycin group	160–163	HCl −103 → −88	—	—	—	—	—	—	—	—	2, 17, 34[d]
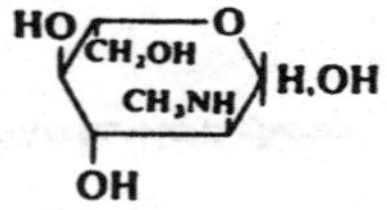		Gum	FB −65 M									
		165–166	N-acetyl −51									

HO CH₂OH   CH₂NH₂   H,OH
OH

Compound and formula	Source	MP	[α]_D	References
Deoxosamine: 3-dimethylamino-3,4,6-trideoxy-D-xylohexose	Antibiotics: erythromycin, griseomycin, methymycin, narbomycin, neomethymycin, oleandomycin, picromycin, plicacetin	189–191	HCl +49.5, +53.4 E	2, 17[d] 35

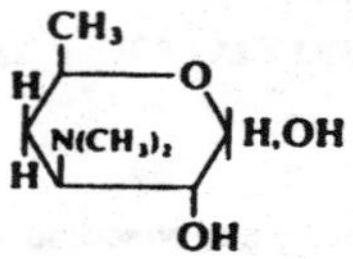

CH₃   N(CH₃)₂   H,OH
H   H   OH

THE NATURALLY OCCURRING AMINO SUGARS (continued)

VI. N-Acetylated[b] and N-Methylated Amino Sugars—(continued)

Compound and formula	Source	Physical constant[a]		R_GlcN values on paper solvent systems[b]					R_GlcN on ion exchange system[c]		References
		MP	[α]_D	A	B	C	D	E	I	II	
Mycaminose: 3-dimethyl-amino-3,6-dideoxy-D-glucose 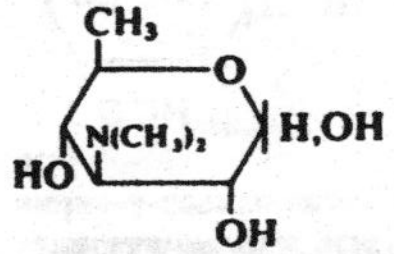	Antibiotics: carbomycin, spiromycin, leucomycin	115–116	HCl +31	—	—	—	—	—	—	—	2, 17[d], 36
Rhodosamine: 3-dimethyl-amino-2,3,6-trideoxy-L-lyxo-hexose 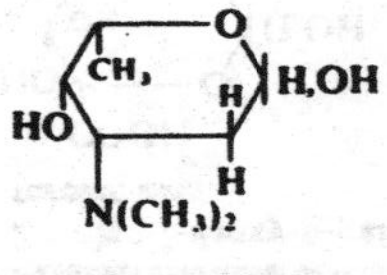	Antibiotics: cinerubins, pyrromycin rhodomycins	152–153	HCl −65.2	—	—	—	—	—	—	—	2, 37
Amosamine: 4-dimethylamino-4,6-dideoxy-D-glucose 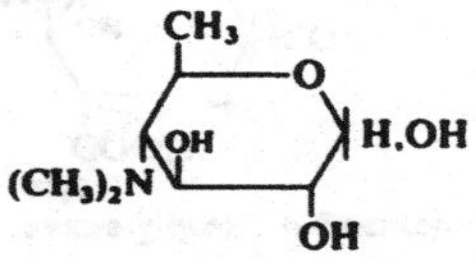	Antibiotics: amicetin	192–193	HCl +45.5	—	—	—	—	—	—	—	2, 17[d], 38
4-Dimethylamino-2,3,4,6-tetradeoxy-hexose 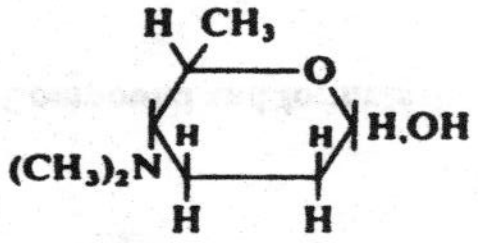	Antibiotics: spiramycins	75	+62.6, +83.9 M	—	—	—	—	—	—	—	2, 39[d]

THE NATURALLY OCCURRING AMINO SUGARS (continued)

Compound and formula	Source	Physical constants[a] MP	Physical constants[a] $[\alpha]_D$	R_{GlcN} values on paper solvent systems[b] A	B	C	D	E	R_{GlcN} on ion exchange system[c] I	II	References
VII. ACIDIC AMINO SUGARS											
Glucosaminuronic acid: 2-amino-2-deoxy-D-glucuronic acid	Polysaccharide of *Haemophilus influenza* type d, *Staphylococcus*	172	+55	0.30 0.35	—	—	0.40	0.46	0.70	—	1[f], 2, 3, 4[e], 40[d]
D-Galactosaminuronic acid: 2-amino-2-deoxy-D-galacturonic acid	Vi antigens: *E. coli, Paracolobacterium ballerup* and *S. typhosa*	160	W-HCl, pH2 +84.5	0.10	0.83	0.58	—	0.54	1.00	—	2–4
Mannosaminuronic acid: 2-amino-2-deoxymannuronic acid	Polysaccharide of *Micrococcus lysodeikticus*, K7 antigen of *E. coli* (D-configuration)	— —	— —	— 0.42	— —	— —	— —	— 0.48	— —	— —	2 52
Gulosaminuronic acid: 2-amino-2-deoxy guluronic acid	Polysaccharide of *Vibrio parahaemolyticus*	—	—	—	—	—	—	—	—	—	59
4-amino-4-deoxy-D-hexuronic acids: Antibiotics: gougeroutin, blasticidins	—	—	—	—	—	—	—	—	—	—	60

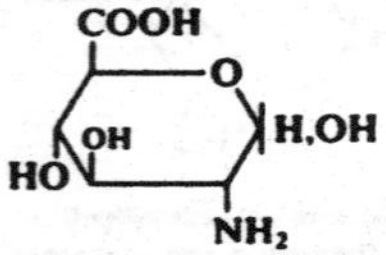

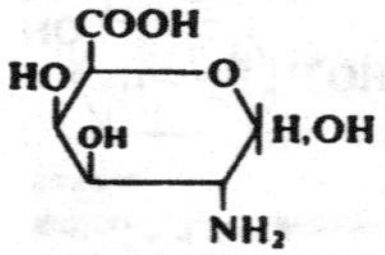

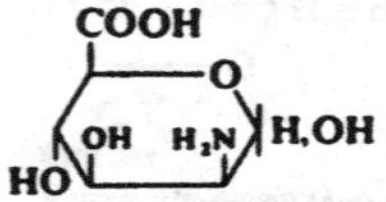

[f]Indicates that the recorded physical properties are for the synthetic compound.

THE NATURALLY OCCURRING AMINO SUGARS (continued)

Compound and formula	Source	Physical constants[a]		R_{GlcN} values on paper solvent systems[b]					R_{GlcN} on ion exchange system[c]		References
		MP	$[\alpha]_D$	A	B	C	D	E	I	II	

VII. Acidic Amino Sugars—(continued)

Compound and formula	Source	MP	$[\alpha]_D$	A	B	C	D	E	I	II	References
Muramic acid	Bacterial cell walls, spores, nucleotide complexes, cell walls of blue-green algae	— —	+109	1.00 1.02	1.86	2.10	0.83	1.11	1.1 1.2	— —	2, 3, 41[d]
Neuraminic acid: 5-amino-3,5-dideoxy-D-glycero-D-galacto nonulosonic acid	Polysaccharide of bacteria, invertebrates, vertebrates	—	—	—	—				—	—	2
Occurs in Nature as:											
N-acetyl-neuraminic acid		185–187	−31 ± 2	0.48	—				—	—	8, 42
N-glycolyl-neuraminic acid		185–187	−32 ± 2	0.33	—				—	—	—
N-4-O-diacetyl-neuraminic acid		200	−61 ± 1	—	—				—	—	—
N-7-O-diacetyl-neuraminic acid		138–140	+6 ± 2	—	—				—	—	—
Bovine N-acetyl-O-diacetylneuraminic acid		130–131	+9 ± 2	—	—				—	—	—

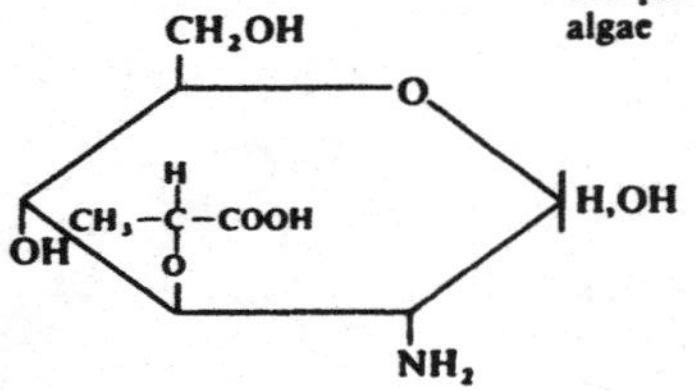

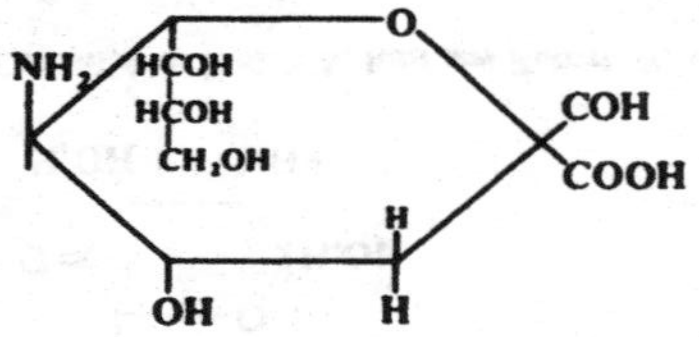

THE NATURALLY OCCURRING AMINO SUGARS (continued)

Compound and formula	Source	Physical constants[a]		R_{GlcN} values on paper solvent systems[b]					R_{GlcN} on ion exchange system[c]		References
		MP	$[\alpha]_D$	A	B	C	D	E	I	II	

VIII. KETO-AMINO SUGARS

2-acetamido-4-keto-2,6-dideoxyhexose 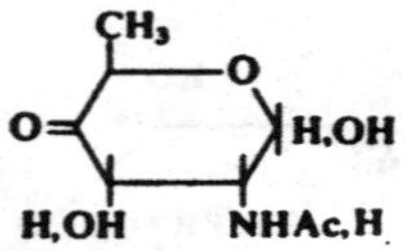	UDP-nucleotide made by enzyme of *D. pneumoniae* type XIV and *Citrobacter freundii* ATCC 10053	—	—	—	—	—	—	—	—	—	31, 43

Compiled by Rudolf A. Raff and Robert W. Wheat.

THE NATURALLY OCCURRING AMINO SUGARS (continued)

REFERENCES

1. Horton, *Advance Carbohyd. Chem.*, 15, 159 (1960).
2. Sharon, in *The Amino Sugars*, Balazo and Jeanloz, Eds., Vol. 2A, Academic Press, New York, 1965, 1.
3. Wheat, *Method Enzymol.*, 8, 60 (1966).
4. Brendel, Roszel, Wheat, and Davidson, *Anal. Biochem.*, 18, 147 (1967); Brendel, Steele, Wheat, and Davidson, *Anal. Biochem.*, 18, 161 (1967).
5. Sharbarova, Buchanan, and Baddiley, *Biochim. Biophys. Acta*, 57, 146 (1962).
6. Lüderitz, Jann, and Wheat, *Comp. Biochem.*, 26, in press.
7. Rüde and Goebel, *J. Expt. Med.*, 116, 73 (1962).
8. Neuberger, Marshall, and Gottschalk, in *Glycoproteins*, Gottschalk, Ed., Elsevier, Amsterdam, 1966, 158.
9. Smith, *Biochem. Biophys. Res. Commun.*, 15, 593 (1964); Colwell, Smith, and Chapman, *Can. J. Microbiol.*, 14, 165 (1968).
10. Raff and Wheat, *J. Biol. Chem.*, 242, 4610 (1967).
11. Wheat, Rollins, and Leatherwood, *Biochem. Biophys. Res. Commun.*, 9, 120 (1962).
12. Smith, Leatherwood, and Wheat, *J. Bacteriol.*, 84, 100 (1962).
13. Crumpton and Davies, *Biochem. J.*, 70, 729 (1958).
14. Wheat, Rollins, and Leatherwood, *Nature*, 202, 492 (1965).
15. Barry and Roark, *Nature*, 202, 493 (1965).
16. Barker, Brimacombe, Horn, and Stacey, *Nature*, 189, 303 (1961).
17. Dutcher, *Advance Carbohyd. Chem.*, 18, 259 (1965).
18. Cron, Forbig, Johnson, Schmitz, Whitehead, Hooper, and Lemieux, *J. Amer. Chem. Soc.*, 80, 2342 (1958).
19. Raff and Wheat, *Fed. Proc.*, 26, 281 (1967).
20. Lüderitz, Ruschmann, Westphal, Raff, and Wheat, *J. Bacteriol.*, 94, 5 (1967).
21. Jann, Jann, and Müller-Seitz, *Nature*, 215, 170 (1967).
22. Ashwell and Volk, *J. Biol. Chem.*, 240, 4549 (1965).
23. Baker, Schaub, and Kissman, *J. Amer. Chem. Soc.*, 77, 5911 (1955).
24. Baer and Fischer, *J. Amer. Chem. Soc.*, 81, 5184 (1959).
25. Stevens, Blumberg, Daniker, Wheat, Kujomoto, and Rollins, *J. Amer. Chem. Soc.*, 85, 3061 (1963).
26. Matsuhashi and Strominger, *J. Biol. Chem.*, 239, 2454 (1964).
27. Rinehart, Jr., Woo, and Argoudelis, *J. Amer. Chem. Soc.*, 80, 6461 (1958).
28. Hichens and Rinehart, Jr., *J. Amer. Chem. Soc.*, 85, 1547 (1963).
29. Zehavi and Sharon, *Israel J. Chem.*, 2, 322 (1964).
30. Sharon and Jeanloz, *J. Biol. Chem.*, 235, 1 (1960).
31. Distler, Kauffman, and Roseman, *Arch. Biochem. Biophys.*, 116, 466 (1966).
32. Ashwell, Brown, and Volk, *Arch. Biochem. Biophys.*, 112, 648 (1965).
33. Walters, Dutcher, and Wintersteiner, *J. Amer. Chem. Soc.*, 79, 5076 (1957).
34. Kuehl, Jr., Flynn, Holly, Mozingo, and Folkers, *J. Amer. Chem. Soc.*, 68, 536 (1946); *J. Amer. Chem. Soc.*, 69, 3032 (1947).
35. Brockman, Konig, and Oster, *Chem. Ber.*, 87, 856 (1954).
36. Hochstein and Regna, *J. Amer. Chem. Soc.*, 77, 3353 (1955).
37. Brockmann, Spohler, and Waehneldt, *Chem. Ber.*, 96, 2925 (1963).
38. Stevens, Gasser, Mukherjee, and Haskell, *J. Amer. Chem. Soc.*, 78, 6212 (1956).
39. Paul and Tchelitcheff, *Bull. Soc. Chim. (France)*, 734 (1957).
40. Hanession and Haskell, *J. Biol. Chem.*, 239, 2758 (1964).
41. Strange and Kent, *Biochem. J.*, 11, 333 (1959).
42. Bourillon and Michon, *Bull. Soc. Chim. Biol.*, 41, 267 (1959).
43. Raff and Wheat, *Fed. Proc.*, 24, 478 (1965).
44. Gardell, *Acta Chem. Scand.*, 7, 207 (1953).
45. Lüderitz, Gmeiner, Kickhofen, Mayer, Westphal, and Wheat, *J. Bacteriol.*, 95, 490 (1968).
46. Weise, Drews, Jann, and Jann, personal communication from Dr. Drews (1969).
47. Livington, *J. Bacteriol.*, 99, 85 (1969).
48. Erler, *Arch. Exp. Veteriarmed*, 22, (6), 1155 (1968).
49. Suziki, *Biochim. Biophys. Acta*, 177, 371 (1969).
50. Jann and Jann, *Eur. J. Biochem.*, 5, 173 (1967).
51. Jann and Jann, *Eur. J. Biochem.*, 2, 26 (1967).
52. Mayer, *Eur. J. Biochem.*, 8, 139 (1969).
53. Sharon, Shif, and Zehavi, *Biochem. J.*, 93, 210 (1964).
54. Mayer and Framberg, *Europ. J. Biochem.*, 44, 181 (1974).

THE NATURALLY OCCURRING AMINO SUGARS (continued)

55.   Jackson, G. D., *University of South Wales, Australia*, personal communication, 1974.
56.   Bowser, Wheat, Foster, and Leong, *Inf. Imm.*, 9, 772 (1974).
57.   Dmitriev, Backinowsky, Kochetkov, and Khomenko, *Europ. J. Biochem.*, 34, 513 (1973).
58.   Weckesser, Drews, Fromme, Mayer, *Arch. Mikrobiol.*, 92, 123 (1973).
59.   Jann and Jann, *Europ. J. Biochem.*, 37, 401 (1973).
60.   Kotick, Klein, Watanabe, and Fox, *Carb. Res.*, 11, 369 (1969).

GLYCOLIPIDS OF BACTERIA

Organism

Acyl Glycoses

Compound	Gram (+)	Photosynthetic	Forms lacking peptidoglycan	Others
Derivatives of D-glucose				
6-Mono-O-acyl glucose[a]	*Corynebacterium*[1] *Mycobacterium*[1] *Mycobacterium*[1] *Brevibacterium*[2]			
Di-O-acyl glucose	*Corynebacterium*[3] *Nocardia*[4]			*Escherichia*[5]
Tri-O-acyl glucose	*Nocardia*[4]			
Tetra-O-acyl glucose	*Corynebacterium*[3] *Streptococcus*[7]		*Mycoplasma*[6]	*Escherichia*[5]
Derivatives of trehalose				
6,6'-Di-O-acyl-α,α'-trehalose (cord factor)	*Mycobacterium*[8] *Corynebacterium*[8] *Nocardia*[4,9] *Micromonospora*[10]			
2,3,6,6'-Tetra-O-acyl trehalose 2'-sulfate	*Mycobacterium*[11,12]			
2,3,6,2',3',6'-Hexa-O-acyl trehalose	*Mycobacterium*[13]			
Derivatives of glucosyl hydroxy acid				
Di-O-acyl-glucosyl-polyhydroxy acid	*Nocardia*[14]			
Derivatives of O-mannosyl-inositol				
1-O-Pentadecanoyl-2-O-(6-O heptadecanoyl-α-D-mannopyranosyl) myoinositol	*Propionibacterium*[15,16]			

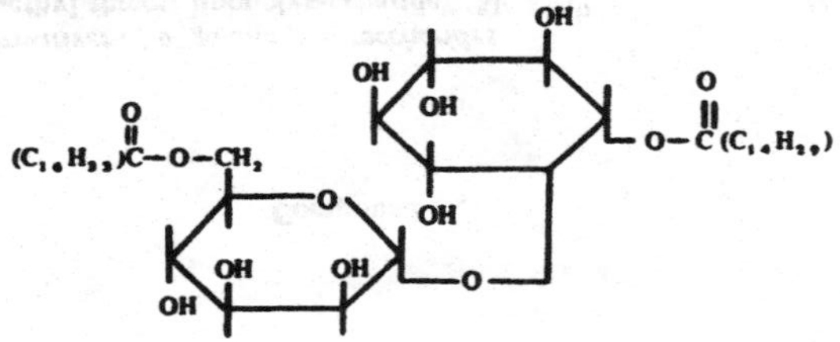

$(C_{14}H_{29})C-O-CH_2$, $O=C(C_{16}H_{33})$

[a]Unless indicated, the sugars are in pyranose forms or their ring structure is unknown.

GLYCOLIPIDS OF BACTERIA (continued)

Organism

Compound	Gram (+)	Photosynthetic	Forms lacking peptidoglycan	Others

Derivatives of oligo-and polysaccharides
"Methyl glucose lipopolysaccharide" (MGLP)[b]

Acyl Glycoses (continued)

Mycobacterium[17-20]

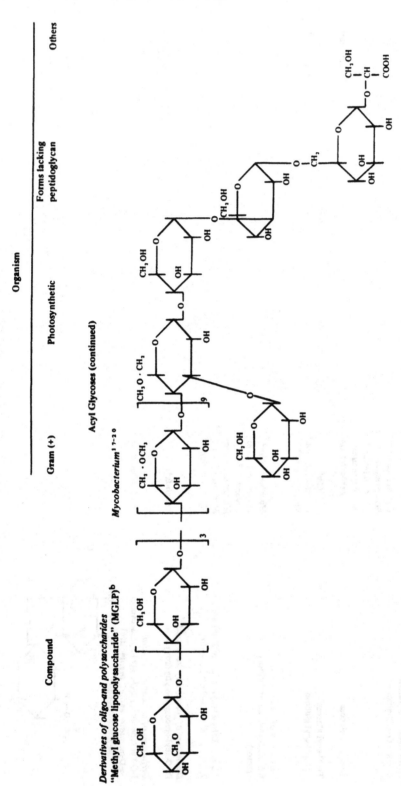

[b]This polysaccharide is acylated by 3 acetate, 1 propionate, 1 isobutyrate, 1 octanoate, and 0 to 3 succinate residues.

GLYCOLIPIDS OF BACTERIA (continued)

	Organism			
Compound	Gram (+)	Photosynthetic	Forms lacking peptidoglycan	Others

Acyl Glycoses (continued)

Mycobacterium[8,12,21]

"Wax D"

R · C · O = mycolyl

(Peptidoglycan fragments)

"Lipopolysaccharide" of gram-negative bacteria (see the separate table)

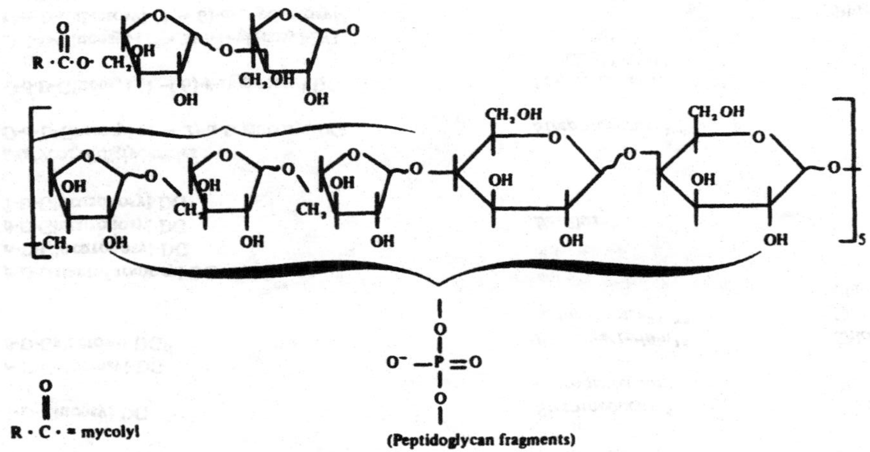

375

GLYCOLIPIDS OF BACTERIA (continued)

Compound	Gram (+)	Photosynthetic	Forms lacking peptidoglycan	Others
		Organism		
Monoglycosyl diglycerides	Glycosyl Diglycerides			
α-D-Glucosyl-DG[c]			Acholeplasma laidlawii[22] Acholeplasma modicum[23]	Pseudomonas[24,25]
?-D-Glucosyl-DG	Streptococcus[26] Mycobacterium[27]	Chromatium[28]		
α-D-Galactosyl-DG β-D-Galactosyl-DG[d]	Bifidobacterium[30] Arthrobacter[31,32]	Chloropseudomonas[33] Chlorobium[34,35] Blue-green algae[36]		Treponema[29]
β-D-Galactofuranosyl-DG α-D-Glucuronosyl-DG β-D-Glucuronosyl-DG ?-D-Glucuronosyl-DG	Bacillus[39]		Mycoplasma mycoides[38] A halophile[40]	Bacteroides[37] Pseudomonas[25] Pseudomonas[24]
Diglycosyl diglycerides				
O-α-D-Glucosyl-(1 → 2)-α-D glucosyl-DG	Streptococcus[41-43]			
O-β-D-Glucosyl-(1 → 6)-β-D glucosyl-DG	Staphylococcus[41,44-47] Bacillus[41,44,48] Nocardia[4]		Acholeplasma laidlawii[22]	
O-?-D-Glucosyl-(1 → ?)-?-D-glucosyl-DG O-α-D-Galactosyl-(1 → 6)-α-D-galactosyl-DG (?)		Blue-green algae[36]		
O-β-D-Galactosyl-(1 →6)-β-D-galactosyl-DG	Arthrobacter[31,32]			
O-?-D-Galactosyl-(1 → ?)-?-D-galactosyl-DG	Bifidobacterium[30]		Mycoplasma pneumoniae[49]	

[c] DG, diglyceride (1,2-di-O-acyl-*sn*-glycerol).
[d] The evidence for the anomeric configuration is not always very strong.
[e] A possibility remains that the lipid was a part of a larger structure.

GLYCOLIPIDS OF BACTERIA (continued)

Compound	Organism			
	Gram (+)	Photosynthetic	Forms lacking peptidoglycan	Others
Glycosyl Diglycerides (continued)				
O-α-Mannosyl-(1 → 3)-α-D mannosyl-DG	*Arthrobacter*[31,32] *Microbacterium*[50,51] *Micrococcus*[52] *Pneumococcus*[53,54] *Lactobacillus*[55,56] *Listeria*[57]			*Pseudomonas*[25]
O-α-D-Galactosyl-(1 → 2)-α-D-glucosyl-DG				
(Galactosyl, glucosyl)-DG				
(Mannosyl, glucosyl)-DG		*Chromatium*[28]	*Mycoplasma pneumoniae*[49]	
O-β-D-Glucosyl-(1 → 4)-α-D-glucuronosyl-DG	*Streptomyces*[58]			
O-α-D-Glucosyl-(1 → 4)-di-O-acyl-α-D-galacturonosyl-DG				
Triglycosyl diglycerides				
O-α-D-Glucosyl-(1 → 2)-O-α-D-glucosyl-(1 → 2)-α-D-glucosyl-DG	*Streptococcus*[59]	*Chromatium*[28] *Chloropseudomonas*[33] *Chlorobium*[34,35]		
(Galactosyl, galactosyl, galactosyl)-DG	*Bifidobacterium*[60] *Arthrobacter*[32] *Lactobacillus*[55,56]			
(Mannosyl, mannosyl, mannosyl)-DG				
O α-D-Glucosyl-(1 → 6)-O-α-D-galactosyl-(1 → 2)-α-D-glucosyl-DG				
(Mannosyl, mannosyl, glucosyl)-DG				
(Galactosyl, rhamnosyl, unknown)-DG				
Tetraglycosyl diglycerides				
(Mannosyl, mannosyl, mannosyl, mannosyl)-DG	*Arthrobacter*[32]			
O-D-Glucosyl-(1 → 6)-O-α-D-glucosyl-(1 → 6)-O-α-D-galactosyl-(1 → 2)-α-D-glucosyl-DG	*Lactobacillus*[56]			
O-D-Galactofuranosyl-(1 → 2)-O-D-galactopyranosyl-(1 → 6)-O-(N-15-methylhexadecanoyl-D-glucosaminyl)-(1 → 2)-D-glucopyranosyl-DG				A thermophilic *Flavobacterium* (?)[60]

GLYCOLIPIDS OF BACTERIA (continued)

	Organism		
Compound	Gram (+)	Photosynthetic	Forms lacking peptidoglycan	Others

Glycosyl Diglycerides (continued)

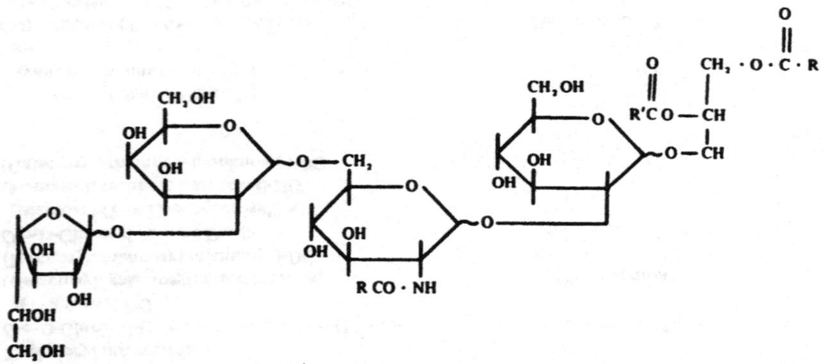

R: CH₃〉 CH—(CH₂)₁₃

R: $CH_3 \rangle CH-(CH_2)_{13}$

Pentaglycosyl diglycerides
O-D-Galactosyl-O-D-galactosyl-O-D-
glycero-D-mannoheptosyl-O-α-D-
glucopyranosyl-(1 → 2)-O-α-D-gluco-
pyranosyl-DG

*Glycosyl diglycerides with substituted
glycosyl units*
6-Deoxy-6-sulfono-α-D-glucosyl
(sulfoquinovosyl)-DG

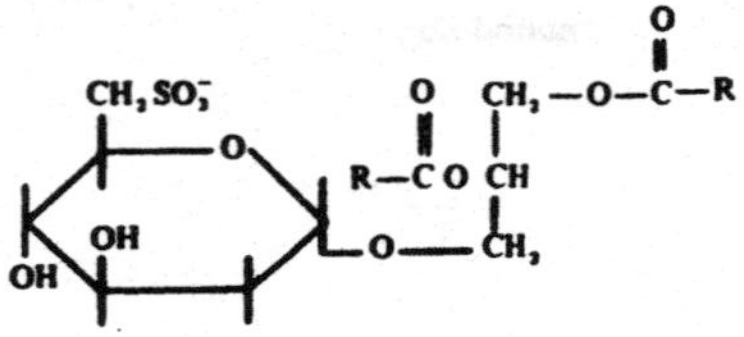

Blue-green algae[3,4]

*Acholeplasma
modicum*[13]

GLYCOLIPIDS OF BACTERIA (continued)

Organism

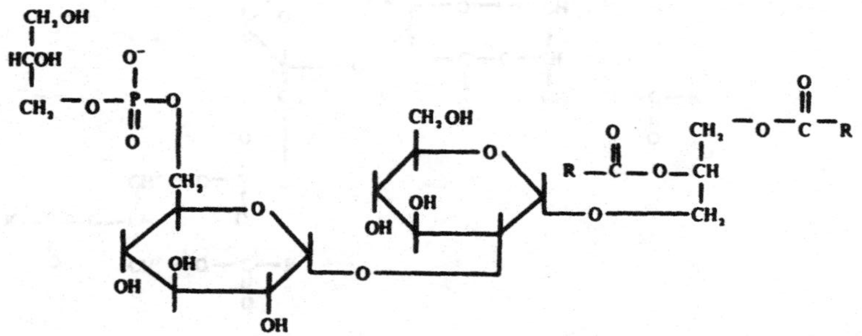

Compound	Gram (+)	Photosynthetic	Forms lacking peptodoglycan	Others
		Glycosyl Diglycerides (continued)		

Glycerophosphoryl diglucosyl diglyceride
(1,2-di-O-acyl-3-O-[6''-(sn-glycero-n-
phosphoryl)-O-α-D-glucopyranosyl-(1 → 2)-
α D-glucopyranosyl] -sn-glycerol)

n = 1

Streptococcus[61]

n = 3

Acholeplasma laidlawii[62,63]

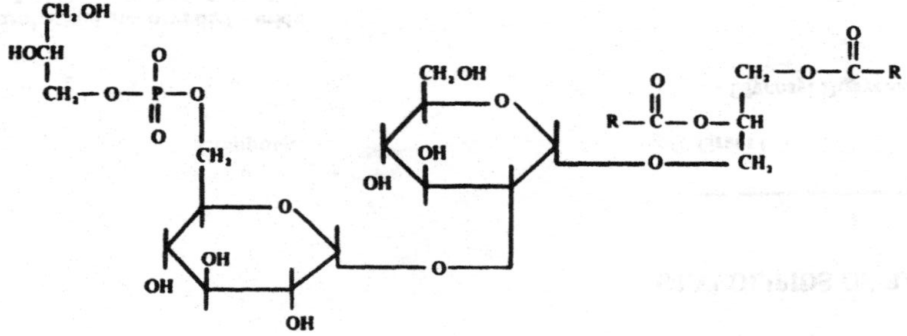

GLYCOLIPIDS OF BACTERIA (continued)

	Organism		
Compound	Gram (+)	Photosynthetic	Forms lacking peptidoglycan	Others
		Glycosyl Diglycerides (continued)		
Phosphatidyl glucosyl diglyceride (1,2-di-O-acyl-3-O-[6'-O-(sn-3-phosphatidyl)-α-D-glucopyranosyl]-sn-glycerol)				Pseudomonas[44]

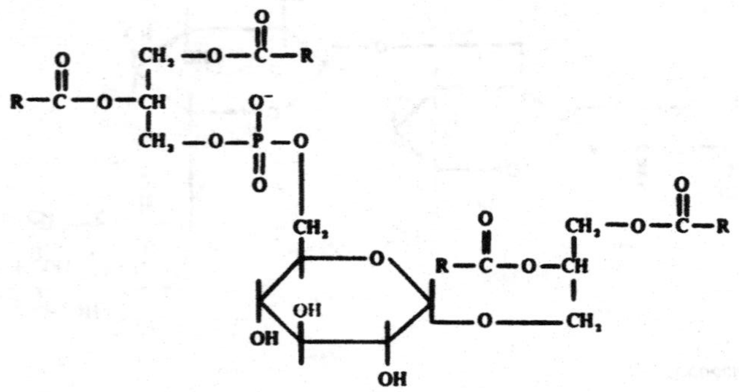

GLYCOLIPIDS OF BACTERIA (continued)

| | Organism | | |
Compound	Gram (+)	Photosynthetic	Forms lacking peptidoglycan	Others
		Glycosyl Diglycerides (continued)		
A similar compound (?) Phosphatidyl diglucosyl diglyceride (1,2-di-O-acyl-3-O-[2'-O-α-D- glucopyranosyl-6'-O-(sn-3- phosphatidyl)-α-D-glucopyranosyl]- sn-glycerol)	Nocardia[4] Streptococcus[45-47]			

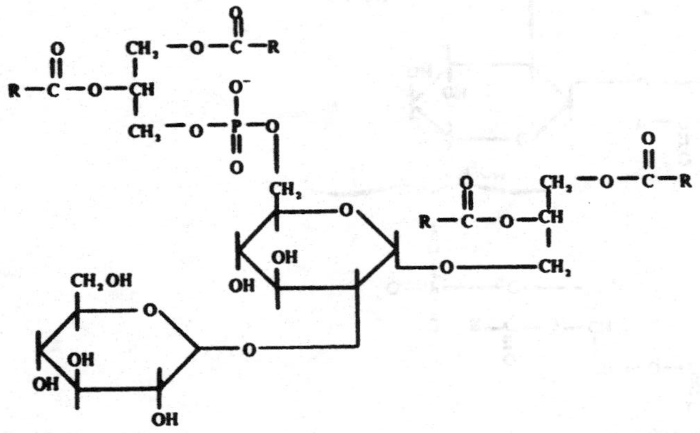

GLYCOLIPIDS OF BACTERIA (continued)

Compound	Organism: Gram (+)	Photosynthetic	Forms lacking peptodoglycan	Others
	Glycosyl Diglycerides (continued)			
"Lipoteichoic acid"	*Streptococcus*[68,69]			

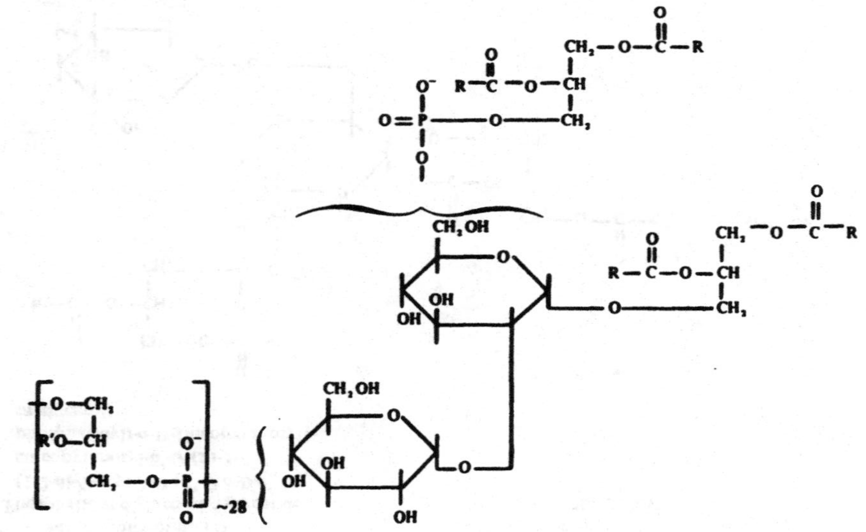

GLYCOLIPIDS OF BACTERIA (continued)

Organism

Compound	Gram (+)	Photosynthetic	Forms lacking peptidoglycan	Others

Glycosyl Diglycerides (continued)

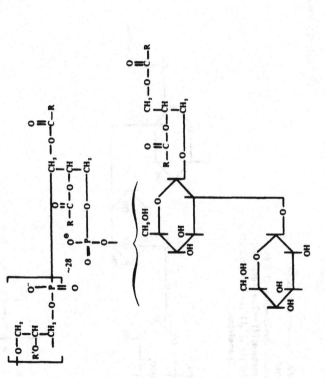

Staphylococcus[70]
Lactobacillus[71]

Compounds with probably similar structure

GLYCOLIPIDS OF BACTERIA (continued)

Compound	Organism: Gram (+)	Organism: Photosynthetic	Organism: Forms lacking peptidoglycan	Organism: Others
	Glycosyl Diglycerides (continued)			
Glyceryl ether analogs of glycosyl diglycerides				
1′[*O*-β-D-Galactosyl-3-sulfate-(1 → 6)-*O*-α-D-mannosyl-(1 → 2)-α-D-glucosyl]-2′,3′-di-*O*-[(3″,7″,11″,15″-tetramethyl)-hexadecyl]-*sn*-glycerol			*Halobacterium*[72,73]	
[*O*-(Glycerophosphoryl)-D-glucosyl]-di-*O*-polyisopranyl-glycerol			*Thermoplasma*[74]	

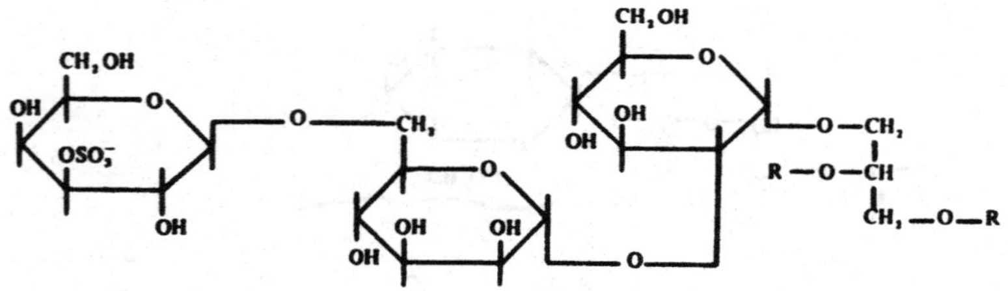

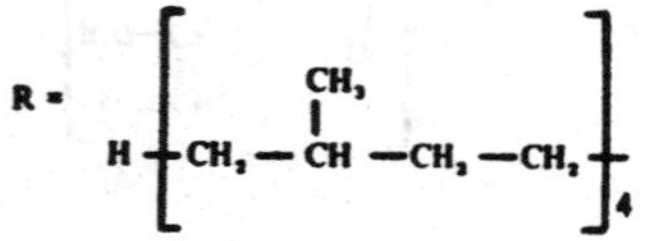

GLYCOLIPIDS OF BACTERIA (continued)

	Organism			
Compound	Gram (+)	Photosynthetic	Forms lacking peptidoglycan	Others

Glycosyl Diglycerides (continued)

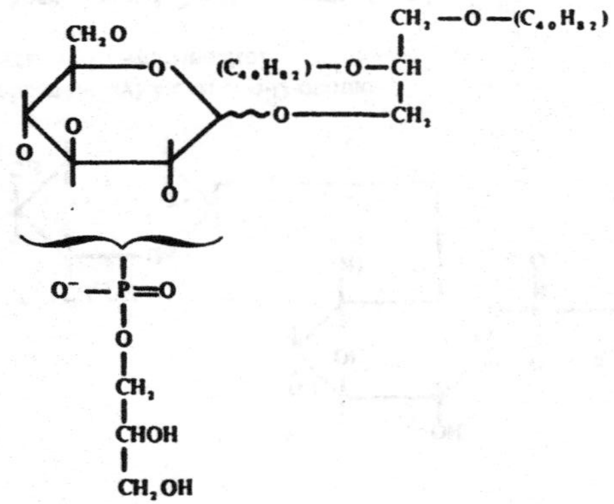

Glycoside Derivatives of Phospholipids

Pseudomonas[7 5]

Glucosaminyl phosphatidyl glycerol
1,2-Di-O-acyl-sn-glycero-3-phosphoryl-1'-(2'-O-α-glucosaminyl)-sn-glycerol

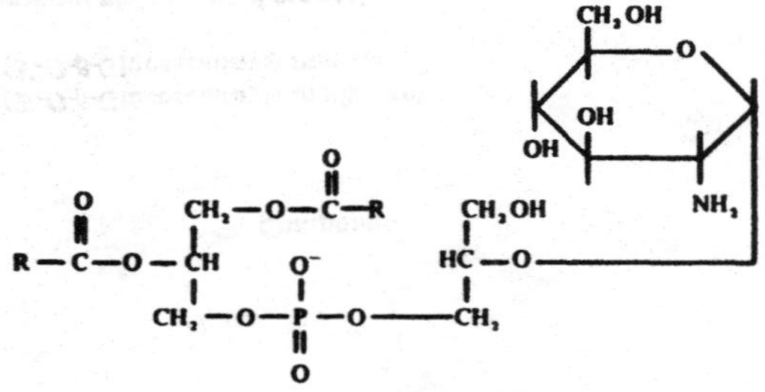

GLYCOLIPIDS OF BACTERIA (continued)

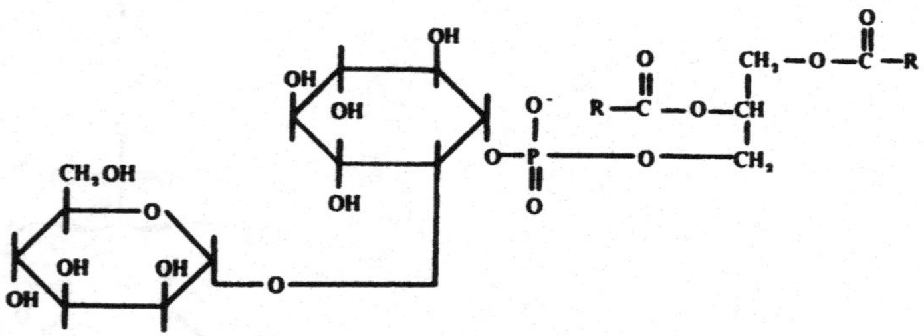

Compound	Organism: Gram (+)	Photosynthetic	Forms lacking peptidoglycan	Others
Glycoside Derivatives of Phospholipids (continued)				
(2'-*O*-β-Glucosaminyl)-*sn*-glycerol (3'-*O*-β-Glucosaminyl)-*sn*-glycerol	*Bacillus*[75,76]			
Mannosyl phosphatidyl inositol 1-Phosphatidyl-2-*O*-α-D-mannopyranosyl-L-*myo*inositol	*Mycobacterium*[77] *Propionibacterium*[78] *Micromonospora*[10] *Nocardia*[79,80] *Streptomyces*[80]			

Compound	Organism: Gram (+)	Photosynthetic	Forms lacking peptidoglycan	Others
1-phosphatidyl-2,6-di-*O*-α-D-mannopyranosyl-L-*myo*inositol	*Mycobacterium*[77,81] *Nocardia*[4] *Corynebacterium*[82]			
1-phosphatidyl-2-*O*-α-D-mannopyranosyl-6-*O*-[*O*-α-D-mannopyranosyl-(1 → 2)-*O*-α-D-mannopyranosyl-(1 → 6)-*O*-α-D-mannopyranosyl-(1 → 6)-α-D-mannopyranosyl]-L-*myo*inositol	*Mycobacterium*[77,81]			

GLYCOLIPIDS OF BACTERIA (continued)

Compound	Organism		
	Gram (+)	Photosynthetic	Forms lacking peptidoglycan	Others

Glycoside Derivatives of Phospholipids (continued)

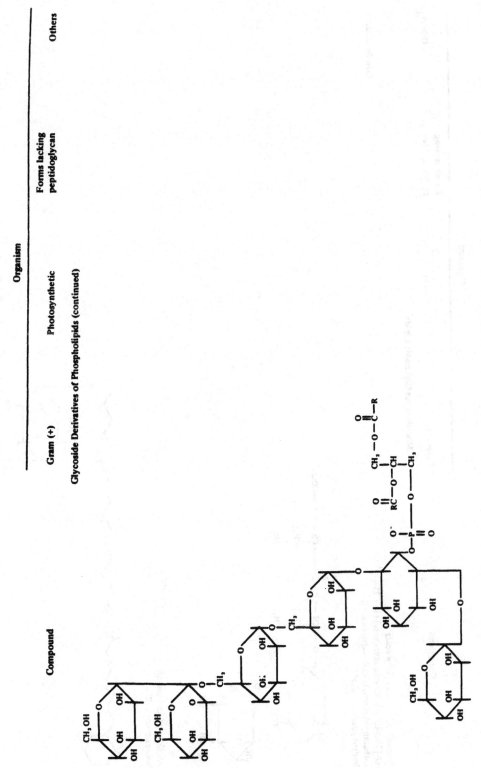

GLYCOLIPIDS OF BACTERIA (continued)

Compound	Organism: Gram (+)	Organism: Photosynthetic	Organism: Forms lacking peptodoglycan	Organism: Others
Miscellaneous Glycosidic Lipids				
Glycoside of hydroxy fatty acids 3-*O*-[3'-*O*-(*O*-α-L-Rhamnopyranosyl-(1 → 2)-α-L-rhamnopyranosyl)-hydroxydecanoyl]-hydroxydecanoic acid				*Pseudomonas*[83]
Glycosides of carotenoids "Phlei-xanthophyll"	*Mycobacterium*[84]			

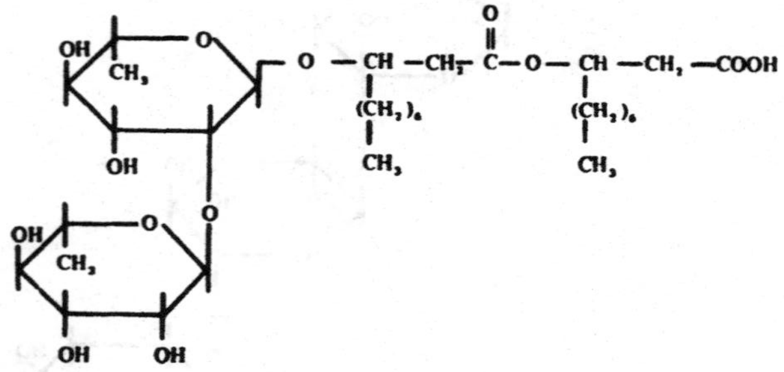

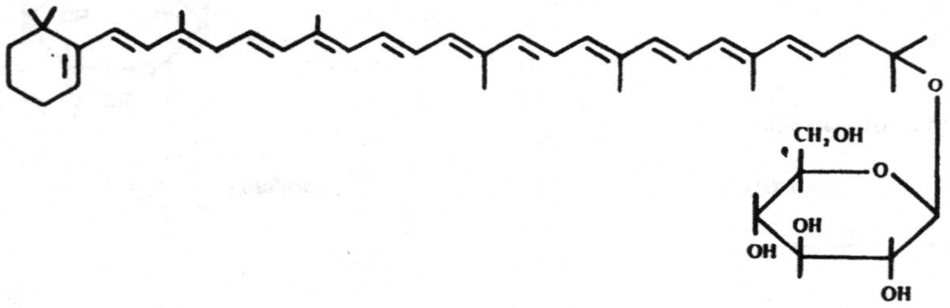

GLYCOLIPIDS OF BACTERIA (continued)

	Organism		
Compound	Gram (+)	Photosynthetic	Forms lacking peptidoglycan	Others

Miscellaneous Glycosidic Lipids (continued)

Glycosides of phenols with side chains

Mycoside A   *Mycobacterium*[9,12,95]

$$RO-\text{⬡}-(CH_2)_n-CH-CH-CH_2-CH-(CH_2)_x-CH$$

with substituents: $\overset{|}{R}$, $\overset{|}{OR''}$, $\overset{|}{OR''}$, and terminal CH_3, CH_2, CH_2, OCH_3

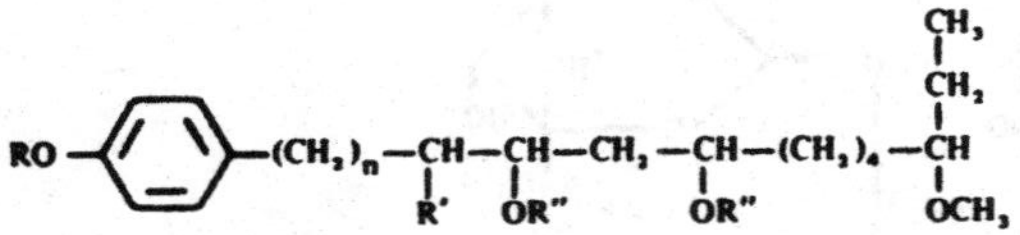

n = 13–17
R = Trisaccharide containing
2-O-methylfucose, 2-O-
methylrhamnose, and 2,4-
di-O-methylrhamnose.
R' = CH₃, sometimes H
R'' = acyl (palmityl, mycocerosyl)

Mycoside B   *Mycobacterium*[9,12,96]

$$-\text{⬡}-(CH_2)_n-CH-CH-CH_2-CH-(CH_2)_x-CH$$

with substituents: $\overset{|}{R}$, $\overset{|}{OR'}$, $\overset{|}{OR'}$, and terminal CH_3, CH_2, CH_2, OCH_3

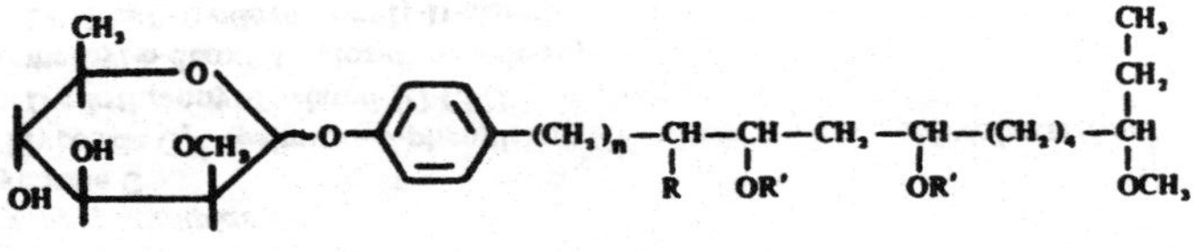

n = 13–17
R = H, sometimes CH₃
R' = acyl (palmityl, mycocerosyl)

GLYCOLIPIDS OF BACTERIA (continued)

	Organism		
Compound	Gram (+)	Photosynthetic	Forms lacking peptidoglycan	Others

Miscellaneous Glycosidic Lipids (continued)

Glycopeptidolipids

Mycoside C

Mycoside C₂ [f] (palmityl-D-phenylalanyl-
D-*allo*threonyl-D-alanyl-[O-(3-O-
methyl-6-deoxy-L-talosyl) or 6-deoxy-
L-talosyl)-D-*allo*threonyl]-D-alanyl-
L-alaninol-(3,4-di-O-methyl-L-α-
rhamnoside)

Mycobacterium[87]

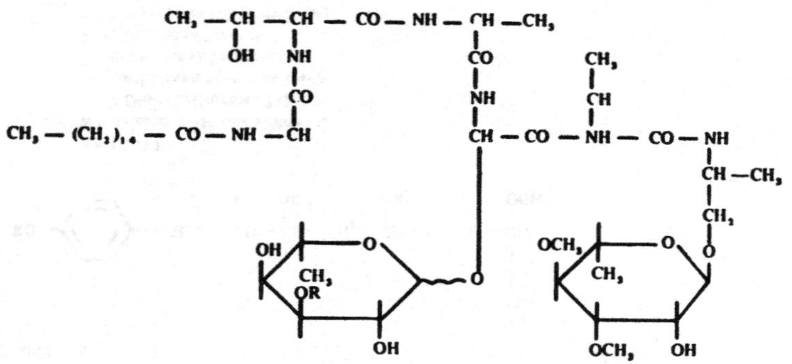

R = H or CH₃

[f]Other mycoside C preparations have slightly different structures.[87,73]

GLYCOLIPIDS OF BACTERIA (continued)

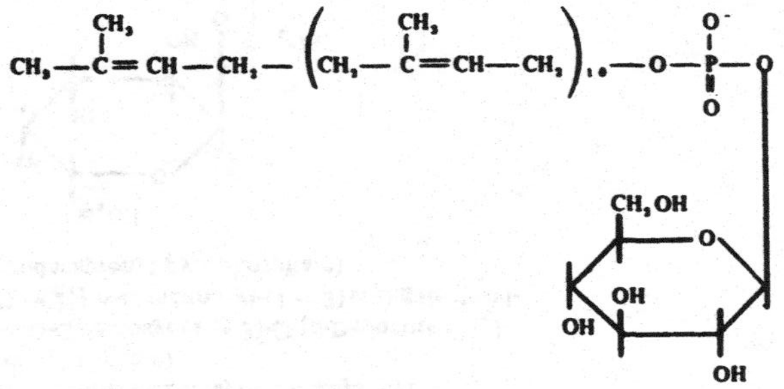

Compound	Organism: Gram (+)	Organism: Photosynthetic	Organism: Forms lacking peptidoglycan	Organism: Others
Glycosyl Esters of Polyisoprenol Phosphate and Pyrophosphate				
Ester of decaprenol phosphate				
D-Mannosyl-(decaprenyl phosphate)	*Mycobacterium*[88]			
Esters of undecaprenol phosphate				
β-D-Glucosyl-(undecaprenyl phosphate)	*Bacillus*[89]			*Salmonella*[90-92] *Shigella*[93]

Compound	Organism: Gram (+)	Organism: Photosynthetic	Organism: Forms lacking peptidoglycan	Organism: Others
6-(*sn*-3′-Glycerophosphoryl)-β-D-glucosyl-(undecaprenyl phosphate)	*Bacillus*[89]			
D-Mannosyl-(undecaprenyl phosphate)	*Micrococcus*[94]			
L-Rhamnosyl-(undecaprenyl phosphate)	*Lactobacillus*[95]			
N-Acetylneuraminyl-(undecaprenol phosphate)				*Escherichia*[96]
Esters of undecaprenol pyrophosphate				
α-D-Galactosyl-(undecaprenyl pyrophosphate)				*Salmonella*[97,98] *Aerobacter*[99]
O-α-L-Rhamnosyl-(1 → 3)-α-D-galactosyl-(undecaprenyl pyrophosphate)				*Salmonella*[100-102]
O-α-D-Mannosyl-(1 → 4)-*O*-α-L-rhamnosyl-(1 → 3)-α-D-galactosyl-(undecaprenol pyrophosphate)				*Salmonella*[103]

GLYCOLIPIDS OF BACTERIA (continued)

Glycosyl Esters of Polyisoprenol Phosphate and Pyrophosphate (continued)

Compound	Organism			
	Gram (+)	Photosynthetic	Forms lacking peptidoglycan	Others
3,6-Dideoxy-*O*-α-D-*xylo*hexosyl (= "abequosyl")-(1 → 3)-*O*-α-D-mannosyl-(1 → 4)-*O*-α-L-rhamnosyl-(1 → 3)-α-D-galactosyl-(undecaprenol pyrophosphate)				*Salmonella*[103]
O-α-D-Mannosyl-(1 → 3)-α-D-galactosyl-l-(undecaprenyl pyrophosphate)				*Aerobacter*[99]
O-β-D-Glucuronosyl-(1 → 2)-*O*-α-D-mannosyl-(1 → 3)-α-D-galactosyl-(undecaprenyl pyrophosphate)				*Aerobacter*[99]
O-α-D-Galactosyl-(1 → 3)-*O*-[β-D-glucuronosyl-(1 → 2)]-α-D-mannosyl-(1 → 3)-α-D-galactosyl-(undecaprenyl pyrophosphate)				*Aerobacter*[99]

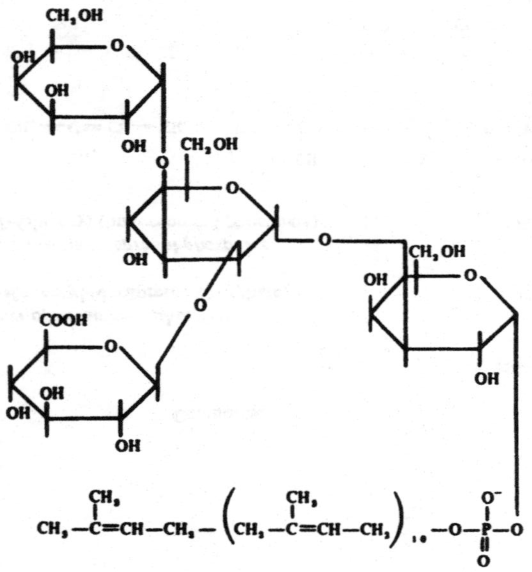

GLYCOLIPIDS OF BACTERIA (continued)

Glycosyl Esters of Polyisoprenol Phosphate and Pyrophosphate (continued)

Compound	Organism			
	Gram (+)	Photosynthetic	Forms lacking peptidoglycan	Others
Peptidyl-N-acetylmuramyl-(undecaprenyl pyrophosphate)	Staphylococcus[104] Micrococcus[105]			
N-acetyl-D-glucosaminyl-(peptidyl)-N-acetylmuramyl-(undecaprenyl pyrophosphate)	Staphylococcus[104]			Escherichia[106]

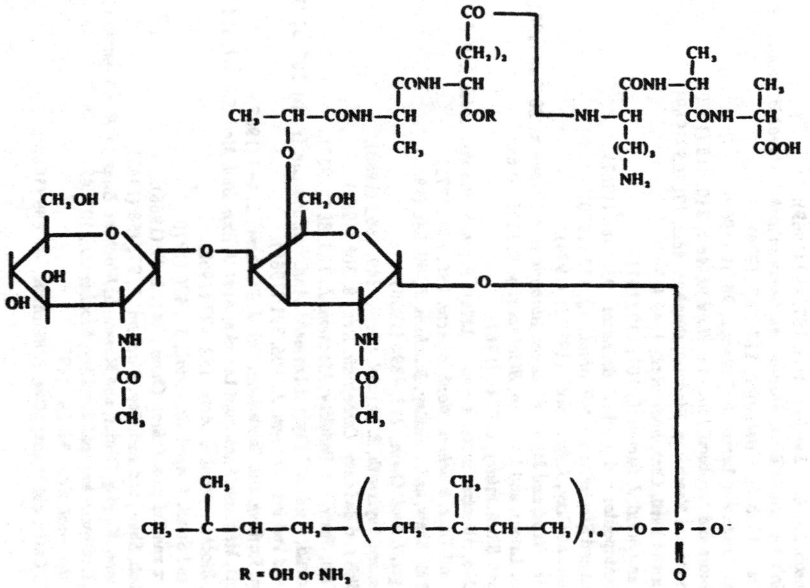

R = OH or NH$_2$

Compiled by Hiroshi Nikaido.

Note: Reviews of this area include References 8, 12, and 56.

GLYCOLIPIDS OF BACTERIA (continued)

REFERENCES

1. Brennan, Lehane, and Thomas, *Eur. J. Biochem.* 13, 117 (1970).
2. Okazaki, Sugino, Kanzaki, and Fukuda, *Agric. Biol. Chem.*, 33, 764 (1969).
3. Brennan and Lehane, *Biochim. Biophys. Acta*, 176, 675 (1969).
4. Khuller and Brennan, *J. Gen. Microbiol.*, 73, 409 (1972).
5. Brennan, Flynn, and Griffin, *FEBS Lett.*, 8, 322 (1970).
6. Smith and Mayberry, *Biochemistry*, 7, 2706 (1968).
7. Welsh, Shaw, and Baddiley, *Biochem. J.*, 107, 313 (1968).
8. Lederer, *Chem. Phys. Lipids*, 1, 294 (1967).
9. Ioneda, Lederer, and Rozanis, *Chem. Phys. Lipids*, 4, 375 (1970).
10. Tabaud, Tisnovska, and Vilkas, *Biochimie*, 53, 55 (1971).
11. Goren, *Biochim. Biophys. Acta*, 210, 127 (1970).
12. Goren, *Bacteriol. Rev.*, 36, 33 (1972).
13. Asselineau, Montrozier, Prome, Savagnac, and Welby, *Eur. J. Biochem.*, 28, 102 (1972).
14. Pommier and Michel, *C. R. Acad. Sci. Ser. Chim.*, 275, 1323 (1972).
15. Prottey and Ballou, *J. Biol. Chem.*, 243, 6196 (1969).
16. Shaw and Dinglinger, *Biochem. J.*, 112, 769 (1969).
17. Saier and Ballou, *J. Biol. Chem.*, 243, 992; 243, 4319; 243, 4332 (1968).
18. Keller and Ballou, *J. Biol. Chem.*, 243, 2905 (1968).
19. Gray and Ballou, *J. Biol. Chem.*, 247, 8129 (1972).
20. Smith and Ballou, *J. Biol. Chem.*, 248, 7118 (1973).
21. Markovits, Vilkas, and Lederer, *Eur. J. Biochem.*, 18, 287 (1971).
22. Shaw, Smith, and Koostra, *Biochem. J.*, 107, 329 (1968).
23. Mayberry, Smith, and Langworthy, *J. Bacteriol.*, 118, 898 (1974).
24. Wilkinson, *Biochim. Biophys. Acta*, 164, 148 (1968).
25. Wilkinson, *Biochim. Biophys. Acta*, 187, 492 (1969).
26. Huis in't Veld and Willers, *Antonie van Leeuwenhoek J. Microbiol. Serol.*, 39, 281 (1973).
27. Schultz and Elbein, *J. Bacteriol.*, 117, 107 (1974).
28. Steiner, Conti, and Lester, *J. Bacteriol.*, 98, 10 (1969).
29. Livermore and Jacobson, *Biochim. Biophys. Acta*, 210, 315 (1970).
30. Exterkate and Veerhamp, *Biochim. Biophys. Acta*, 176, 65 (1969).
31. Walker and Bastl, *Carbohydr. Res.*, 4, 49 (1967).
32. Shaw and Stead, *J. Bacteriol.*, 107, 130 (1971).
33. Constantopoulos and Bloch, *J. Bacteriol.*, 93, 1788 (1967).
34. Cruden and Stanier, *Arch. Mikrobiol.*, 72, 115 (1970).
35. Kenyon and Gray, *J. Bacteriol.*, 119, 131 (1974).
36. Nichols, Harris, and James, *Biochem. Biophys. Res. Commun.*, 20, 256 (1965).
37. Reeves, Latour, and Lousteau, *Biochemistry*, 3, 1248 (1964).
38. Plackett, *Biochemistry*, 6, 2746 (1967).
39. Minnikin, Abdolrahimzadeh, and Baddiley, *Biochim. Biophys. Acta*, 249, 651 (1971).
40. Stern and Tietz, *Biochim. Biophys. Acta*, 296, 130 (1973).
41. Brundish, Shaw, and Baddiley, *Biochem. J.*, 99, 546 (1966).
42. Pieringer, *J. Biol. Chem.*, 243, 4894 (1968).
43. Fischer and Seyfreuth, *Z. Physiol. Chem.*, 349, 1662 (1968).
44. Brundish and Baddiley, *Carbohydr. Res.*, 8, 308 (1968).
45. Brundish, Shaw, and Baddiley, *Biochem. J.*, 105, 885 (1967).
46. Polonovski, Wald, and Paysant-Diament, *Ann. Inst. Pasteur*, (Paris), 103, 32 (1962).
47. Ward and Perkins, *Biochem. J.*, 106, 391 (1968).
48. Bishop, Rutberg, and Samuelson, *Eur. J. Biochem.*, 2, 448 (1967).
49. Plackett, Marmion, Shaw, and Lemcke, *Aust. J. Exp. Biol. Med. Sci.*, 47, 171 (1969).
50. Shaw, *Biochim. Biophys. Acta*, 152, 427 (1968).
51. Shaw and Stead, *J. Appl. Bacteriol.*, 33, 470 (1970).
52. Lennarz and Talamo, *J. Biol. Chem.*, 241, 2707 (1966).
53. Brundish, Shaw, and Baddiley, *Biochem. J.*, 97, 158 (1965).
54. Kaufmann, Kundig, Distler, and Roseman, *Biochem. Biophys. Res. Commun.*, 18, 312 (1965).
55. Shaw, Heatherington, and Baddiley, *Biochem. J.*, 107, 491 (1968).
56. Shaw, *Bacteriol. Rev.*, 34, 365 (1970).
57. Carroll, Cutts, and Murray, *Can. J. Biochem.*, 46, 899 (1968).

58. Bergelson, Batrakov, and Pilipenko, *Chem. Phys. Lipids*, 4, 181 (1970).
59. Ishizuka and Yamakawa, *J. Biochem.* (Tokyo), 64, 13 (1968).
60. Oshima and Yamakawa, *Biochemistry*, 13, 1140 (1974).
61. Fischer, Ishizuka, Landgraf, and Herrmann, *Biochim. Biophys. Acta*, 296, 527 (1973).
62. Shaw, Smith, and Verheij, *Biochem. J.*, 129, 167 (1972).
63. Shaw and Stead, *FEBS Lett.*, 21, 249 (1972).
64. Wilkinson and Bell, *Biochim. Biophys. Acta*, 248, 293 (1971).
65. Ambron and Pieringer, *J. Biol. Chem.*, 246, 4216 (1971).
66. Pieringer, *Biochem. Biophys. Res. Commun.*, 49, 502 (1972).
67. Fischer, Landgraf, and Herrmann, *Z. Physiol. Chem.*, 353, 1513 (1972).
68. Toon, Brown, and Baddiley, *Biochem. J.*, 127, 399 (1972).
69. Knox and Wicken, *Bacteriol. Rev.*, 37, 215 (1973).
70. Fiedler and Glaser, *J. Biol. Chem.*, 249, 2684 (1974).
71. Wicken, Gibbens, and Knox, *J. Bacteriol.*, 113, 365 (1973).
72. Kates, Palameta, Perry, and Adams, *Biochim. Biophys. Acta*, 137, 213 (1967).
73. Kates and Deroo, *J. Lipid Res.*, 14, 438 (1973).
74. Langworthy, Smith, and Mayberry, *J. Bacteriol.*, 112, 1193 (1972).
75. MacDougall and Phizackerley, *Biochem. J.*, 114, 361 (1969).
76. Op den Kamp, Bonsen, and van Deenen, *Biochim. Biophys. Acta*, 176, 298 (1969).
77. Lee and Ballou, *J. Biol. Chem.*, 239, 1316 (1964); *Biochemistry*, 4, 1395 (1965).
78. Brennan and Ballou, *Biochem. Biophys. Res. Commun.*, 30, 69 (1968).
79. Yano, Furukawa, and Kusunose, *J. Bacteriol.*, 98, 124 (1969).
80. Kataoka and Nojima, *Biochim. Biophys. Acta*, 144, 681 (1967).
81. Brennan and Ballou, *J. Biol. Chem.*, 242, 3046 (1967).
82. Brennan and Lehane, *Lipids*, 6, 401 (1971).
83. Edwards and Hayashi, *Arch. Biochem. Biophys.*, 111, 415 (1965).
84. Hertzberg and Liaaen-Jensen, *Acta Chem. Scand.*, 21, 15 (1967).
85. Gastambide-Odier, Sarda, and Lederer, *Tetrahedron Lett.*, p. 3135 (1965).
86. Demarteau-Ginsburg and Lederer, *Biochim. Biophys. Acta*, 70, 442 (1963).
87. Voiland, Bruneteau, and Michel, *Eur. J. Biochem.*, 21, 285 (1971).
88. Takayama and Goldman, *J. Biol. Chem.*, 245, 6251 (1970).
89. Hancock and Baddiley, *Biochem. J.*, 127, 27 (1972).
90. Nikaido and Nikaido, *J. Biol. Chem.*, 246, 3912 (1971).
91. Wright, *J. Bacteriol.*, 105, 927 (1971).
92. Sasaki, Uchida, and Kurahashi, *J. Biol. Chem.*, 249, 761 (1974).
93. Jankowski, Chojnacki, and Janczura, *J. Bacteriol.*, 112, 1420 (1972); Jankowski, Mańkowski, and Chojnacki, *Biochim. Biophys. Acta*, 337, 153 (1974).
94. Scher, Lennarz, and Sweeley, *Proc. Natl. Acad. Sci. USA*, 59, 1313 (1968).
95. Thorne, *J. Bacteriol.*, 116, 235 (1972).
96. Troy, Vijay, and Tesche, *J. Biol. Chem.*, in press.
97. Osborn and Yuan Tze-Yuen, *J. Biol. Chem.*, 243, 5145 (1968).
98. Osborn, Cynkin, Gilbert, Müller, and Singh, *Methods Enzymol.*, 28, 583 (1972).
99. Troy, Frerman, and Heath, *J. Biol. Chem.*, 246, 118 (1971); Yurewicz, Ghalambor, and Heath, *J. Biol. Chem.*, 246, 5596 (1971).
100. Wright, Dankert, and Robbins, *Proc. Natl. Acad. Sci. USA*, 54, 235 (1965).
101. Weiner, Higuchi, Rothfield, Saltmarsh-Andrew, Osborn, and Horecker, *Proc. Natl. Acad. Sci. USA*, 54, 228 (1965).
102. Wright, Dankert, Fennessey, and Robbins, *Proc. Natl. Acad. Sci. USA*, 57, 1798 (1967).
103. Osborn and Weiner, *J. Biol. Chem.*, 243, 2631 (1968).
104. Anderson, Matsuhashi, Haskin, and Strominger, *Proc. Natl. Acad. Sci. USA*, 53, 881 (1965); *J. Biol. Chem.*, 242, 3180 (1967).
105. Higashi, Strominger, and Sweeley, *Proc. Natl. Acad. Sci. USA*, 57, 1878 (1967); *J. Biol. Chem.*, 245, 3697 (1970).
106. Umbreit and Strominger, *J. Bacteriol.*, 112, 1306 (1972).

LIPOPOLYSACCHARIDES OF GRAM-NEGATIVE BACTERIA

Table 1
SUGAR COMPOSITION

Chemo-type[a]	Sugar composition[b]					Other sugars	Isolated from					
	Glucosamine	KDO	L-Glycero-D-mannoheptose	Galactose	Glucose		E. coli O-type	Salmonella O-group	Arizona O-group	Shigella	Citrobacter O-group	Others
							Bacteria Belonging to *Enterobacteriaceae*					
I	+	+	+	+	+		24, 28, 30, 42, 56, 64, 82, 83, 85, 118, 141 (1)[c]	V, X, Y (2)	8, 19, 26, 29 (2, 3)	S. boydii 3, 7, 8, 15 (4)	9, 10, 13, 14, 29, 33 (3, 5)	*Klebsiella* 1, 2, 6, 8, 9 (6); *Yersinia pestis* (7); *Proteus morganii* (8)
II	+	+	+	+	+	GalN	21–23, 27, 33, 37, 46, 61, 76, 81, 87 (1)	L, P, 51 (2)	16 (2, 3)	S. boydii 16 (4); S. dysenteriae 3, 6 (9)	5, 12, 16, 17, 29, 30, 42 (5)	
III	+	+	+	+	+	Man	8, 9, 40, 58, 73, 78 (1)	C₁, C₄, H (2)	30 (2, 3)	S. dysenteriae 5, 7 (9)	21, 48 (5)	*Klebsiella* 3 (6); *P. rettgeri* (8)
IV	+	+	+	+	+	GalN, Man	6 (1)	K, R (2)			2, 28 (5)	
V	+	+	+	+	+	Fuc	41, 52 (1)	W (2)		S. dysenteriae 5 (9)	31 (5)	
VI	+	+	+	+	+	GalN, Fuc	80, 86, 90, 127, 128 (1)	G, N, U (2)	21, 25 (2, 3)		6 (5)	

[a] Chemotypes I through XLIII are those found in *E. coli*, *Shigella*, or *Salmonella*. CC-, CY-, and CK- chemotypes are those found in *Citrobacter*, *Yersinia*, and *Klebsiella*.

[b] Sugars present either in trace amounts or only in some of the strains examined are shown in parentheses. Systematic names of uncommon sugars are shown in brackets.

[c] *E. coli* O14, which had been thought to belong to this chemotype, turned out to be an encapsulated R strain (1a).

Table 1 (continued)
SUGAR COMPOSITION

Chemotype[a]	Sugar composition[b]						Isolated from					
	Glucosamine	KDO	L-glycero-D-mannoheptose	Galactose	Glucose	Other sugars	E. coli O-type	Salmonella O-group	Arizona O-group	Shigella	Citrobacter O-group	Others
						Bacteria Belonging to *Enterobacteriaceae* (continued)						
VII	+	+	+	+	+	Rha	1, 13, 18, 19, 31, 35, 39, 50, 53, 54, 60, 69, 99, 100, 102, 119, 129 (1, 10)[d]	59 (2)	6 (2, 3)	*S. flexneri* (11); *S. boydii* 1, 2, 4, 9, 10, 11 14(4)		*Klebsiella* 12 (6)
VIII	+	+	+	+	+	GalN, Rha	48, 49, 51, 117 (1)	53, 57 (2)			1, 7, 12, 15, 18 (5)	
IX	+	+	+	+	+	GalN, Rib		56 (2)				
X	+	+	+	+	+	Colitose[3,6-dideoxy-L-xylo-hexose]	111 (1)	O (2)	9a, c, 20 (2, 3, 3a)			
XI	+	+	+	+	+	GalN, colitose	55 (1)	Z (2)				*Y. pseudotuberculosis* VI (13)
XII	+	+	+	+	+	GalN, Man, Fuc	11, 43, 125 (1)	I (2)				*Y. pseudotuberculosis* VB (13)
XIII	+	+	+	+	+	Man, Rha	34, 68, 75, 79 (1)	E, F, 54 (2)	17 (2, 3)	*S. boydii* 5, 12 (4)	3, 8 (5)	
XIV	+	+	+	+	+	Man, Rha, abequose[3,6-dideoxy-D-xylo-hexose]		B,C$_1$, C$_3$ (2)			22, 38 (5, 14)	
XV	+	+	+	+	+	Man, Rha, paratose[3,6-dideoxy-D-ribo-hexose]		A (2)				
XVI	+	+	+	+	+	Man, Rha, tyvelose[3,6-dideoxy-D-arabino-hexose]		D$_1$, D$_2$ (2)				
XVII	+	+	+	+	+	Man	44, 59, 77 (1)					
XVIII	+	+	+	+	+	Man, Fuc	126 (1)					

[d] *E. coli* K12 (an R strain) belongs to this chemotype (12).

Table 1 (continued)
SUGAR COMPOSITION

Chemo-type[a]	Sugar composition[b]: Glucosamine	KDO	L-Glycero-D-mannoheptose	Galactose	Glucose	Other sugars	Isolated from: *E. coli* O-type	*Salmonella* O-group	*Arizona* O-group	*Shigella*	*Citrobacter* O-group	Others
						Bacteria Belonging to *Enterobacteriaceae* (continued)						
XIX	+	+	+		+	Man, Rha	17 (1)					
XX	+	+	+	+	+	FucN	12, 15, 29, 57 (1)					
XXI	+	+	+	+	+	FucN, Rha	4, 6, 25, 26 (1)					
XXII	+	+	+	+	+	FucN, 6-deoxytalose	45 (1)					
XXIII	+	+	+	+	+	2-Amino-2,6-dideoxymannose	3 (1)					
XXIV	+	+	+	+	+	Fuc, Rha	36 (1)					
XXV	+	+	+	+	+	Rib		52 (2)	15 (2, 3)			*Klebsiella* 4, 11 (6)
XXVI	+	+	+	+	+	Man, 6-deoxytalose	66, 88 (1)					
XXVII	+	+	+	+	+	Fuc, 6-deoxytalose	84 (1)					
XXVIII	+	+	+	+	+	3-Amino-3,6-dideoxy-D-galactose	74 (1)					
XXIX	+	+	+	+	+	Rha, 3-amino-3,6-dideoxy-D-galactose	2 (1)					
XXX	+	+	+	+	+	GalN, 3-amino-3,6-dideoxy-D-glucose	5, 65 (1)					
XXXI	+	+	+	+	+	GalN, Fuc, 3-amino-3,6-dideoxy-D-glucose	70 (1)					
XXXII	+	+	+	+	+	GalN, Rha, 3-amino-3,6-dideoxy-D-glucose	71 (1)	M (2, 15)			20 (3, 5, 15)	
XXXIII	+	+	+	+	+	Rib, 3-amino-3,6-dideoxy-D-glucose	114 (1)					
XXXIV	+	+	+	+	+	ManN		J (2, 16)				
XXXV	+	+	+	+	+	ManN, Rha		T (2, 16)				
XXXVI	+	+	+	+	+	Quinovosamine[2-amino-2,6-dideoxy-D-glucose]		58 (2, 16)	1, 33 (3, 16)			
XXXVII	+	+	+	+	+	Man, quinovosamine		S (2, 16)				

Table 1 (continued)
SUGAR COMPOSITION

Chemo-type[a]	Glucosamine	KDO	L-glycero-D-mannoheptose	Galactose	Glucose	Other sugars	E. coli O-type	Salmonella O-group	Arizona O-group	Shigella	Citrobacter O-group	Others
	Glucosamine	KDO	L-glycero-D-mannoheptose	Galactose	Glucose							
						Bacteria Belonging to Enterobacteriaceae (continued)						
XXXVIII	+	+	+	+	+	GalN, 3-amino-3,6-dideoxy-D-galactose		55 (2, 15)	24 (3, 15)			
XXXIX	+	+	+	+	+	GalN, Rib, 3-amino-3,6-dideoxy-D-glucose		M (2, 15)				
XL	+	+	+	+	+	GalN, Man, Fuc, 3-amino-3,6-dideoxy-D-glucose		Q (2, 15)				
XLI	+	+	+	+	+	Rha, 4-amino-4,6-dideoxy-D-galactose	10 (16a)					
XLII	+	+	+	+	+	Rha, 4-amino-4,6-dideoxy-D-glucose	7 (16a)					
XLIII	+	+	+	+	+	GalN, 2-aminohexuronic acid				S. sonnei I (17)		
CC-A	+	+	+	+	+	GalN, Fuc, Rha					26 (5)	
CC-B	+	+	+	+	+	GalN, FucN, Man					11 (5)	
CC-C	+	+	+	+	+	GalN, 3-amino-3,6-dideoxy-D-glucose, 6-deoxytalose					19 (5)	
CC-D	+	+	+	+	+	GalN, 3-amino-3,6-dideoxy-D-galactose, 6-deoxytalose					36, 41 (5)	
CC-E	+	+	+	+	+	Man, Xyl, Rha					8 (5)	
CC-F	+	+	+	+	+	GalN, Xyl, Rha					25, 32 (5)	
CC-G	+	+	+	+	+	GalN, 4-deoxy-arabino-hexose					4, 27, 36 (5)	
CC-H	+	+	+	+	+	GalN, Man, 4-deoxy-arabino-hexose					23 (5)	
CC-K	+	+	+	+	+	Fuc, Rha, unknown sugar					35 (5)	
CC-L	+	+	+	+	+	Rha, 3-amino-3,6-dideoxyglucose					C. freundii strain 8090 (18)	
CY-A	+	+	+	+	+	Pantose, 6-deoxy-D-manno-heptose						Y. pseudotuberculosis IA (13)

Table 1 (continued)
SUGAR COMPOSITION

Bacteria Belonging to Enterobacteriaceae (continued)

Chemo-type[a]	Sugar composition[b]						Isolated from					
	Glucosamine	KDO	L-Glycero-D-mannoheptose	Galactose	Glucose	Other sugars	E. coli O-type	Salmonella O-group	Arizona O-group	Shigella	Citrobacter O-group	Others
CY-B	+	+	+	+	+	Abequose, 6-deoxy-D-manno-heptose						Y. pseudotuberculosis IIA (13)
CY-C	+	+	+	+	+	Tyvelose, 6-deoxy-D-manno-heptose						Y. pseudotuberculosis IVB (13)
CY-D	+	+	+	(+)	+	GalN, Man, Fuc, paratose						Y. pseudotuberculosis III (13)
CY-E	+	+	+	+	+	GalN, Man, Fuc, abequose						Y. pseudotuberculosis IIB (13)
CY-F	+	+	+	(+)	+	Man, Fuc, paratose						Y. pseudotuberculosis IB (13)
CY-G	+	+	+		+	GalN, Man, Fuc, tyvelose						Y. pseudotuberculosis IVA (13)
CY-H	+	+	+		+	GalN, Man, Fuc, ascarylose-[3,6-dideoxy-L-arabino-hexose]						Y. pseudotuberculosis VA (13)
CK-A	+	+	+	+	+	Rib, Rha						Klebsiella 7 (6)
CK-B	+	+	+	+	+	Rib, Rha, 3-O-Me-Rha						Klebsiella 10 (6)
CK-C	+	+	+	+	+	Man, 3-O-Me-Man						Klebsiella 5 (6)
CO-A	+	+	+	+	+	GalN, quinovosamine						Proteus vulgaris (16)
CO-B	+	+	+	(+)	+	GalN, (GlcUA), GalUA, D-glycero-D-manno-heptose						Proteus mirabilis (19)

SUGAR COMPOSITION

Chemotype	Sugar composition					Other sugars	Found in
	Glucosamine	KDO	L-glycero-D-manno-heptose	Galactose	Glucose		
						Bacteria Not Belonging to Enterobacteriaceae	
CP-A	+	+	+	+	+	GalN, Rha	Pseudomonas alcaligenes (19a)
CP-B	+	+	+		+	GalN, Rha, Rib, quinovosamine	Pt. syncyanea (20)
CP-C	+	+	+		+	GalN, Rha, FucN	Pt. aeruginosa (21)
CP-D	+	+	+		+	GalN, Rha, quinovosamine	Pt. stutzeri (20)
CP-E	+	+	+		+	Man	Pt. dilimuta (20)
CP-F	+	+		+	+	(GalN), (FucN)	Pt. rubescens (20)
CP-G	+	+		+	(+)		Pt. pavonaceae (20)
CX-A	+	+			+	Man, Rha, GalUA, Xyl	Xanthomonas (22)
CX-B	+	+			+	Man, Fuc, Rha, GalUA	Xanthomonas (22)
CX-C	+	+			+	Man, Rha, GalUA^e	Xanthomonas (22)
CR-A	+	+	+		+	Fuc, GlcUA	Rhizobium trifolii[f] (24)
CR-B	+	+	+		+	Fuc, GlcUA	Rhizobium trifolii[f] (24)
CN-A	+	+		+	+	GalN, Rha	Neisseria perflava (26)
CN-B	+	+			+	GalN	N. sicca (27)
CN-C	+	+			+	GalN	Branhamella catarrhalis (28)
							Moraxella duplex (28)
							Actinobacter calcoaceticus (28)
CI-A	+	+	+	+	+	Quinovosamine, fructose	Vibrio cholerae (29–31)
CS-A	+	?		+	+	GalN, Rha, Ketose?	Treponema pallidum (32)
CM-A	+	+			+	Man, Rib, Ara, (3-O-Me-Xyl)	Cytophaga (33)
CM-B	+	+		+	+	(GalN), Man, (Rha), Rib, Ara, (3-O-Me-Xyl)	Cytophaga (33)
CM-C	+	+			+	Man, Rib, (Xyl), Ara, (3-O-Me-Xyl)	Sporocytophaga (33)
CM-D	+	+			+	Man, Rha, Rib, (Xyl), Ara, (3-O-Me-Xyl)	Polyangium (33)
							Stigmatella (33)
CM-E	+	+		+	(+)	GalN, (Man), (Rha), Rib, (Xyl), Ara, (3-O-Me-Xyl)	Myxococcus (33, 34)
							Sorangium (33)
CA-A	+	+		+	+	Man, Fuc, Rha, 2-amino-2-deoxyheptose	Anacystis nidulans (35)

a One of the strains also produces a "phenol-soluble" lipopolysaccharide, which contains GlcN, Glc, Rha, GalUA, 3-amino-3,6-dideoxy-D-galactose but not KDO or heptose (23).

f In another investigation on 22 strains of Rhizobium and Agrobacterium species, Glc and Rha were found in all strains whereas GlcN, Man, Fuc, Gal, and 4-O-methylglucuronic acid were present in many strains. A few strains also contained Xyl or Ara. The presence of heptose or KDO was not examined (25).

Table 1 (continued)
SUGAR COMPOSITION

Sugar composition

Bacteria Not Belonging to *Enterobacteriaceae* (continued)

Chemotype	Glucosamine	KDO	L-glycero-D-manno-heptose	Galactose	Glucose	Other sugar	Found in
CA-B	+			+	+	Man, Rha, 3-O-Me-Rha	*Anabaena variabilis* (35a)
CH-A	+	+		+	+	Rha, 3-O-Me-Rha, neuraminic acid	*Rhodopseudomonas capsulata* (35b)
CH-B	+	+		+	+	Quinovosamine, Man, 2,3-diamino-dideoxy-hexose, 3-O-Me-Man, 3-O-Me-Xyl, GalNUA	*R. viridis* (36)
CH-C	+	+	+	+		Quanovosamine, Man, 2,3-diamino-dideoxy-hexose, 4-O-Me-Xyl, unidentified amino sugar	*R. palustris* (37)
CH-D	+		+	+		Quinovosamine, Man, 2,3-diamino-dideoxy-hexose, 6-deoxytalose, Xyl, 3-O-Me-6-deoxytalose	*R. palustris* (37)
CH-E	+	+	+	+	+	Quinovosamine, Man, 2,3-diamino-dideoxy-hexose, GalN, Rha, Xyl, 6-O-Me-GlcN	*R. palustris* (37)
CV-A	+	+	+	+		GalN	*Veillonella* (38)
CV-B	+	+	+		+	GalN	*Veillonella* (38)
CV-C	+	+	+		+	GalN, Rha	*Veillonella* (38)
CV-D	+	+	+	+	+	GalN	*Veillonella* (38)

Compiled by Hiroshi Nikaido

Table 2
SUGAR SEQUENCES

General Structure of Lipopolysaccharide

$$(\text{Repeating unit})_n \rightarrow (\text{Core oligosaccharide}) \rightarrow (\text{Lipid A})$$

"O side chain"	"R core"

Organism	Structure[a]	Reference

O Side Chain Repeating Unit

Salmonella paratyphi A
(O-antigen: 2, 12) — Reference 39

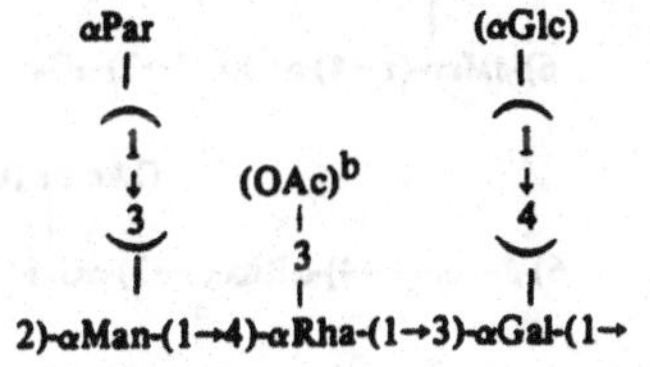

```
   αPar              (αGlc)
    |                  |
    1      (OAc)[b]    1
    ↓        |         ↓
    3        3         4
    |        |         |
2)-αMan-(1→4)-αRha-(1→3)-αGal-(1→
```

S. typhimurium
(O-antigen: 4, 5, 12) — Reference 40

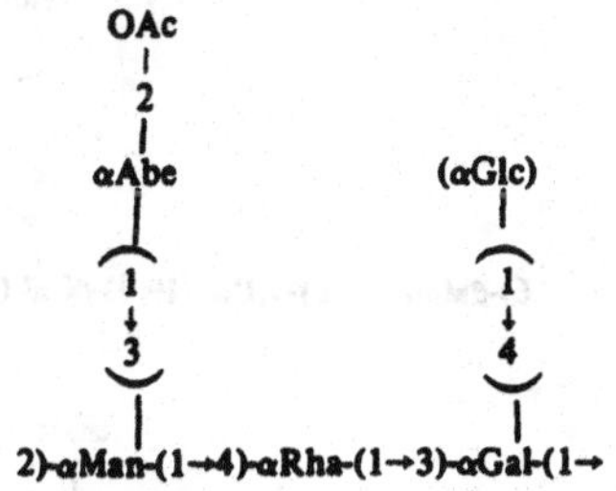

```
   OAc
    |
    2
    |
   αAbe              (αGlc)
    (                  (
    1                  1
    ↓                  ↓
    3                  4
    )                  )
    |                  |
2)-αMan-(1→4)-αRha-(1→3)-αGal-(1→
```

S. bredeney
(O-antigen: 1, 4, 12) — Reference 41

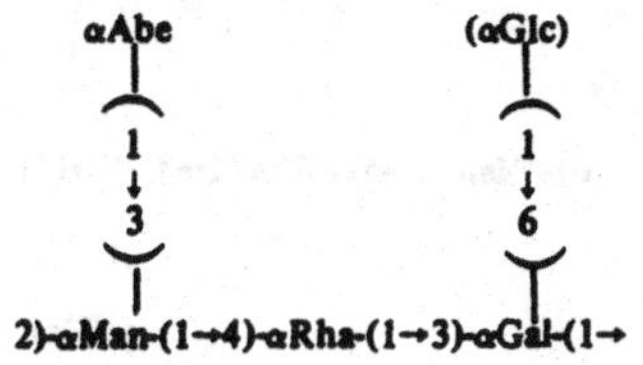

```
   αAbe              (αGlc)
    (                  (
    1                  1
    ↓                  ↓
    3                  6
    )                  )
    |                  |
2)-αMan-(1→4)-αRha-(1→3)-αGal-(1→
```

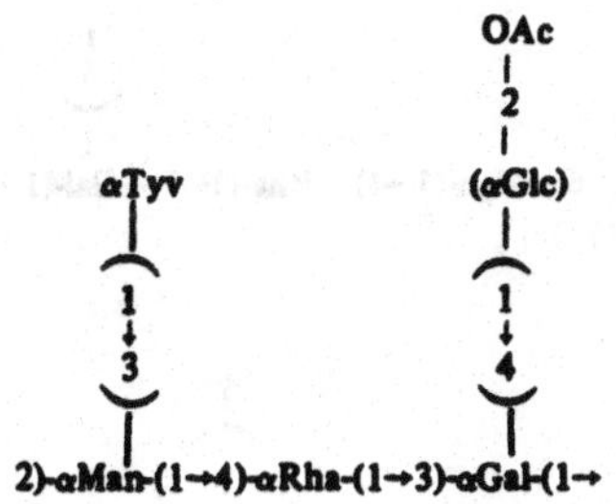

S. typhi
(O-antigen: 9, 12) — Reference 42

```
                      OAc
                       |
                       2
                       |
   αTyv               (αGlc)
    (                  (
    1                  1
    ↓                  ↓
    3                  4
    )                  )
    |                  |
2)-αMan-(1→4)-αRha-(1→3)-αGal-(1→
```

[a]Except for L-rhamnose (Rha), L-fucose (Fuc), and colitose, sugar residues in this table presumably belong to the D-series.
[b]Substitutions which are not always present are shown in parentheses.

Table 2 (continued)
SUGAR SEQUENCES

Organism	Structure[a]	Reference

O Side Chain Repeating Unit (continued)

Organism	Structure[a]	Reference
S. strasbourg (O-antigen: (9), 46)	αTyv (αGlc) 1 1 ↓ ↓ 3 4 6)-βMan-(1→4)-αRha-(1→3)-αGal-(1→	43
S. anatum and *S. muenster* (O-antigen: 3, 10)	OAc or (Glc) | 6)-βMan-(1→4)-αRha-(1→3)-αGal-(1→	44, 45
S. newington (O-antigen: 3, 15)	(Glc) | 1 ↓ 4 | 6)-βMan-(1→4)-αRha-(1→3)-βGal-(1→	44, 46
S. minneapolis (O-antigen: 3, (15), 34)	αGlc | 1 ↓ 4 | 6)-βMan-(1→4)-αRha-(1→3)-βGal-(1→	44
S. senftenberg (O-antigen: 1, 3, 19)	(αGlc) | 1 ↓ 6 | 6)-βMan-(1→4)-αRha-(1→3)-αGal-(1→	47, 48
S. cholerae suis (O-antigen: 6_2, 7)	Glc | 1 ↓ 3 | ?)-Man-(1→2)-Man-(1→2)-Man-(1→2)-Man-(1→3)-GlcNAc-(1→	49, 50

Table 2 (continued)
SUGAR SEQUENCES

Organism	Structure[a]	Reference

O Side Chain Repeating Unit (continued)

S. newport
(O-antigen: 6₁, 8)

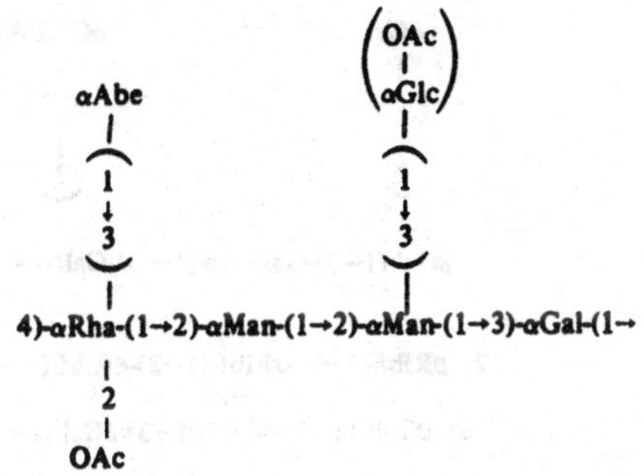

51, 52

```
                                    ⎛ OAc  ⎞
                                    ⎜  |   ⎟
           αAbe                     ⎝ αGlc ⎠
            |                          |
           ⎛1⎞                        ⎛1⎞
           ⎜↓⎟                        ⎜↓⎟
           ⎝3⎠                        ⎝3⎠
            |                          |
4)-αRha-(1→2)-αMan-(1→2)-αMan-(1→3)-αGal-(1→
            |
            2
            |
           OAc
```

S. kentucky
(O-antigen: 8, 20)

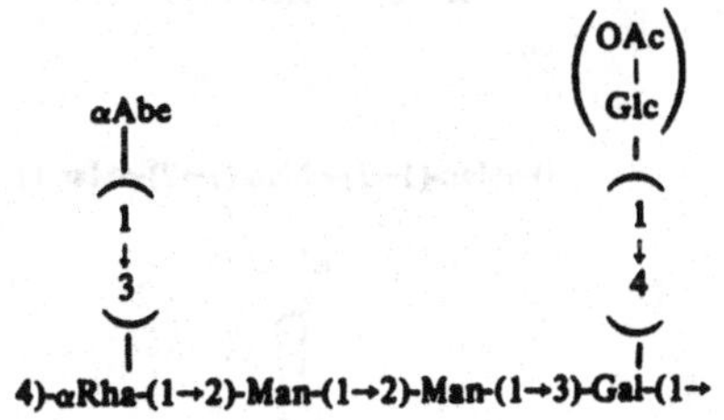

51

```
                                    ⎛ OAc ⎞
                                    ⎜  |  ⎟
           αAbe                     ⎝ Glc ⎠
            |                          |
           ⎛1⎞                        ⎛1⎞
           ⎜↓⎟                        ⎜↓⎟
           ⎝3⎠                        ⎝4⎠
            |                          |
4)-αRha-(1→2)-Man-(1→2)-Man-(1→3)-Gal-(1→
```

S. friedenau
(O-antigen: 13, 22)

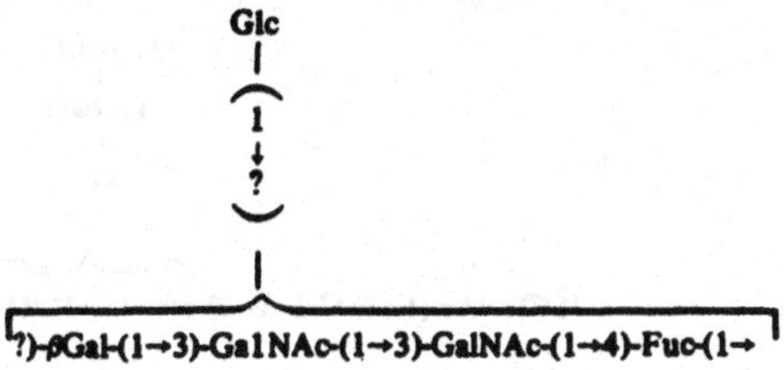

53

```
           Glc
            |
           ⎛1⎞
           ⎜↓⎟
           ⎝?⎠
            |
⎡?)-βGal-(1→3)-GalNAc-(1→3)-GalNAc-(1→4)-Fuc-(1→⎤
```

S. godesberg
(O-antigen: 30)

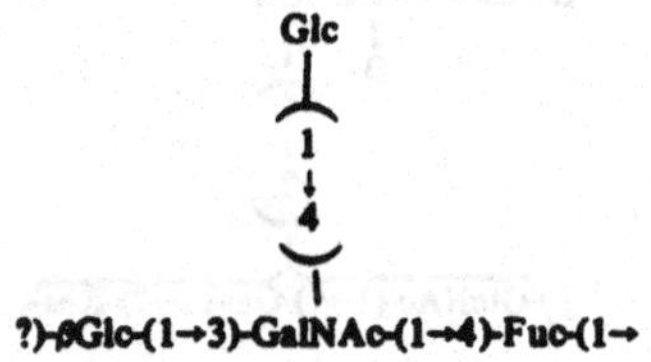

53

```
           Glc
            |
           ⎛1⎞
           ⎜↓⎟
           ⎝4⎠
            |
?)-βGlc-(1→3)-GalNAc-(1→4)-Fuc-(1→
```

S. milwaukee
(O-antigen: 43)

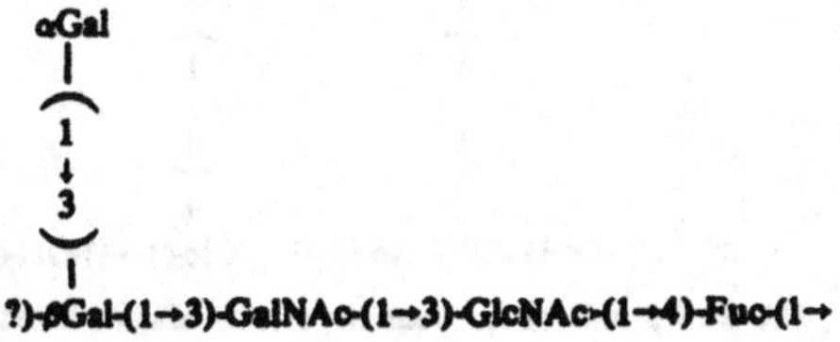

53

```
           αGal
            |
           ⎛1⎞
           ⎜↓⎟
           ⎝3⎠
            |
?)-βGal-(1→3)-GalNAc-(1→3)-GlcNAc-(1→4)-Fuc-(1→
```

Table 2 (continued)
SUGAR SEQUENCES

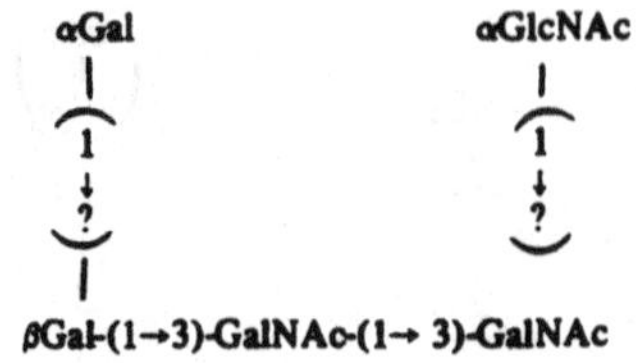

Organism	Structure[a]	Reference

O Side Chain Repeating Unit (continued)

S. minnesota
(O-antigen: 21)

```
   αGal              αGlcNAc                          54
    |                  |
   ⌒                  ⌒
   1                  1
   ↓                  ↓
   ?                  ?
   |                  |
βGal-(1→3)-GalNAc-(1→ 3)-GalNAc
```

Salmonella T$_1$-form
(T$_1$-antigen instead
of O-antigen)

2) βRibf-(1→2)-βRibf-(1→2)-βRibf-(1→   55
and
6) βGalf-(1→3)-βGalf-(1→3)-βGal-(1→

Salmonella T$_2$-form
(T$_2$-antigen instead
of O-antigen)

X-3 or 4)-GlcNAc (1→[c]   56

Escherichia coli O8

3)-αMan-(1→2)-αMan-(1→2)-αMan-(1→   57

E. coli O86

```
   αFuc                                           58
    |
   ⌒
   1
   ↓
   ?
   |
?)-αGal-(1→3)-βGal-(1→3 or 4)-GalNAc-(1→
```

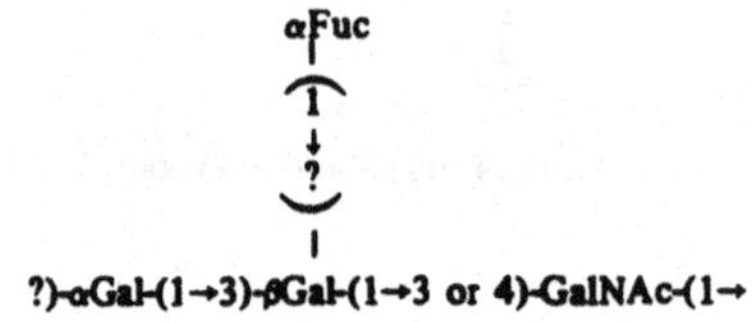

E. coli O100   59

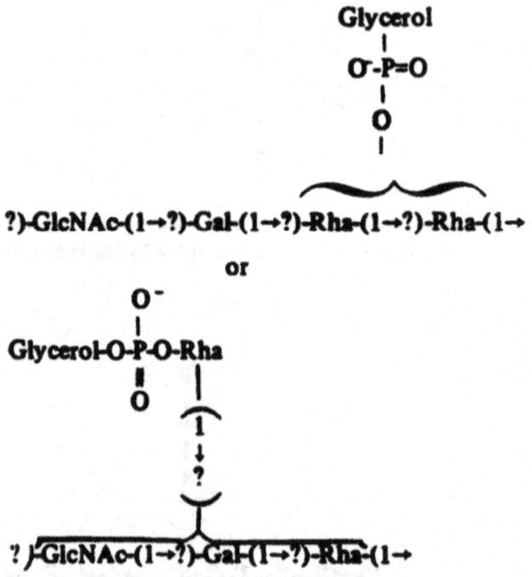

```
                Glycerol
                   |
                O⁻-P=O
                   |
                   O
                   |
              ⏜⏜⏜⏜
?)-GlcNAc-(1→?)-Gal-(1→?)-Rha-(1→?)-Rha-(1→

              or

           O⁻
           |
Glycerol-O-P-O-Rha
           ‖         |
           O        ⌒
                    1
                    ↓
                    ?
                    |
? )-GlcNAc-(1→?)-Gal-(1→?)-Rha-(1→
```

E. coli O111

```
   αCol              αCol                          60
    |                  |
   ⌒                  ⌒
   1                  1
   ↓                  ↓
   6                  4
   |                  |
3 or 4)-βGlcNAc-(1→2)-αGlc-(1→4)-Gal-(1→
```

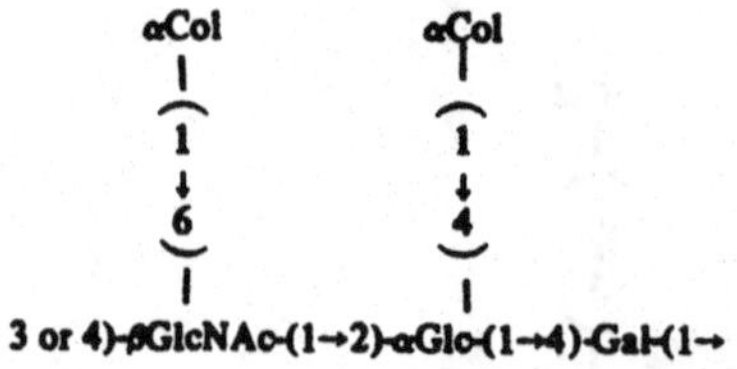

[c]X: unknown substitution. The entire side chain consists of this single, substituted *N*-acetylglucosamine residue; this structure strictly is not a *repeating* unit.

Table 2 (continued)
SUGAR SEQUENCES

Organism	Structure[a]	Reference

O Side Chain Repeating Unit (continued)

Shigella flexneri Y

3)-GlcNAc-(1→2)-Rha-(1→2)-Rha-(1→3)-Rha-(1→
or
3)-GlcNAc-(1→2)-Rha-(1→3)-Rha-(1→2)-Rha-(1→

61

Sh. flexneri 2a[d]

αGlc
|
⌒
1
↓
4
⌣
|
3)-GlcNAc-(1→2)-Rha-(1→2)-Rha-(1→3)-Rha-(1→

61, 62

Sh. flexneri 3a[d]

αGlc
|
⌒
1
↓
3
⌣
|
3)-GlcNAc-(1→2)-Rha-(1→2)-Rha-(1→3)-Rha-(1→

61, 62

Sh. flexneri 4a[d]

αGlc
|
⌒
1
↓
6
⌣
|
3)-GlcNAc-(1→2)-Rha-(1→2)-Rha-(1→3)-Rha-(1→

61, 62

Citrobacter O22 (strain 1026)

αAbe
|
⌒
1
↓
3
⌣
|
2)-αMan-(1→4)-Rha-(1→3)-αGal-(1→

62a

Citrobacter O22 (strain 86/57)

αAbe
|
⌒
1
↓
3
⌣
|
6)-αMan-(1→4)-αRha-(1→3)-αGal-(1→

62a

[d]These side chains correspond to glucosylated forms of *Sh. flexneri* Y O side chain. Here only the structures corresponding to the first of the two possible structures of *Sh. flexneri* Y are shown. Alternative structures, generated by the glucosylation of the second structure for *Sh. flexneri* Y chain, are equally possible.

Table 2 (continued)
SUGAR SEQUENCES

Organism	Structure[a]	Reference

O Side Chain Repeating Unit (continued)

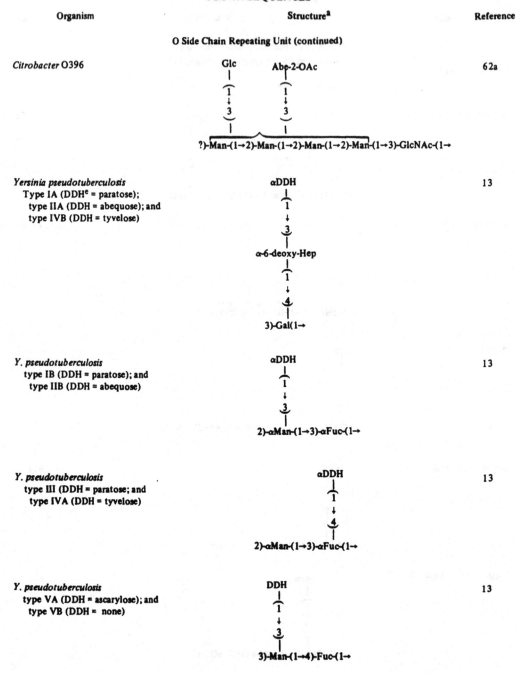

Citrobacter O396 — 62a

Yersinia pseudotuberculosis
    Type IA (DDH[e] = paratose);
    type IIA (DDH = abequose); and
    type IVB (DDH = tyvelose) — 13

Y. pseudotuberculosis
    type IB (DDH = paratose); and
    type IIB (DDH = abequose) — 13

Y. pseudotuberculosis
    type III (DDH = paratose; and
    type IVA (DDH = tyvelose) — 13

Y. pseudotuberculosis
    type VA (DDH = ascarylose); and
    type VB (DDH = none) — 13

[e]DDH = 3,6-dideoxyhexose

Table 2 (continued)
SUGAR SEQUENCES

Organism	Structure[a]	Reference

Core Oligosaccharide

Salmonella typhimurium
and S. minnesota

63—71

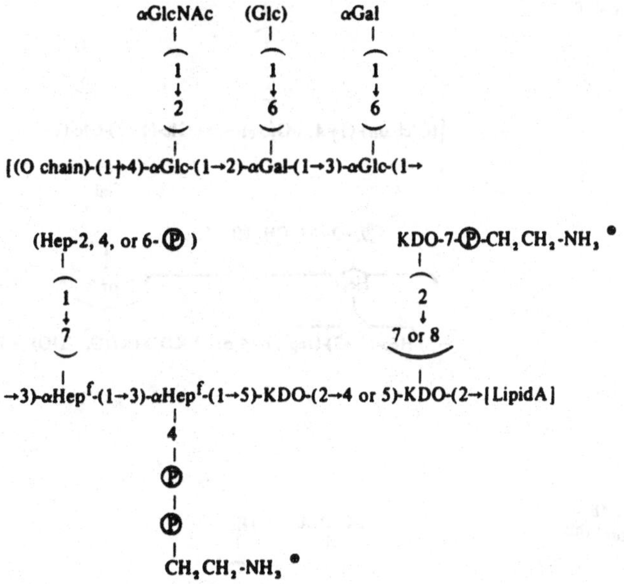

```
        αGlcNAc      (Glc)        αGal
          |            |            |
         ⌒            ⌒            ⌒
          1            1            1
          ↓            ↓            ↓
          2            6            6
         ⌣            ⌣            ⌣
          |            |            |
[(O chain)-(1→4)-αGlc-(1→2)-αGal-(1→3)-αGlc-(1→
```

```
   (Hep-2, 4, or 6-Ⓟ )                    KDO-7-Ⓟ-CH₂CH₂-NH₂ •
          |                                     |
         ⌒                                      2
          1                                     ↓
          ↓                                   7 or 8
          7
         ⌣                                    ⌣
          |                                     |
→3)-αHep^f-(1→3)-αHep^f-(1→5)-KDO-(2→4 or 5)-KDO-(2→[LipidA]
          |
          4
          |
          Ⓟ
          |
          Ⓟ
          |
     CH₂CH₂-NH₂ •
```

E. coli strain B

71a

```
                    Hep
                     |
                    ⌒
                     1
                     ↓
                     6                 Ⓟ-Ⓟ-CH₂CH₂-NH₂ •
                    ⌣                        |
                     |                       6
Glc-(1→3)-Glc-(1→3)-Hep-(1→3)-Hep-(1→5)-KDO-(2→
                     |
                     Ⓟ
                     |
          KDO-7-Ⓟ- CH₂CH₂-NH₂ •
                     |
                     2
                     ↓
                     4
                     |
         →7 or 8)-KDO
```

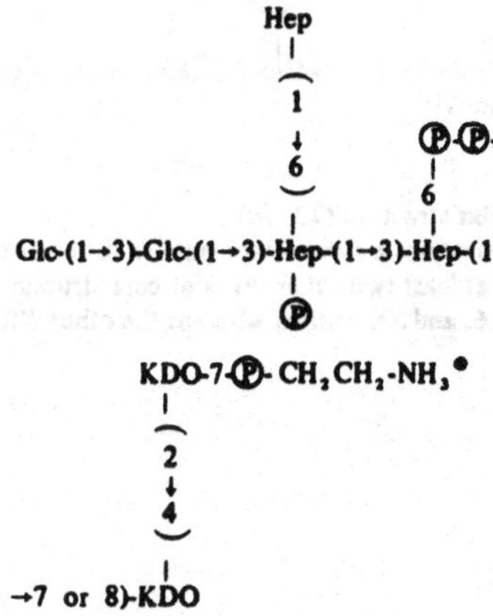

[f]The anomeric configuration of these heptosyl residues can be expressed as L-*glycero*-α-D-*manno*pyranosyl (British-American Rules of Carbohydrate Nomenclature) or β-L-*glycero*-D-*manno*pyranosyl (IUPAC-IUB Rules).

Table 2 (continued)
SUGAR SEQUENCES

Organism	Structure[a]	Reference

Core Oligosaccharide (continued)

Escherichia coli O100
("R2-type core")[g]

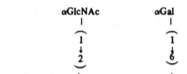

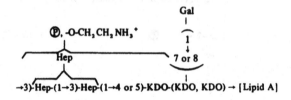

[(O chain)-(1→4)-αGlc-(1→2)-αGlc-(1→3)-Glc-(1→

72

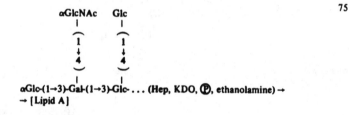

®, -O-CH₂CH₂NH₃⁺

Gal
|
1
↓
7 or 8
|
→3)-Hep-(1→3)-Hep-(1→4 or 5)-KDO-(KDO, KDO) → [Lipid A]

Shigella flexneri 4b
("R3-type core")[h,i]

αGlcNAc   Glc
| |
1   1
↓   ↓
4   4
| |
αGlc-(1→3)-Gal-(1→3)-Glc- . . . (Hep, KDO, ®, ethanolamine) →
→ [Lipid A]

75

[g]*E. coli* O8:K42 produces a core of very similar structure (73, 74).
[h]*E. coli* O111:K58 and *Citrobacter* O10, 9b produce a core of very similar structure (74, 76).
[i]Immunological data suggest the presence of at least two other types of core structure in *E. coli-Shigella* group. One, "R1," is found in *E. coli* O8:K27, *Sh. boydii* 3 and 6, and *Sh. sonnei*, whereas the other, "R4," is found in *E. coli* O14:K7 as well as *Sh. dysenteriae* type 4 (73, 74, 76).

Table 2 (continued)
SUGAR SEQUENCES

Organism	Structure[a]	Reference

Core Oligosaccharide (continued)

E. coli O111[j]   77

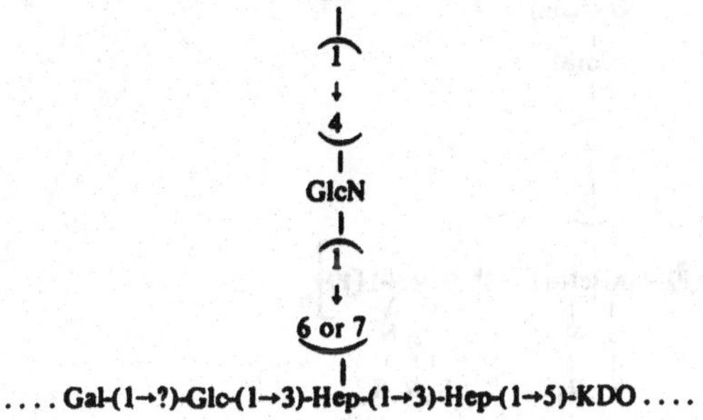

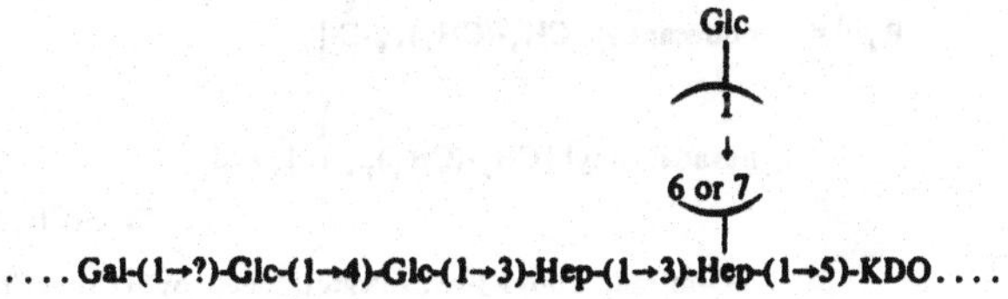

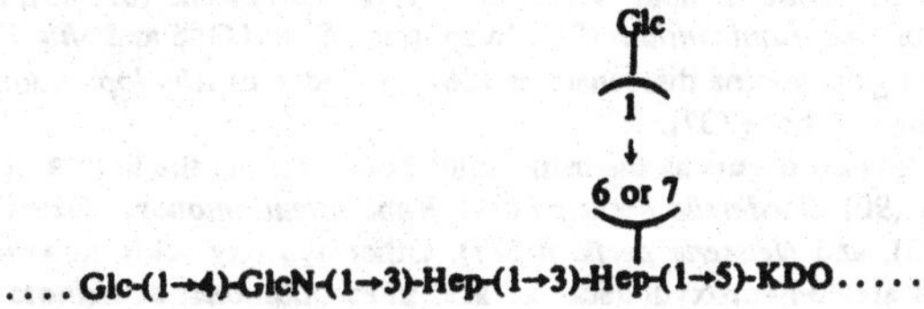

```
            Glc
             |
           ↑ 1
             |
           ↓ 4
             |
           GlcN
             |
           ↑ 1
             |
          ↓ 6 or 7
             |
.... Gal-(1→?)-Glc-(1→3)-Hep-(1→3)-Hep-(1→5)-KDO ....
```

```
                            Glc
                             |
                           ↓ 1
                             |
                          6 or 7
                             |
.... Gal-(1→?)-Glc-(1→4)-Glc-(1→3)-Hep-(1→3)-Hep-(1→5)-KDO ....
```

```
                          Glc
                           |
                         ↓ 1
                           |
                        6 or 7
                           |
.... Glc-(1→4)-GlcN-(1→3)-Hep-(1→3)-Hep-(1→5)-KDO .....
```

[j]The three structures shown were all found in a single strain. This strain lacks UDP-galactose 4-epimerase, and the core produced is incomplete in its structure.

Table 2 (continued)
SUGAR SEQUENCES

Organism	Structure[a]	Reference

Lipid A

Salmonella minnesota   (O chain)   78–81

$$R_1{}^l = \text{3-hydroxytetradecanoyl } [CH_3\text{-}(CH_2)_{10}\text{-CHOH-CH}_2\text{-}\overset{\overset{\textstyle O}{\|}}{C}\text{-}]$$

$$R_2{}^m = \text{dodecanoyl } [CH_3\text{-}(CH_2)_{10}\text{-}\overset{\overset{\textstyle O}{\|}}{C}\text{-}],$$

$$\text{hexadecanoyl } [CH_3\text{-}(CH_2)_{14}\text{-}\overset{\overset{\textstyle O}{\|}}{C}\text{-}], \text{ and}$$

$$\overset{\displaystyle CH_3\text{-}(CH_2)_{12}\text{-}\overset{\overset{\textstyle O}{\|}}{C}\text{-O}}{}$$

$$\text{3-}O\text{-tetradecanoyl-3-hydroxytetradecanoyl } [CH_3\text{-}(CH_2)_{10}\text{-CH-CH}_2\text{-CO-}]$$

[k]βGlcN-(1→6)-βGlcN is the backbone of lipid A also in *Serratia marcescens* (82, 83), *Pseudomonas aeruginosa* (84), *Ps. alcaligenes* (84), and *Selenomonas ruminantium* (85). In contrast, *E. coli* O86 and *Shigella flexneri* are reported to produce lipid A with β-(1→4)-linked glucosamine disaccharides (86). In lipid A of *Rhodopseudomonas* glucosamine is absent and a 2,3-diaminohexose forms the backbone (37).

[l]3-Hydroxytetradecanoic acid also occurs as the main amide-bound acid in the lipid A of *E. coli* (87, 88), *Proteus mirabilis* (89), *Aerobacter aerogenes* (90), *Bordetella pertussis* (91), *Rhodopseudomonas palustris* (35), *Acinetobacter calcoaceticus* (20), *Moraxella duplex* (20), and *Neisseria perflava* (27). Other hydroxy acids, however, occur in this position in some other organisms. Examples are: 3-hydroxydodecanoic acid in *Pseudomonas aeruginosa* (92, 93), *Ps. alcaligenes* (12), *Ps. syncyanea* (25), *Ps. diminuta* (25), *Ps. pavonacea* (25), and *Azotobacter agilis* (94); 3-hydroxyhexadecanoic acid in *Branhamella catarrhalis* (20) and *Rhizobium trifolii* (95); 3-hydroxytridecanoic and 3-hydroxypentadecanoic acids in *Veillonella* (28) and *Selenomonas ruminantium* (85); 3-hydroxy-*iso*pentadecanoic and heptadecanoic acids in *Myxococcus, Polyangium, Flexibacter,* and *Cytophaga* (34); and 3-hydroxy-*iso*tridecanoic acid in *Ps. rubescens* (25). The lipid A of *Brucella* does not contain any hydroxy fatty acids (96, 97).

[m]Other fatty acids occur in lipid A of other bacteria. These include *iso*-pentadecanoic and *iso*-heptadecanoic acids in myxobacteria (34), octadecanoic acid in *Anacystis* (29) and *Brucella* (96, 97), docosanoic acid in *Anacystis* (31), and 2-hydroxydodecanoic acid in *Ps. aeruginosa* (92, 93) and *Ps. syncyanea* (25).

Compiled by Hiroshi Nikaido, who acknowledges the advice and help received from Otto Lüderitz, K. Jann, and H. Mayer. Earlier results have been tabulated in References 98 and 99.

Table 2 (continued)
SUGAR SEQUENCES

REFERENCES

1. Ørskov, Ørskov, Jann, Jann, Müller-Seitz, and Westphal, *Acta Pathol. Microbiol. Scand.*, 71, 339 (1967).
1a. Schmidt, Jann, and Jann, *Eur. J. Biochem.*, 42, 303 (1974).
2. Kauffmann, Lüderitz, Stierlin, and Westphal, *Zentralbl. Bakteriol. Parasitenkd. Infektionskr. Hyg. Abt. 1 Orig.*, 178, 442 (1960); Kauffmann, Jann, Krüger, Lüderitz, and Westphal, *Zentralbl. Bakteriol. Parasitenkd. Infektionskr. Hyg. Abt. 1 Orig.*, 186, 509 (1962).
3. Westphal, Kauffmann, Lüderitz and Stierlin, *Zentralbl. Bakteriol. Parasitenkd. Infektionskr. Hyg. Abt. 1 Orig.*, 179, 336 (1960).
3a. Schwarzmüller, Mayer, and Westphal, *Abstr. Joint Meet. Eur. Soc. Immunol.*, Strasbourg, 1974.
4. Seltmann and Hofmann, *Zentralbl. Bakteriol. Parasitenkd. Infektionskr. Hyg. Abt. 1 Orig.*, 199, 497 (1966); Seltmann, *Arch. Immunol. Ther. Exp.*, 16, 367 (1968).
5. Keleti, Lüderitz, Mlynarčik, and Sedlák, *Eur. J. Biochem.*, 20, 237 (1971); Keleti, Mayer, Fromme, and Lüderitz, *Eur. J. Biochem.*, 16, 284 (1970).
6. Nimmich and Korten, *Pathol. Microbiol.*, 36, 179 (1970).
7. Hartley, Adams, and Tornabene, *J. Bacteriol.*, 118, 848 (1974).
8. Checcacci, Nava, Garofano, and Bo, *G. Microbiol.*, 5, 87 (1958); Lüderitz, unpublished data, 1969.
9. Dimitriev, Backinowsky, Lvov, Kochetkov, and Hofman, *Eur. J. Biochem.*, 40, 355 (1973).
10. Lopes and Innis, *Can. J. Microbiol.*, 16, 1117 (1970).
11. Simmons, *Biochem. J.*, 84, 353 (1962); 98, 903 (1966).
12. Rapin and Mayer, *Experientia*, 29, 756 (1973).
13. Samuelson, Lindberg, and Brubaker, *J. Bacteriol.*, 117, 1010 (1974).
14. Yuan and Horecker, *J. Bacteriol.*, 95, 2242 (1968).
15. Lüderitz, Ruschmann, Westphal, Raff, and Wheat, *J. Bacteriol.*, 93, 1681 (1967).
16. Lüderitz, Gmeiner, Kickhöfen, Mayer, Westphal, and Wheat, *J. Bacteriol.*, 95, 490 (1968).
16a. Jann and Jann, *Eur. J. Biochem.*, 2, 26 (1967).
17. Romanowska and Mulczyk, *Biochim. Biophys. Acta*, 136, 312 (1967); Romanowska and Reinhold, *Eur. J. Biochem.*, 36, 160 (1973).
18. Raff and Wheat, *J. Biol. Chem.*, 242, 4610 (1967); *J. Bacteriol.*, 95, 2035 (1968).
19. Kotelko, Lüderitz, and Westphal, *Biochem. Z.*, 343, 227 (1965); Bagdian, Dröge, Kotelko, Lüderitz, Westphal, Yamakawa, and Ueta, *Biochem. Z.*, 344, 197 (1966); Sidorczyk and Kotelko, *Arch. Immunol. Ther. Exp.*, 21, 829 (1973); Kotelko, Fromme, and Sidorczyk, *Bull. Acad. Polon. Sci.*, 23, 249 (1975).
19a. Key, Gray, and Wilkinson, *Biochem. J.*, 120, 559 (1970).
20. Wilkinson, Galbraith, and Lightfoot, *Eur. J. Biochem.*, 33, 158 (1973).
21. Chester, Gray, and Wilkinson, *Biochem. J.*, 126, 395 (1972).
22. Volk, *J. Bacteriol.*, 91, 39 (1966); 95, 980 (1968).
23. Hickman and Ashwell, *J. Biol. Chem.*, 241, 1424 (1966).
24. Humphrey and Vincent, *J. Gen. Microbiol.*, 59, 411 (1969).
25. Graham and O'Brien, *Antonie van Leeuwenhoek J. Microbiol. Serol.*, 34, 326 (1965).
26. Adams, Kates, Shaw, and Yaguchi, *Can. J. Biochem.*, 46, 1175 (1968).
27. Adams, *Can. J. Biochem.*, 49, 243 (1971).
28. Adams, Tornabene, and Yaguchi, *Can. J. Microbiol.*, 15, 365 (1969); Adams, Quadling, Yaguchi, and Tornabene, *Can. J. Microbiol.*, 16, 1 (1970).
29. Jackson and Redmond, *FEBS Lett.*, 13, 117 (1971).
30. Redmond, Korsch, and Jackson, *Aust. J. Exp. Biol. Med. Sci.*, 51, 229 (1973).
31. Jann, Jann, and Beyaert, *Eur. J. Biochem.*, 37, 531 (1973).
32. Nell and Hardy, *Immunochemistry*, 3, 233 (1966).
33. Sutherland and Smith, *J. Gen. Microbiol.*, 74, 259 (1973).
34. Rosenfelder, Lüderitz, and Wesphal, *Eur. J. Biochem.*, 44, 411 (1974).
35. Weise, Drews, Jann, and Jann, *Arch. Mikrobiol.*, 71, 89 (1970).
35a. Weckesser, Katz, Drews, Mayer, and Fromme, *J. Bacteriol.*, 120, 672 (1974).
35b. Weckesser, Drews, and Fromme, *J. Bacteriol.*, 109, 1106 (1972); Weckesser, Mayer, and Drews, *Eur. J. Biochem.*, 16, 158 (1970).
36. Weckesser, Rosenfelder, Mayer, and Lüderitz, *Eur. J. Biochem.*, 24, 112 (1971); Weckesser, Mayer, and Fromme, *Biochem. J.*, 135, 293 (1973); Weckesser, Drews, Roppel, Mayer, and Fromme, *Arch. Mikrobiol.*, 101, 233 (1974); Roppel, Mayer, and Weckesser, *Carbohydr. Res.*, 40, 31 (1975).

Table 2 (continued)
SUGAR SEQUENCES

37. Weckesser, Drews, Fromme, and Mayer, *Arch. Mikrobiol.*, 92, 123 (1973); Mayer, Framberg, and Weckesser, *Eur. J. Biochem.*, 44, 181 (1974).
38. Hewett, Knox, and Bishop, *Eur. J. Biochem.*, 19, 169 (1971).
39. Hellerqvist, Lindberg, Samuelsson, and Lindberg, *Acta Chem. Scand.*, 25, 955 (1971).
40. Hellerqvist, Lindberg, Svensson, Holme, and Lindberg, *Carbohydr. Res.*, 8, 43 (1968); 9, 237 (1969).
41. Hellerqvist, Larm, Lindberg, Holme, and Lindberg, *Acta Chem. Scand.*, 23, 2217 (1969).
42. Hellerqvist, Lindberg, Svensson, Holme, and Lindberg, *Acta Chem. Scand.*, 23, 1588 (1969).
43. Hellerqvist, Lindberg, Pilotti, and Lindberg, *Acta Chem. Scand.*, 24, 1168 (1970).
44. Robbins and Uchida, *Biochemistry*, 1, 323 (1962).
45. Hellerqvist, Lindberg, Lönngrenn, and Lindberg, *Carbohydr. Res.*, 16, 289 (1971).
46. Hellerqvist, Lindberg, Lönngrenn, and Lindberg, *Acta Chem. Scand.*, 25, 939 (1971).
47. Staub and Girard, *Bull. Soc. Chim. Biol.*, 47, 1245 (1965).
48. Hellerqvist, Lindberg, Pilotti, and Lindberg, *Carbohydr. Res.*, 16, 297 (1971).
49. Fuller and Staub, *Eur. J. Biochem.*, 4, 286 (1968).
50. Hellerqvist, Lindberg, Svensson, Lindberg, and Holme, personal communication, 1968.
51. Hellerqvist, Lindberg, Svensson, Holme, and Lindberg, *Carbohydr. Res.*, 14, 17 (1970).
52. Hellerqvist, Lindberg, Lönngrenn, and Lindberg, *Acta Chem. Scand.*, 25, 601 (1971).
53. Simmons, Lüderitz, and Westphal, *Biochem. J.*, 97, 807, 815, 820 (1965).
54. Lüderitz, Galanos, Risse, Ruschmann, Schlecht, Schmidt, Schulte-Holthausen, Wheat, Westphal, and Schlosshardt, *Ann. N.Y. Acad. Sci.*, 133, 349 (1966).
55. Berst, Lüderitz, and Westphal, *Eur. J. Biochem.*, 18, 361 (1971).
56. Bruneteau, Volk, Singh, and Lüderitz, *Eur. J. Biochem.*, 43, 501 (1974).
57. Reske and Jann, *Eur. J. Biochem.*, 31, 320 (1972).
58. Springer, Wang, Nichols, and Shear, *Ann. N.Y. Acad. Sci.*, 133, 566 (1966).
59. Jann, Jann, Shmidt, Ørskov, and Ørskov, *Eur. J. Biochem.*, 15, 29 (1970).
60. Edstrom and Heath, *J. Biol. Chem.*, 242, 4125 (1967).
61. Lindberg, Lönngrenn, Rudén, and Simmons, *Eur. J. Biochem.*, 32, 15 (1973).
62. Simmons, *Eur. J. Biochem.*, 11, 554 (1969).
62a. Jann, personal communication.
63. Osborn, Rosen, Rothfield, Zeleznick, and Horecker, *Science*, 145, 783 (1964).
64. Sutherland, Lüderitz, and Westphal, *Biochem. J.*, 96, 439 (1965).
65. Nikaido, *J. Biol. Chem.*, 244, 2835 (1969); *Eur. J. Biochem.*, 15, 57 (1970).
66. Hämmerling, Lüderitz, and Westphal, *Eur. J. Biochem.*, 15, 48 (1970).
67. Hellerqvist and Lindberg, *Carbohydr. Res.*, 16, 39 (1971).
68. Dröge, Lüderitz, and Westphal, *Eur. J. Biochem.*, 4, 126 (1968).
69. Dröge, Lehmann, Lüderitz, and Westphal, *Eur. J. Biochem.*, 14, 175 (1970).
70. Lehmann, Lüderitz, and Westphal, *Eur. J. Biochem.*, 21, 339 (1971).
71. Hämmerling, Lehmann, and Lüderitz, *Eur. J. Biochem.*, 38, 453 (1973).
71a. Prehm, Jann, Stirm, and Jann, *Eur. J. Biochem.*, in press.
72. Hämmerling, Lüderitz, Westphal, and Mäkelä, *Eur. J. Biochem.*, 22, 331 (1971).
73. Schmidt, Jann, and Jann, *Eur. J. Biochem.*, 10, 501 (1969).
74. Schmidt, Fromme, and Mayer, *Eur. J. Biochem.*, 14, 357 (1970).
75. Johnston, Johnston, and Simmons, *Biochem. J.*, 105, 79 (1967).
76. Mayer and Schmidt, *Zentralbl. Bakteriol. Parasitenkd. Infektionskr. Hyg. Abt. 1 Orig. A*, 224, 345 (1973).
77. Fuller, Wu, Wilkinson, and Heath, *J. Biol. Chem.*, 248, 7938 (1973).
78. Gmeiner, Lüderitz, and Westphal, *Eur. J. Biochem.*, 7, 370 (1969).
79. Gmeiner, Simon, and Westphal, *Eur. J. Biochem.*, 21, 355 (1971).
80. Rietschel, Gottert, Lüderitz, and Westphal, *Eur. J. Biochem.*, 28, 166 (1973).
81. Lüderitz, Galanos, Lehmann, Nurminen, Rietschel, Rosenfelder, Simon, and Westphal, *J. Infect. Dis.*, 128, S17 (1973).
82. Adams and Singh, *Can. J. Biochem.*, 48, 55 (1970).
83. Bundle and Shaw, *Carbohydr. Res.*, 21, 211 (1972).
84. Drewry, Lomax, Gray, and Wilkinson, *Biochem. J.*, 133, 563 (1973).
85. Kamio, Kim, and Takahashi, *J. Biochem.* (Tokyo) 70, 189 (1971).
86. Adams and Singh, *Biochim. Biophys. Acta*, 202, 553 (1970).
87. Ikawa, Koepfli, Mudd, and Niemann, *J. Am. Chem. Soc.*, 75, 1035 (1953).
88. Burton and Carter, *Biochemistry*, 3, 411 (1964).
89. Nesbitt and Lennarz, *J. Bacteriol.*, 89, 1020 (1965).

Table 2 (continued)
SUGAR SEQUENCES

90. Gallin and O'Leary, *J. Bacteriol.*, 96, 660 (1968).
91. Kasai, *Ann. N.Y. Acad. Sci.*, 133, 486 (1966).
92. Fensom and Gray, *Biochem. J.*, 114, 185 (1969).
93. Hancock, Humphreys, and Meadow, *Biochim. Biophys. Acta*, 202, 389 (1970).
94. Kaneshiro and Marr, *Biochim. Biophys. Acta*, 70, 271 (1963).
95. Russa and Lorkiewicz, *J. Bacteriol.*, 119, 771 (1974).
96. Lacave, Asselineau, Serre, and Roux, *Eur. J. Biochem.*, 9, 189 (1969).
97. Berger, Fukui, Ludwig, and Rosselet, *Proc. Soc. Exp. Biol. Med.*, 131, 1376 (1969).
98. Lüderitz, Jann, and Wheat, in *Comparative Biochemistry*, Vol. 26, Florkin and Stotz, Eds., Elsevier, Amsterdam, 1968, 105.
99. Lüderitz, Westphal, Staub, and Nikaido, in *Microbial Toxins*, Vol. IV, Weinbaum, Kadis, and Ajl, Eds., Academic Press, New York, 1971, 145.

THE TABLE OF GLYCOLIPIDS

Sen-itiroh Hakomori and Ineo Ishizuka

CLASSIFICATION AND NOMENCLATURE OF GLYCOLIPIDS

Glycolipids can be classified into sphingoglycolipids and glyceroglycolipids, depending on whether they contain N-acylsphingosine (ceramide) or diacylglyceride (diglyceride) as aglycon. Classification of sphingoglycolipids could be either (1) neutral sphingoglycolipids, sulfatides, and gangliosides, depending on the presence or absence of sulfate and sialic acid, or (2) a series of differing oligosaccharide names plus *osyl*ceramide, which distinguishes the backbone structure of carbohydrate chain in glycolipids. According to the second classification, which is more feasible to indicate exact structure of glycolipids, five classes of basic oligosaccharide chain can be distinguished:

Galα1→4Galβ1→4Glc	Globotriaosylceramide	Gb3a
GalNAcβ1→3Galα1→4Galβ1→4Glc	Globotetraosylceramide	Gb4a
Galα1→3Galβ1→4Glc	Globoisotriaosylceramide	Gb3b
GalNAcβ1→3Galα1→3Galβ1→4Glc	Globoisotetraosylceramide	Gb4b
Galβ1→4Galβ1→4Glc	Mucotriaosylceramide	Mu3
Galβ1→3Galβ1→4Galβ1→4Glc	Mucotetraosylceramide	Mu4
GlcNAcβ1→3Galβ1→4Glc	Lactinotriaosylceramide	Lc3
Galβ1→3GlcNAcβ1→3Galβ1→4Glc	Lactinotetraosylceramide	Lc4a
Galβ1→4GlcNAcβ1→3Galβ1→4Glc	Laneotetraosylceramide	Lc4b
GalNAcβ1→4Galβ1→4Glc	Gangliotriaosylceramide	Gg3
Galβ1→3GalNAcβ1→4Galβ1→4Glc	Gangliotetraosylceramide	Gg4
Galα1→4Gal	Galabiosylceramide	Ga2
Gal1→4Galα1→4Gal	Galatriaosylceramide	Ga3
GalNAc1→3Gal1→4Galα1→4Gal	Galatetraosylceramide	Ga4

Glycolipids can be named by adding the name of the oligosaccharide plus the ending *osyl*ceramide. Symbols for those structures should be expressed by signifying these classifications, plus arabic numbers indicating the number of carbohydrate residues, and the letters that indicate positional isomers. For example, globoside is globotetraosylceramide and can be abbreviated as Gb4a. Cytolipin R could be called globoisotetraosylceramide and its symbol should be Gb4b. Blood group H_1-glycolipids should be lactofucopentaosyl-(IV)-ceramide, which could be symbolized as Lc5a. H_3-glycolipids could be symbolized as Lc10.

THE TABLE OF GLYCOLIPIDS

I. Sphingoglycolipids

A. Neutral sphingoglycolipid

  1. Monoglycosylceramide

    Galβ1→1Cer

Isolation: Thudicum,[1-4] Thierfelder and Klenk;[5] structure: Carter et al.[6]

    Glcβ1→1Cer

Occurrence, Gaucher spleen: Lieb,[7] Halliday et al;[8] liver, spleen, serum: Svennerholm[9]

  2. Diglycosylceramide

    Galβ1→4Glcβ1→1Cer

Occurrence: Klenk and Rennkampf;[10] as human tumor hapten ("cytolipin H"): Rapport et al;[11] identity of cytolipin H with ceramide dihexoside of bovine kidney: Rapport and Graf;[12] isolation from erythrocytes: Yamakawa et al;[13] kidney: Makita and Yamakawa;[14] structure: Yamakawa et al.[15]

    Galα1→4Galβ1→1Cer

In mouse kidney showing sex hormone response: Gray;[16] in Fabry kidney: Sweeley and Klionsky;[17] structure: Handa et al;[18] Li et al.[19]

  3. Triglycosylceramide

    Galα1→4Galβ1→4Glcβ1→1Cer

In Fabry kidney: Sweeley and Klionsky;[17] erythrocyte: Vance and Sweeley;[20] structure: Hakomori et al.,[21] Li and Li,[22] Handa et al.[18]

    GalNAcβ1→3Gal1→4Glcβ1→1Cer

Isolation and structure from guinea pig erythrocytes: Yamakawa et al;[13] structure: Yamakawa,[23] Seyama and Yamakawa;[24] Tay-Sach's brain: Makita and Yamakawa[14]

  4. Tetraglycosylceramide

    GalNAcβ1→3Galα1→4Galβ1→4Glc→Cer
    (globoside)

Occurrence: Klenk and Lauenstein,[25] Yamakawa and Suzuki;[26] structure: Yamakawa et al.,[27] Hakomori et al.[21]

    GalNAcβ1→3Galα1→3Galβ1→4Glc→Cer
    (cytolipin R)

Occurrence and isolation: Rapport et al;[28] structure: Laine et al.,[29] Siddiqui et al.[30]

    Galβ1→4GlcNAcβ1→3Galβ1→4Glc→Cer
    (paragloboside)

Isolation and structure (human erythrocytes): Siddiqui and Hakomori,[31] Wiegandt,[32] Ando and Yamakawa[33]

    L-Fucα1→2Galα1→4Galβ1→4Glc→Cer

Isolation and characterization from hog gastric mucosa: Slomiany et al.[34]

  5. Pentaglycosylceramide

    GalNAcα1→GalNAcβ1→3Galα1→4Galβ1→4Glc1→Cer
    (Forssman glycolipid)

Occurrence: Brunius,[35] Yamakawa et al,[13] isolation: Makita et al;[36] structure: Siddiqui and Hakomori[37]

THE TABLE OF GLYCOLIPIDS (continued)

I. Sphingoglycolipids (continued)

5. Pentaglycosylceramide (continued)

Galα1→3Galβ1→4GlcNAcβ1→3Galβ1→4Glc1→1Cer (rabbit B-active glycolipid)

Isolation and structure (rabbit erythrocyte) Eto et al.,[38] Stellner et al.[39]

Galβ1→3Galβ1→4GlcNAcβ1→3Galβ1→4Glc1→1Cer

Isolation and structure of human erythrocytes: Stellner and Hakomori[40]

Fucα1→2Galβ1→4GlcNAcβ1→3Galβ1→4Glc→Cer (H₁ glycolipid)

Isolation and structure from human erythrocytes: Stellner et al.[41]

Galβ1→3GlcNAcβ1→3Galβ1→4Glc→Cer
4
↑
Fucα1
(Leᵃ active glycolipid)

Isolation and structure from adenocarcinoma: Hakomori and Jeanloz[42]

Galβ1→4GlcNAcβ1→3Galβ1→4Glc→Cer
3
↑
Fucα1
(X-hapten)

Isolation and structure from adenocarcinoma: Yang and Hakomori[43]

6. Hexaglycosylceramide

GalNAcα1→3Galβ1→4GlcNAcβ1→3Galβ1→4Glc→Cer
2
↑
Fuc1
(A glycolipid)

Isolation and structure from human erythrocytes: Hakomori et al.[44]

Galα1→3Galβ1→3GlcNAcβ1→3Galβ1→4Glc→Cer
2
↑
Fuc1
(B glycolipid of human)

Isolation and structure (from Fabry's pancreas): Wherrett and Hakomori[45]

Gal1→3 or 4GlcNAcβ1→3Galβ1→4Glc→Cer
2   2
↑   ↑
Fuc1   Fuc1
(Leᵇ glycolipid)

Isolation and structure: Hakomori and Andrews[46]

GalNAcα1→3Gal1→3Gal1→4Gal→Glc→Cer
2
↑
Fuc1

Isolation and characterization from hog gastric mucosa: Slomiany et al.[47]

7. Heptaglycosylceramide

Fuc1→2Galβ1→4GlcNAcβ1→3Galβ1→4GlcNAcβ1→
3Galβ1→4Glc→Cer

Isolation and characterization: Koscielak et al.,[48] Stellner et al.[41]

GalNAc→Gal→GlcNAc→Gal→Gal→Glc→Cer
↑
Fuc

Isolation and characterization from hog gastric mucosa: Slomiany and Horowitz[49]

THE TABLE OF GLYCOLIPIDS (continued)

I. Sphingoglycolipids (continued)

8. Octaglycosylceramide

GalNAcα1→3Galβ1→4GlcNAcl→3Galβ1→4GlcNAcl→3Galβ1→4Glcβ1→4Glc→Cer
2
↑   Isolation and structure: Hakomori et al.[44]
L-Fuc1

Fuc1→2Gal1→4GlcNAcl→3Gal1→4GlcNAcl→3Gal1→4Glc→Cer
↑   Isolation and characterization: Hakomori
Fuc   and Andrews[46]

9. Further complex megaloglycosylceramides

Fucα1→2Galβ1→4GlcNAc
$\searrow$ 3Gal1→4GlcNAcl→3Gal1→4Glc→Cer
Fucα1→2Gal1→4GlcNAcl $\nearrow$ 6   Watanabe et al.[50]

Fuc
1
↓
2
GalNAcl→3Gal1→4GlcNAcl
$\searrow$ 3Gal1→4GlcNAcl→3Gal1→4Glc→Cer
Gal1→4GlcNAcl $\nearrow$ 6
(A^c glycolipid)   Hakomori et al.[44]

B. Sulfatides

HSO$_3$→3Galβ1→1Cer   Occurrence and isolation: Blix;[51]
structure: Yamakawa et al.,[15] Stoffyn and
Stoffyn[52]

HSO$_3$→3Galβ1→4Glcβ1→1Cer   Occurrence and isolation: Martensson;[53]
structure: Stoffyn et al.[54]

HSO$_3$→3Gal1→4Gal1→4Glc1→1Cer   Occurrence and isolation from hog gastric
mucosa[54a]

C. Gangliosides (sialylglycolipid)

GM$_4$ NANA2→3Gal→Cer   Isolation and structure: Siddiqui and
McCluer[55]

GM$_3$ NGNA2→3Galβ1→4Glc→Cer   Occurrence: Yamakawa and Suzuki;[56] structure:
Klenk and Padberg[57]

NANA2→3Galβ1→4Glc→Cer   Occurrence: Svennerholm,[58] Klenk and Heuer;[59]
structure: Puro,[60] Handa and Yamakawa[61]

NGNA2→3Galβ1→4Glc→Cer   Isolation and structure: Hakomori and Saito[62]
↑
AcO

GD$_3$ NGNA2→8NGNA2→3Galβ1→4Glc→Cer   Isolation and structure: Handa and Handa,[63]
Handa and Yamakawa[61]

NANA2→8NANA2→3Galβ1→4Glc→Cer   Isolation and structure: Puro,[60] Puro and
Keränen[64]

THE TABLE OF GLYCOLIPIDS (continued)

I. Sphingoglycolipids (continued)

C. Gangliosides (sialylglycolipid) (continued)

GM$_2$ GalNAcβ1→4Galβ1→4Glc→Cer
                           3
                           ↑
                           2
                       NANA

       Tay-Sach's ganglioside — occurrence and isolation: Klenk;[65] structure: Makita and Yamakawa,[14] Ledeen and Salzman[66]

GM$_1$ Gal1→3GalNAcβ1→4Galβ1→4Glc→Cer
                                3
                                ↑
                                2
                            NANA

       Occurrence and isolation: Klenk;[67] structure: Kuhn and Wiegandt,[68] Svennerholm[69]

GD$_{1a}$ Gal1→3GalNAcβ1→4Galβ1→4Glc→Cer
     3   3
     ↑   ↑
     2   2
   NANA   NANA

       Occurrence and isolation: Klenk,[67] structure: Kuhn and Wiegandt,[68] Svennerholm,[69] Johnson and McCluer[70]

GD$_{1b}$ Gal→3GalNAcβ1→4Galβ1→4Glc→Cer
                             3
                             ↑
                           2
              NANA2→8NANA

       Isolation and structure: Kuhn and Wiegandt[68]

GT   Gal1→3GalNAcβ1→4Galβ1→4Glc→Cer
     3   3
     ↑   ↑
     2   2
  NANA   NANA
  Ga   3
                     ↑
                     2
                NANA

       Isolation and structure: Kuhn and Wiegandt[68]

GQ   Gal1→3GalNAc1→4Gal1→4Glc→Cer
GP   ↑   ↑
  NANA   NANA
  ↑   ↑
 (NANA)   NANA
                     ↑
                NANA

       Isolation and structure of fish brain: Ishizuka et al.,[71] Wiegandt,[32] Ishizuka and Wiegandt[72]

GalNAcβ1→4Galβ1→3GalNAcβ1→4Galβ1→4Glc→Cer
               3   3
               ↑   ↑
           NANA2   NANA2

       Isolation and characterization from human brain: Svennerholm et al.[73]

Fucα1→2Galβ1→3GalNAcβ1→4Galβ1→4Glc
                          3
                          ↑
                          2
                     NANA

       Isolation and characterization from bovine liver: Wiegandt[74]

NANA2→3Galβ1→4GlcNAcβ1→3Galβ1→4Glc→Cer

       Isolation and structure: Wiegandt,[75] Siddiqui and Hakomori,[31] Li et al.,[76] Wherrett[77]

THE TABLE OF GLYCOLIPIDS (continued)

I. Sphingoglycolipids (continued)

C. Gangliosides (sialylglycolipid) (continued)

NGNA2→3Galβ1→4GlcNAcβ1→3Galβ1→4Glc→Cer

Isolation and structure: Wiegandt[75]

NANAα2→6Galβ1→4GlcNAcβ1→3Galβ1→4Glc→Cer

Isolation and characterization from spleen and kidney: Wiegandt[74]

NANAα2→3Galβ1→3Galβ1→3GlcNAcβ1→3Galβ1→4Glcp1→Cer

Isolation and structure: Stellner et al.[40] and Watanabe et al.[50]

II. Glyceroglycolipids

A. Monoglycosyl diglycerides

Galpβ1→3 sn-Gly

Higher plants: 18:3, Carter et al.[77a]
Chlorella vulgaris: 18:3, 16:2, Konstantopoulos[77b]
Runner bean leaves: 16.6%, 18:3, Sastry and Kates[77c]
Bovine spinal cord: 15%, 16:0, 18:1, Steim[78]
Bovine brain white matter: 0.4% A, Norton and Brotz[79]
Sheep brain: B, Rumsby[80]
Boar and human testis: 16:0, Ishizuka et al.,[81] Ishizuka and Yamakawa,[82] Kornblatt et al[83]
Rat brain: Wenger et al.[84]

Acyl-O-6Galpβ1→3 sn-Gly

Spinach leaf homogenate: Heinz and Tulloch[85]

Galfβ1→3 sn-Gly

Bacteroides symbiosus: Reeves et al.[86]
Mycoplasma mycoides: 1.3%, 18:0, 18:1, 16:0, Plackett[87]

Galpα1→3Gly

Treponema pallidum Kazan 5: 49%, 16:0, 18:1, Livermore and Johnson[88]
Streptococcus faecalis: Pieringer[89]

H₂SO₄→3Galpβ1→3(1) sn-Gly

Mammalian testis and sperm: ca.3%, 16:0, Ishizuka et al.,[81] Ishizuka and Yamakawa,[82] Suzuki et al.,[90] Handa et al.,[91] Kornblatt et al.[83]

Glcpα1→3 sn-Gly

Pseudomonas diminuta: 5%, 18:1, 16:0, Wilkinson[92]
Mycoplasma laidlawlii: Shaw et al.[93]
Pneumococcus type XIV: Kaufman et al.[94]

Glcpβ1→3 sn-Gly

Pseudomonas rubescens: 16:1, 18:1, Wiklinson[95]

GlcUpβ1→3 sn-Gly

Pseudomonas rubescens: 16:1, 18:1, Wilkinson[95,96]

GlcUpα1→3 sn-Gly

Pseudomonas diminuta: Wilkinson[92]

H₂SO₃→6 Quinovosepα1→3 sn-Gly

Plants: Benson[97]
Sea urchin: 12:0, 14:0, Nagai and Isono[98]

GlcNAcα1→3(1) sn-Gly

Streptococcus hemolyticus: Ishizuka and Yamakawa[99]

GlcNAcβ1→3 sn-Gly

Bacillus megaterium: Phizackerley and MacDougall[100]

THE TABLE OF GLYCOLIPIDS (continued)

II. Glyceroglycolipids (continued)

B. Diglycosyl diglycerides

Galpα1→6Galpβ1→3 *sn*-Gly

Plants: 18:3, Carter et al.,[77a] Konstantopoulos,[77b] Sastry and Kates[77c]
Arthrobacter globiformis: 0.6% *anteiso*-15:0, Walker and Bastle[101]
Rat brain: Wenger et al.,[102] Subba Rao et al.,[103] Inoue et al.[104]

Acyl-*O*-6Galpα1→6Galpβ1→3 *sn*-Gly

Spinach leaf homogenate D: Heinz et al.[105]

Galpα1→2Glcpα1→3 *sn*-Gly

Pneumococcus I-R: 32%, 16:0, 16:1, Brundish et al.[106]
Lactobacillus casei: 16:0, 18:1, 19cy, Shaw et al.[107]
Pneumococcus type XIV: Fischer and Seyferth[108]

Glcpα1→2Glcpα1→3 *sn*-Gly

Streptococcus lactis: Ishizuka and Yamakawa[109]
Streptococcus hemolyticus: Fischer et al.[110]
Mycoplasma laidlawlii: Shaw et al.[93]
Streptococcus faecalis: Pieringer[89]
S. faecalis var. *faecalis*: 18:1, 16:0, 19cy, Fischer et al.[110]

Glcpβ1→6Glcpβ1→3 *sn*-Gly

Staphylococcus lactis: Brundish et al.,[111] Brundish and Baddiley[112]
Staphylococcus aureus: Brundish and Baddiley.,[112] Polonovsky et al.,[113] Ward and Perkins[114]
Bacillus subtilis: Brundish and Baddiley[112]
Bacillus cereus: Saito and Mukoyama[115]

Manpα1→3Manpα1→3 *sn*-Gly

Micrococcus lysodeikticus: 7.5−15%, *iso*- and *anteiso*-15:0, Lennarz and Talamo[116]
Microbacterium lacticum: 46%, Shaw[117]

Glcpβ1→4GlcUpα1→3 *sn*-Gly

Pseudomonas diminuta: 0.1%, 18:1, 16:0, 19:1, Wilkinson[92]

Glcpα1→4GalUp1→3(1) *sn*-Gly

Streptomyces LA 7017: 6%, 15:0, Bergelson et al.[118]

C. Triglycosyl diglycerides

H₂SO₄→3Galpβ1→6Manpα1→2Glcpα1→1 *sn*-Gly

Halobacterium cutirubrum: phytanol, Kates and Deroo[119]

Glcpα1→2Glcpα1→2Glcpα1→3(1) *sn*-Gly

Streptococcus hemolyticus: 0.9%, 16:0, 18:1, Ishizuka and Yamakawa[109]
Streptococcus faecalis var. *faecalis*: Fischer et al.[120]

Glcpα1→6Galpα1→2Glcpα1→3 *sn*-Gly

Lactobacillus casei: less than 17%, 16:0, 18:1 19cy, Shaw et al.[107]

Galpα1→6Galpα1→6Galpβ1→3 *sn*-Gly

Potato tuber: 1%, Galliard[121]

D. Polyglycosyl diglycerides

Galfl→2Galpα1→6GlcNA₂p1→2Glcp1→3(1) *sn*-Gly

Flavobacterium stearothermophilis: 70%, 15- and 17-*anteiso*, Oshima and Yamakawa[122] (G)

THE TABLE OF GLYCOLIPIDS (continued)

II. Glyceroglycolipids (continued)

D. Polyglycosyl diglycerides (continued)

(Manpα1→2Manpα1→2Manpα1→3)$_n$ Glcp1→1(3) sn-Gly — *Thermoplasma acidophilum*: H, Mayberry-Carson et al.[123]

E. Phosphoglyceroglycolipids

3-Phosphatidyl-6Glcpα1→3(1) sn-Gly — *Pseudomonas diminuta*: Wilkinson and Bell[124]

Glcpα1→2(3-phosphatidyl-6)Glcpα1→3(1) sn-Gly — *Streptococcus faecalis* var. *faecalis*: 18:1, 16:0, 19cy, Fischer et al.[120] *Streptococcus lactis, S. faecalis* var. *zymogenes*: Fischer et al.[120] *S. faecalis*: Ambron and Pieringer[125]

1-sn-Glycerophosphoryl-6-Glcpα1→2Glcpα1→3(1) sn-Gly — *Streptococcus hemolyticus*: 1.8%, 18:1, 16:0, Ishizuka and Yamakawa,[109] Fischer et al.[110] *Streptococcus lactis*: Fischer and Seyferth,[108] Fischer et al.[120] *Streptococcus faecalis* var. *faecalis*, *S. faecalis* var. *zymogenes*, Fischer et al.[120]

1-sn-Glycoerphosphoryl-6Galfα1→3 sn-Gly — *Bifidobacterium bifidum* var. *Pennsylvanicus*: Veerkamp and Van Schaik[126]

1-sn-Glycerophosphoryl-6Glcpα1→2(3-phosphatidyl)Glcpα1→3(1) sn-Gly — *Streptococcus hemolyticus*: Fischer and Landgraf,[127] Fischer[128]

Compiled by Sen-itroh Hakamori and Ineo Ishizuka.

REFERENCES

1. Thudicum, *Report of the Medical Officer Privy Council and Local Government Board*, London, No. III, 113 (1874).
2. Thudicum, *Report of the Medical Officer Privy Council and Local Government Board*, London, No. VIII, 117 (1876).
3. Thudicum, *A Treatise on the Chemical Constitution of the Brain*, Archon Books, Hamden, Conn., 1962.
4. Thudicum, *Die Chemische Konstitution des Gehirns des Menschen und Tiere*, Grantz Pietscher, Tubingen, 1904.
5. Thierfelder and Klenk, *Die Chemie der Cerebroside und Phosphatide*, Julius Springer, Berlin, 1930.
6. Carter, Greenwood, and Humiston, *Fed. Am. Soc. Exp. Biol.*, 9, 159 (1950).
7. Lieb, *Z. Physiol. Chem.*, 140, 305 (1924).
8. Halliday, Duel, Tragerman, and Ward, *J. Biol. Chem.*, 132, 171 (1940).
9. Svennerholm, *Acta Chem. Scand.*, 17, 860 (1963).
10. Klenk and Rennkampf, *Z. Physiol. Chem.*, 273, 253 (1942).
11. Rapport, Graf, Skipski, and Alonzo, *Cancer* 12, 348 (1959).
12. Rapport and Graf, *Cancer Res.*, 21, 1225 (1961).
13. Yamakawa, Irie, and Iwanaga, *J. Biochem.* (Tokyo), 48, 490 (1960).
14. Makita and Yamakawa, *Jap. J. Exp. Med.*, 33, 361 (1963).
15. Yamakawa, Kiso, Handa, Makita, and Yokoyama, *J. Biochem.* (Tokyo), 52, 226 (1962).
16. Gray, *Biochim. Biophys. Acta*, 239, 494 (1971).
17. Sweeley and Klionsky, *J. Biol. Chem.*, 238, 3148 (1963).
18. Handa, Ariga, Miyatake, and Yamakawa, *J. Biochem.* (Tokyo), 69, 625 (1971).
19. Li, Li, and Dawson, *Biochim. Biophys. Acta*, 88, 92 (1972).
20. Vance and Sweeley, *J. Lipid Res.*, 8, 621 (1967).
21. Hakomori, Siddiqui, Hellerqvist, Li, and Li, *J. Biol. Chem.*, 246, 2271 (1971).
22. Li and Li, *J. Biol. Chem.*, 246, 3769 (1971).
23. Yamakawa, *Lipoide, 16 Colloquium der Gesellschaft Physiologische Chemie*, Mosbach/Baden, Springer-Verlag, Berlin, 1966.
24. Seyama and Yamakawa, *J. Biochem.* (Tokyo), 75, 837 (1974).
25. Klenk and Lauenstein, *Z. Physiol. Chem.*, 291, 249 (1951).

THE TABLE OF GLYCOLIPIDS (continued)

26. Yamakawa and Suzuki, *J. Biochem.* (Tokyo), 38, 199 (1951).
27. Yamakawa, Nishimura, and Kamimura, *Jap. J. Exp. Med.*, 35, 201 (1965).
28. Rapport, Schneider, and Graf, *Biochim. Biophys. Acta*, 137, 409 (1967).
29. Laine, Sweeley, Kisic, and Rapport, *J. Lipid Res.*, 13, 519 (1972).
30. Siddiqui, Kawanami, Li, and Hakomori, *J. Lipid Res.*, 13, 657 (1972).
31. Siddiqui and Hakomori, *Biochim. Biophys. Acta*, 330, 147 (1973).
32. Wiegandt, in *Glycolipids, Glycoproteins, and Mucopolysaccharides of the Nervous System*, Zambotti, Ed., Plenum Press, New York, 1972.
33. Ando and Yamakawa, *Chem. Phys. Lipids*, 5, 91 (1970).
34. Sloimiany, Slomiany, and Horowitz, *Eur. J. Biochem.*, 3, 161 (1974).
35. Brunius, *Chemical Studies on the True Forssman Hapten*, Aktiebolaget Fahlencrantz, Stockholm, 1936.
36. Makita, Suzuki, and Yosizawa, *J. Biochem.* (Tokyo), 60, 502 (1966).
37. Siddiqui and Hakomori, *J. Biol. Chem.*, 246, 5766 (1971).
38. Eto, Ichikawa, Nishimura, Ando, and Yamakawa, *J. Biochem.* 64, 205 (1968).
39. Stellner, Saito, and Hakomori, *Arch. Biochim. Biophys.*, 155, 464 (1973).
40. Stellner and Hakomori, *J. Biol. Chem.*, 249, 1022 (1974).
41. Stellner, Watanabe, and Hakomori, *Biochemistry*, 12, 656 (1973).
42. Hakomori and Jeanloz, *Blood and Tissue Antigens*, Aminoff, Ed., Academic Press, New York 1970, 149.
43. Yang and Hakomori, *J. Biol. Chem.*, 246, 1192 (1971).
44. Hakomori, Stellner, and Watanabe, *Biochem. Biophys. Res. Commun.*, 49, 1061 (1972).
45. Wherrett and Hakomori, *J. Biol. Chem.*, 248, 3046 (1973).
46. Hakomori and Andrews, *Biochim. Biophys. Acta*, 202, 255 (1970).
47. Slomiany, Slomiany, and Horowitz, *Biochim. Biophys. Acta*, in press.
48. Koscielak, Piasek, Gorniak, and Gardas, *Eur. J. Biochem.*, 37, 214 (1973).
49. Slomiany and Horowitz, *J. Biol. Chem.*, 248, 6232 (1973).
50. Watanabe, Stellner, Yogeeswaran, and Hakomori, *Fed. Proc.*, 33, 1225 Abstr. #3 (1974).
51. Blix, *Z. Physiol. Chem.*, 219, 82 (1933).
52. Stoffyn and Stoffyn, *Biochim. Biophys. Acta*, 70, 218 (1963).
53. Martensson, *Biochim. Biophys. Acta*, 116, 521 (1966).
54. Stoffyn, Stoffyn, and Martensson, *Biochim. Biophys. Acta*, 152, 533 (1968).
54a. Slomiany, Slomiany, and Horowitz, *Biochim. Biophys. Acta*, 348, 388 (1974).
55. Siddiqui and McCluer, *J. Lipid Res.*, 9, 366 (1968).
56. Yamakawa and Suzuki, *J. Biochem.* (Tokyo), 38, 199 (1951).
57. Klenk and Padberg, *Z. Physiol. Chem.*, 327, 249 (1962).
58. Svennerholm, *Acta Chem. Scand.*, 17, 239 (1963).
59. Klenk and Heuer, *Z. Verdau. Stoffwechsel.*, 20, 180 (1960).
60. Puro, *Biochim. Biophys. Acta*, 189, 401 (1969).
61. Handa and Yamakawa, *Jap. J. Exp. Med.*, 34, 293 (1964).
62. Hakomori and Saito, *Biochemistry*, 8, 5082 (1969).
63. Handa and Handa, *Jap. J. Exp. Med.*, 35, 331 (1965).
64. Puro and Keinen, *Biochim. Biophys. Acta*, 187, 393 (1969).
65. Klenk, *Z. Physiol. Chem.*, 262, 128 (1939).
66. Ledeen and Salzman, *Biochemistry*, 4, 2225 (1965).
67. Klenk, *Z. Physiol. Chem.*, 273, 76 (1942).
68. Kuhn and Wiegandt, *Chem. Ber.*, 96, 866 (1963).
69. Svennerholm, *J. Neurochem.*, 10, 613 (1963).
70. Johnson and McCluer, *Biochim. Biophys. Acta*, 70, 487 (1963).
71. Ishizuka, Kloppenburg, and Wiegandt, *Biochim. Biophys. Acta*, 210, 299 (1970).
72. Ishizuka and Wiegandt, *Biochim. Biophys. Acta*, 260, 279 (1972).
73. Svennerholm, Mansson, and Li, *J. Biol. Chem.*, 248, 740 (1973).
74. Wiegandt, *Z. Physiol. Chem.*, 354, 1049 (1973).
75. Wiegandt, *Chem. Phys. Lipids*, 5, 198 (1970).
76. Li, Mansson, Vanier, and Svennerholm, *J. Biol. Chem.*, 248, 2634 (1973).
77. Wherrett, *Biochim. Biophys. Acta*, 326, 63 (1973).
77a. Carter, Johnson, and Weber, *Annu. Rev. Biochem.*, 34, 109 (1965).
77b. Konstantopoulos, *J. Biol. Chem.*, 242, 3538 (1967).
77c. Sastry and Kates, *Biochemistry*, 3, 1271 (1964).
78. Steim, *Biochim. Biophys. Acta*, 137, 80 (1967).
79. Norton and Brotz, *Biochem. Biophys. Res. Commun.*, 12, 198 (1963).

THE TABLE OF GLYCOLIPIDS (continued)

80. Rumsby, *J. Neurochem.*, 14, 733 (1967).
81. Ishizuka, Suzuki, and Yamakawa, *J. Biochem.* (Tokyo), 73, 77 (1973).
82. Ishizuka and Yamakawa, *J. Biochem.* (Tokyo), 76, 221 (1974).
83. Kornblatt, Knapp, Levine, and Schachter, *Can. J. Biochem.*, 52, 689 (1974).
84. Wenger, Petitpas, and Pieringer, *Biochemistry*, 7, 3700 (1968).
85. Heinz and Tulloch, *Z. Physiol. Chem.*, 350, 439 (1969).
86. Reeves, Latour, and Lostaeau, *Biochemistry*, 3, 1284 (1964).
87. Plackett, *Biochemistry*, 6, 2746 (1967).
88. Livermore and Johnson, *Biochim. Biophys. Acta*, 152, 314 (1970).
89. Pieringer, *J. Biol. Chem.*, 243, 4894 (1968).
90. Suzuki, Ishizuka, Ueta, and Yamakawa, *Jap. J. Exp. Med.*, 43, 435 (1973).
91. Handa, Yamato, Ishizuka, Suzuki, and Yamakawa, *J. Biochem.* (Tokyo), 75, 77 (1974).
92. Wilkinson, *Biochim. Biophys. Acta*, 187, 492 (1969).
93. Shaw, Smith, and Koostra, *Biochem. J.*, 107, 329 (1968).
94. Kaufman, Kundig, and Roseman, *Biochem. Biophys. Res. Commun.*, 18, 312 (1965).
95. Wilkinson, *Biochim. Biophys. Acta*, 164, 148 (1968).
96. Wilkinson, *Biochim. Biophys. Acta*, 152, 227 (1968).
97. Benson, *Adv. Lipid Res.*, 1, 387 (1963).
98. Nagai and Isono, *Jap. J. Exp. Med.*, 35, 315 (1965).
99. Ishizuka and Yamakawa, *Jap. J. Exp. Med.*, 39, 321 (1969).
100. Phizackerley and MacDougall, *Biochem. J.*, 126, 499 (1972).
101. Walker and Bastle, *Carbohydr. Res.*, 4, 49 (1967).
102. Wenger, Subba Rao, and Pieringer, *J. Biol. Chem.*, 245, 2513 (1970).
103. Subba Rao, Wenger, and Pieringer, *J. Biol. Chem.*, 245, 2520 (1970).
104. Inoue, Deshmukh, and Pieringer, *J. Biol. Chem.*, 246, 5688 (1971).
105. Heinz, Rullkotter, and Budzikiewicz, *Z. Phys. Chem.*, 355, 612 (1974).
106. Brundish, Shaw, and Baddiley, *Biochem. J.*, 97, 158 (1965).
107. Shaw, Heatherington, and Baddiley, *Biochem. J.*, 107, 491 (1965).
108. Fischer and Seyferth, *Z. Physiol. Chem.*, 349, 1662 (1968).
109. Ishizuka and Yamakawa, *J. Biochem.* (Tokyo), 64, 13 (1968).
110. Fischer, Ishizuka, Landgraf, and Herrmann, *Biochim. Biophys. Acta*, 296, 527 (1973).
111. Brundish, Shaw, and Baddiley, *Biochem. J.*, 105, 885 (1967).
112. Brundish and Baddiley, *Carbohydr. Res.*, 8, 308 (1968).
113. Polonovsky, Wald, and Paysant-Diament, *Ann. Inst. Pasteur* (Paris), 103, 302 (1962).
114. Ward and Perkins, *Biochem. J.*, 106, 391 (1968).
115. Saito and Mukoyama, *J. Biochem.* (Tokyo), 69, 83 (1970).
116. Lennarz and Talamo, *J. Biol. Chem.*, 241, 2707 (1966).
117. Shaw, *Biochim. Biophys. Acta*, 152, 427 (1968).
118. Bergelson, Batrakov, and Pilipenko, *Chem. Phys. Lipids*, 4, 181 (1970).
119. Kates and Deroo, *J. Lipid Res.*, 14, 438 (1973).
120. Fischer, Landgraf, and Herrmann, *Biochim. Biophys. Acta*, 306, 353 (1973).
121. Galliard, *Biochem. J.*, 115, 335 (1969).
122. Oshima and Yamakawa, *Biochemistry*, 13, 1140 (1974).
123. Mayberry-Carson, Langworthy, Mayberry, and Smith, *Biochim. Biophys. Acta*, 360, 217 (1974).
124. Wilkinson and Bell, *Biochim. Biophys. Acta*, 248, 293 (1971).
125. Ambron and Pieringer, *J. Biol. Chem.*, 246, 4216 (1971).
126. Veerkamp and Van Schaik, *Biochim. Biophys. Acta*, 348, 370 (1974).
127. Fischer and Landgraf, *Biochim. Biophys. Acta*, in press.
128. Fischer, *Proc. 12th Int. Congr. Fat Research*, Raven Press, New York, in press.

GLYCOHYDROLASES

Table 1
α-D-MANNOSIDE MANNOHYDROLASE (3.2.1.24)

Sources	pH optimum	pH stability	K_m (mM)	V_{max}	Substrate used[a]	Specificity and remarks[a]	Reference
Almond emulsin	4.5	—	4.2 23.8 88.7	— — —	pNPh-α-Man Ph-α-Man Me-α-Man	Hydrolyze glycopeptide from ovalbumin pineapple bromelain, α-amylase of *Asp. oryzae*	1
Arthrobacter species	6.5–7	—	0.5–2	—	di-, tri-, tetra-, penta- and hexasaccharides	Hydrolyze yeast mannan and oligosaccharides derived from yeast mannan; low activity with synthetic α-mannosides	2
Aspergillus niger	4.8	5–8	2.0	μmol/mg/min 1.3	2-O-α-Man₂	Hydrolyze 2-O-α-Man₂, 2-O-α-Man, specific for 1.2-α-D-mannosidic bonds	3
	4.2	5–7	1.2 8.2	μmol/mg/h 41.3 12.3	pNPh-α-Man 4-O-α-Man₂	Specific for 1,4-α-and 1,6-α-mannosidic bonds, hydrolyze 4-O-α- and 6-O-α-mannosidic linkages to D-mannose or GlcNAc, glycopeptides from α₁-acid glycoprotein, fetuin, human chorionic gonadotropin; low activity with synthetic substrate	4
Baker's yeast	6.8	—	1.0	—	pNPh-α-Man	Low activity on yeast mannan	5

[a] Abbreviations: pNPh = *p*-nitrophenyl; Ph = phenyl; Man = D-mannopyranose; Me = methyl; NeuAc = *N*-acetylneuraminic acid; Gal = D-galactopyranose; GlcNAc = 2-acetamido-2-deoxy-D-glucopyranose; MeUmb = 4-methylumbelliferyl.

Table 1 (continued)
α-D-MANNOSIDE MANNOHYDROLASE (3.2.1.24)

Sources	pH optimum	pH stability	K_m (mM)	V_{max}	Substrate used[a]	Specificity and remarks[a]	Reference
				μmol/mg/h			
Cerebral cortex	4.1	—	0.4	0.4	pNPh-α-Man	Inhibited by Hg^{2+}, inactivated above 40°C	6
			0.027	0.4	Fetuin (minus NeuAc.Gal, GlcNAc)		
			0.82	1.6	Ovalbumin		
			0.002	0.3	Ovalbumin (minus GlcNAc)		
Charonia lampas (Marine gastropod)	4.0	—	4.3	—	pNPh-α-Man	Activated by Na^+, inactivated by freeze-drying, hydrolyze ovalbumin glycopeptide	7
Dictyostelium discoideum (Slime mold)	3.5;5	—	1.0	—	pNPh-α-Man	Lysosomal enzyme	8
Epididymis, rat	5.0	5—6.5	13.0	—	pNPh-α-Man	Specifically and competitively inhibited by lactone; Zn^{2+}-enzyme	9
			57.0	—	Ph-α-Man		10
				μmol/mg/min			
Kidney, hog	4.6	—	0.91	19.0	pNPh-α-Man	Inactivated by freeze-drying; Zn^{2+}-enzyme; hydrolyze glycopeptides from ovalbumin, Taka®-amylase and stem bromelain	11
Jack bean	4—4.5	—	2.5	—	pNPh-α-Man	Inhibited by 1,4- and 1,5-lactone; hydrolyze α-1,2-Man$_2$, Man$_3$, and glycopeptides, Zn^{2+}-enzyme; crystalline enzyme	12
			31.0	—	Benzyl-α-Man		13
			120.0	—	Me-α Man		14
				μmol/mg/h			
Leukocytes, human	4.3—4.6	5—7	0.65—1.8	0.45	pNPh-α-Man	Zn^{2+}-enzyme; inhibited by lactone	15
Liver, rat lysosomal	4.5	6.0	8.5	—	pNPh-α-Man	Stable at 55°C, Zn^{2+}-enzyme	16
			3.2	—	MeUmb-α-Man		

Table 1 (continued)
α-D-MANNOSIDE MANNOHYDROLASE (3.2.1.24)

Sources	pH optimum	pH stability	K_m (mM)	V_{max} (μmol/mg/min)	Substrate used[a]	Specificity and remarks[a]	Reference
Glogi	5.5	6.5–8.0	2.8 7.4	— —	pNPh-α-Man MeUmb-α-Man	Moderately stable at 55°C, not effected by Zn^{2+} but by Cu^{2+}, tightly bound to membranes	17
cytoplasmic	6.5	8.0	0.16 0.11	— —	pNph-α-Man MeUmb-α-Man	Unstable at 55°C	
Milk, bovine	2.9	—	1.2	—	pNPh-α-Man	Require Zn^{2+} and Mn^{2+}; inhibited by zwitterions	18
Oviduct, hen	4.6	—	2.9	—	pNPh-α-Man	Hydrolyze Me-α-Man; inhibited by Ag^+, Hg^{2+}, and lactone	
Patella vulgata (limpet)	3.5–4	5–6	4.5	—	pNPh-α-Man	Require Zn^{2+} and Cl^- for full activity	19
Phaseolus vulgaris (pinto bean)	3.8–4.0	6–7	1.17	—	pNPh-α-Man	Hydrolyze Me-α-Man	20
	4.6	—	1.6	—	pNPh-α-Man	Zn^{2+}-enzyme	21
Small intestine, monkey	3.8	4–6	0.28	0.1	pNPh-α-Man	Hydrolyze Me-α-Man; Zn^{2+}-enzyme	22
Soy bean	3.6–4.6	—	1.6	—	pNPh-α-Man	Hydrolyze Taka®-amylase glycopeptide	23
Streptomyces griseus	8.0	—	<0.1	—	Ph-α-Man	Hydrolyze mannosidostreptomycin	24
Sweet almond emulsin	4.0–5.0	—	88.7 23.8 4.2	— — —	Me-α-Man Ph-α-Man pNPh-α-Man	Rapidly hydrolyze oligosaccharide; low activity for glycopeptides; inhibited by mannolactone	25
Thyroid, sheep	4–4.8	—	0.85	—	pNPh-α-Man	Hydrolyze thyroglobulin glycopeptides	26
Turbo cornutus (Marine gastropod)	3.5–4.5	—	2.3	—	pNPh-α-Man	Hydrolyze glycopeptide from ovalbumin, Taka®-amylase A; activated by Cl^-; inactivated by freeze-drying	27

Compiled by Su-Chen Li and Yu-Teh Li.

Table 1 (continued)
α-D-MANNOSIDE MANNOHYDROLASE (3.2.1.24)

REFERENCES

1. Schwartz, Slaon, and Lee, *Arch. Biochem. Biophys.*, 137, 122 (1970).
2. Jones and Ballou, *J. Biol. Chem.*, 244, 1043 (1969).
3. Swaminathan, Matta, Donoso, and Bahl, *J. Biol. Chem.*, 247, 1775 (1972).
4. Matta and Bahl, *J. Biol. Chem.*, 247, 1780 (1972).
5. Kaya and Kutsumi, *J. Biochem.* (Tokyo), 73, 181 (1973).
6. Bosmann and Hemsworth, *Biochim. Biophys. Acta*, 242(1), 152 (1971).
7. Muramatsu, *J. Biochem.* (Tokyo), 62, 487 (1967).
8. Loomis, *J. Bacteriol.*, 103, 375 (1970).
9. Conchie and Hay, *Biochem. J.*, 73, 327 (1959).
10. Snaith, Hay, and Levvy, *J. Endocrinol.*, 50, 659 (1971).
11. Okumura and Yamashina, *J. Biochem.* (Tokyo), 68, 561 (1970).
12. Li, *J. Biol. Chem.*, 242, 5474 (1967).
13. Snaith and Levvy, *Biochem. J.*, 110, 663 (1968).
14. Li and Li, *Methods Enzymol.*, 28, 702 (1972).
15. Avila and Convit, *Clin. Chim. Acta*, 47, 335 (1973).
16. Dewald and Touster, *J. Biol. Chem.*, 248, 7223 (1973).
17. Mellors and Harwalkar, *Can. J. Biochem.*, 46, 1351 (1968).
18. Sukeno, Tarentino, Plummer, and Maley, *Methods Enzymol.*, 28, 777 (1972).
19. Snaith, Levvy, and Hay, *Biochem. J.*, 117, 129 (1970).
20. Agrawal and Bahl, *J. Biol. Chem.*, 243, 103 (1968).
21. Paus and Christensen, *Eur. J. Biochem.*, 25, 308 (1972).
22. Seetharam and Radhakrishnan, *Indian J. Biochem. Biophys.*, 9, 59 (1972).
23. Saita, Ikenaka, and Matsushima, *J. Biochem.* (Tokyo), 70, 827 (1971).
24. Hockenhull, Ashton, Fantes, and Whitehead, *Biochem. J.*, 57, 93 (1954).
25. Lee, *Methods Enzymol.*, 28, 699 (1972).
26. Chabaud, Bouchilloux, and Ferrand, *Biochim. Biophys. Acta*, 227, 154 (1971).
27. Muramatsu and Egami, *J. Biochem.* (Tokyo), 62, 700 (1967).

Table 2
β-2-ACETYLAMINO-2-DEOXY-D-GLUCOSIDE ACETYLAMINODEOXYGLUCOHYDROLASE (3.2.1.30)

Sources	pH optimum	pH stability	K_m (mM)	V_{max}	Substrate used[a]	Specificity and remarks[a]	Reference
Aorta, human				nmol/mg/min			
Hexosaminidase A	4.3	—	1.04	11.0	pNPh-β-GlcNAc	Enzyme A, but not B, is activated by NaCl; the same enzyme hydrolyzes both pNPh-β-GlcNAc and pNPh-β-GalNAc; inhibited by GlcNAc lactone	1
Hexosaminidase B	4.0	—	0.54	1.56	pNPh-β-GalNAc		
		—	1.74	10.4	pNPh-β-GlcNAc		
			1.48	1.9	pNPh-β-GalNAc		
Aspergillus niger	3.9–4.6	3.5–7.0	0.66	μmol/mg/min 71.4	pNPh-β-GlcNAc	Hydrolyze both β-glucosaminide and β-galactosaminide, also glycopeptides from ovalbumin, fetuin and α₁-acid glycoprotein	2
Aspergillus oryzae	5.2	—	1.8	μmol/mg/min 330.0	Phβ-GlcNAc	The same enzyme hydrolyzes both pNPh-β-GlcNAc and pNPh-β-GalNAc; rapidly hydrolyze N-acetyl chitopentaose	3
			4.9	350.0	Ph-3-O-Me-β-GlcNAc		
			4.8	16.0	Ph-6-O-Me β-GlcNAc		
Bacillus subtilis B	5.9	8.5	0.15	μmol/mg/h 14.5	pNPh-β-GlcNAc	No detectable activity on galactosaminide; hydrolyze α₁-acid glycoprotein (minus NeuAc, Gal); inhibited by glucosamino-1,5-lactone	4
			0.11	5.2	MeUmb-β-GlcNAc		
			0.31	1.22	Chitobiose		
			0.39	1.31	Chitotriose		
			0.38	1.05	Chitotetraose		
Brain, calf	3.8	—	0.6	μmol/mg/h 0.5	GalNAc-Gal-Glc-Cer	Require detergent for hydrolysis of glycolipids; hydrolyze GalNAc-Gal-Glu-Cer, globoside; low activity with Tay-Sach's ganglioside	5
			0.2	0.35	Globoside		

[a] Abbreviations: pNPh = P-nitrophenyl; GlcNAc = 2-acetamido-2-deoxy-D-glucopyranose; GalNAc = 2-acetamido-2-deoxy-D-galactopyranose; MeUmb = 4-methylumbelliferyl; Ph = phenyl; Me = methyl; NeuAc = N-acetylneuraminic acid; Gal = D-galactopyranose; G_{M2} = GalNAcβ1→4(NeuAcα2→3)Galβ1→4Glcβ1→1 ceramide; G_{A2} = GalNAcβ1→4Galβ1→4Glcβ1→1 ceramide; GlcUA = D-glucuronic acid; Asn = L-asparagine.

Table 2 (continued)

β-2-ACETYLAMINO-2-DEOXY-D-GLUCOSIDE ACETYLAMINODEOXYGLUCOHYDROLASE (3.2.1.30)

Sources	pH optimum	pH stability	K_m (mM)	V_{max}	Substrate used[a]	Specificity and remarks[a]	Reference
β-Hexosaminidase	4.2 3.8	— —	0.8 0.54	19.0 3.0	pNPh-β-GlcNAc pNPh-β-GalNAc	Hydrolyze both pNPh-β-GlcNAc and GalNAc, particulate enzyme	6
β-Galactosaminidase	5.5	—	0.35	0.67	pNPh-β-GalNAc	Low activity with pNPh-β-GlcNAc; not inhibited by acetate	
β-Glucosaminidase	5.2	—	0.72	2.5	pNPh-β-GlcNAc	Low activity with pNPh-GalNAc; inhibited by acetate	
Brain, rat	5.1	—	0.083	nmol/mg/h 0.336	G_{M_2}	Inactivated by freezing and thawing; low activity with G_{M_2}	7
Diplococcus pneumoniae	5.3	—	0.22	µmol/mg/min 0.26	pNPh-β-GlcNAc	Hydrolyze α1-acid glycoprotein (minus NeuAc, Gal)	8
Epididymis, hog	4.3 4.1–4.2	—	2.2 3.7	— —	Ph-β-GlcNAc Globoside I	Hydrolyze both pNPh-β-Glc-NAc and pNPh-β-Gal-NAc; require detergent for hydrolysis of glycolipids, globoside, asialo G_{M2}	9
Epididymis, pig	4.2	3–7.5	1.8–2.1	—	pNPh-β-GlcNAc	Stabilized and activated by albumin	10
Epididymis, ram	5.1–5.6 4.5–4.9	— —	0.5 0.086	— —	MeUmb-β-GlcNAc MeUmb-β-GalNAc	Several enzymic components shown by isoelectric focusing	11
Jack bean	5.0–6.0 3.5–4.0	7–8 7–8	0.64 0.31	µmol/mg/min 137.2 70.9	pNPh-β-GlcNAc pNPh-β-GalNAc	Crystalline enzyme, MW about 100,000; hydrolyze ovalbumin, chitobiose, α1-acid glycoprotein (minus NeuAc, Gal) The same enzyme hydrolyzes pNPh-β-GlcNAc and pNPh-β-GalNAc	12

Table 2 (continued)

β-2-ACETYLAMINO-2-DEOXY-D-GLUCOSIDE ACETYLAMINODEOXYGLUCOHYDROLASE (3.2.1.30)

Sources	pH optimum	pH stability	K_m (mM)	V_{max}	Substrate used[a]	Specificity and remarks[a]	Reference
Kidney, rat	4.3	—	1.32 1.02 0.72 0.40	0.087 0.017 0.156 0.016	Ph-β-GlcNAc Ph-β-GalNAc pNPh-β-GlcNAc pNPh-β-GalNAc	No separation of β-GlcNAc and β-GalNAc activities was achieved	13
	4.5						14
Liver, beef	4.5 4.2	— —	1.02 15.40	mmol/mg/h 7.02 0.19	pNPh-β-GlcNAc GlcNAc-β-GlcUA-β-GlcNAc	Hydrolyze GlcNAc-β-GlcUA-β-GlcNAc derived from hyaluronic acid	15
Liver, human Hexosaminidase A	3.8–4.5	—	0.83 1.11 0.4	— — —	MeUmb-β-GlcNAc G_{A_2} Globoside	Require detergent for hydrolysis of glycolipids; the same enzyme hydrolyzes both pNPh-β-GlcNAc and pNPh-β-GalNAc; degree of hydrolysis was small on G_{M_2}	16
Hexosaminidase B	3.8–4.5	—	0.83 1.11 0.12	— — —	MeUmb-β-GlcNAc G_{A_2} Globoside		
Milk, bovine	4.2	—	1.0	μmol/mg/min —	pNPh-β-GlcNAc	No activation by albumin	17
Oviduct, hen	4.2 3.0	4.6–7.1	0.56	218.0	pNPh-β-GlcNAc	The enzyme hydrolyzes both pNPh-β-GlcNAc and pNPh-β-GalNAc; multiforms of enzyme was observed; hydrolyze Asn(GlcNAc)$_2$ but not G_{M2}	18
Phaseolus vulgaris	4.6–4.8	4.6–8	0.47	—	pNPh-β-GlcNAc	Hydrolyze pNPh-β-GlcNAc and pNPh-β GalNAc, also hydrolyze fetuin (minus NeuAc, Gal), glycopeptide from orosomucoid	19
Placenta, human Hexosaminidase A	4.4	—	1.1 0.4	mmol/mg/h 173.0 19.0	MeUmb-β-GlcNAc MeUmb-β-GalNAc	Require taurocholate for hydrolysis of glycolipids, both enzyme A and B hydrolyze G_{M2}	20
Hexosaminidase B	4.4	—	1.0 0.45	158.0 17.0	MeUmb-β-GlcNAc MeUmb-β-GalNAc		
Sclerotinia fructigena	5.4 4.4	4–11 —	2.0 2.0	μmol/mg/h 45.0 —	pNPh-β-GlcNAc pNPh-β-GalNAc	No noticeable chitin degradation; MW 141,000	21

Table 2 (continued)

β-2-ACETYLAMINO-2-DEOXY-D-GLUCOSIDE ACETYLAMINODEOXYGLUCOHYDROLASE (3.2.1.30)

Sources	pH optimum	pH stability	K_m (mM)	V_{max}	Substrate used[a]	Specificity and remarks[a]	Reference
Saliva, human parotid	4.5 3.8	10.0 10.0	1.02 2.27 0.30 1.56	μmol/μg/h 2.333 0.310 0.204 0.029	pNPh-β-GlcNAc Ph-β-GlcNAc pNPh-β-GalNAc Ph-β-GalNAc	Homogeneous enzyme; the same enzyme catalyzes both glucosaminidase and galactosaminidase activities, MW 155,000	22
Serum, pregnant Hexosaminidase A Hexosaminidase P	4.5 4.5	— —	0.65 0.55	— —	MeUmb-β-GlcNAc MeUmb-β-GlcNAc	Form P enzyme is more pH and heat stable; exist only in pregnant serum, not in amniotic fluid or cord serum	23
Spleen, beef Hexosaminidase A Hexosaminidase B	4.5 4.5	— —	0.87 0.15 0.85 0.08	— — — —	pNPh-β-GlcNAc pNPh-β-GalNAc pNPh-β-GlcNAc pNPh-β-GalNAc	MW of enzyme A, 136,900; enzyme B, 139,700; both enzymes are strongly inhibited by metal ions	24
Taka®-diastase	— 5.0 4.5	— — —	0.85 1.8 5.8	μmol/mg/min 0.037 0.026 0.012	pNPh-β-GlcNAc Ph-β-GlcNAc Ph-β-GalAc	MW about 140,000; glycoprotein in nature	25
Testis, ram	5.5–5.9 4.9–5.3	— —	0.26–1.43 0.097–0.11	— —	MeUmb-β-GlcNAc MeUmb-β-GalNAc	Multiforms of enzyme existed, MW all about 140,000	10 26
Thyroid, sheep	3.5–5.2	—	0.9	—	pNPh-β-GlcNAc	Hydrolyze the glycopeptide from thyroglobulin (minus NeuAc, Gal)	27
Turbo cornutus (marine gastropod)	4.0 4.0	— —	1.16 0.442	μmol/mg/min 0.683 0.178	Ph-β-GlcNAc Ph-β-GalNAc	Same enzyme hydrolyzes both Ph-β-GlcNAc and Ph-β-GalNAc; NaCl activates the enzyme; hydrolyze ovomucoid	28
Uterus, bovine	4.5	—	1.25	μmol/mg/min 7.7	pNPh-β-GlcNAc	Strongly inhibited by Ag⁺ and Hg²⁺, activated by albumin	29

Compiled by Su-Chen Li and Yu-Teh Li.

Table 2 (continued)

β-2-ACETYLAMINO-2-DEOXY-D-GLUCOSIDE ACETYLAMINODEOXYGLUCOHYDROLASE (3.2.1.30)

REFERENCES

1.   Hayase, Reisher, and Miller, *Prep. Biochem.*, 3, 221 (1973).
2.   Bahl and Agrawal, *J. Biol. Chem.*, 244, 2970 (1969).
3.   Mega, Ikenaka, and Matsushima, *J. Biochem.* (Tokyo), 71, 107 (1972).
4.   Berkeley, Brewer, Ortiz, and Gillespie, *Biochim. Biophys. Acta*, 309, 157 (1973).
5.   Frohwein and Gatt, *Biochemistry*, 6, 2783 (1967).
6.   Frohwein and Gatt, *Biochemistry*, 6, 2775 (1967).
7.   Tallman and Brady, *J. Biol. Chem.*, 247, 7570 (1972).
8.   Hughes and Jeanloz, *Biochemistry*, 3, 1543 (1964).
9.   Abe, Handa, and Yamakawa, *J. Biochem.* (Tokyo), 70, 1027 (1971).
10.   Findlay and Levvy, *Biochem. J.*, 77, 170 (1960).
11.   Winchester, *Biochem. J.*, 124, 929 (1971).
12.   Li and Li, *J. Biol. Chem.*, 245, 5153 (1970).
13.   Pugh, Leaback, and Walker, *Biochem. J.*, 65, 464 (1957).
14.   Walker, Woollen, and Heyworth, *Biochem. J.*, 79, 288 (1961).
15.   Weissmann, Hadjiioannou, and Tornheim, *J. Biol. Chem.*, 239, 59 (1964).
16.   Wenger, Okada, and O'Brien, *Arch. Biochem. Biophys.*, 153, 116 (1972).
17.   Mellors, *Can. J. Biochem.*, 46, 451 (1968).
18.   Tarentino and Maley, *Arch. Biochem. Biophys.*, 147, 446 (1971).
19.   Agrawal and Bahl, *J. Biol. Chem.*, 243, 103 (1968).
20.   Tallman, Brady, Quirk, Villalba, and Gal, *J. Biol. Chem.*, 249, 3489 (1974).
21.   Reyes and Byrde, *Biochem. J.*, 131, 381 (1973).
22.   Watanabe, Nakamura, Iwamoto, and Tsunemitsu, *J. Dent. Res.*, 52, 782 (1973).
23.   Stirling, *Biochim. Biophys. Acta*, 271, 154 (1972).
24.   Verpoorte, *J. Biol. Chem.*, 247, 4787 (1972).
25.   Mega, Ikenaka, and Matsushima, *J. Biochem.* (Tokyo), 68, 109 (1970).
26.   Bullock and Winchester, *Biochem. J.*, 133, 593 (1973).
27.   Chabaud, Bouchilloux, and Ferrand, *Biochim. Biophys. Acta*, 227, 154 (1971).
28.   Muramatsu, *J. Biochem.* (Tokyo), 64, 521 (1968).
29.   Coleman, Scroggs, and Whittington, *Biochim. Biophys. Acta*, 146, 290 (1967).

Table 3
β-D-GALCTOSIDE GALACTOHYDROLASE (3.2.1.23)

Sources	pH optimum	pH stability	K_m (mM)	V_{max}	Substrate used[a]	Specificity and remarks[a]	Reference
Aerobacter cloacae	6.6	—	0.22	—	oNPh-β-Gal	Induced enzyme; homogeneous enzyme; composed of tetramer	1
Aspergillus niger	3.2–4.0	2.8–3.9	1.0	μmol/mg/min 55.5	pNPh-β-Gal	Hydrolyze Me-β-Gal, lactose, asialo fetuin, gonadotropin and α_1-acid glycoprotein	2
Brain, rat	4.5	—	0.022	—	Galactosylceramide	Activated by taurocholate; inhibited by Gal lactone, sphingosine; hydrolyze galactocerebroside	3
Brain, calf rat	4.5 3.1	— —	— 0.4	μmol/mg/h 1.4 1.76	pNPh-β-Gal pNPh-β-Gal	Inhibited by Gal lactone and Gal; hydrolyze lactose	4
Brain, rabbit	3.6 4.25	— —	0.143 0.4	μmol/mg/h 66.6 83.3	MeUmb-β-Gal MeUmb-β-Gal	Inhibited by Gal 1,4-lactone; purified enzyme does not hydrolyze glycolipids	5
Brain, rat	4.2–4.5	—	0.011	—	Psychosine	Activated by oleic acid and taurocholate, inhibited by galactosyl ceramide	6
Corticium rolfsii IFO 6146	2.0–2.5	2.0–8.0	0.38	μmol/mg/min 6.9	pNPh-β-Gal	Relatively inactive towards lactose	7
Diplococcus pneumoniae type I	6.3–6.5	5.3–8.0	4.5 1.9 4.4	mol/mg/min 3.9 1.6 2.4	oNPh-β-Gal pNPh-β-Gal *N*-Acetyllactosamine	Inhibited by metal ions; hydrolyze asialo α_1-acid glycoprotein	8
Epididymis, rat	2.9 2.9; 3.5	3.0–6.5	0.38 1.6	—	oNPh-β-Gal Ph-β-Gal	Inhibited by metal ions, aldonolactone	9
Escherichia coli ML 308	7.0	—	—	mol/mol/sec 1.81×10^3	oNPh-β-Gal	Crystalline enzyme, MW 3.65×10^5; required no Mg^{2+} for activation	10

[a] Abbreviations: oNPh = o-nitrophenyl; pNPh = p-nitrophenyl; Ph = phenyl; Gal = D-galactopyranose; Glc = D-glucopyranose; MeUmb = 4-methylumbelliferyl; Me = methyl; ClHgBzO⁻ = p-chloromercuric benzoate.

Table 3 (continued)
β-D-GALCTOSIDE GALACTOHYDROLASE (3.2.1.23)

Sources	pH optimum	pH stability	K_m (mM)	V_{max}	Substrate used[a]	Specificity and remarks[a]	Reference
Escherichia coli K-12	7.2–7.3	6.0–8.0	0.18 0.093 0.73	nmol/ml/min 32.0 5.8 5.0	oNPh-β-Gal pNPh-β-Gal ph-β-Gal	Activated by Na⁺, to a lesser extent by K⁺	11
Helix pomatia β-Galactosidase-1	5.4	—	8.0 10.0 2.0 0.5	μmol/mg/min 10.0 10.0 10.0 6.0	oNPh-β-Gal Lactose Cellobiose pNPh-β-Gal	Homogeneous enzyme, glycoprotein in nature; evidences showed that the same enzyme has both β-galactosidase and β-glucosidase activities.	12
β-Galactosidase-2	5.2	—	2.0 6.0 2.0 0.3	11.0 4.5 24.0 13.0	oNPh-β-Gal Lactose Cellobiose pNPh-β-Gal		
Intestine, mucosa human	4.0–4.5	—	2.5–2.9	—	Ph-β-Gal	Multiform enzyme	13
Intestine, hog	5.0–6.0	—	0.33 0.9	— —	pNPh-β-Gal oNPh-β-Gal	Multiform enzymes; enzyme Ca-I-2 and Ca-II-2 have high activity for synthetic substrate, low activity for lactose; enzyme T-Ca-II and Ca-I-1 have high activity for lactose	14
Intestine, monkey (*Macaca mulatta*) particulate	4.5	—	2.5 3.0 9.0	μmol/mg/min 0.02 0.096 0.039	oNPh-β-Gal Ph-β-Gal Ph-β-Glc	Inhibited by Cu²⁺, Ag⁺, Glc and Gal lactone; these two enzymes are found besides lactase	15
soluble	7.0	—	4.0 3.0 3.0	0.63 0.06 0.5	oNPh-β-Gal Ph-β-Gal Ph-β-Glc		
Intestine, rabbit	6.0–6.5	—	2.2	—	oNPh-β-Gal	Multiform enzymes; hydrolyze both synthetic β-galactoside and β-glucoside; little activity toward lactose	16

Table 3 (continued)
β-D-GALCTOSIDE GALACTOHYDROLASE (3.2.1.23)

Sources	pH optimum	pH stability	K_m (mM)	V_{max}	Substrate used[a]	Specificity and remarks[a]	Reference
Intestine, rat and human lysosomal brush border	3.0 6.0	— —	— —	— —	oNPh-β-Gal oNPh-β-Gal	At least two β-galactosidases existed in intestinal mucosa; lysosomal enzyme is relatively heat stable and not inhibited by ClHgBzO⁻	17
Intestine, rat fraction I	3.0—4.0	—	10.2 0.21	— —	Lactose pNPh-β-Gal	The purified enzyme is unstable upon storage	19
fraction II	3.0—4.0	—	9.8 0.21	— —	Lactose pNPh-β-Gal		
fraction III	5.6—5.8	—	25.0 21.0	— —	Lactose pNPh-β-Gal		
Jack bean	3.5—4.5	—	—	—	pNPh-β-Gal	Hydrolyze asialo α₁-acid glycoprotein, glycopeptide from ovalbumin, other glycopeptides and glycolipids	20
Liver, human	3.5	—	0.2	—	pNPh-β-Gal	Stabilized by Cl⁻; inhibited by ClHgBzO⁻, Gal lactone	21
Neurospora crassa 74-OR 23-1A	4.2	—	4.5	—	oNPh-β-Gal	Not inhibited by ClHgBzO⁻; homogeneous in disc gel electrophoresis	22
Phaseolus vulgaris (pinto bean)	3.8	4.6—8	0.91	—	pNPh-β-Gal	Hydrolyze lactose, asialo fetuin and its glycopeptide	23
Saccharomyces fragilis KY5463	6.8	—	4.0 21.0	— —	oNPh-β-Gal Lactose	Crystalline and homogeneous enzyme; MW 2.03×10^5; activated by K⁺ but not Na⁺; inhibited by ClHgBzO⁻	24
				μmol/ml/15 min			
Saccharomyces fragilis Y-1109	6.3—6.5	6.0—7.0	24.0 2.5	11.6 9.9	Lactose oNPh-β-Gal	Stabilized by Mn²⁺, activated by K⁺	25
Saccharomyces lactis M-12	7.2	—	1.18	—	oNPh-β-Gal	Required Mg²⁺ for maximal activity	26

Table 3 (continued)
β-D-GALCTOSIDE GALACTOHYDROLASE (3.2.1.23)

Sources	pH optimum	pH stability	K_m (mM)	V_{max}	Substrate used[a]	Specificity and remarks[a]	Reference
Skin fibroblast, human	4.0–4.5	—	0.41 0.05	— —	MeUmb-β-Gal MeUmb-β Gal	Activated by NaCl; the enzyme has low and high affinity forms; inhibited by Gal lactone	27
Spinach, leaf	4.2	—	0.4	—	pNPh-β-Gal	Hydrolyze lactose, monogalactosyldiglyceride	28
Sporobolomyces singularis	3.9–4.0	—	5.0	μmol/mg/min 41.2	oNPh-β-Gal	Hydrolyze β-1,4 linkage in both lactose and cellobiose; homogeneous on electrophoresis	29
Testis, bovine	4.3	—	0.029 0.028 4.4 18.0	nmol/U/min 1.0 0.74 0.98 0.94	pNPh-β-Gal oNPh-β-Gal Lactosamine Lactose	Readily hydrolyze 1,3- and 1,4-linked lactosamine; slowly hydrolyze 1,6-linked isomer; also hydrolyze glycopeptides and glycolipids; activated by Glc	30
Testis, ram	3.5	—	0.67	—	oNPh-β-Gal pNPh-β-Gal		31
Thermus aquaticus	5.0	—	2.0	—	oNPh-β-Gal	This thermophilic enzyme has optimum temperature at 80°C; activated by Na⁺, Mn²⁺ and cysteine; MW about 5.7×10^5	32
Thyroid, sheep	3.5–5.2	—	0.14 0.15	— —	oNPh-β-Gal pNPh-β-Gal	Strongly inhibited by ClHgBzO⁻	33
Verticillium albo-atrum V3H	7.0	—	80.0 2.0	— —	Lactose oNPh-β-Gal	Stabilized by Mg²⁺, Mn²⁺, glucose and glycerol; inhibited by iodoacetate and ClHgBzO⁻	34

Compiled by Su-Chen Li and Yu-Teh Li.

Table 3 (continued)
β-D-GALCTOSIDE GALACTOHYDROLASE (3.2.1.23)

REFERENCES

1. Erickson and Steers, Jr., *Arch. Biochem. Biophys.*, 137, 399 (1970).
2. Bahl and Agrawal, *J. Biol. Chem.*, 244, 2970 (1969).
3. Radin, *Methods Enzymol.*, 28, 834 (1972).
4. Gatt and Rapport, *Biochim. Biophys. Acta*, 113, 567 (1966).
5. Jungalwala and Robins, *J. Biol Chem.*, 243, 4258 (1968).
6. Miyatake and Suzuki, *J. Biol. Chem.*, 247, 5398 (1972).
7. Kaji, Sato, Shinmyo, and Yasuda, *Agric. Biol. Chem.*, 36, 1729 (1972).
8. Hughes and Jeanloz, *Biochemistry*, 3, 1535 (1964).
9. Conchie and Hay, *Biochem. J.*, 73, 327 (1959).
10. Hu, Wolfe, and Reithel, *Arch. Biochem. Biophys.*, 81, 500 (1959).
11. Kuby and Lardy, *J. Am. Chem. Soc.*, 75, 890 (1952).
12. Got and Marnay, *Eur. J. Biochem.*, 4, 240 (1968).
13. Asp, *Biochem. J.*, 121, 299 (1971).
14. Sato and Yamashina, *J. Biochem.* (Tokyo), 70, 683 (1971).
15. Swaminathan and Radhakrishnan, *Arch. Biochem. Biophys.*, 135, 288 (1969).
16. Johnson, *Biochim. Biophys. Acta*, 302, 382 (1973).
17. Alpers, *J. Biol. Chem.*, 244, 1238 (1969).
18. Kraml, Kolinska, Ellederova, and Hirsova, *Biochim. Biophys. Acta*, 258, 520 (1972).
19. Asp and Dahlqvist, *Biochem. J.*, 110, 143 (1968).
20. Li and Li, *Methods Enzymol.*, 28, 702 (1972).
21. Meisler, *Methods Enzymol.*, 28, 820 (1972).
22. Johnson and DeBusk, *Arch. Biochem. Biophys.*, 138, 408 (1970).
23. Agrawal and Bahl, *J. Biol. Chem.*, 243, 103 (1968).
24. Uwajima, Yagi, and Terada, *Agric. Biol. Chem.*, 36, 570 (1972).
25. Wendorff and Amundson, *J. Milk Food Technol.*, 34, 300 (1971).
26. Biermann and Glantz, *Biochim. Biophys. Acta*, 167, 373 (1968).
27. Kanfer and Spielvogel, *Biochim. Biophys. Acta*, 289, 359 (1972).
28. Gatt and Baker, *Biochim. Biophys. Acta*, 206, 125 (1970).
29. Blakely and MacKenzie, *Can. J. Biochem.*, 47, 1021 (1969).
30. Distler and Jourdian, *J. Biol. Chem.*, 248, 6772 (1973).
31. Caygill, Roston, and Jevons, *Biochem. J.*, 98, 405 (1966).
32. Ulrich, McFeters, and Temple, *J. Bacteriol.*, 110, 691 (1972).
33. Chabaud, Bouchilloux, and Ferrand, *Biochim. Biophys. Acta*, 227, 154 (1971).
34. Keen, *Physiol. Plant.*, 23, 878(1970).

Table 4
α-D-GALACTOSIDE GALACTOHYDROLASE (3.2.1.22)

Sources	pH optimum	pH stability	K_m (mM)	V_{max}	Substrate used[a]	Specificity and remarks[a]	Reference
Aspergillus niger	3.8–4.2	3.8–5.8	0.35	μmol/mg/min 58.8	pNPh-α-Gal	Very active toward melibiose, raffinose, stachyose and oligosaccharide	1
Corticium rolfsii IFO 6146	2.5–4.5	4.0–7.0	0.16 / 0.26	μmol/mg/min 26.6 / 28.6	pNPh-α-Gal / oNPh-α-Gal	The enzyme is active at pH 1.1–2.0.	2
Fig	2–5.5	–	0.5	–	pNPh-α-Gal	Rapidly hydrolyze glycolipids as well as oligosaccharide	3
Intestine, monkey	4.2	–	4.1 / 2.5 / 12.0 / 14.0	μmol/mg/min 0.074 / 0.114 / 0.001 / 0.003	pNPh-α-Gal / Ph-α-Gal / Melibiose / Raffinose	Inhibited by metal ions; no inhibition by Gal was observed for hydrolyzing synthetic substrates	4
Intestine, rat	5.0	–	0.37	–	Gal₁-Glc-Cer	Activated by sodium taurocholate; specific to hydrolyze Gal₂-Glc-Cer; inhibited by glucosylsphingosine; not active toward synthetic substrate	5
Mortierella vinacea	4.0–6.0 / 3.5–5.0	7–10.6	0.36 / 0.43 / 0.39 / 1.83	mol/mg/min 299.9 / 143.5 / 33.9 / 19.2	oNPh-α-Gal / pNPh-α-Gal / Melibiose / Raffinose	Crystalline enzyme; glycoprotein in nature; no hydrolysis on glyco-peptide or glycoprotein	6
Phaseolus vulgaris (pinto bean)	6.5–6.7	4.6–8.0	0.657	–	pNPh-α-Gal	Rapidly hydrolyze oligosaccharide	7
Placenta, human Galactosidase A	4.5	–	3.4 / 40.6	–	MeUmb-α-Gal / Melibiose	Enzyme B does not hydrolyze melibiose; enzyme A is relatively heat labile	8
Galactosidase B	4.5	–	–	–	MeUmb-α-Gal		
Placenta, human	4.4; 4.8	4.0; 5.8	0.84 / 1.9	μmol/mg/h 13.4 / 80.0	Gal₂-Glc-Cer / MeUmb-α-Gal	Inhibited by ionic detergents	9

Abbreviations: pNPh = *p*-nitrophenyl; oNPh = *o*-nitrophenyl; Ph = phenyl; Gal = D-galactopyranose; Cer = ceramide.

Table 4 (continued)
α-D-GALACTOSIDE GALATOHYDROLASE (3.2.1.22)

Sources	pH optimum	pH stability	K_m (mM)	V_{max}	Substrate used[a]	Specificity and remarks[a]	Reference
Spinach leaf	5.3	—	0.3	—	pNPh-α-Gal	Hydrolyze melibiose at 1.5% of the rate of pNPh-α-Gal	10
Streptococcus bovis	5.6–6.3	—	—	—	pNPh-α-Gal	Hydrolyze α(1,6) linked Gal; not hydrolyze 4-O-α-Gal₂	11
Sweet almond	5.5–5.7	—	2.4 7.6	μmol/mg/min 2.0 35.0	pNPh-α-Gal Melibiose	MW about 33,000	12
Urine, human	4.6	—	6.7–9.3	—	pNPh-α-Gal	Hydrolyze Gal₂-Glc-Cer	13
Vicia faba							
Galactosidase I	6.3	—	0.38 4.0	μmol/mg/min 25.53 28.4	pNPh-α-Gal Raffinose	Enzyme I and II contain 25% and 2.8% carbohydrate, respectively. Enzyme I was inhibited by oligosaccharide with terminal nonreducing Gal	14
Galactosidase II	5.3 4.0	—	0.45	2.39	pNPh-α-Gal Raffinose		15
Vicia sativa	6.3	—	0.97 3.8 58.0	—	pNPh-α-Gal Ph-α-Gal Raffinose	Homogeneous enzyme; MW 30,000; does not hydrolyze galactomannans	16

Compiled by Su-Chen Li and Yu-Teh Li.

Table 4 (continued)
α-D-GALACTOSIDE GALATOHYDROLASE (3.2.1.22)

REFERENCES

1.   Bahl and Agrawal, *J. Biol. Chem.*, 244, 2970 (1969).
2.   Kaji and Yoshihara, *Agric. Biol. Chem.*, 36, 1335 (1972).
3.   Li and Li, *Methods Enzymol.*, 28, 714 (1972).
4.   Seetharam and Radhakrishnan, *Indian J. Biochem. Biophys.*, 9, 59 (1972).
5.   Brady, Gal, Bradley, and Martensson, *J. Biol. Chem.*, 242, 1021 (1967).
6.   Suzuki, Li, and Li, *J. Biol. Chem.*, 245, 781 (1970).
7.   Agrawal and Bahl, *J. Biol. Chem.*, 243, 103 (1968).
8.   Beutler and Kuhl, *J. Biol. Chem.*, 247, 7195 (1972).
9.   Johnson and Brady, *Methods Enzymol.*, 28, 849 (1972).
10.   Gatt and Baker, *Biochim. Biophys. Acta*, 206, 125 (1970).
11.   Bailey, *Biochem. J.*, 86, 509 (1963).
12.   Malhotra and Dey, *Biochem. J.*, 103, 508 (1967).
13.   Rietra, Tager, and Borst, *Biochim. Biophys. Acta*, 279, 436 (1972).
14.   Dey and Pridham, *Biochem. J.*, 113, 49 (1969).
15.   Dey and Pridham, *Biochem. J.*, 115, 47 (1969).
16.   Petek, Villarroya, and Courtois, *Eur. J. Biochem.*, 8, 395 (1969).

Table 5
MISCELLANEOUS GLYCOHYDROLASES

Sources	pH optimum	pH stability	K_m (mM)	V_{max} (μmol/mg/min)	Substrate used[a]	Specificity and remarks[a]	Reference
α-Acetylaminodeoxyglucosidase							
Liver, pig	4.7	5–6	0.30 0.08	— —	pNPh-α-GlcNAc oNPh-α-GlcNAc	The enzyme is very labile and insoluble at pH4; inhibited by GlcNAc and ManNAc but not GalNAc	1 2
Turbo cornutus (marine gastropod)	4.0	—	0.45	—	Ph-α-GlcNAc	Activated by NaCl; inhibited by ClHgBzO$^-$	3
α-Acetylaminodeoxygalactosidase							
Aspergillus niger	4.0–4.2	—	6.99	0.5	Ph-α-GalNAc	Specific for α-GalNAc bonds	4
Clostridium perfringens	5.8	—	3.3 0.4	—	Ph-α-GalNAc Ov. sub. mucin	Activated by Ni^{2+}, Co^{2+}, Mn^{2+}, Mg^{2+}, Ca^{2+}; inhibited by heavy metal ions	5
Liver, beef	4.7	6.0	25.0	—	Ph-α-GalNAc	Hydrolyze blood group A substance and Ov. sub. mucin; inhibited by GalNAc	6
Liver, human	4.3	—	3.5	—	pNPh-α-GalNAc	Relatively thermostable at 50°C; inhibited by GalNAc	7
β-D-Mannoside Mannohydrolase (3.2.1.25)							
Achatina fulica (snail)	4.5	—	6.5	—	Ph-β-Man	Hydrolyze the glycopeptide from Taka®-amylase and Man-(GlcNAc)$_2$-Asn	8, 9
Oviduct, hen	4.6	—	4.5 16.9	— —	pNPh-βMan Man-(GlcNAc)$_2$-Asn	Hydrolyze Man-(GlcNAc)$_2$-Asn; inhibited by Man (1,5)-lactone,MW 10^5	10

[a]Abbreviations: pNPh = p-nitrophenyl; Ph = phenyl; GlcNAc = 2-acetamido-2-deoxy-D-glucopyranose; Man = D-mannopyranose; Asn = L-asparagine; Me = methyl; Fu = L-fucopyranose; Gal = D-galactopyranose; ClHgBzO$^-$ = p-chloromercuric benzoate.

Table 5 (continued)
MISCELLANEOUS GLYCOHYDROLASES

Sources	pH optimum	pH stability	K_m (mM)	V_{max}	Substrate used[a]	Specificity and remarks[a]	Reference
β-D-Mannoside Mannohydrolase (3.2.1.25) (continued)							
Pineapple	3.4	3–6	—	—	pNPh-β-Man	Hydrolyze Man-(GlcNAc)₂-Asn	11
Synovial fluid human	4.0	—	3.4	—	pNPh-β-Man	Inhibited by Man (1,4)-lactone	12
Turbo cornutus (marine gastropod)	4.0	—	7.1	—	Ph-β-Man	Inhibited by iodoacetate, activated by NaCl	13
α-L-Fucoside Fucohydrolase				μmol/mg/h			
Aspergillus niger	1.3	—	8.3	16.0	Me-α-Fu-β-Gal	Specific to 1→2α linkage; no activity on pNPh-α-Fu or lacto-N-Fu₃, II and III from human milk	14, 15
Aspergillus oryzae	4.5–5.0	—	3.7	—	pNPh-α-Fu	Inhibited by ClHgBzO⁻, also hydrolyze pNPh-α-Gal	16
				μmol/mg/h			
Cerebral cortex, rat	4.3	—	1.33	3.33	pNPh-α-Fu	Inhibited by Hg²⁺	17
Clostridium perfringens	6.0	—	0.175	—	Hog H submaxillary glycoprotein	Specific to 1→2α linkage; no activity on Me-α-Fu or pNPh-α-Fu; lost activity in lyophilization	18, 19
Epididymis, rat	6.3	—	—	—	pNPh-α-Fu	Active toward the glycopeptide of bovine luteinizing hormone and horse immunoglobulin G; mol wt 216,000	20
Hallotis giganta (abalone)	5.0–5.6	3–5	—	—	pNPh-α-Fu	Hydrolyze pNPh-α-Fu, not on porcine submaxillary mucin	21
	2.0	—	—	—	pNPh-α-Fu	Hydrolyze both pNPh-α-Fu and porcine submaxillary mucin	

Table 5 (continued)
MISCELLANEOUS GLYCOHYDROLASES

Sources	pH optimum	pH stability	K_m (mM)	V_{max}	Substrate used[a]	Specificity and remarks[a]	Reference
					α-L-Fucoside Fucohydrolase (continued)		
Mammalian tissues	5.6	4.0–7.0	0.21	—	pNPh-α-Fu	Not inhibited by Gal 1,4-lactone or Fu 1,4-lactone	22
Trichomonas foetus	6.0–7.0	5.0–9.0	—	—	α-L-Fu-(1,2)-D-Gal, Lacto-N-Fu$_3$ II.	Stable at 55°C for 30 min	23

Compiled by Su-Chen Li and Yu-Teh Li.

REFERENCES

1. Weissman, Rowin, Marshall, and Friederici, *Biochemistry*, 6, 207 (1967).
2. Weissman, *Methods Enzymol.*, 28, 796 (1972).
3. Muramatsu, *J. Biochem.* (Tokyo), 64, 521 (1968).
4. McDonald and Bahl, *Methods Enzymol.*, 28, 734 (1972).
5. McGuire, Chipowsky, and Roseman, *Methods Enzymol.*, 28, 755 (1972).
6. Weissman, *Methods Enzymol.*, 28, 801 (1972).
7. Callahan, Lassila, Tandt, and Philippart, *Biochem. Med.*, 7, 424 (1973).
8. Sugahara, Okumura, and Yamashina, *Biochim Biophys. Acta*, 268, 488 (1972).
9. Sugahara and Yamashina, *Methods Enzymol.*, 28, 769 (1972).
10. Sukeno, Tarentino, Pulmmer, and Maley, *Methods Enzymol.*, 28, 777 (1972).
11. Li and Lee, *J. Biol Chem.*, 247, 3677 (1972).
12. Bartholomew and Perry, *Biochim. Biophys. Acta*, 315, 123 (1973).
13. Muramatsu and Egami, *J. Biochem.* (Tokyo), 62, 700 (1967).
14. Bahl, *J. Biol. Chem.*, 245, 299 (1970).
15. Bahl, *Methods Enzymol.*, 28, 738 (1972).
16. Iwashita and Egami, *J. Biochem.* (Tokyo), 73, 1217 (1973).
17. Bosmann and Hemsworth, *Biochim. Biophyx Acta*, 242, 152 (1971).
18. Aminoff and Furukawa, *J. Biol. Chem.*, 245, 1659 (1970).
19. Aminoff, *Methods Enzymol.*, 28, 763 (1972).
20. Carlsen and Pierce, *J. Biol. Chem.*, 247, 23 (1972).
21. Tanaka, Nakano, Noguchi, and Pigman, *Arch. Biochem. Biophys.*, 126, 624 (1968).
22. Levvy and McAllen, *Biochem. J.*, 80, 435 (1961).
23. Watkins, *Biochem. J.*, 71, 261 (1959).

ISOLATION AND ENZYMATIC SYNTHESIS OF SUGAR NUCLEOTIDES

Sugar	Nucleotide	Isolation	Enzymic synthesis
Triose			
Dihydroxyacetone	UDP	Bacteria[1]	—
Pentoses			
D-Xylose	UDP	Plants,[2] animals,[3] fungus[4]	UDP-D-xylose pyrophosphorylase; plants[5]; UDP-D-glucuronic acid decarboxylase; plants;[6-9] animal;[10] bacteria[11]
L-Arabinose	GDP, UDP	Plants[1,2]; Plants[2]	UDP-L-arabinose pyrophosphorylase; plants[5]; UDP-D-xylose 4-epimerase; plants[13,15]
?-Arabinose	GDP, ADP	Animals; Alga (*Chlorella*)[15]	—
D-Ribose	dTDP	Bacteria (*Streptomyces*)[16]	—
Hexose			
D-Glucose	UDP	Yeast,[17] other fungi,[18-20] bacteria,[21,22] plants,[3,19,21] algae,[23] animals[24-33]	UDP-D-glucose pyrophosphorylase; yeast,[34,35] bacteria,[21,36,37] plants,[5,38,41] animals[43-50]
	GDP	Fungi,[11,52] plants[12,53] animals,[14,54]	GDP-D-glucose pyrophosphorylase; animals,[54,55] plants[56]
	CDP	Bacteria,[57] fungus[58]	CDP-D-glucose pyrophosphorylase; bacteria,[59-61] plant[62]
	ADP	Plants;[53,63-67] algae;[63] bacteria;[57] animal?[68]	ADP-D-glucose pyrophosphorylase; plants,[69-73] bacteria[74-79]
	dTDP	Plant;[30] bacteria[31]	dTDP-D-glucose pyrophosphorylase; bacteria,[41,82-85] plants[83]
D-Galactose	UDP	Yeast,[64] other fungi,[18] bacteria,[87-89] plants,[2,34,26] animals[24-33]	UDP-D-glucose 4-epimerase; yeast;[90-98] bacteria,[99-105] plants;[5] animals[106,107]; Galactose-1-P uridyl transferase; yeast;[108] bacteria,[36,109,110] plants;[111] animals[112-114]; UDP-D-galactose pyrophosphorylase;[a] plants,[5] animals[115,116]

aModified and updated from Ginsburg, *Handbook of Biochemistry*, 2nd ed., Sober, Ed., CRC Press, Cleveland, 1970, D-82.

ISOLATION AND ENZYMATIC SYNTHESIS OF SUGAR NUCLEOTIDES (continued)

Sugar	Nucleotide	Isolation	Enzymic synthesis
D-Galactose (continued)	GDP	Plants,[12,53] animals,[14,23] algae[15]	—
	ADP	Plants,[117] algae[118]	AI,P-D-galactose pyrophosphorylase; plants[119]
	dTDP	Bacteria[91]	dTDP-D-galactose pyrophosphorylase; bacteria;[120,121] plants[122]; dTP-D glucose 4-epimerase; bacteria;[120,123] plants[122]
	dUDP	—	dUDP-D-galactose pyrophosphorylase; plants[122]
L-Galactose	GDP	Alga,[123] animals[124]	Isomerization of GDP-D-mannose[125]
D-Mannose	UDP	Animal[68]	—
	GDP	Yeast,[126,127] other fungi,[18,51] plants,[12,23] animals,[30,32,33,54,128] bacteria[21]	GDP-D-mannose pyrophosphorylase; yeast,[192] bacteria,[130-133] algae,[134] animals[54,135,136]
	ADP	Plants[17]	ADP-D-mannose pyrophosphorylase; plant[119]
			GDP-D-hexose pyrophosphorylase; animal[135]
D-Fructose	dTDP	Bacteria[137]	dTDP-D-glucose 2-epimerase; bacteria[16]
	UDP	Plants[138-140]	—
	GDP	Fungi[1,141]	—
	ADP	Plants[53]	—
D-Galactofuranose	UDP	—	Isomerization of UDP-D-galacto(pyrano)se; fungus[142,143]
Heptoses D-*glycero*-D-*manno*-heptose	GDP	Yeast[144]	GDP-D-*glycero*-D-*manno*-heptose pyrophosphorylase; yeast[130]
Uronic acids D-Glucuronic acid	UDP	Bacteria,[21,22,145,146] algae,[15,23] plant,[147] animals[24-28,148-150]	UDP-D-glucose dehydrogenase; bacteria,[151-153] plants,[154-156] animals[157-162]; UDP-D-glucuronic acid pyrophosphorylase; plants[163]
	dTDP	—	dTDP-D-glucose dehydrogenase; plants[164]

ISOLATION AND ENZYMATIC SYNTHESIS OF SUGAR NUCLEOTIDES (continued)

Sugar	Nucleotide	Isolation	Enzymic synthesis
D-Galacturonic acid	UDP	Bacteria,[145] plants[165]	UDP-D-glucuronic acid-4-epimerase; bacteria,[11,166] plants,[6] blue-green algae[167,168]
	dTDP	—	UDP-D-galacturonic acid pyrophosphorylase; plants[163]
			dTDP-D-galactose dehydrogenase; plants[164]
D-Mannuronic acid	GDP	Algae[169]	GDP-D-mannose dehydrogenase; bacteria[131,170]
L-Iduronic acid	dTDP UDP	Plants[80]	
L-Guluronic acid	GDP	Algae[169]	UDP-D-glucuronic acid 5-epimerase[171,172]
Branched sugars			
3-C-Hydroxymethyl-D-erythrofuranose (apiose)	UDP	Plants[173]	From UDP-D-glucuronic acid; plants[174-178]
5-Deoxy-3-formyl-L-lyxose (streptose)	dTDP	—	From dTDP-D-glucose; bacteria (*Streptomyces*)[179]
6-Deoxy-3-O-methyl-2-O-methyl-L-aldohexose (vinelose)	CDP	Bacteria[180]	From CDP-D-glucose[181]
4-O-(O-methylglycolyl)-vinelose	CDP	Bacteria[180]	—
Deoxy sugars			
6-Deoxy-L-galactose (L-fucose)	GDP	Bacteria;[182] animals[14,30,183]	Reduction of GDP-D-mannose; bacteria,[184-186] plants,[187] animals[188] GDP-L-fucose pyrophosphorylase; animals[189]
6-Deoxy-L-mannose	UDP	Bacteria;[57] alga;[190] plants[173,191]	Reduction of UDP-D-glucose; plants[192,193]
	dUDP		
	dTDP	Bacteria[137,194-196]	Reduction of dUDP-D-glucose; bacteria[192] Reduction of dTDP-D-glucose; bacteria[16,83,196-208]
6-Deoxy-D-mannose (D-rhamnose)	GDP	—	Reduction of GDP-D-mannose; plants,[209] bacteria[210,211]
6-Deoxy-D-talose	GDP		
2,6-Dideoxy-D-ribo-hexose (digitoxose)	UDP	Plants[213]	Reduction of GDP-D-mannose; bacteria[210-212]

ISOLATION AND ENZYMATIC SYNTHESIS OF SUGAR NUCLEOTIDES (continued)

Sugar	Nucleotide	Isolation	Enzymic synthesis
3,6-Dideoxy-L-xylo-hexose (colitose)	GDP	Bacteria[214]	Reduction of GDP-D-mannose; bacteria[215,216]
3,6-Dideoxy-D-arabino-hexose (tyvelose)	CDP	Bacteria[217]	Epimerization of CDP-paratose[218-222]
3,6-Dideoxy-D-xylo-hexose (abequose)	CDP	Bacteria[217]	Reduction of CDP-D-glucose[218,220,221,223,224]
3,6-Dideoxy-D-ribo-hexose (paratose)	CDP	Bacteria[225]	Reduction of CDP-D-glucose[218,220,221,223,224]
3,6-Dideoxy-L-manno-hexose	CDP	—	Reduction of CDP-D-glucose[220,221]
Polyols			
Glycerol	CDP	Bacteria[226,227]	CDP-(D-1)(=sn-3)-glycerol pyrophosphorylase; yeast, bacteria, plants[214]
Glycerophosphoryl-glycerol	CDP	Bacteria[229]	—
Ribitol	CDP	Bacteria[229-232]	CDP-(L-1)-ribitol pyrophosphorylase; yeast, bacteria, plants[228]
Ribitol-phosphate-ribitol	CDP	Bacteria[229]	—
D-Mannitol	ADP	Bacteria[233]	—
Amino sugars			
D-Glucosamine	UDP	—	UDP-D-glucosamine pyrophosphorylase; animals[234,235]
N-Acetyl-D-glucosamine	dTDP		dTDP-D-glucosamine pyrophosphorylase[236]
	UDP	Yeast,[237] other fungi,[18-20] bacteria,[21,22,233,238,239] plants,[138,147] animals[26-33,126,240-242]	UDP-N-acetyl-D-glucosamine pyrophosphorylase, yeast,[243] bacteria,[244] animals[42,244,245]
	ADP	Plants[117]	
	dTDP	—	Acetylation of dTDP-D-glucosamine; bacteria[236]
D-Galactosamine	UDP	—	dTDP-N-acetyl-D-glucosamine pyrophosphorylase; animals[246]
N-Acetyl-D-galactosamine	UDP	Bacteria,[236] plants,[134,147] animals[30,126,240,248]	UDP-D-glucosamine 4-epimerase: animals[233,147] UDP-N-acetyl-D-glucosamine 4-epimerase; bacteria,[236] animals[172,247]
	dTDP	—	dTDP-N-acetyl-D-glucosamine 4-epimerase: bacteria,[236]

ISOLATION AND ENZYMATIC SYNTHESIS OF SUGAR NUCLEOTIDES (continued)

Sugar	Nucleotide	Isolation	Enzymic synthesis
4-Acetylamino-4,6-dideoxy-D-galactose and -D-glucose	dTDP	Bacteria[81,249]	Reduction, amination, and acetylation of dTDP-D-glucose; bacteria[249-252]
3-Acetylamino-3,6-dideoxyhexose	dTDP	—	Reduction, amination, and acetylation of dTDP-D-glucose; bacteria[253]
2-Acetylamino-4-amino-2,4,6-trideoxyhexose	UDP	—	Reduction and amination of UDP-N-acetyl-D-glucosamine; bacteria[254]
Aminouronic acids			
N-Acetyl-D-glucosaminuronic acid	UDP	Bacteria[255,256]	UDP-N-acetyl-D-glucosamine dehydrogenase; bacteria[257]
N-Acetyl-D-mannosaminuronic acid	UDP	Bacteria[258]	—
Keto acids			
N-Acetylneuraminic acid	CMP	Bacteria[259]	CMP-N-acetylneuraminic acid pyrophosphorylase; bacteria,[260,261] animals,[260-264]
N-Glycolylneuraminic acid	CMP	—	CMP-N-glycolylneuraminic acid pyrophosphatase; animals[261]
2-Keto-3-deoxyoctonic acid	CMP	—	CMP-2-keto-3-deoxyoctonic acid pyrophosphorylase; bacteria[265,266]
Complex sugars			
Cellobiose	UDP	Plants[53]	—
Lactose and other oligosaccharides	GDP	Animals[14]	—
N-Acetyl-D-glucosamine (β1 → 4) D-galactose	UDP	Animals[3,267]	—
N-Acetyl-D-glucosamine (α1 → 4) L-fucose	UDP	Animals[268]	—

ISOLATION AND ENZYMATIC SYNTHESIS OF SUGAR NUCLEOTIDES (continued)

Sugar	Nucleotide	Isolation	Enzymic synthesis
N-Acetyl-D-glucosamine (β1 → 4) and (β1 → 6) D-galactose (2 → 6) N-acetyl and N-glycolyl neuraminic acid	UDP	Animals[269]	Transglycosylation by β-galactosidase, followed by sialyl transfer; animals[270]
N-Acetyl-D-glucosamine (β1 → 4) D-galactose (α1 → 2) L-fucose	UDP	Animals[267,271,272]	—
N-Acetyl-D-galactosamine (1 → 3) D-galactose (2 → 6) N-acetyl- and N-glycolyl-neuraminic acid	UDP	Animals[273]	—
D-Galactose-2(or 4)-sulfate	UDP	Animal[274]	Sulfation of UDP-D-galactose; animals[274]
N-Acetyl-D-galactosamine-4-sulfate	UDP	Animal[128,136]	Sulfation of UDP-N-acetyl-D galactosamine; animals[274]
N-Acetyl-D-galactosamine-4,6-disulfate	UDP	Animal[274]	Sulfation of UDP-N-acetyl-D-galactosamine 4-sulfate; animals[274]
N-Acetyl-D-galactosamine-4-sulfate-6-phosphate	UDP	Animal[274]	—
N-Acetyl-D-galactosamine-6-phosphate (α1 → P) D-galactose	UDP	Animals[128,275,276]	
N-Acetyl-D-galactosamine-6-phosphate (α1 → P) D-galactose-2 (or 4)-sulfate	UDP	Animal[274]	—

ISOLATION AND ENZYMATIC SYNTHESIS OF SUGAR NUCLEOTIDES (continued)

Sugar	Nucleotide	Isolation	Enzymic synthesis
N-Acetylmuramic acid	UDP	Bacteria[232,277,278]	Addition of phosphoenolpyruvate to UDP-N-acetyl-D-glucosamine, followed by reduction; bacteria[279-281]
N-Acetylmuramyl peptides	UDP	Bacteria[277,278,283-296]	Stepwise addition of amino acids[297-302]
N-Glycolylmuramyl peptides	UDP	Bacteria[306,307]	

Compiled by Hiroshi Nikaido.

453

ISOLATION AND ENZYMATIC SYNTHESIS OF SUGAR NUCLEOTIDES (continued)

REFERENCES

1. Smith, Galloway, and Mills, *Biochem. Biophys. Res. Commun.*, 5, 148 (1961).
2. Ginsburg, Stumpf, and Hassid, *J. Biol. Chem.*, 223, 977 (1956).
3. Kobata and Suzuoki, *Biochim. Biophys. Acta*, 107, 405 (1965).
4. Ankel, Farrell, and Feingold, *Biochim. Biophys. Acta*, 90, 397 (1964).
5. Neufeld, Ginsburg, Putman, Fanshier, and Hassid, *Arch. Biochem. Biophys.*, 69, 602 (1957).
6. Feingold, Neufeld, and Hassid, *J. Biol. Chem.*, 235, 910 (1960).
7. Ankel and Feingold, *Fed. Proc.*, 24, 478 (1965).
8. Ankel and Feingold, *Biochemistry*, 4, 2468 (1965).
9. Wellman, Baron, and Grisebach, *Biochim. Biophys. Acta*, 244, 1 (1971).
10. Bdolah and Feingold, *Biochem. Biophys. Res. Commun.*, 21, 543 (1965).
11. Fan and Feingold, *Arch. Biochem. Biophys.*, 148, 576 (1972).
12. Selvendran and Isherwood, *Biochem. J.*, 105, 723 (1967).
13. Aspinall, Cottrell, and Matheson, *Can. J. Biochem.*, 50, 574 (1972).
14. Denamur, Fauconneau, and Guntz, *Ann. Biol. Anim. Biochem. Biophys.*, 1, 74 (1961).
15. Sanwal and Preiss, *Phytochemistry*, 8, 707 (1969).
16. Baddiley, Blumson, Girolamo, and Girolamo, *Biochim. Biophys. Acta*, 50, 391 (1961).
17. Caputto, Leloir, Cardini, and Leloir, *J. Biol. Chem.*, 184, 333 (1950).
18. Ballio, Casinovi, and Serlupi-Crescenzi, *Biochim. Biophys. Acta*, 20, 414 (1956).
19. Bergkvist, *Acta Chem. Scand.*, 10, 1303 (1956); 11, 1457 (1957); 12, 1549, (1958).
20. Smith and Wheat, *Arch. Biochem. Biophys.*, 86, 267 (1960).
21. Smith, Mills, and Harper, *J. Gen. Microbiol.*, 16, 426 (1957).
22. Cifonelli and Dorfman, *J. Biol. Chem.*, 228, 547 (1957).
23. Su and Hassid, *Biochemistry*, 1, 474 (1962).
24. Carey and Wyatt, *Biochim. Biophys. Acta*, 41, 178 (1960).
25. Rutter and Hansen, *J. Biol. Chem.*, 202, 323 (1953).
26. Smith and Mills, *Biochim. Biophys. Acta*, 13, 386, 587 (1954).
27. Hurlbert and Potter, *J. Biol. Chem.*, 209, 1 (1954).
28. Hansen, Freeland, and Scott, *J. Biol. Chem.*, 219, 391 (1956).
29. Manson, *Biochim. Biophys. Acta*, 19, 398 (1956).
30. Denamur, Fauconneau, and Guntz, *C.R. Seances Soc. Biol.* (Paris), 246, 492, 652 (1958); 248, 2531 (1959); *Rev. Fsp. Fisiol.*, 15, 301 (1959).
31. Mandel and Klethi, *Biochim. Biophys. Acta*, 28, 199 (1958); Klethi and Mandel, *Biochim. Biophys. Acta*, 51, 379 (1962).
32. Kempf and Mandel, *C.R. Seances Soc. Biol.*, (Paris), 253, 2155 (1961).
33. Mills and Jones, *Tex. Rep. Biol. Med.*, 21, 57 (1963).
34. Munch-Petersen, Kalckar, Cutolo, and Smith, *Nature* (Lond.), 172, 1037 (1953).
35. Munch-Petersen, *Acta Chem. Scand.*, 9, 1523 (1955).
36. Kurahashi, *Science*, 125, 115 (1957).
37. Nakae and Nikaido, *J. Biol. Chem.*, 246, 4386 (1971); Nakae, *J. Biol. Chem.*, 246, 4404 (1971).
38. Burma and Mortimer, *Arch. Biochem. Biophys.*, 62, 16 (1956).
39. Ginsburg, *J. Biol. Chem.*, 232, 55 (1958).
40. Turner and Turner, *Biochem. J.*, 69, 448 (1958).
41. Ganguli, *J. Biol. Chem.*, 232, 337 (1958).
42. Smith, Munch-Petersen, and Mills, *Nature* (Lond.), 172, 1038 (1953).
43. Smith and Mills, *Biochim. Biophys. Acta*, 18, 152 (1955).
44. Villar-Palasi and Larner, *Arch. Biochem. Biophys.*, 86, 61 (1960).
45. Oliver, *Biochim. Biophys. Acta*, 52, 75 (1961).
46. Kornfeld and Brown, *J. Biol. Chem.*, 238, 1604 (1963).
47. Albrecht, Bass, Seifert, and Hansen, *J. Biol. Chem.*, 241, 2968 (1966).
48. Tsuboi, Fukunaga, and Petricciani, *J. Biol. Chem.*, 244, 1008 (1969).
49. Knop and Hansen, *J. Biol. Chem.*, 245, 2499 (1970).
50. Hopper and Dickinson, *Biochim. Biophys. Acta*, 309, 307 (1973).
51. Pontis and Baddiley, *Biochem. J.*, 75, 428 (1960).
52. Kawaguchi, Tanida, Matsuda, Tani, and Ogata, *Agric. Biol. Chem.*, 37, 75 (1973).
53. Cumming, *Biochem. J.*, 116, 189 (1970).
54. Carlson and Hansen, *J. Biol. Chem.*, 237, 1260 (1962).
55. Danishefsky and Heritier-Watkins, *Biochim. Biophys. Acta*, 139, 349 (1967).

ISOLATION AND ENZYMATIC SYNTHESIS OF SUGAR NUCLEOTIDES (continued)

56. Péaud-Lenoël and Axelos, *Eur. J. Biochem.*, 4, 561 (1968).
57. Ginsburg, *J. Biol. Chem.*, 241, 3750 (1966).
58. Elnaghy and Nordin, *Arch. Biochem. Biophys.*, 110, 593 (1965).
59. Ginsburg, O'Brien, and Hall, *Biochem. Biophys. Res. Commun.*, 7, 1 (1962).
60. Kimata and Suzuki, *J. Biol. Chem.*, 241, 1099 (1966).
61. Mayer and Ginsburg, *J. Biol. Chem.*, 240, 1900 (1965).
62. Vidla and Loerch, *Biochim. Biophys. Acta*, 159, 551 (1968).
63. Kauss and Kandler, *Z. Naturforsch.*, 17B, 858 (1962).
64. Recondo, Dankert, and Leloir, *Biochem. Biophys. Res. Commun.*, 12, 204 (1963).
65. Murata, Mikaminawa, and Akazawa, *Biochem. Biophys. Res. Commun.*, 13, 439 (1963).
66. Jenner, *Plant Physiol.*, 43, 41 (1968).
67. Cassells and Harmez, *Arch. Biochem. Biophys.*, 126, 485 (1968).
68. Cantore, Leoni, Leveroni, and Recondo, *Biochim. Biophys. Acta*, 230, 423 (1971).
69. Espada, *J. Biol. Chem.*, 237, 3577 (1962).
70. Ghosh and Preiss, *J. Biol. Chem.*, 241, 4491 (1966).
71. Sanwal, Greenberg, Hardie, Camerson, and Preiss, *Plant Physiol.*, 43, 417 (1968).
72. Huber, de Fekete, and Ziegler, *Plants* (Berlin), 87, 360 (1969).
73. Dickinson and Preiss, *Arch. Biochem. Biophys.*, 130, 119 (1969).
74. Shen and Preiss, *J. Biol. Chem.*, 240, 2334 (1965).
75. Shen and Preiss, *Arch. Biochem. Biophys.*, 116, 375 (1966).
76. Preiss, Shen, Greenberg, and Gentner, *Biochemistry*, 5, 1833 (1966).
77. Ribereau-Gayon, Sabraw, Lammel, and Preiss, *Arch. Biochem. Biophys.*, 142, 675 (1971).
78. Lapp and Elbein, *J. Bacteriol.*, 112, 327 (1972).
79. Paule and Preiss, *J. Biol. Chem.*, 246, 4602 (1971).
80. Katan and Avigad, *Isr. J. Chem.*, 3, 110 (1966).
81. Matsuhashi and Strominger, *J. Bacteriol.*, 93, 2017 (1967).
82. Kornfeld and Glaser, *J. Biol. Chem.*, 236, 1791 (1961).
83. Pazur and Shuey, *J. Biol. Chem.*, 236, 1791 (1961).
84. Bernstein and Robbins, *J. Biol. Chem.*, 240, 391 (1965).
85. Melo and Glaser, *J. Biol. Chem.*, 240, 398 (1965).
86. Mills, Smith, and Lochhead, *Biochim. Biophys. Acta*, 25, 521 (1957).
87. Nikaido, *Biochim. Biophys. Acta*, 48, 460 (1961).
88. Wiesmeyer and Jordan, *Anal. Biochem.*, 2, 281 (1961).
89. Morikawa, Imae, and Nikaido, *J. Biochem.* (Tokyo), 56, 145 (1964).
90. Maxwell, Robichon-Szulmajster, and Kalckar, *Arch. Biochem. Biophys.*, 78, 407 (1958).
91. Maxwell and Robichon-Szulmajster, *J. Biol. Chem.*, 235, 308 (1960).
92. Leloir, *Arch. Biochem.*, 33, 186 (1951).
93. Bertland, Bugge, and Kalcker, *Arch. Biochem. Biophys.*, 116, 280 (1966).
94. Creveling, Darrow, Kalckar, Randerath, Randerath, and Rodstrom, *Science*, 146, 424 (1964).
95. Creveling, Bhaduri, Christensen, and Kalckar, *Biochem. Biophys. Res. Commun.*, 21, 624 (1965).
96. Bhaduri, Christensen, and Kalckar, *Biochem. Biophys. Res. Commun.*, 21, 631 (1965).
97. Darrow and Rodstrom, *Biochemistry*, 7, 1645 (1968).
98. Salo, Nordin, Peterson, Bevill, and Kirkwood, *Biochim. Biophys. Acta*, 151, 484 (1968).
99. Hansen and Craine, *J. Biol. Chem.*, 208, 293 (1954).
100. Wilson and Hogness, *J. Biol. Chem.*, 239, 2469 (1964); 244, 2132 (1969).
101. Nelsestuen and Kirkwood, *J. Biol. Chem.*, 246, 7533 (1971).
102. Davis and Glaser, *Biochem. Biophys. Res. Commun.*, 43, 1429 (1971).
103. Maitra and Ankel, *Proc. Natl. Acad. Sci. USA*, 68, 2660 (1971).
104. Wee and Frey, *J. Biol. Chem.*, 248, 33 (1973).
105. Adair, Gabriel, Ullrey, and Kalckar, *J. Biol. Chem.*, 248, 4635 (1973).
106. Maxwell, *J. Biol. Chem.*, 229, 139 (1957); in *The Enzymes*, Vol 6, Boyer, Landy, and Myrbäck, Eds., Academic Press, New York, 1962, 443.
107. Langer and Glaser, *J. Biol. Chem.*, 249, 426 (1974).
108. Kalckar, Braganca, and Munch-Petersen, *Nature* (Lond.), 172, 1038 (1953).
109. Kurahashi and Sugimura, *J. Biol. Chem.*, 235, 940 (1960).
110. Wong and Frey, *J. Biol. Chem.*, 249, 2322 (1974).
111. Pazur and Shadaksharaswamy, *Biochem. Biophys. Res. Commun.*, 5, 130 (1961).
112. Maxwell, Kalckar, and Burton, *Biochim. Biophys. Acta*, 18, 444 (1955).
113. Kurahashi and Anderson, *Biochim. Biophys. Acta*, 29, 498 (1958).

ISOLATION AND ENZYMATIC SYNTHESIS OF SUGAR NUCLEOTIDES (continued)

114. Bertoli and Segal, *J. Biol. Chem.*, 241, 4023 (1966).
115. Isselbacher, *Science*, 126, 652 (1957).
116. Abraham and Howell, *J. Biol. Chem.*, 244, 545 (1969).
117. Dankert, Passeron, Recondo, and Leloir, *Biochem. Biophys. Res. Commun.*, 14, 358 (1964).
118. Pakhomova, Zaitzeva, and Albitzkaya, *Biokhimiya*, 30, 1204 (1965).
119. Passeron, Recondo, and Dankert, *Biochim. Biophys. Acta*, 89, 372 (1964).
120. Pazur, Kleppe, and Cepure, *Biochem. Biophys. Res. Commun.*, 7, 157 (1962).
121. Pazur and Anderson, *J. Biol. Chem.*, 238, 3155 (1963).
122. Neufeld, *Biochem. Biophys. Res. Commun.*, 7, 461 (1962).
123. Tinelli, Michelson, and Strominger, *J. Bacteriol.*, 86, 246 (1963).
124. Goudsmit and Neufeld, *Biochim. Biophys. Acta*, 19, 417 (1965).
125. Goudsmit and Neufeld, *Biochem. Biophys. Res. Commun.*, 26, 730 (1967).
126. Cabib and Leloir, *J. Biol. Chem.*, 206, 779 (1954).
127. Kawaguchi, Tanida, Mugibayashi, Tani, and Ogata, *J. Ferment. Technol.*, 59, 195 (1971).
128. Strominger, *Biochim. Biophys. Acta*, 17, 283 (1955); *J. Biol. Chem.*, 237, 1388 (1962).
129. Munch-Petersen, *Acta Chem. Scand.*, 10, 298 (1956); *Methods Enzymol.*, 5, 171 (1962).
130. O'Brien and Ginsburg, *Fed. Proc.*, 21, 155 (1962).
131. Preiss, *Biochem. Biophys. Res. Commun.*, 9, 235 (1962).
132. Preiss and Wood, *J. Biol. Chem.*, 239, 3119 (1964).
133. Lieberman and Markovitz, *J. Bacteriol.*, 101, 965 (1970).
134. Zetsche, *Planta*, 64, 129 (1965).
135. Verachtert, Rodriguez, Bass, and Hansen, *J. Biol. Chem.*, 241, 2007 (1966).
136. Donovan, Davis, and Park, *Arch. Biochem. Biophys.*, 122, 17 (1967).
137. Baddiley and Blumson, *Biochim. Biophys. Acta*, 39, 376 (1960).
138. Gonzalez and Pontis, *Biochim. Biophys. Acta*, 69, 179 (1963).
139. Unemura, Nakamura, and Funahashi, *Arch. Biochem. Biophys.*, 199, 240 (1967).
140. Brown and Mangat, *Biochim. Biophys. Acta*, 148, 350 (1967).
141. Saviova and Miettinen, *Acta Chem. Scand.*, 20, 2444 (1966).
142. Trejo, Chittendin, Buchanan, and Baddiley, *Biochem. J.*, 117, 637 (1970).
143. Garcia, *Eur. J. Biochem.*, 43, 93 (1974).
144. Ginsburg, O'Brien, and Hall, *J. Biol. Chem.*, 237, 497 (1962).
145. Smith, Mills, and Harper, *Biochim. Biophys. Acta*, 23, 662 (1957).
146. Lieberman, Shaparis, and Markovitz, *J. Bacteriol.*, 101, 959 (1970).
147. Solms and Hassid, *J. Biol. Chem.*, 228, 357 (1957).
148. Dutton, *Biochem. J.*, 71, 141 (1959).
149. Simonart, Salo, and Kirkwood, *Biochem. Biophys. Res. Commun.*, 24, 113 (1966).
150. Fan and Troen, *Metab. Clin. Exp.*, 23, 125 (1974).
151. Smith, Mills, Bernheimer, and Austrian, *J. Gen. Microbiol.*, 20, 654 (1959).
152. Markovitz, Cifonelli, and Dorfman, *J. Biol. Chem.*, 234, 2343 (1959).
153. Bdolah and Feingold, *J. Bacteriol.*, 96, 1144 (1968).
154. Strominger and Mapson, *Biochem. J.*, 66, 567 (1957).
155. Davis and Dickinson, *Arch. Biochem. Biophys.*, 152, 53 (1972).
156. Ruberg, *Planta*, 103, 188 (1972).
157. Strominger, Maxwell, Axelrod, and Kalckar, *J. Biol. Chem.*, 224, 79 (1957).
158. Jacobson and Davidson, *J. Biol. Chem.*, 237, 635 (1962).
159. Neufeld and Hall, *Biochem. Biophys. Res. Commun.*, 19, 456 (1965).
160. Zalitis and Feingold, *Arch. Biochem. Biophys.*, 132, 457 (1969); Zalitis, Uram, Bowser, and Feingold, *Methods Enzymol.*, 28, 430 (1972).
161. Balduini, Brovelli, DeLuca, Galligani, and Castellani, *Biochem. J.*, 133, 243 (1973).
162. Schiller, Bowser, and Feingold, *Carbohydr. Res.*, 21, 249 (1972).
163. Feingold, Neufeld, and Hassid, *Arch. Biochem. Biophys.*, 78, 401 (1958).
164. Katan and Avigad, *Biochem. Biophys. Res. Commun.*, 24, 18 (1966).
165. Neufeld and Feingold, *Biochim. Biophys. Acta*, 53, 589 (1961).
166. Smith, Mills, Bernheimer, and Austrian, *Biochim. Biophys. Acta*, 29, 640 (1958).
167. Ankel and Tischer, *Biochim. Biophys. Acta*, 178, 415 (1969); Gaunt, Ankel, and Schutzbach, *Methods Enzymol.*, 28, 426 (1972).
168. Gaunt, Maitra, and Ankel, *J. Biol. Chem.*, 249, 2366 (1974).
169. Lin and Hassid, *J. Biol. Chem.*, 241, 3283 (1966).
170. Preiss, *J. Biol. Chem.*, 239, 3127 (1964).

ISOLATION AND ENZYMATIC SYNTHESIS OF SUGAR NUCLEOTIDES (continued)

171. Jacobson and Davidson, *J. Biol. Chem.*, 237, 638 (1962).
172. Jacobson and Davidson, *Biochim. Biophys. Acta*, 73, 145 (1963).
173. Sandermann, Jr. and Grisebach, *Eur. J. Biochem.*, 6, 404 (1968).
174. Sandermann, Jr., Tisue, and Grisebach, *Biochim. Biophys. Acta*, 165, 550 (1968).
175. Gustine and Kindel, *J. Biol. Chem.*, 244, 1382 (1969).
176. Wellmann and Grisebach, *Biochim. Biophys. Acta*, 235, 389 (1971).
177. Kindel and Watson, *Biochem. J.*, 133, 227 (1973).
178. Grisebach, Baron, Sandermann, and Wellmann, *Methods Enzymol.*, 28, 439 (1972).
179. Ortmann, Matern, Grisebach, Stadler, Sinnwell, and Paulsen, *Eur. J. Biochem.*, 43, 265 (1974).
180. Okuda, Suzuki, and Suzuki, *J. Biol. Chem.*, 242, 958 (1967); 243, 6353 (1969).
181. Eguchi, Takagi, Uda, Kimata, Okuda, Suzuki, and Suzuki, *J. Biol. Chem.*, 248, 3341 (1973).
182. Ginsburg and Kirkman, *J. Am. Chem. Soc.*, 80, 3481 (1958).
183. Denamur, Fauconneau, and Guntz, *C.R. Seances Soc. Biol.* (Paris), 246, 2820 (1958).
184. Ginsburg, *J. Biol. Chem.*, 235, 2196 (1960); 236, 2389 (1961).
185. Kornfeld and Ginsburg, *Biochim. Biophys. Acta*, 117, 79 (1966).
186. Markovitz, *Proc. Natl. Acad. Sci. USA*, 51, 239 (1964).
187. Liao and Barber, *Biochim. Biophys. Acta*, 230, 64 (1971).
188. Foster and Ginsburg, *Biochim. Biophys. Acta*, 54, 376 (1961).
189. Ishiwara and Heath, *J. Biol. Chem.*, 243, 1110 (1968); *Methods Enzymol.*, 28, 403 (1972).
190. Kauss, *Biochem. Biophys. Res. Commun.*, 18, 170 (1965).
191. Kampe and Gonzalez, *Biochim. Biophys. Acta*, 148, 566 (1967).
192. Barber, *Biochem. Biophys. Res. Commun.*, 8, 204 (1962).
193. Barber and Chang, *Arch. Biochem. Biophys.* 118, 659 (1967).
194. Smith, Galloway, and Mills, *Biochim. Biophys. Acta*, 3, 276 (1959).
195. Okazaki, *Biochim. Biophys. Acta*, 4, 478 (1960).
196. Okazaki, Okazaki, Strominger, and Michelson, *J. Biol. Chem.*, 237, 3014 (1962).
197. Glaser and Kornfeld, *J. Biol. Chem.*, 236, 1795 (1961).
198. Gabriel and Ashwell, *J. Biol. Chem.*, 240, 4128 (1965).
199. Gabriel, *J. Biol. Chem.*, 241, 924 (1966).
200. Gabriel and Lindquist, *J. Biol. Chem.*, 243, 1479 (1968).
201. Melo, Elliot, and Glaser, *J. Biol. Chem.*, 243, 1467 (1968).
202. Melo and Glaser, *J. Biol. Chem.*, 243, 1475 (1968).
203. Herrmann and Lehmann, *Eur. J. Biochem.*, 3, 369 (1968).
204. Zarkowsky and Glaser, *J. Biol. Chem.*, 244, 4750 (1969).
205. Wang and Gabriel, *J. Biol. Chem.*, 244, 3420 (1969); *J. Biol. Chem.*, 245, 8 (1970).
206. Zarkowsky, Lipkin, and Glaser, *Biochem. Biophys. Res. Commun.*, 38, 787 (1970); *J. Biol. Chem.*, 245, 6599 (1970).
207. Lehmann and Pfeiffer, *FEBS Lett.*, 7, 314 (1970).
208. Glaser, Zarkowsky, and Ward, *Methods Enzymol.*, 28, 446 (1972).
209. Barber, *Biochim. Biophys. Acta*, 165, 68 (1968).
210. Markovitz, *Biochem. Biophys. Res. Commun.*, 6, 250 (1961); *J. Biol. Chem.*, 239, 2091 (1964).
211. Winkler and Markovitz, *J. Biol. Chem.*, 246, 5868 (1971).
212. Gabriel, *Methods Enzymol.*, 28, 454 (1972); Gangler and Gabriel, *J. Biol. Chem.*, 248, 6041 (1973).
213. Franz and Meyer, *Biochim. Biophys. Acta*, 184, 658 (1969).
214. Heath, *Biochim. Biophys. Acta*, 39, 377 (1960).
215. Elbein and Heath, *J. Biol. Chem.*, 240, 1926 (1965).
216. Heath and Elbein, *Proc. Natl. Acad. Sci. USA*, 48, 1209 (1962).
217. Nikaido and Jokura, *Biochem. Biophys. Res. Commun.*, 6, 304 (1961).
218. Nikaido and Nikaido, *J. Biol. Chem.*, 241, 1376 (1966).
219. Matsuhashi, *J. Biol. Chem.*, 241, 4275 (1966).
220. Matsuhashi, Matsuhashi, and Strominger, *J. Biol. Chem.*, 241, 4267 (1966).
221. Matsuhashi, Matsuhashi, Brown, and Strominger, *J. Biol. Chem.*, 241, 4283 (1966).
222. Elbein, *Proc. Natl. Acad. Sci. USA*, 53, 803 (1965).
223. Pape and Strominger, *J. Biol. Chem.*, 244, 3598 (1969).
224. Gonzalez-Porqué and Strominger, *Proc. Natl. Acad. Sci. USA*, 69, 1625 (1972); *J. Biol. Chem.*, 247, 6748 (1972); *Methods Enzymol.*, 28, 461 (1972).
225. Mayer and Ginsburg, *Biochem. Biophys. Res. Commun.*, 15, 334 (1964).
226. Baddiley, Buchanan, Mathias, and Sanderson, *J. Chem. Soc.* (England), 4186 (1956).
227. Clarke, Glover, and Mathias, *J. Gen. Microbiol.*, 20, 156 (1959).

228. Shaw, *Biochem. J.*, 82, 297 (1962).
229. Ito and Sato, *Seikagaku*, 34, 403 (1962).
230. Baddiley, Buchanan, Carss, and Mathias, *J. Chem. Soc.* (England), 4583 (1956).
231. Baddiley, Buchanan, and Carss, *J. Chem. Soc.* (England), 1869 (1956).
232. Strominger, *J. Biol. Chem.*, 234, 1520 (1959).
233. Scher and Ginsburg, *J. Biol. Chem.*, 243, 2385 (1968).
234. Maley, Maley, and Lardy, *J. Am. Chem. Soc.*, 78, 5303 (1956).
235. Silbert and Brown, *Biochim. Biophys. Acta*, 54, 590 (1961).
236. Kornfeld and Glaser, *J. Biol. Chem.*, 237, 3052 (1962).
237. Cabib, Leloir, and Cardini, *J. Biol. Chem.*, 203, 1055 (1953).
238. Glaser, *Biochim. Biophys. Acta*, 31, 575 (1959).
239. Akamatsu, *J. Biochem.* (Tokyo), 59, 613 (1966).
240. Pontis, *J. Biol. Chem.*, 216, 195 (1955).
241. Lunt and Kent, *Biochem. J.*, 78, 128 (1961).
242. Wylie and Smith, *Can. J. Biochem.*, 42, 1347 (1964).
243. Glaser and Brown, *Proc. Natl. Acad. Sci. USA*, 41, 253 (1955).
244. Strominger and Smith, *J. Biol. Chem.*, 234, 1822 (1959).
245. Maley and Lardy, *Science*, 124, 1297 (1956).
246. Kornfeld, Kornfeld, and Ginsburg, *Biochem. Biophys. Res. Commun.*, 17, 578 (1964).
247. Maley and Maley, *Biochim. Biophys. Acta*, 31, 577 (1959).
248. Strominger and Smith, *J. Biol. Chem.*, 234, 1828 (1959).
249. Matsuhashi and Strominger, *J. Biol. Chem.*, 239, 2454 (1964).
250. Gilbert, Matsuhashi, and Strominger, *J. Biol. Chem.*, 240, 1305 (1965).
251. Matsuhashi and Strominger, *J. Biol. Chem.*, 241, 4738 (1966).
252. Ohashi, Matsuhashi, and Matsuhashi, *J. Biol. Chem.*, 246, 2325 (1971).
253. Volk and Ashwell, *Biochem. Biophys. Res. Commun.*, 12, 116 (1963).
254. Distler, Kaufman, and Roseman, *Arch. Biochem. Biophys.*, 116, 466 (1966).
255. Smith, *Biochim. Biophys. Acta*, 158, 470 (1968).
256. Bieley and Jeanloz, *J. Biol. Chem.*, 244, 4929 (1969).
257. Fan, John, Zalitis, and Feingold, *Arch. Biochem. Biophys.*, 135, 49 (1969).
258. Rosenthal and Sharon, *Biochim. Biophys. Acta*, 83, 378 (1964).
259. Comb, Shimizu, and Roseman, *J. Am. Chem. Soc.*, 81, 5513 (1959).
260. Warren and Blacklow, *J. Biol. Chem.*, 237, 3527 (1962).
261. Roseman, *Proc. Natl. Acad. Sci. USA*, 48, 437 (1962).
262. Kean and Roseman, *Methods Enzymol.*, 8, 208 (1966).
263. Kean, *J. Biol. Chem.*, 245, 2301 (1970).
264. Kean, *Methods Enzymol.*, 28, 413 (1972).
265. Ghalambor and Heath *Biochem. Biophys. Res. Commun.*, 10, 346 (1963).
266. Ghalambor and Heath, *J. Biol. Chem.*, 241, 3216 (1966).
267. Kobata, *J. Biochem.* (Tokyo), 53, 167 (1963).
268. Nakanishi, Shimizu, Takahashi, Sugiyama, and Suzuki, *J. Biol. Chem.*, 242, 967 (1967).
269. Jourdian, Shimizu, and Roseman, *Fed. Proc.*, 20, 161 (1961).
270. Jourdian and Distler, *J. Biol. Chem.*, 248, 6781 (1973).
271. Kobata, *Biochem. Biophys. Res. Commun.*, 7, 346 (1962).
272. Kobata, *J. Biochem.* (Tokyo), 59, 63 (1966).
273. Denamur and Gaye, *Eur. J. Biochem.*, 19, 23 (1971).
274. Harada, Shimizu, Nakanishi, and Suzuki, *J. Biol. Chem.*, 242, 2288 (1967); Nakanishi, Sonohara, and Suzuki, *J. Biol. Chem.*, 245, 6046 (1970); Tsuji, Shimizu, Nakanishi, and Suzuki, *J. Biol. Chem.*, 245, 6039 (1970).
275. Gabriel and Ashwell, *J. Biol. Chem.*, 237, 1400 (1962).
276. Suzuki, *J. Biol. Chem.*, 237, 1393 (1962).
277. Park, *J. Biol. Chem.*, 194, 877 (1952).
278. Strominger, *J. Biol. Chem.*, 224, 509 (1957).
279. Strominger, *Biochim. Biophys. Acta*, 30, 645 (1958).
280. Gunetilke and Anwar, *J. Biol. Chem.*, 241, 5740, 5771 (1966).
281. Taku, Gunetilke, and Anwar, *J. Biol. Chem.*, 245, 5012 (1970).
282. Reynolds, *Biochim. Biophys. Acta*, 52, 403 (1961).
283. Plapp and Kandler, *Arch. Mikrobiol.*, 50, 171, 282 (1965).
284. Plapp and Kandler, *Biochem. Biophys. Res. Commun.*, 28, 141 (1967).
285. Strominger and Threnn, *Biochim. Biophys. Acta*, 36, 83 (1959).

ISOLATION AND ENZYMATIC SYNTHESIS OF SUGAR NUCLEOTIDES (continued)

286. Saito, Ishimoto, and Ito, *J. Biochem.* (Tokyo), 54, 273 (1963).
287. Strominger, Threnn, and Scott, *J. Am. Chem. Soc.*, 81, 3803 (1959).
288. Strominger and Birge, *J. Bacteriol.*, 89, 1124 (1965).
289. Neuhaus and Struve, *Biochemistry*, 4, 120 (1965).
290. Comb, Chin, and Roseman, *Biochim. Biophys. Acta*, 46, 394 (1961).
291. Anwar, Roy, and Watson, *Can. J. Biochem. Physiol.*, 41, 1065 (1963).
292. Nakatani, Araki, and Ito, *Biochim. Biophys. Acta*, 156, 210 (1968).
293. Miller, Plapp, and Kandler, *Z. Naturforsch.*, 23B, 217 (1968).
294. Mandelstam, Loercher, and Strominger, *J. Biol. Chem.*, 237, 2683 (1962).
295. Strominger, Scott, and Threnn, *Fed. Proc.*, 18, 334 (1959).
296. Chatterjee and Perkins, *Biochem. Biophys. Res. Commun.*, 24, 489 (1966).
297. Ito and Strominger, *J. Biol. Chem.*, 237, 2689 (1962); 239, 210 (1964); 248, 3131 (1973).
298. Nathenson, Strominger, and Ito, *J. Biol. Chem.*, 239, 1773 (1964).
299. Ito, Nathenson, Dietzler, Anderson, and Strominger, *Methods Enzymol.*, 8, 324 (1966).
300. Mizuno and Ito, *J. Biol. Chem.*, 243, 2665 (1968).
301. Comb, *J. Biol. Chem.*, 237, 1601 (1962).
302. Egan, Lawrence, and Strominger, *J. Biol. Chem.*, 248, 3122 (1973).
303. Neuhaus, *J. Biol. Chem.*, 237, 778 (1962).
304. Neuhaus, Carpenter, Moller, Lee, Gragg, and Stickgold, *Biochemistry*, 8, 5119 (1969).
305. Carpenter and Neuhaus, *Biochemistry*, 11, 2594 (1972).
306. Takayama, David, Wang, and Goldman, *Biochem. Biophys. Res. Commun.*, 39, 7 (1970).
307. Petit, Adam, and Wietzerbin Falszpan, *FEBS Lett.*, 6, 55 (1970).

OPTICAL ACTIVITY OF SUGARS[a]

Table 1
OPTICAL ROTATORY DISPERSION

	Extrema		Reference
	λ	$[\phi]_\lambda$	
Mono- and Oligosaccharides[b]			
D-Glucose	300	+492[c]	1
	200	+2,380[c]	1
	190	+3,600[c]	1
	190	+3,500[c]	2
D-Mannose	200	+1,700[c]	1
D-Allose	200	+900[c]	1
D-Altrose	200	+2,600[c]	1
	190	+5,500[c]	1
D-Galactose	205	+1,580	1
	200	+1,440[c]	1
	190	+650[c]	1
	208	+1,200	2
D-Glucose	200	−2,100[c]	1
D-Talose	204	+520	1
	200	+400[c]	1
6-Deoxy-D-galactose (D-fucose)	205	+1,280	1
6-Deoxy-L-galactose (L-fucose)	208	−1,050	2
2-Deoxy-D-galactose	200	+1,500[c]	1
D-Sorbitol	190	+500[c]	2
2-Deoxy-D-glucose	200	+2,300[c]	1
3-O-Methyl-D-glucose	200	+2,100[c]	1
6-Deoxy-D-mannose	260	−100	1
	200	+800[c]	1
2,6-Dideoxy-D-ribohexose	200	+1,700	1
D-Xylose	300	+250[c]	1
	200	+800[c]	1
D-Lyxose	300	−100[c]	1
	200	+300[c]	1
D-Ribose	300	−130[c]	1
	200	−460[c]	1
	300	−100[c]	3
	200	−450[c]	3
D-Arabinose	300	−400[c]	1
	200	−1,550[c]	1
	300	-550[c]	3
	200	−1,700[c]	3
2-Deoxy-D-ribose	300	-650[c]	1
	200	-1,950[c]	1

[a]List includes naturally occurring carbohydrates and some common derivatives.
[b]Data are expressed in terms of molecular rotation $[\phi]_\lambda$ which is defined from the relationship

$$[\phi]_\lambda = \frac{[\alpha]_\lambda M}{100} \quad (\text{deg cm}^2 \times 10^{-2})$$

where

$[\alpha]$ = the specific rotation;
M = the molecular weight (or mean residue weight of an oligomer and polymer).

[c]These data were not recorded at extrema of optical activity.

Table 1 (continued)
OPTICAL ROTATORY DISPERSION

	Extrema		
	λ	$[\phi]_\lambda$	Reference

Mono- and Oligosaccharides[b] (continued)

	λ	$[\phi]_\lambda$	Reference
2-Deoxy-D-ribose (continued)	300	-330[c]	3
	200	-1,500[c]	3
Methyl-α-D-glucopyranoside	200	+5,240[c]	1
	190	+6,790[c]	1
	–	+3,940[c]	4
Methyl-α-D-galactopyranoside	200	+6,100[c]	1
	190	+6,900[c]	1
	–	+5,330[c]	4
Methyl-α-D-mannopyranoside	200	+2,600[c]	1
	190	+4,660[c]	1
Methyl-α-D-xylopyranoside	200	+3,800[c]	1
Methyl-α-D-arabinopyranoside	250	-180	1
	200	+1,100[c]	1
Methyl-β-D-glucopyranoside	200	-960	1
	190	-970	1
	–	-775	4
Methyl-β-D-galactopyranoside	200	-2,800[c]	1
	190	-4,750[c]	1
	–	-225[c]	4
Methyl-β-D-xylopyranoside	200	-1,700[c]	1
Methyl-β-D-arabinopyranoside	200	-6,000[c]	1
D-Fructose	300	-750[c]	5
	200	-2,000[c]	5
Methyl-β-D-fructofuranoside	300	-400[c]	5
	201	-1,250	5
Ethyl-β-D-galactofuranoside	300	-1,000[c]	5
	201	-4,850	5
Levan	300	-350[c]	5
	201	-1,250	5
Inulin	300	-370[c]	5
	201	-1,250	5
D-Mannoheptulose	300	+300[c]	5
	200	+1,700[c]	5
D-Glucoheptulose	300	+750[c]	5
	200	+1,950[c]	5
D-Galactoheptulose	300	+800[c]	5
	210	+1,580	5
	200	+1,400[c]	5
D-Sorbose	300	+350[c]	5
	215	+680	5
	200	+490[c]	5
D-Glycero-D-gulooctulose	300	+400[c]	5
	200	+950	5
	190	+500[c]	5
D-Glycero-D-guloheptose	300	-220[c]	5
	200	-1,750	5
	190	-1,600[c]	5
D-Glycero-L-mannoheptose	300	-250[c]	5
	200	-3,500[c]	5
D-Glycero-L-galactoheptose	300	-550[c]	5
	200	-3,500[c]	5
D-Erythro-L-galactooctose	300	-500[c]	5
	200	-1,800[c]	5

Table 1 (continued)
OPTICAL ROTATORY DISPERSION

	Extrema		
	λ	[φ]$_\lambda$	Reference

Mono- and Oligosaccharides[b] (continued)

	λ	[φ]$_\lambda$	Reference
D-Glycero-tetrulose	295	−940	6
	254	+1,270	6
	220	+960	6
L-Glycero-tetrulose	295	+940	6
	254	−1,260	6
	230	−1,000	6
	220	−11,500	6
D-Erythro-pentulose	295	−390	6
	257	+30	6
	220	−240	6
L-Erythro-pentulose	295	+390	6
	256	−190	6
	220	+150	6
D-Threo-pentulose	290	−10	6
	250	−600	6
	240	−570	6
D-Threo-3-pentulose	305	−390	6
	260	+440	6
	220	+280	6
β-D-Fructofuranosyl-α-D-glucopyranoside (sucrose)	300[c]	+1,160	7
	200[c]	+4,580	7
β-D-Fructofuranosyl-α-D-galactopyranoside (galsucrose)	300[c]	+1,330	7
	200[c]	+4,510	7
6-O-α-D-Glucopyranosyl-D-glucose (isomaltose)	300[c]	+1,810	7
	200[c]	+7,700	7
4-O-α-D-Glucopyranosyl-D-glucose (maltose)	300[c]	+2,380	7
	200[c]	+8,640	7
6-O-β-D-Glucopyranosyl-D-glucose (gentibiose)	300[c]	+123	7
	200[c]	+1,190	7
3-O-β-D-Glucopyranosyl-D-glucose (laminaribiose)	300[c]	+305	7
	200[c]	+923	7
6-O-α-D-Galactopyranosyl-D-glucose (melibiose)	300[c]	+2,490	7
	200[c]	+9,260	7
4-O-β-D-Galactopyranosyl-D-glucose (lactose)	300[c]	+828	7
	200[c]	+936	7
α-D-Glucopyranosyl-α-D-glucopyranoside (α,α-trehalose)	300[c]	+3,550	7
	200[c]	+14,700	7
O-α-D-Glucopyranosyl-(1 → 3)-O-β-D-fructofuranosyl-α-D-glucopyranoside (melezitose)	300[c]	+2,260	7
	200[c]	+9,040	7
O-α-D-Galactopyranosyl-(1 → 6)-O-α-D-glucopyranosyl-β-D-fractofuranoside (raffinose)	300[c]	+3,030	7
	200[c]	+10,200	7
O-α-D-Galactopyranosyl-(1 → 6)-O-β-D-fructofuranosyl-α-D-glucopyranoside (planteose)	300[c]	+3,530	7
	200[c]	+12,300	7
O-α-D-Galactopyranosyl-(1 → 6)-O-α-D-galactopyranosyl-(1 → 6)-O-α-D-glucopyranosyl-β-D-fructofuranoside (stachyose)	300[c]	+4,400	7
	200[c]	+18,000	7
N-Acetyl-D-galactosamine (pH 6.6)	224	+640	8
	208	+9,940[c]	8
(pH 1.2)	224	+635	8
	208	+10,000[c]	8
	225	+700	9
	200	+13,600	9

Table 1 (continued)
OPTICAL ROTATORY DISPERSION

	Extrema		
	λ	$[\phi]_\lambda$	Reference

Mono- and Oligosaccharides[b] (continued)

	λ	$[\phi]_\lambda$	Reference
N-Acetyl-D-galactosamine (continued)	240	+1,250	10
	225	+640	10
	200	+10,400	10
N-Acetyl-D-glucosamine	222.5	−1,700	9
	196	+7,000	9
	260	+400	10
	220	−1,200	10
	197	+4,700	10
N-Acetyl-D-mannosamine	220	+1,300	10
Methyl-α-2-acetamido-2-deoxy-D-glucopyranoside	201	+12,800	11
	190	+5,600[c]	11
	–	+3,100	4
Methyl-β-2-acetamido-2-deoxy-D-glucopyranoside	220	−2,260	11
	201	+3,800	11
	190	+1,500[c]	11
	–	−2,690	4
Methyl-α-2-acetamido-2-deoxy-D-galactopyranoside	201	+18,900	11
	190	+8,400	11
	–	+5,360	4
Ethyl-β-2-acetamido-2-deoxy-D-galactopyranoside	225	−700	11
	202	+7,900	11
	190	+380[c]	11
	–	−336	4
N-Acetylneuraminic acid	220	+1,400	12
N-Acetylneuraminyl lactose	280	+600	12
	215	+4,700	12
Glucuronic acid (pH 6.6)	225	−19.6	8
	216	+2,234	8
(pH 1.2)	250	+4,704	8
	207	+1,400	8
(pH 7.0)	218	+1,560	10
	200	−570	10
Galacturonic acid (pH 7.0)	223	+2,180	10
	200	−2,600[c]	10
Methyl-α-D-glucopyranosiduronic acid (pH 3.0)	212	+4,500	11
(pH 7.0)	205	+4,400	11
Propyl-β-D-glucopyranosiduronic acid (pH 3.0)	242	−1,160	11
	223	−1,020	11
	200	−4,900[c]	11
	190	−11,100[c]	11
Cyclohexyl-β-D-glucopyranosiduronic acid (pH 3.0)	230	+2,100	10
	195	+4,900[c]	10
Benzyl-β-D-glucopyranosiduronic acid (pH 3.0)	220	+5,450	10
	200	+8,990	10
	190	+3,080[c]	10
Methyl-α-D-glucopyranosiduronic acid (pH 3.0)	228	+3,800	11
	200	+910[c]	11
(pH 7.0)	215	−3,760	11
Methyl-α-D-mannopyranosiduronic acid (pH 3.0)	212	+2,780	11
(pH 7.0)	205	+2,900	11

Table 1 (continued)
OPTICAL ROTATORY DISPERSION

	Extrema		
	λ	$[\phi]_\lambda$	Reference
Polysaccharides			
Polygalacturonic acid (pH 6.5)	211	+150[d]	13
(pH 3.0)	217	+145[d]	13
(pH 2.5)	220	+7,350	10
	200	+4,510[c]	10
(pH 8.0)	210	+7,600	10
	195	+6,400	10
Heparin	198	+9,200	14
	230	+2,500	9
	200	+8,900	9
(pH 7.0)	200	+8,100	8
	190	+3,200	8
(pH 2.6)	195	+11,500	8
Hyaluronic acid	220	−11,800	9
	199	−7,700	9
(pH 1.0)	220	−9,600	15
(pH 1.5)	220	−10,400	15
(pH 2.1)	220	−11,000	15
(pH 2.5)	220	−11,800	15
(pH 3.2)	220	−12,300	15
(pH 3.8)	220	−12,800	15
(pH 4.5)	220	−13,100	15
(pH 5.1)	220	−13,500	15
(pH 6.7)	220	−13,800	15
Chondroitin-4-sulfate	218	−4,000	9
	205	+100	9
	218	−1,600[d]	16
	220	−1,180	17
Chondroitin-6-sulfate	220	−850[d]	16
	216.5	−5,900	9
	202	+250	9
(c = 0.3%)	221	−957[d]	18
	205	+366[d]	18
(c = 0.6%)	222	−1,170[d]	18
	205	+461[d]	18
(c = 1.22%)	222	−1,200[d]	18
	204	+361[d]	18
(c = 2.45%)	221	−1,240[d]	18
	204	+228[d]	18
(c = 0.6 in 0.03 M HCl)	225	−498[d]	18
	205	+596[d]	18
(c = 0.6 in 0.8 M Na⁺)	220	−958[d]	18
	205	+293[d]	18
(c = 0.6 in .27 M Ca)	220	−953[d]	18
	204	+296[d]	18
Sulfated chondroitin-6-sulfate	220	−6,100	14
	216.5	−6,300	9, 19
	202	+400	9, 19
Dermatan sulfate	220	−2,200[d]	16
	222	−8,000	9
	199	−14,800	9
	200	−13,000	9, 19

[d]Data presented as observed rotation specific rotation or units not given.

Table 1 (continued)
OPTICAL ROTATORY DISPERSION

	Extrema		
	λ	[φ]$_\lambda$	Reference

Polysaccharides (continued)

	λ	[φ]$_\lambda$	Reference
Desulfated dermatan sulfate	220	−1,600[d]	16
Dermatan sulfate, disaccharide	220	−1,300[d]	16
Dermatan sulfate, tetrasaccharide	220	−1,500[d]	16
Heparan sulfate	210	−3,600	20
	212.5	−5,500	19
	196	+9,400	19
Dermatan sulfate	210	−10,240	20
Keratin sulfate	222	−4,800	9
	198.5	+18,600	9
	222	−4,700	19
	198.5	+18,600	19
S-Keratin sulfate	220	−4,800	9
	198	+7,900	9
Colominic acid	250	−3,500	12
	215	+12,000	12
Type IV pneumococcal polysaccharide	220	−770	4

Compiled by Irving Listowsky.

Note: References follow Table 2.

Table 2
CIRCULAR DICHROISM

	Extrema		
	λ	$[\theta]_\lambda$	Reference
Mono- and Oligosaccharides[a]			
D-Glucose	169	+10,000	21
D-Galactose	178	−4,000	21
D-Xylose	167	+7,300	21
Methyl-α-D-glucopyranoside	190	+200[b]	22
Methyl-β-D-glucopyranoside	190	+200[b]	22
Methyl-α-D-galactopyranoside	190	−170[b]	22
Methyl-β-D-galactopyranoside	190	−660[b]	22
α-D-Glucopyranosyl-α-D-glucopyranoside	190	+330[b]	22
4-O-α-D-Glucopyranosyl-D-glucose	190	+70[b]	22
4-O-β-D-Glucopyranosyl-D-glucose	190	+260[b]	22
4-O-β-D-Galactopyranosyl-D-glucose	190	−720[b]	22
4-O-β-D-Galactopyranosyl-D-fructose	190	−700[b]	22
6-Deoxy-D-galactose	190	−520[b]	22
D-Mannose	190	+1,200[b]	22
Methyl-α-D-mannopyranoside	190	+560[b]	22
D-Talose	190	+90[b]	22
D-Erythrose	278	−3,200	23
D-Arabinose	290	+13.2	23
L-Arabinose	287	−11.5	23
D-Lyxose	288	+11.5	23
D-Ribose	288	−21.5	23
D-Xylose	292	−6.6	23
L-Xylose	294	+6.6	23
2-Deoxy-D-erythropentose	287	−49.5	23
D-Ribose	195	−180[b]	3
2-Deoxy-D-ribose	195	+15	3
	192	−95[b]	3
D-Arabinose	195	+280[b]	3
	192	+510[b]	3
D-Fructose	275	+33	24
Fructose-1-phosphate	275–285	+26	24
Fructose-6-phosphate	275	+280	24
Fructose-1,6-diphosphate	275–280	+106	24
L-Sorbose	273	−12.3	24
D-Tagatose	282	+16.8	24
D-threo-2,5-Hexodiulose	295	−47	24
D-Glucose-6-phosphate	305	−0.11	24
	275	+3.7	24

[a]Data are expressed in terms of molar ellipticity $[\theta]_\lambda$ which is defined from the relationship

$$[\theta]_\lambda = \frac{\theta \text{obs}}{1 \times 10 \times C} M \left(\frac{\text{deg cm}^2}{\text{d mole}} \right)$$

where

θobs	=	the observed ellipticity (degrees);
M	=	the molecular weight (or mean residue weight);
l	=	the path length, in cm;
C	=	the concentration in g|ml.

Occasionally data were expressed in terms of $[\alpha]_\lambda$ or $\Delta\epsilon$ in the original references. These were converted to molecular rotation or molar ellipticity ($[\phi]_\lambda = \Delta\epsilon_\lambda \cdot 3300$) wherever possible.
[b]These data were not recorded at extrema of optical activity.

Table 2 (continued)
CIRCULAR DICHROISM

	Extrema		
	λ	$[\theta]_\lambda$	Reference
Mono- and Oligosaccharides[a] (continued)			
6-*O*-α-D-Glucopyranosyl-D-fructose	275	+95	24
4-*O*-α-D-Galactopyranosyl-D-fructose	273	+10	24
3-*O*-α-D-Glucopyranosyl-D-fructose	285	+56	24
1-*O*-β-D-Glucopyranosyl-D-fructose	275	+5	24
N-Acetyl-D-glucosamine (pH 2.5)	211	−5,900	25
(pH 6.5)	211	−6,300	25
(pH 1.2)	212	−5,040	18
(pH 6.6)	212	−5,040	18
	210	−4,000	12
	210	−5,700	11
	211	−6,500	9, 19
	210	−5,600	26
	190	+3,400[b]	26
	212.5	−5,800	26
N-Acetyl-D-galactosamine	212.5	−4,800	26
	190	+11,600[b]	26
	210	−4,700	26
	190	+10,500[b]	26
	212	−3,050	12
	210	−5,900	11
	212	−4,800	9,19
	189	+12,200[b]	9, 19
N-Acetyl-D-mannosamine	212	+1,050	11
Methyl-α-2-acetamido-2-deoxy-D-glucose	210	−4,100	12
Methyl-β-2-acetamido-2-deoxy-D-glucose	215	−6,100	12
Methyl-α-2-acetamido-2-deoxy-D-galactose	215	−3,050	12
Ethyl-β-2-acetamido-2-deoxy-D-galactose	218	−4,500	12
N-Acetylneuraminic acid	197.5	+10,600	26
	196	+10,600	9, 19
	220	+1,000[b]	12
	216	+400[b]	27
	210	+500[b]	27
	198	+8,100	27
Methyl-(methyl-β-D-neuraminid)ate	221	+2,800	27
β-Methoxyneuraminic acid	217	−5,000	27
	189	+10,100	27
(2→3)*N*-Acetylneuraminyl lactose	220	−3,000	27
	207	−2,200	27
	199	+10,900	27
(2→6)*N*-Acetylneuraminyl lactose	226	−500	27
	211	+800	27
	199	+3,800	27
β-D-gal(1→6)D-glu NAc	218	−4,840	12
β-D-gal(1→4)D-glu NAc	218	−5,000	12
β-D-gal(1→3)D-glu NAc	218	−5,360	12
Lacto-*N*-neotetraose[c]	212	−7,500	12
Lacto-*N*-tetraose[c]	211	−9,300	12
Lacto-*N*-fucopentaose I[c]	212	−19,200	12
Lacto-*N*-fucopentaose II[c]	210	+13,400	12
Lacto-*N*-difucohexaose[c]	214	−24,200	12

[c]Structures of these compounds are shown in the reference.

Table 2 (continued)
CIRCULAR DICHROISM

	Extrema		
	λ	$[\theta]_\lambda$	Reference
Mono- and Oligosaccharides[a] (continued)			
β-L-Fucosyl(1→3)D-glu NAc	205	−8,000	12
N-Acetylneuraminic acid	216	+400	12
	210	+500	12
	198	+8,100	12
Galacturonic acid (pH 2.5)	210	+3,920	28
Glucuronic acid (in 95% dioxane, 5% H_2O)	230	−1,180	28
(pH 6.6)	215	−770	18
	202	+601	18
(pH 1.2)	234	−502	18
	210	+2,560	18
Glucuronic acid (pH 2.8)	235	−390	28
	205	+1,840	28
(in ethylene glycol)	220	−504	10
	200	+1,660	10
(in 50% dioxane)	235	−630	28
	208	+720	28
Methyl-α-D-glucopyranosiduronic acid	235	−520	28
	208	+2,140	28
(pH 6.5)	215	−1,110	10
	200	+400	10
Methyl-α-D-galactopyranosiduronic acid	210	+3,360	28
N-Propyl-β-D-glucopyranosiduronic acid	235	−430	28, 33
(pH 2.5)	205	+2,380	28, 33
(pH 6.5)	215	−760	10
	203	+830	10
Methyl-α-D-mannopyranosiduronic acid (pH 2.5)	231	−740	28, 33
	207	+1,840	28, 33
(pH 6.5)	210	−1,580	10
Methyl-2,3,4-tri-O-methyl-β-D-glucopyranosiduronic	236	−480	28, 33
acid (pH 2.5)	209	+4,530	28, 33
(pH 6.5)	215	−680	10
	202	+1,210	10
(in hexane)	225	−1,560	28
	205	−860	28
	195	−1,700[b]	28
Muramic acid (pH 2.5)	275	−14	25, 33
	244	+40	25, 33
	208	−5,200	25, 33
(pH 6.5)	275	−5	25
	225	+260	25
	201	−4,700	25
Isomuramic acid (pH 2.5)	207	+1,800	25, 33
(pH 6.5)	221	−250	25, 33
	203	+800	25, 33
D-Glucosamine (pH 2.5)	200	−290[b]	25
(pH 6.5)	200	−130[b]	25
N-Acetylmuramic acid (pH 2.5)	245	+49	25, 33
	209	−12,600	25, 33
(pH 6.5)	204	−15,500	25, 33
β-Xylose tetraacetate	213	+3,200	31
β-Xylobiose tetraacetate	213	+1,500	31
β-Xylotriose octaacetate	214	+400	31

Table 2 (continued)
CIRCULAR DICHROISM

	Extrema		
	λ	$[\theta]_\lambda$	Reference

Mono- and Oligosacchraides[a] (continued)

β-Xylotetraose decaacetate	210	−200	31
White birch xylan diacetate	210	−650	31
Esparto grass xylan diacetate	210	−1,050	31
α-D-Glucose pentaacetate	210	−2,800	31
β-D-Glucose pentaacetate	220	+1,150	31
α-Cellobiose octaacetate	210	−2,350	31
β-Cellobiose octaacetate	212	−850	31
Cellulose acetate (DS = 0.9)	210	−500	31
(DS = 2.0)	210	−1,250	31
(DS = 2.44)	210	−1,350	31
Cellulose triacetate	210	−1,600	31
α-1,6-Glucan triacetate	210	−4,100	32
β-Isomaltose octaacetate	213	−1,500	32
β-Gentiobiose octaacetate	210	−1,100	32
β-Maltose octaacetate	220	+250	32
Cellobiose octaacetate	213	−900	32
β-D-Glucose pentaacetate	220	+1,150	32
β-D-Maltose pentaacetate	220	+250	32
β-Maltotriose hendecaacetate	210	−300	32
Amylose triacetate	208	−400	32
Amylose acetate (DS = 2.44)	220	+150	32

Polysaccharides

Polygalacturonic acid	200	+3,600	26
(pH 2.5)	210	+4,110	28
(pH 6.5)	200	+3,290	28
Colominic acid	230	−5,100	12
Sodium alginate	213	−1,600	29
Calcium alginate (film)	202	+450[d]	29
Sodium alginate (film)	213	−500[d]	29
Pectic acid (pH 7.0)	200	+185[d]	30
Pectic acid methylated	210	+230[d]	30
Alginic acid	215	−290[d]	30
	201	−150[d]	30
(M blocks)	204	+495[d]	30
(G blocks)	206	−680[d]	30
Calcium alginate (G blocks, initial)	208	−705[d]	30
	199	−580[d]	30
(G, 10-day gel)	206	+3,750	30
(M blocks, initial)	215	−480	30
	201	−170	30
(M, 10-day gel)	218	−80	30
	204	+100	30
Hyaluronic acid (pH 1.0)	210	−9,600	15
	191.5	+7,200	15
(pH 1.5)	210	−9,900	15
	190	+9,800	15
(pH 2.1)	210	−10,700	15
	188	+10,900	15

[d]Data presented as observed rotation specific rotation or units not given.

Table 2 (continued)
CIRCULAR DICHROISM

	Extrema		
	λ	$[\theta]_\lambda$	Reference

Polysaccharides (continued)

	λ	$[\theta]_\lambda$	Reference
(pH 2.5)	210	−11,200	15
	187.5	+12,200	15
(pH 3.2)	210	−11,200	15
	187	+5,900	15
(pH 3.8)	210	−11,300	15
	187	+3,200	15
(pH 4.5)	210	−11,500	15
	186	+2,000	15
(pH 5.1)	210	−11,500	15
	186	+3,800	15
(pH 6.7)	210	−11,500	15
	186	+5,200	15
(pH 8.1)	210	−11,300	15
	185	+4,500	15
	208	−10,700	9
	201.5	−11,100	26
Heparin	210	−1,280	26
	190	+2,580	26
	210	−1,800	26
	192.5	+3,280	26
	210	−1,300	9, 19
	192	+2,600	9, 19
	210	−1,800	20
	191	+3,600	20
(High mol wt)	210	−1,400	20
	192	+3,000	20
Heparan sulfate-1	209	−4,600	9, 19
	190	+11,500	9, 19
Heparan sulfate-2	240	+2,400	9, 19
	202.5	−12,800	9, 19
	210	−4,300	26
	190	+11,500	26
Heparan sulfate	209	−4,300	20
	190	+11,500	20
Heparan sulfate (Sanfilippo)	212	−4,800	20
	195	+2,300	20
(Sanfilippo in 1 M NaCl)	210	−4,800	20
	190	+9,600	20
(Sanfilippo 1.3 M NaCl)	210	−3,100	20
	190	+4,600	20
(Hurler)	209	−4,700	20
	189	−10,900	20
Keratan sulfate	210	−8,900	26
	190	+11,500	26
	210	−9,300	9, 19
	190	+7,900	9, 19
S-Keratan sulfate	207.5	−9,500	9, 19
	189	+5,900	9, 19
	205	−9,500	26
	190	+5,900	26
Chondroitin-4-sulfate	207.5	−7,300	26
	208.5	−7,300	9, 19
	210	−1,190[b]	17

Table 2 (continued)
CIRCULAR DICHROISM

| | Extrema | | |
	λ	$[\theta]_\lambda$	Reference
Polysaccharides (continued)			
Chondroitin-6-sulfate (C = 0.3)	211	−3,280	18
(C = 0.6)	211	−3,370	18
(C = 1.2)	211	−3,590	18
(C = 2.4)	210.5	−3,620	18
(C = 0.6 in 0.03 *M* HCl)	213	−2,250	18
(C = 0.6 in 0.8 *M* Na⁺)	210	−3,300	18
(C = 0.6 in .266 *M* Ca⁺⁺)	237	−3,180	18
Sulfated chondroitin-6-sulfate	207.5	−11,200	26
	195	−7,400	26
	208	−11,300	9, 19
Dermatan sulfate	207.5	−3,500	26
	190	−16,000	26
	212	−3,300	9, 19
	188	−16,500	9, 19
	212	−3,900	26
	189	−16,500	26

Compiled by Irving Listowsky.

REFERENCES

1. Listowsky, Avigad, and Englard, *J. Am. Chem. Soc.*, 87, 1765 (1965).
2. Pace, Tanford, and Davidson, *J. Am. Chem. Soc.*, 86, 3160 (1964).
3. Adler, Grossman, and Fasman, *Biochemistry*, 7, 3836 (1968).
4. Beychok and Kabat, *Biochemistry*, 12, 2565 (1965).
5. Listowsky, Englard, and Avigad, *Carbohydr. Res.*, 2, 261 (1966).
6. Sticzay, Peciar, Babor, Fedoronko, and Linek, *Carbohydr. Res.*, 6, 418 (1968).
7. Englard, Avigad, and Listowsky, *Carbohydr. Res.*, 2, 380 (1975).
8. Stone, *Nature*, 216, 551 (1967).
9. Stone, *Biopolymers*, 7, 173 (1969).
10. Listowsky, unpublished results.
11. Listowsky, Avigad, and Englard, *Carbohydr. Res.*, 8, 205 (1968).
12. Kabat, Lloyd, and Beychok, *Biochemistry*, 8, 747 (1969).
13. Stoddart, Spires, and Tipton, *Biochem. J.*, 114, 863 (1969).
14. Stone, *Biopolymers*, 3, 617 (1965).
15. Chakrabarti and Balazs, *J. Mol. Biol.*, 78, 135 (1973).
16. Davidson, *Biochim. Biophys. Acta*, 101, 121 (1965).
17. Eyring and Yang, *J. Biol. Chem.*, 243, 1306 (1968).
18. Eyring and Yang, *Biopolymers*, 6, 691 (1968).
19. Stone, in *Structure and Stability of Macromolecules*, Vol. 2, Timasheff and Fasman, Eds., Marcel Dekker, New York, 1969, 353.
20. Stone, Constantopoulos, Sotsky, and Dekaban, *Biochim. Biophys. Acta*, 222, 79 (1970).
21. Nelson and Johnson, *J. Am. Chem. Soc.*, 94, 3343 (1972).
22. Listowsky and Englard, *Biochem. Biophys. Res. Commun.*, 30, 329 (1968).
23. Totty, Hudec and Hayward, *Carbohydr. Res.*, 23, 152 (1972).
24. Avigad, Englard, and Listowsky, *Carbohydr. Res.*, 14, 365 (1970).
25. Listowsky, Avigad, and Englard, *Biochemistry*, 9, 2186 (1970).
26. Stone, *Biopolymers*, 10, 739 (1971).
27. Dickinson and Bush, *Biochemistry*, 14, 2299 (1975).
28. Listowsky, Englard, and Avigad, *Biochemistry*, 8, 1781 (1969).
29. Bryce, McKinnon, Morris, Rees, and Thom, *Faraday Discuss. Chem. Soc.*, 57, 221 (1974).

Table 2 (continued)
CIRCULAR DICHROISM

30. Morris and Sanderson, in *New Techniques in Biophysics and Cell Biology*, Pain and Smith, Eds., John Wiley & Sons, 1973, 113.
31. Mukherjee, Marchessault, and Sarko, *Biopolymers*, 11, 291 (1972).
32. Mukherjee, Sarko, and Marchessault, *Biopolymers*, 11, 303 (1972).
33. Listowsky, Englard, and Avigad, *Trans. N.Y. Acad. Sci.*, 34, 218 (1972).

AVERAGE DIMENSIONS OF A MONOSACCHARIDE UNIT

V.S.R. Rao

X-Ray crystal structure data of various monosaccharides and disaccharides have been compiled, and the weighted average of the bond lengths and bond angles for a sugar unit are computed; these are shown in the figure. The bond lengths and bond angles involving hydrogen atoms have not been considered in the present compilation because of the nonavailability of sufficient, accurate data. Wherever more than one study has been made on the same molecule, the data have been individually considered. Also, whenever the data on a disaccharide or trisaccharide is available, they are considered as individual units while computing the average dimensions. The weighted average standard deviations are not given here. Only the values of the bond lengths and bond angles computed have been reported here, and no attempt has been made to bring out any conclusions. The references for the various data compiled here follow the figure.

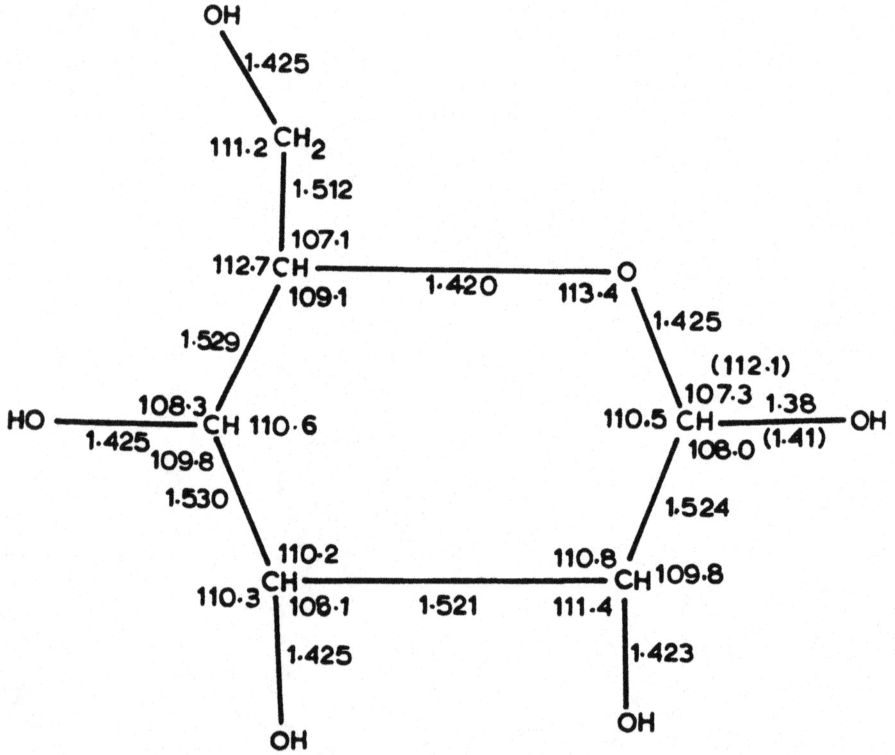

Averaged bond lengths in (A) and bond angles (degrees) in a sugar unit. [Values in the bracket correspond to the axial orientation of the hydroxyl group.]

REFERENCES

1. Chu and Jeffrey, *Acta Crystallogr.*, 23, 1038 (1967).
2. Ham and Williams, *Acta Crystallogr.*, B26, 1373 (1970).
3. Chu and Jeffrey, *Acta Crystallogr.*, B24, 830 (1968).
4. Berman and Kim, *Acta Crystallogr.*, B24, 897 (1968).
5. Brown and Levy, *Science*, 147, 1038 (1965).
6. Berman, *Acta Crystallogr.*, B26, 290 (1970).
7. Brown, Cox, and Llewellyn, *J. Chem. Soc. A*, p. 922 (1966).
8. Fries, Rao, and Sundaralingam, *Acta Crystallogr.*, B27, 994 (1971).
9. Gatehouse and Poppleton, *Acta Crystallogr.*, B26, 1761 (1970).
10. Killiam, Sharma, and Lawrence, *Acta Crystallogr.*, B27, 1707 (1971).
11. Snyder and Rosenstein, *Acta Crystallogr.*, B27, 1969 (1971).
12. Park, Kim, and Jeffrey, *Acta Crystallogr.*, B27, 220 (1971).
13. Kim and Jeffrey, *Acta Crystallogr.*, 22, 537 (1967).
14. Jacobson, Wunderlich, and Lipscomb, *Acta Crystallogr.*, 14, 598 (1961).
15. Park, Kim, and Jeffrey, *Acta Crystallogr.*, B27, 1323 (1971).
16. Gatehouse and Poppleton, *Acta Crystallogr.*, B27, 871 (1971).
17. Brown, *J. Chem. Soc. A*, p. 927 (1966).
18. Quigley, Sarko, and Marchessault, *J. Am. Chem. Soc.*, 92, 5834 (1970).

ELECTRONIC CHARGE DISTRIBUTION IN MONOSACCHARIDES AND SOME OF THEIR DERIVATIVES AND POLYSACCHARIDES

V.S.R. Rao

The electronic charge distributions in monosaccharides, their derivatives, and polysaccharides have been compiled. The MO-LCAO method of DelRe was used for evaluating the σ-charges, and the Huckel method was used for the π charges in the original literature.

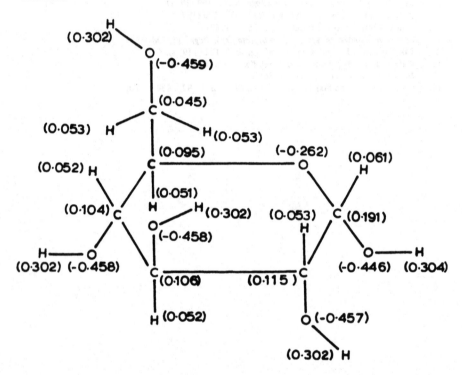

CHARGE DISTRIBUTION IN ALDOHEXOPYRANOSES

FIGURE 1.

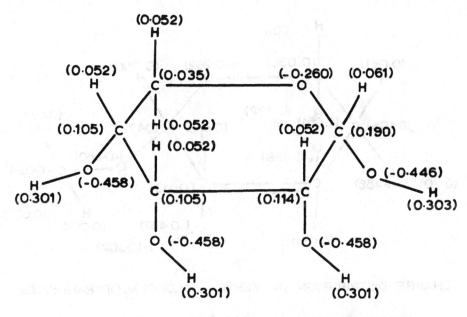

CHARGE DISTRIBUTION IN ALDOPENTOPYRANOSES

FIGURE 2.

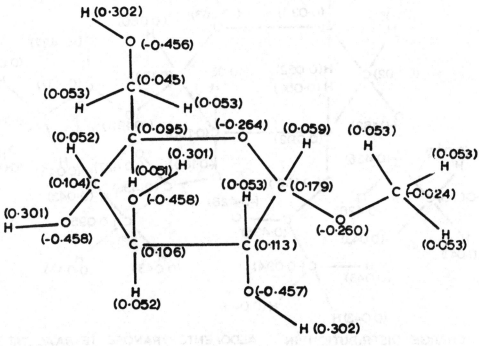

CHARGE DISTRIBUTION IN METHYL ALDOHEXOPYRANOSIDES

FIGURE 3.

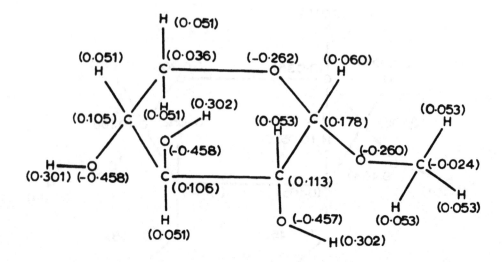

CHARGE DISTRIBUTION IN MEHYL   ALDOPENTOPYRANOSIDES

FIGURE 4.

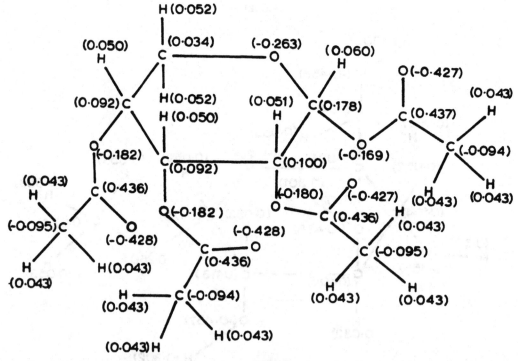

CHARGE DISTRIBUTION IN   ALDOPENTOPYRANOSE TETRA ACETATE

FIGURE 5.

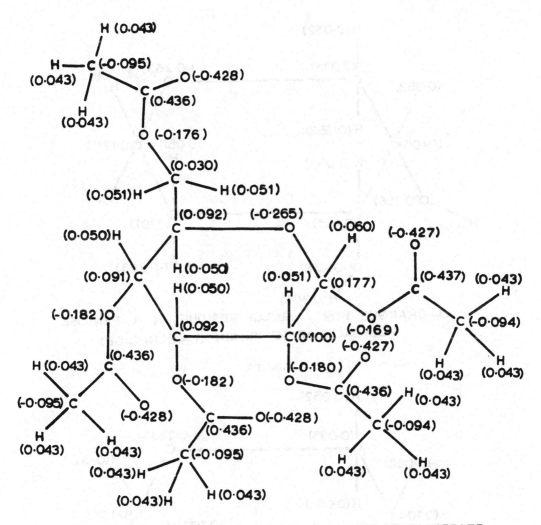

CHARGE DISTRIBUTION IN ALDOHEXOPYRANOSE PENTAACETATE

FIGURE 6.

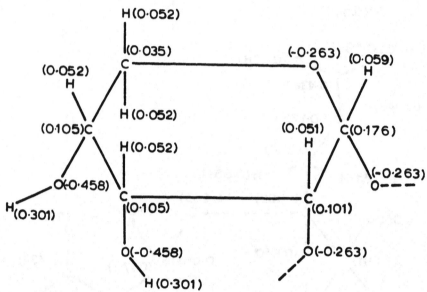

σ- CHARGES FOR A SUGAR RESIDUE IN A PENTOSE
POLYSACCHARIDE CHAIN (1→2 LINKAGE)

FIGURE 7.

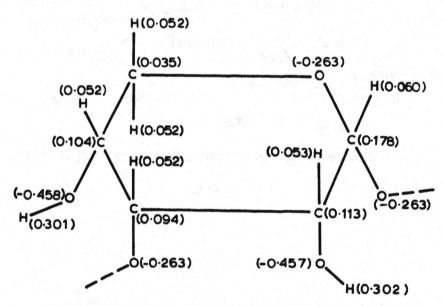

σ-CHARGES FOR A SUGAR RESIDUE IN A PENTOSE
POLYSACCHARIDE CHAIN (1→3 LINKAGE)

FIGURE 8.

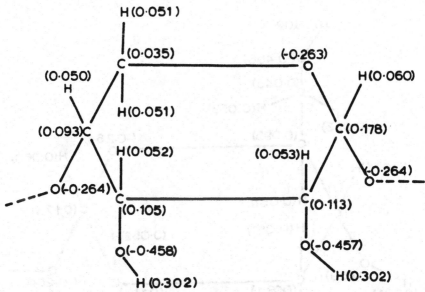

σ-CHARGES FOR A SUGAR RESIDUE IN A PENTOSE
POLYSACCHARIDE CHAIN (1→4 LINKAGE)

FIGURE 9.

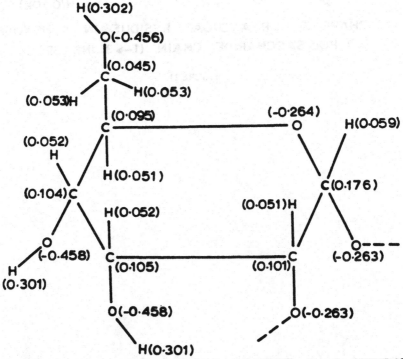

σ-CHARGES FOR A SUGAR RESIDUE IN A HEXOSE
POLYSACCHARIDE CHAIN (1→2 LINKAGE)

FIGURE 10.

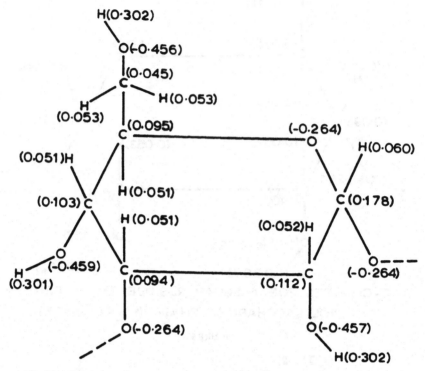

σ- CHARGES FOR A SUGAR RESIDUE IN A HEXOSE
POLYSACCHARIDE CHAIN (1→3LINKAGE)

FIGURE 11.

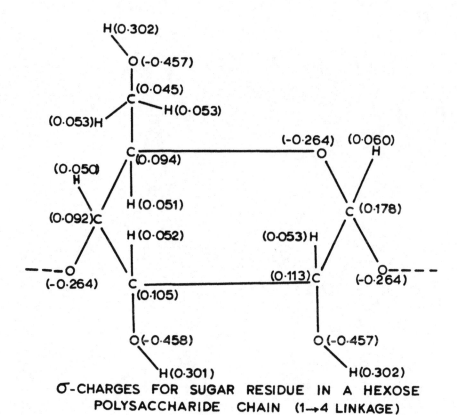

σ-CHARGES FOR SUGAR RESIDUE IN A HEXOSE
POLYSACCHARIDE CHAIN (1→4 LINKAGE)

FIGURE 12.

REFERENCES

1. Rao, Vijayalakshmi, and Sundararajan, *Carbohydr. Res.*, 17, 341 (1971).
2. Yathindra and Rao, *Carbohydr. Res.*, 25, 256 (1972).
3. Vijayalakshmi and Rao *Carbohydr. Res.*, 22, 413 (1972).
4. Vijayalakshmi, Yathindra, and Rao, *Carbohydr. Res.*, 31, 197 (1973).
5. Vijayalakshmi and Rao, *Carbohydr. Res.*, 29, 427 (1973).
6. Yathindra and Rao, *J. Polym. Sci.*, A2, 10, 1369 (1972).
7. Rao and Vijayalakshmi, *Carbohydr. Res.*, 33, 363 (1974).

Lipids

FATTY ACIDS: PHYSICAL AND CHEMICAL CHARACTERISTICS

No	Acid — Systematic name	Acid — Common name	Chemical formula	Molecular weight	Melting point °C	Boiling point °C/mm[a]
			SATURATED FATTY ACIDS			
1	**Methanoic**	Formic	$HCOOH$	46.0	8.4	100.5
2	**Ethanoic**	Acetic	CH_3COOH	60.1	16.7	118.2
3	**Propanoic**	Propionic	C_2H_5COOH	74.1	−22.0	141.1
4	**Butanoic**	Butyric	C_3H_7COOH	88.1	−7.9	163.5
5	**Pentanoic**	Valeric	C_4H_9COOH	102.1	−34.5	187
6	**Hexanoic**	Caproic	$C_5H_{11}COOH$	116.2	−3.4	205.8
7	**Heptanoic**	Heptylic[g]	$C_6H_{13}COOH$	130.2	−10.5	223.0
8	**Octanoic**	Caprylic	$C_7H_{15}COOH$	144.2	16.7	239.7
9	**Nonanoic**	Pelargonic	$C_8H_{17}COOH$	158.2	12.5	255.6
10	**Decanoic**	Capric	$C_9H_{19}COOH$	172.3	31.6	270[-]
11	**Undecanoic**[h]	Undecylic	$C_{10}H_{21}COOH$	186.3	29.3	284
12	**Dodecanoic**	Lauric	$C_{11}H_{23}COOH$	200.3	44.2	225/100
13	**Tridecanoic**	Tridecylic	$C_{12}H_{25}COOH$	214.3	41.5	236/100
14	**Tetradecanoic**	Myristic	$C_{13}H_{27}COOH$	228.4	53.9	250/100
15	**Pentadecanoic**	Pentadecylic	$C_{14}H_{29}COOH$	242.2	52.3	202.5/10
16	**Hexadecanoic**	Palmitic	$C_{15}H_{31}COOH$	256.4	63.1	268/100
17	**Heptadecanoic**	Margaric	$C_{16}H_{33}COOH$	270.4	61.3	220/10
18	**Octadecanoic**	Stearic	$C_{17}H_{35}COOH$	284.5	69.6	213.5
19	**Nonadecanoic**	Nonadecyclic	$C_{18}H_{37}COOH$	298.5	68.6	299/10
20	**Eicosanoic**	Arachidic	$C_{19}H_{39}COOH$	312.5	76.5	204/1
21	**Docosanoic**	Behenic	$C_{21}H_{43}COOH$	340.6	81.5	306/60
22	**Tetracosanoic**	Lignoceric	$C_{23}H_{47}COOH$	368.6	86.0	272/10
23	**Hexacosanoic**	Cerotic	$C_{25}H_{51}COOH$	396.7	88.5	—
24	**Octacosanoic**	Montanic	$C_{27}H_{55}COOH$	424.7	90.9	—
25	**Triacontanoic**	Melissic	$C_{29}H_{59}COOH$	452.8	93.6	—
26	**Dotriacontanoic**	Lacceroic	$C_{31}H_{63}COOH$	480.0	96.2	—
27	**Tetratriacontanoic**	Gheddic	$C_{33}H_{67}COOH$	508.9	98.4	—
28	**Pentatriacontanoic**	Ceroplastic	$C_{34}H_{69}COOH$	522.9	98.4	—
			UNSATURATED FATTY ACIDS (MONOETHENOIC)			
29	*trans*-**2-Butenoic**	Crotonic	$C_4H_6O_2$	86.1	72	189.0
30	*cis*-**2-Butenoic**	Isocrotonic	$C_4H_6O_2$	86.1	15.5	169.3
31	**2-Hexenoic**	Isohydrosorbic	$C_6H_{10}O_2$	114.1	32	217
32	**4-Decenoic**	Obtusilic	$C_{10}H_{18}O_2$	170.2	—	149/13
33	**9-Decenoic**	Caproleic	$C_{10}H_{18}O_2$	170.2	—	142/4
34	**4-Dodecenoic**	Linderic	$C_{12}H_{22}O_2$	198.3	1.0–1.3	171/13
35	**5-Dodecenoic**	Denticetic	$C_{12}H_{22}O_2$	198.3	—	—
36	**9-Dodecenoic**	Lauroleic	$C_{12}H_{22}O_2$	198.3	—	142/4
37	**4-Tetradecenoic**	Tsuzuic	$C_{14}H_{26}O_2$	226.4	18.0–18.5	185–188/13
38	**5-Tetradecenoic**	Physeteric	$C_{14}H_{26}O_2$	226.4	—	190–195/15
39	**9-Tetradecenoic**	Myristoleic	$C_{14}H_{26}O_2$	226.4	−4	—
40	**9-Hexadecenoic**	Palmitoleic	$C_{16}H_{30}O_2$	254.4	−0.5 to +0.5	131/0.06
41	**6-Octadecenoic**	Petroselinic	$C_{18}H_{34}O_2$	282.5	32–33	237.5/18
42	*cis*-**9-Octadecenoic**	Oleic	$C_{18}H_{34}O_2$	282.5	13.4(α), 16.3(β)	234/15
43	*trans*-**9-Octadecenoic**	Elaidic	$C_{18}H_{34}O_2$	282.5	44.5	288/100
44	*trans*-**11-Octadecenoic**	Vaccenic	$C_{18}H_{34}O_2$	282.5	44	—
45	**9-Eicosenoic**	Gadoleic	$C_{20}H_{38}O_2$	310.5	24–24.5	220/6
46	**11-Eicosenoic**	Gondoic	$C_{20}H_{38}O_2$	310.5	23.5–24	267/15
47	**11-Docosenoic**	Cetoleic	$C_{22}H_{42}O_2$	338.6	32.5–33	—
48	**13-Docosenoic**	Erucic	$C_{22}H_{42}O_2$	338.6	34.7	242/5
49	**15-Tetracosenoic**	Nervonic[i]	$C_{24}H_{46}O_2$	366.6	42.5–43.0	—
50	**17-Hexacosenoic**	Ximenic	$C_{26}H_{50}O_2$	394.7	45–45.5	—
51	**21-Triacontenoic**	Lumequeic	$C_{30}H_{58}O_2$	450.8	—	—
			UNSATURATED FATTY ACIDS (DIENOIC)			
52	**2,4-Pentadienoic**	β-Vinylacrylic	$C_5H_6O_2$	98.1	80	110 d.
53	**2,4-Hexadienoic**	Sorbic	$C_6H_8O_2$	112.1	134.5	228 d.
54	**2,4-Decadienoic**	Stillingic	$C_{10}H_{16}O_2$	168.2	—	—
55	**2,4-Dodecadienoic**	—	$C_{12}H_{20}O_2$	196.3	—	—
56	**9,12-Hexadecadienoic**	—	$C_{16}H_{28}O_2$	252.4	—	—
57	*cis*-**9,***cis***-12-Octadecadienoic**	α-Linoleic	$C_{18}H_{32}O_2$	280.5	−5.2 to −5.0	202/1.4

FATTY ACIDS: PHYSICAL AND CHEMICAL CHARACTERISTICS (continued)

No	Specific gravity[b]	Refractive index[c] n_D^c	Neutral-ization value[d]	Iodine value (calcu-lated)[e]	Solubility[f]	Reference	No
				SATURATED FATTY ACIDS			
1	$1.220^{20°}$	$1.3714^{20°}$	1.219		s.w.	13, 28, 29	1
2	$1.049^{20°}$	$1.3718^{20°}$	934.2		s.w.	15, 28, 29	2
3	$0.992^{20°}$	$1.3874^{20°}$	757.3		s.al., chl., eth., w.	28, 29	3
4	$0.9587^{20°}$	$1.33906^{20°}$	636.8		s.al., eth., w.	13, 29, 36	4
5	$0.942^{20°}$	$1.4086^{20°}$	549.3		s.al., eth.; sl.s.w.	29, 36	5
6	$0.929^{20°}$	$1.41635^{20°}$	483.0		s.al., eth.; sl.s.w.	29, 36	6
7	$0.92215^{20°}$	$1.4230^{20°}$	431.0		s.al., eth.; v.sl.s.w.	29, 36	7
8	$0.910^{20°}$	$1.4285^{20°}$	389.1		s.al., bz., eth.; v.sl.s.w.	13, 29, 36	8
9	$0.907^{20°}$	$1.4322^{20°}$	354.6		s.al., chl., eth.; v.sl.s.w.	29, 36	9
10	$0.8858^{40°}$	$1.42855^{40°}$	325.7		s.al., eth., pet.eth.; v.sl.s.w.	13, 29, 36	10
11	$0.9905^{25°}$	$1.4202^{70°}$	301.2		s.al., chl., eth., pet.eth.	29, 36	11
12	$0.8690^{50°}$	$1.4261^{60°}$	280.1		s.acet., al., eth., pet.eth.	13, 29, 36	12
13	$0.8458^{80°}$	$1.4286^{60°}$	261.8		s.acet., al., eth., pet.eth.	14, 29, 31, 36	13
14	$0.8622^{54°}$	$1.4273^{70°}$	245.7		s.acet., al., eth., pet.eth.	13, 29, 36	14
15	$0.8423^{80°}$	$1.4292^{70°}$	231.5		s.acet., al., eth., pet.eth.	29, 36	15
16	$0.8487^{70°}$	$1.4309^{70°}$	218.8		s.acet., h.al., eth., pet.eth.	29, 36	16
17	$0.853^{60°}$	$1.4324^{70°}$	207.5		s.acet., h.al., eth., pet.eth.	29, 36	17
18	$0.8390^{80°}$	1.4337^{70}	197.2		s.acet., h.al., eth., pet.eth.	13, 29, 36	18
19	$0.8771^{24°}$	$1.4512^{25°}$	188.0		s.acet., h.al., eth., pet.eth.	29	19
20	$0.8240^{100°}$	$1.4250^{100°}$	179.5		s.bz., chl., eth., pet.eth.	13, 29, 36	20
21	$0.8221^{100°}$	$1.4270^{100°}$	164.7		sl.s.al., eth.	13, 29, 36	21
22	$0.8207^{100°}$	$1.4287^{100°}$	152.2		s.ac.a., bz., CS_2, eth.	28, 29, 36, 39	22
23	$0.8198^{100°}$	$1.4301^{100°}$	141.4		s.h.acet., h.chl., h.me.al.	13, 29, 36	23
24	$0.8191^{100°}$	$1.4313^{100°}$	132.1		s.h.ac.a., h.bz., h.me.al.	13, 29, 36	24
25		$1.4323^{100°}$	123.9		s.chl., CS_2, h.me.al.	13, 29, 36	25
26			116.7		s.h.acet., h.bz., chl.	13, 17, 29, 36	26
27			110.2		s.h.acet., h.bz., chl.	13, 29, 32, 36	27
28			107.3		s.h.acet., h.bz., chl.	13, 29, 32, 36	28
				UNSATURATED FATTY ACIDS (MONOETHENOIC)			
29	$0.964^{80°}$	$1.4228^{80°}$	651.7	294.9	s.acet., al., tol., w.	29	29
30	$1.0312^{15°}$	$1.4457^{20°}$	651.7	294.9	s.al., pet.eth., w.	29	30
31	$0.965^{20°}$	$1.4460^{40°}$	491.5	222.5	s.CS_2, eth.	29, 36	31
32	$0.9197^{20°}$	$1.4497^{20°}$	329.6	149.1	s.bz., eth.	2, 13, 29, 36	32
33	$0.9238^{15°}$	$1.4507^{15°}$	329.6	149.1	s.al., eth.	13, 29, 36, 37	33
34	$0.9081^{20°}$	$1.4529^{20°}$	282.9	128.0	s.bz., chl., eth.	13, 29, 36	34
35	$0.9130^{15°}$	$1.4535^{15°}$	282.9	128.0	s.bz., chl., eth.	13, 29, 36, 39	35
36			282.9	128.0	s.bz., chl., eth.	13, 29, 36	36
37	$0.9024^{20°}$	$1.4557^{20°}$	247.9	112.2	s.bz., pet.eth.	2, 13, 29, 36	37
38	$0.9046^{20°}$	$1.4552^{20°}$	247.9	112.2	s.bz., eth., pet.eth.	13, 29, 36, 39	38
39	$0.9018^{20°}$	$1.4519^{20°}$	247.9	112.2	s.bz., eth., pet.eth.	2, 13, 29, 36	39
40			220.5	99.8	s.bz., eth., pet.eth.	2, 13, 18, 29	40
41	$0.8824^{35°}$	$1.4533^{40°}$	198.6	89.9	s.al., eth., pet.eth.	13, 21, 22, 29, 36	41
42	$0.8905^{20°}$	$1.45823^{20°}$	198.6	89.9	s.acet., eth., me.al.	13, 29, 36	42
43	$0.851^{70°}$	$1.4468^{50°}$	198.6	89.9	s.al., chl., eth., pet.eth.	29	43
44	$0.8563^{70°}$	$1.4406^{70°}$	198.6	89.9	s.acet., me.al.	13, 29, 36	44
45	$0.8882^{25°}$	$1.4597^{25°}$	180.7	81.8	s.acet., me.al., pet.eth.	13, 16, 21, 29	45
46			180.7	81.8	s.al., me.al.	13, 16, 29	46
47			165.7	75.0	s.al.	13, 21, 29, 39	47
48	$0.85321^{70°}$	$1.4444^{70°}$	165.7	75.0	v.s.eth., me.al.	13, 29, 30, 36	48
49			153.0	69.2	s.acet., al., eth.	13, 21, 29, 36	49
50			142.2	64.3	s.bz., chl., eth., pet.eth.	13, 29	50
51			124.5	56.3	s.bz., chl., eth., pet.eth.	13, 29	51
				UNSATURATED FATTY ACIDS (DIENOIC)			
52			572.0	517.5	v.s.al., eth.; s.h.w.	29, 36	52
53			500.4	452.7	s.al., eth.; sl.s.w.	29, 36	53
54			333.5	301.7	s.acet., eth., hex.	29	54
55			285.8	258.6	s.acet., eth., pet.eth.	29	55
56			222.3	201.1	s.acet., eth., pet.eth.	7	56
57	$0.9038^{18°}$	$1.4699^{20°}$	200.1	181.0	s.acet., al., eth., pet.eth.	13, 29, 36	57

FATTY ACIDS: PHYSICAL AND CHEMICAL CHARACTERISTICS (continued)

No	Acid — Systematic name	Acid — Common name	Chemical formula	Molec- ular weight	Melting point °C	Boiling point °C/mm[a]
	UNSATURATED FATTY ACIDS (DIENOIC)					
58	*trans*-9,*trans*-12-Octadeca-dienoic	Linolelaidic	$C_{18}H_{32}O_2$	280.5	28–29	—
59	*trans*-10,*trans*-12-Octadeca-dienoic	—	$C_{18}H_{32}O_2$	280.5	55.5–56	—
60	11,14-Eicosadienoic	—	$C_{20}H_{36}O_2$	308.4	—	—
61	13,16-Docosadienoic	—	$C_{22}H_{40}O_2$	336.6	—	—
62	17,20-Hexacosadienoic	—	$C_{26}H_{48}O_2$	392.7	61	—
	UNSATURATED FATTY ACIDS (TRIENOIC)					
63	6,10,14-Hexadecatrienoic	Hiragonic	$C_{16}H_{26}O_2$	250.4	—	180–190/15
64	7,10-13-Hexadecatrienoic	—	$C_{16}H_{26}O_2$	250.4	—	—
65	*cis*-6,*cis*-9,*cis*-12-Octadeca-trienoic	γ-Linolenic	$C_{18}H_{30}O_2$	278.4	—	—
66	*trans*-8,*trans*-10,*cis*-12-Octa-decatrienoic	α-Calendic	$C_{18}H_{30}O_2$	278.4	40–40.5	—
67	*trans*-8,*trans*-10,*trans*-12-Octa-decatrienoic	β-Calendic	$C_{18}H_{30}O_2$	278.4	77–78	—
68	*cis*-8,*trans*-10,*cis*-12-Octa-decatrienoic	—	$C_{18}H_{30}O_2$	278.4	—	—
69	*cis*-9,*cis*-12,*cis*-15-Octadeca-trienoic	α-Linolenic	$C_{18}H_{30}O_2$	278.4	−10 to −11.3	157/0.001
70	*trans*-9,*trans*-12,*trans*-15-Octa-decatrienoic	Linolenelaidic	$C_{18}H_{30}O_2$	278.4	29–30	—
71	*cis*-9,*trans*-11,*trans*-13-Octa-decatrienoic	α-Eleostearic	$C_{18}H_{30}O_2$	278.4	48–49	235/15
72	*trans*-9,*trans*-11,*trans*-13-Octadecatrienoic	β-Eleostearic	$C_{18}H_{30}O_2$	278.4	71.5	—
73	*cis*-9,*trans*-11,*cis*-13-Octadeca-trienoic	Punicic	$C_{18}H_{30}O_2$	278.4	43.5–44	—
74	*trans*-9,*trans*-11,*trans*-13-Octa-decatrienoic	—	$C_{18}H_{30}O_2$	278.4	—	—
75	5,8,11-Eicosatrienoic	—	$C_{20}H_{34}O_2$	306.5	—	—
76	8,11,14-Eicosatrienoic	—	$C_{20}H_{34}O_2$	306.5	—	—
	UNSATURATED FATTY ACIDS (TETRAENOIC)					
77	4,8,11,14-Hexadecatetraenoic	—	$C_{16}H_{24}O_2$	248.4	—	—
78	6,9,12,15-Hexadecatetraenoic	—	$C_{16}H_{24}O_2$	248.4	—	—
79	4,8,12,15-Octadecatetraenoic	Moroctic	$C_{18}H_{28}O_2$	276.4	—	208–213/15
80	6,9,12,15-Octadecatetraenoic	—	$C_{18}H_{28}O_2$	276.4	−57.4 to −56.6	—
81	9,11,13,15-Octadecatetraenoic	α-Parinaric	$C_{18}H_{28}O_2$	276.4	85–86	—
82	9,11,13,15-Octadecatetraenoic	β-Parinaric	$C_{18}H_{28}O_2$	276.4	95–96	—
83	9,12,15,18-Octadecatetraenoic	—	$C_{18}H_{28}O_2$	276.4	—	—
84	4,8,12,16-Eicosatetraenoic	—	$C_{20}H_{32}O_2$	304.5	—	217–220/10
85	5,8,11,14-Eicosatetraenoic	Arachidonic	$C_{20}H_{32}O_2$	304.5	−49.5	163/1
86	6,10,14,18-Eicosatetraenoic?	—	$C_{20}H_{32}O_2$	304.5	—	—
87	4,7,10,13-Docosatetraenoic	—	$C_{22}H_{36}O_2$	332.5	—	—
88	7,10,13,16-Docosatetraenoic	—	$C_{22}H_{36}O_2$	332.5	—	—
89	8,12,16,19-Docosatetraenoic	—	$C_{22}H_{36}O_2$	332.5	—	—
	UNSATURATED FATTY ACIDS (PENTA- AND HEXA-ENOIC)					
90	4,8,12,15,18-Eicosapentaenoic	Timnodonic?	$C_{20}H_{30}O_2$	302.5	—	—
91	5,8,11,14,17-Eicosapentaenoic	—	$C_{20}H_{30}O_2$	302.5	−54.4 to −53.8	—
92	4,7,10,13,16-Docosapentaenoic	—	$C_{22}H_{34}O_2$	330.5	—	—
93	4,8,12,15,19-Docosapentaenoic	Clupanodonic	$C_{22}H_{34}O_2$	330.5	—	207–212/2
94	7,10,13,16,19-Docosapentaenoic	—	$C_{22}H_{34}O_2$	330.5	—	—
95	4,7,10,13,16,19-Docosahexaenoic	—	$C_{22}H_{32}O_2$	328.5	−44.5 to −44.1	—
96	4,8,12,15,18,21-Tetracosahexa-enoic	Nisinic	$C_{24}H_{36}O_2$	356.6	—	—

FATTY ACIDS: PHYSICAL AND CHEMICAL CHARACTERISTICS (continued)

No	Specific gravity[b]	Refractive index[c] n_D^c	Neutral- ization value[d]	Iodine value (calcu- lated)[e]	Solubility[f]	Reference	No
UNSATURATED FATTY ACIDS (DIENOIC)							
58	–	---	200.1	181.0	s.al., eth., me.al., pet.eth.	29, 36	58
59	--	--	200.1	181.0	s.acet., cyc., eth.	23	59
60	-	–	181.9	164.5	s.acet., eth., pet.eth.	29	60
61	-	- -	166.7	150.8	s.acet., eth.	29	61
62	--	-	142.9	129.3	s.eth., pet.eth.	29	62
UNSATURATED FATTY ACIDS (TRIENOIC)							
63	0.9296^{20°	1.4850^{50°	224.1	304.1	s.al., eth.	13, 29, 36, 38	63
64	–	---	224.1	304.1	s.al., eth.	29	64
65	–	–	201.5	273.5	s.acet., eth., me.al.	29, 36	65
66	--	--	201.5	273.5	s.acet., pent.	8, 29, 36	66
67	--	--	201.5	273.5	s.me.al., pet.eth.	8	67
68	-	–	201.5	273.5	v.s.acet., al., pent., pet.eth.	10, 29	68
69	0.914^{20°	1.4678^{50°	201.5	273.5	s.acet., al., eth., pet.eth.	13, 29, 36	69
70	--		201.5	273.5	s.me.al., pet.eth.	29, 36	70
71	--	1.5112^{50°	201.5	273.5	s.al., cyc., eth., pet.eth.	13, 28, 29, 36	71
72	-	1.5002^{-5°	201.5	273.5	s.al., eth., me.al., pet.eth.	13, 29, 36	72
73	0.9027^{50°	1.5114^{50°	201.5	273.5	s.al., pent., pet.eth.	13, 29, 36	73
74	--	....	201.5	273.5	s.acet., al., CS_2, pent.	9, 29	74
75	--	---	183.1	248.3	s.CS_2, hept., me.al.	29	75
76	–	--	183.1	248.3	s.CS_2, hept., me.al.	29	76
UNSATURATED FATTY ACIDS (TETRAENOIC)							
77	--	–	225.9	408.8	s.acet., al., eth., pet.eth.	29	77
78	–	1.4870^{29°	225.9	408.8	s.acet., al., CS_2, eth., pent.	29	78
79	0.9297^{20°	1.4911^{20°	203.0	367.3	s.acet., al., eth., pet.eth.	13, 29, 36, 38	79
80	-	1.4888^{16°	203.0	367.3	s.CS_2, me.al.	29	80
81	- -	--	203.0	367.3	s.acet., al., eth., pet.eth.	13, 29, 36	81
82	--	---	203.0	367.3	s.eth., pet.eth.	13, 29, 36	82
83	--	----	203.0	367.3	s.CS_2, me.al.	29	83
84	0.9263^{20°	1.4915^{20°	184.3	333.4	s.acet., eth.	13, 29, 36	84
85	0.9082^{20°	1.4824^{20}	184.3	333.4	s.acet., eth., me.al., pet.eth.	13, 29, 36	85
86	0.9263^{20°	1.4935^{20°	184.3	333.4	s.acet., me.al., pent., pet.eth.	29	86
87	–	--	168.7	305.4	s.acet., me.al., pet.eth.	24, 29	87
88	–	-	168.7	305.4	s.CS_2, hept., me.al.	1, 29	88
89	–	--	168.7	305.4	s.acet., me.al., pet.eth.		89
UNSATURATED FATTY ACIDS (PENTA- AND HEXA-ENOIC)							
90	0.9399^{15°	1.5109^{15°	185.5	419.6	s.bz., chl., eth., pet.eth.	13, 29, 36	90
91	--	1.4977^{23°	185.5	419.6	s.hept., me.al.	25	91
92	--	--	169.8	384.0	s.chl., hept., me.al.	24, 29	92
93	0.9356^{20°	1.5014^{20}	169.8	384.0	s.acet., eth., pet.eth.	13, 29, 36	93
94	-	--	169.8	384.0	s.bz., chl., me.al., pet.eth.	26, 29	94
95	--	1.5017^{26°	170.8	463.6	s.bz., chl., me.al., pet.eth.	19, 24, 29	95
96	0.9452^{20}	1.5122^{20°	157.4	427.1	s.bz., chl., eth., pet.eth.	13, 29, 36	96

FATTY ACIDS: PHYSICAL AND CHEMICAL CHARACTERISTICS (continued)

No	Acid — Systematic name	Acid — Common name	Chemical formula	Molecular weight	Melting point °C	Boiling point °C/mm[a]
HYDROXYALKANOIC ACIDS						
97	2-Hydroxydodecanoic	2-Hydroxylauric	$C_{12}H_{24}O_3$	216.3	73–74	—
98	12-Hydroxydodecanoic	Sabinic	$C_{12}H_{24}O_3$	216.3	84	—
99	2-Hydroxytetradecanoic	2-Hydroxymyristic	$C_{14}H_{28}O_3$	244.4	81.5–82	—
100	11-Hydroxypentadecanoic	Convolvulinolic	$C_{15}H_{30}O_3$	258.4	63.5–64	—
101	2-Hydroxyhexadecanoic	2-Hydroxypalmitic	$C_{16}H_{32}O_3$	272.4	86–87	—
102	11-Hydroxyhexadecanoic	Jalapinolic	$C_{16}H_{32}O_3$	272.4	68–69	—
103	16-Hydroxyhexadecanoic	Juniperic	$C_{16}H_{32}O_3$	272.4	95	—
104	2-Hydroxyoctadecanoic	2-Hydroxystearic	$C_{18}H_{36}O_3$	300.5	91	—
105	23-Hydroxydocosanoic	Phellonic	$C_{22}H_{44}O_3$	356.6	95–96	—
106	2-Hydroxytetracosanoic	Cerebronic	$C_{24}H_{48}O_3$	384.6	99.5–100.5	—
107	3,11-Dihydroxytetradecanoic	Ipurolic	$C_{14}H_{28}O_4$	260.4	100–101	—
108	2,15-Dihydroxypentadecanoic	Dihydroxypentade-cyclic	$C_{15}H_{30}O_4$	274.4	102–103	—
109	15,16-Dihydroxyhexadecanoic	Ustilic A	$C_{16}H_{32}O_4$	288.4	112–113	-
110	9,10-Dihydroxyoctadecanoic	9,10-Dihydroxy-stearic	$C_{18}H_{36}O_4$	316.5	141[9]	—
111	9,10-Dihydroxyoctadecanoic	9,10-Dihydroxy-stearic	$C_{18}H_{36}O_4$	316.5	90[10]	—
112	11,12-Dihydroxyeicosanoic	11,12-Dihydroxy-arachidic	$C_{20}H_{40}O_4$	344.5	130[9]	—
113	2,15,16-Trihydroxyhexadecanoic	Ustilic	$C_{16}H_{32}O_5$	304.4	140	—
114	9,10,16-Trihydroxyhexadecanoic	Aleuritic	$C_{16}H_{32}O_5$	304.4	100	—
KETO, EPOXY, AND CYCLO FATTY ACIDS						
115	4-Ketopentanoic	Levulinic	$C_5H_8O_3$	116.1	37.2	154/15
116	6-Ketooctadecanoic	Lactarinic	$C_{18}H_{34}O_3$	298.5	87	—
117	4-Keto-9,11,13,octadecatrienoic	α-Licanic	$C_{18}H_{28}O_3$	292.4	74–75	—
118	4-Keto-*trans*-9,-*trans*-11,-*trans*-13-octadecatrienoic	β-Licanic	$C_{18}H_{28}O_3$	292.4	99.5	—
119	*cis*-12,13-Epoxy-*cis*-9-octa-decenoic	Vernolic	$C_{18}H_{32}O_3$	296.5	31–32	—
120	*cis*-9,10-Epoxyoctadecanoic	Epoxystearic	$C_{18}H_{34}O_3$	298.5	57.5–58	—
121	ω-(2-*n*-Octylcycloprop-1-enyl)-octanoic	Sterculic	$C_{19}H_{34}O_2$	294.5	18	—
122	ω-(2-*n*-Octylcyclopropyl)-octanoic	Lactobacillic	$C_{19}H_{36}O_2$	296.5	28–29	—
123	13-(2-Cyclopentenyl)-tridecanoic	Chaulmoogric	$C_{18}H_{32}O_2$	280.2	68.5	247.5/20
124	11-(2-Cyclopentenyl)-hendec-anoic	Hydnocarpic	$C_{16}H_{28}O_2$	252.2	60.5	—
125	9-(2-Cyclopentenyl)-nonanoic	Alepric	$C_{14}H_{24}O_2$	224.2	48.0	—
126	7-(2-Cyclopentenyl)-heptanoic	Aleprylic	$C_{12}H_{20}O_2$	196.2	32.0	—
127	5-(2-Cyclopentenyl)-pentanoic	Aleprestic	$C_{10}H_{16}O_2$	168.1	Liquid	—
128	2-Cyclopentenyl-1-oic	Aleprolic	$C_6H_8O_2$	112.1	Liquid	—
129	13-(2-Cyclopentenyl)-6-tri-decenoic	Gorlic	$C_{18}H_{30}O_2$	278.2	6.0	232.5
HYDROXY UNSATURATED ACIDS						
130	16-Hydroxy-7-hexadecenoic	Ambrettolic	$C_{16}H_{30}O_3$	270.5	25	—
131	9-Hydroxy-12-octadecenoic		$C_{18}H_{34}O_3$	298.5	—	—
132	d-12-Hydroxy-*cis*-9-octadecenoic	Ricinoleic	$C_{18}H_{34}O_3$	298.5	5, 7.7, & 16	225/10
133	d-12-Hydroxy-*trans*-9-octa-decenoic	Ricinelaidic	$C_{18}H_{34}O_3$	298.5	52–53	—
134	2-Hydroxy-15-tetracosenoic	Hydroxynervonic	$C_{24}H_{46}O_3$	382.6	65	—
135	9-Hydroxy-10,12-octadeca-dienoic		$C_{18}H_{32}O_3$	296.5	—	—
136	13-Hydroxy-9,11-octadeca-dienoic		$C_{18}H_{32}O_3$	296.5	—	—
137	18-Hydroxy-*cis*-9,*trans*-11,-*trans*-13-octadecatrienoic	α-Kamlolenic	$C_{18}H_{30}O_3$	294.4	77–78	—
138	18-Hydroxy-*trans*-9,*trans*-11,-*trans*-13-octadecatrienoic	β-Kamlolenic	$C_{18}H_{30}O_3$	294.4	88–89	—

FATTY ACIDS: PHYSICAL AND CHEMICAL CHARACTERISTICS (continued)

No	Specific gravity[b]	Refractive index[c] n_D[c]	Neutral-ization value[d]	Iodine value (calcu-lated)[e]	Solubility[f]	Reference	No
					HYDROXYALKANOIC ACIDS		
97	—	—	259.4	—	s.al., me.al.	29	97
98	—	—	259.4	—	s.al., h.bz.	3, 13, 29	98
99	—	—	229.1	—	s.al., chl., eth.	29	99
100	—	—	217.1	—	s.al., chl., eth.	13, 29, 34	100
101	—	—	206.0	—	s.al., me.al.	29, 40	101
102	—	—	206.0	—	s.al., eth.	13, 29, 33	102
103	—	—	206.0	—	s.al., bz., eth.	13, 21, 29, 36	103
104	—	—	186.7	—	s.al., me.al.	29, 40	104
105	—	—	157.3	—	s.acet., chl., eth., glac.ac.a., pyr.	5, 13, 29, 36	105
106	—	—	145.9	—	s.acet., h.al., eth., pyr.	13, 29, 36	106
107	—	—	215.5	—	s.chl., eth.	13, 29, 33	107
108	—	—	204.5	—	s.me.al.	29	108
109	—	—	194.5	—	s.me.al.	29	109
110	—	—	177.3	—	s.h.al.; sl.s.eth.	13, 29	110
111	—	—	177.3	—	s.al., eth., h.w.	29	111
112	—	—	162.9	—	s.acet., eth.	13, 29	112
113	—	—	184.3	—	s.me.al.	29	113
114	—	—	184.3	—	s.me.al.	29	114
					KETO, EPOXY, AND CYCLO FATTY ACIDS		
115	1.1395[20°]	1.442[15.8°]	483.2	—	v.s.al., eth., w.	29	115
116	—	—	188.0	—	s.h.al., chl., eth.	13, 21, 29, 36	116
117	—	—	191.9	260.4	s.h.pet.eth.	4, 15, 29, 36	117
118	—	—	191.9	260.4	s.h.pet.eth.	4, 15, 29, 36	118
119	—	—	189.3	85.6	s.acet., al., hex.	27, 29	119
120	—	—	188.0	—	s.acet., al., hex.	6	120
121	—	—	190.5	86.2	s.eth.	29	121
122	—	—	189.2	—	s.acet., eth., pet.eth.	29	122
123	—	—	200.1	90.5	s.acet., chl., eth.	12, 13, 21, 29, 36	123
124	—	—	222.3	100.6	s.al., chl., pet.eth.	21, 29, 36	124
125	—	—	250.1	113.1	s.al., eth., pet.eth.	29	125
126	—	—	285.8	129.3	s.acet., eth., pet.eth.	29	126
127	—	—	333.5	150.8	s.acet., eth., pet.eth.	29	127
128	—	—	500.4	226.4	s.acet., eth., pet.eth.	29	128
129	0.9436[25°]	1.4782[25°]	201.5	182.5	s.h.al.	11, 13, 29, 36	129
					HYDROXY UNSATURATED ACIDS		
130	—	—	207.5	93.9	s.al., eth.	29, 36	130
131	—	—	188.0	85.0	s.acet., al., eth.	29	131
132	0.940[27.4°]	1.4716[20°]	188.0	85.0	s.acet., al., eth.	13, 29, 36	132
133	—	—	188.0	85.0	s.acet., al., eth.	13, 29, 36	133
134	—	—	146.6	66.3	s.acet., al., chl., eth., pyr.; sl.s.pet.eth.	13, 29, 36	134
135	—	—	189.2	171.2	s.acet., al., pent.	8	135
136	—	—	189.2	171.2	s.acet., al., pent.	8	136
137	—	—	190.5	258.6	—	29	137
138	—	—	190.5	258.6	—	29	138

FATTY ACIDS: PHYSICAL AND CHEMICAL CHARACTERISTICS (continued)

	Acid		Chemical formula	Molecular weight	Melting point °C	Boiling point °C/mm[a]
No	Systematic name	Common name				

BRANCHED-CHAIN FATTY ACIDS

No	Systematic name	Common name	Chemical formula	Molecular weight	Melting point °C	Boiling point °C/mm[a]
139	3-Methylbutanoic	Isovaleric	$C_5H_{10}O_2$	102.1	−37.6	176.7
140	d-6-Methyloctanoic	—	$C_9H_{18}O_2$	158.2	--	—
141	8-Methyldecanoic	—	$C_{11}H_{22}O_2$	186.3	−18.5	—
142	10-Methylhendecanoic	Isolauric	$C_{12}H_{24}O_2$	200.3	41.2	—
143	d-10-Methyldodecanoic	—	$C_{13}H_{26}O_2$	214.3	6.2-6.5	—
144	11-Methyldodecanoic	Isoundecylic	$C_{13}H_{26}O_2$	214.3	39.4-40	—
145	12-Methyltridecanoic	Isomyristic	$C_{14}H_{28}O_2$	228.4	53.6	—
146	d-12-Methyltetradecanoic	—	$C_{15}H_{30}O_2$	242.4	25.8	—
147	13-Methyltetradecanoic	Isopentadecylic	$C_{15}H_{30}O_2$	242.4	52.2	—
148	14-Methylpentadecanoic	Isopalmitic	$C_{16}H_{32}O_2$	256.4	62.4	—
149	d-14-Methylhexadecanoic	—	$C_{17}H_{34}O_2$	270.4	38.0	—
150	15-Methylhexadecanoic	—	$C_{17}H_{34}O_2$	270.4	60.5	—
151	10-Methylheptadecanoic	—	$C_{18}H_{36}O_2$	284.5	33.5	—
152	16-Methylheptadecanoic	Isostearic	$C_{18}H_{36}O_2$	284.5	69.5	—
153	l-D-10-Methyloctadecanoic	Tuberculostearic	$C_{19}H_{38}O_2$	298.5	13.2	175-178/0.7
154	d-16-Methyloctadecanoic	—	$C_{19}H_{38}O_2$	298.5	49.9-50.7	—
155	18-Methylnonadecanoic	Isoarachidic	$C_{20}H_{40}O_2$	312.5	75.3	—
156	d-18-Methyleicosanoic	—	$C_{21}H_{42}O_2$	326.6	55.6	—
157	20-Methylheneicosanoic	Isobehenic	$C_{22}H_{44}O_2$	340.6	79.5	—
158	d-20-Methyldocosanoic	—	$C_{23}H_{46}O_2$	354.6	62.1	—
159	22-Methyltricosanoic	Isolignoceric	$C_{24}H_{48}O_2$	368.6	83.1	—
160	d-22-Methyltetracosanoic	—	$C_{25}H_{50}O_2$	382.7	67.8	—
161	24-Methylpentacosanoic	Isocerotic	$C_{26}H_{52}O_2$	396.7	86.9	—
162	d-24-Methylhexacosanoic	—	$C_{27}H_{54}O_2$	410.7	72.9	—
163	26-Methylheptacosanoic	Isomontanic	$C_{28}H_{56}O_2$	424.7	89.3	—
164	d-28-Methyltriacontanoic	—	$C_{31}H_{62}O_2$	466.8	80.7	—
165	2,4,6-(D)-Trimethyloctacosanoic	Mycoceranic(myco-cerosic)	$C_{31}H_{62}O_2$	466.8	27-28	—
166	2-Methyl-cis-2-butenoic	Angelic	$C_5H_8O_2$	100.1	45	185
167	2-Methyl-trans-2-butenoic	Tiglic	$C_5H_8O_2$	100.1	65.5	198.5
168	4-Methyl-3-pentenoic	Pyroterebic	$C_6H_{10}O_2$	114.1	—	207
169	d-2,4(L),6(L)-Trimethyl-trans-2-tetracosenoic	C_2--Phthienoic (mycolipenic)	$C_{27}H_{52}O_2$	408.7	39.5-41	—

These data were compiled originally for the *Biology Data Book* by Klare S. Markley (1964) pp. 370–80. Data are reproduced here in modified form by permission of the copyright owners of the above publication, the Federation of American Societies for Experimental Biology, Washington, D.C.

[a]Boiling Point: d. = decomposes; 760 mm of mercury (atmospheric pressure), unless otherwise specified.
[b]At temperature indicated in superscript, referred to water at 4°C.
[c]Refractive index (*n*) is given for the sodium D-line at temperature shown in superscript.
[d]Milligrams KOH required to neutralize one gram of acid.
[e]Grams of iodine absorbed by 100 grams of acid.
[f]Solubility: a. = acid; acet. = acetone; ac. = acetic; al. = alcohol; bz. = benzene; chl. = chloroform; cyc. = cyclohexane; eth. = ether; glac. = glacial; hept. = heptane; hex. = hexane; h. = hot; me. = methyl; pent. = pentane; pet. = petroleum; pyr. = pyridine; s. = soluble; sl. = slightly; tol. = toluene; v. = very; w. = water.
[g]Also called enanthic acid.
[h]Also called hendecanoic acid.
[i]Also called selacholeic acid.

FATTY ACIDS: PHYSICAL AND CHEMICAL CHARACTERISTICS (continued)

No	Specific gravity[b]	Refractive index[c] n_D^c	Neutral-ization value[d]	Iodine value (calculated)[e]	Solubility[f]	Reference	No
					BRANCHED-CHAIN FATTY ACIDS		
139	0.937¹⁵°	1.40178²²·⁴°	549.3		s.al., chl., eth.; sl.s.w.	13, 28, 29, 36	139
140			354.6		s.acet., eth., me.al., pet.eth.	13, 29, 36, 40	140
141			301.2		s.acet., eth., me.al., pet.eth.	13, 29, 36, 40	141
142			280.1		s.acet., eth., me.al., pet.eth.	13, 29, 36, 40	142
143		1.4424²⁵°	261.8		s.bz., chl., me.al., pet.eth.	13, 29, 36, 40	143
144		1.4293⁶⁰°	261.8		s.acet., al., me.al., pet.eth.	29	144
145			245.7		s.acet., me.al., pet.eth.	13, 29, 36, 40	145
146		1.4327⁵⁹°	231.5		s.chl., eth., me.al., pet.eth.	13, 29, 36, 40	146
147		1.4312⁵⁹°	231.5		s.me.al., pet.eth.	29	147
148		1.4293⁷⁰°	218.8		s.acet., eth., me.al., pet.eth.	13, 29, 36, 40	148
149			207.5		s.acet., eth., me.al., pet.eth.	13, 29, 36, 40	149
150		1.4315⁷⁰°	207.5		s.acet., eth., pet.eth.	13, 29, 36, 40	150
151			197.2		s.acet., glac.ac.a.	20	151
152			197.2		s.acet., eth., pet.eth.	13, 29, 36, 40	152
153	0.887²⁵°	1.4512²⁵°	188.0		s.acet., al., me.al., pent.	13, 29, 36	153
154			188.0		s.acet., me.al., pet.eth.	13, 29, 35, 36, 40	154
155			179.5		s.al., eth., pet.eth.	13, 29, 36, 40	155
156			171.8		s.acet., chl., pet.eth.	13, 29, 36, 40	156
157			164.7		s.chl., eth., me.al., pet.eth.	13, 29, 36, 40	157
158			158.2		s.acet., chl., eth., pet.eth.	13, 29, 36, 40	158
159			152.2		s.acet., chl., pet.eth.	13, 29, 36, 40	159
160			146.6		s.al., bz., chl., pet.eth.	13, 29, 36, 40	160
161			141.4		s.acet., chl., glac.ac.a	13, 29, 36, 40	161
162			136.6		s.bz., chl., glac.ac.a., pet.eth.	13, 29, 36, 40	162
163			132.1		s.bz., chl., glac.ac.a., pet.eth.	13, 29, 36, 40	163
164			120.2		s.bz., chl., glac.ac.a., pet.eth.	13, 29, 36, 40	164
165			120.2		s.ch., pet.eth.	13, 29	165
166	0.983⁴·⁷°	1.4434⁴·⁷°	560.4	253.6	v.s.eth.; s.al.; sl.s.w.	29	166
167		1.4342⁸¹°	560.4	253.6	v.s.h.w.; s.al., eth.	29	167
168			491.6	222.4	s.al., chl., eth.	29	168
169		1.4598²⁵°	137.3	62.1	s.acet., me.al., pet.eth.	29	169

REFERENCES

1. Baudert, *Bull. Soc. Chim. Fr. Ser. 5,* 9, 922 (1942).
2. Bosworth and Brown, *J. Biol. Chem.,* 103, 115 (1933).
3. Bougault and Bourdier, *J. Pharm. Chim. Ser. 6,* 30, 10 (1909).
4. Brown and Farmer, *Biochem. J.,* 29, 631 (1935).
5. Chibnall, Piper, and Williams, *Biochem. J.,* 30, 100 (1936).
6. Chisholm and Hopkins, *Chem. Ind.* (London), p. 1154 (1959).
7. Chisholm and Hopkins, *Can. J. Chem.,* 38, 805 (1960).
8. Chisholm and Hopkins, *Can. J. Chem.,* 38, 2500 (1960).
9. Chisholm and Hopkins, *J. Chem. Soc.,* p. 573 (1962).
10. Chisholm and Hopkins, *J. Org. Chem.,* 27, 3137 (1962).
11. Cole and Cardoss, *J. Am. Chem. Soc.,* 60, 612 (1938).
12. Cole and Cardoss, *J. Am. Chem. Soc.,* 61, 2349 (1939).
13. Deuel, *The Lipids; Their Chemistry and Biochemistry,* Interscience, New York, 1951–57.
14. Dorinson, McCorkle, and Ralston, *J. Am. Chem. Soc.,* 64, 2739 (1942).
15. Dyson, *A Manual of Organic Chemistry,* Vol. I, Longmans, Green, London, 1950.
16. Foreman and Brown, *Oil Soap* (Chicago), 21, 183 (1944).
17. Francis and Piper, *J. Am. Chem. Soc.,* 61, 577 (1939).
18. Gupta, Grollman, and Niyogy, *Proc. Nat. Inst. Sci.* (India), 19, 519 (1953).
19. Hammond and Lundberg, *J. Am. Oil Chem. Soc.,* 30, 438 (1953).
20. Hansen, Shorland, and Cooke, *Chem. Ind.* (London), p. 839 (1951).
21. Heilbron, *Dictionary of Organic Compounds.* Eyre and Spottiswoods, Eds., London, 1934.

FATTY ACIDS: PHYSICAL AND CHEMICAL CHARACTERISTICS (continued)

22. Hilditch and Jones, *Biochem. J.*, 22, 326 (1928).
23. Hopkins and Chisholm, *Chem. Ind.* (London), p. 2064 (1962).
24. Klenk and Bongard, *Z. Phys. Chem.*, 291, 104 (1952).
25. Klenk and Montag, *Ann. Chem.*, 604, 4 (1957).
26. Klenk and Tomuschat, *Z. Phys. Chem.*, 308, 165 (1957).
27. Krewson, Ard, and Riemenschneider, *J. Am. Oil Chem. Soc.*, 39, 334 (1962).
28. Lange, *Handbook of Chemistry*, 6th ed., Handbook Publications, Sandusky, Ohio, 1946.
29. Markley, *Fatty Acids*, 2nd ed., Interscience, New York, 1960–61.
30. Noller and Talbot, *Organic Synthesis Collection*, Vol. 12, John Wiley & Sons, New York, 1943.
31. Nunn, *J. Chem. Soc.*, p. 313 (1952).
32. Piper et al., *Biochem. J.*, 28, 2175 (1934).
33. Power and Rogerson, *J. Am. Chem. Soc.*, 32, 106 (1910).
34. Power and Rogerson, *J. Chem. Soc.*, 101(T), 1 (1912).
35. Prout, Cason, and Ingersoll, *J. Am. Chem. Soc.*, 69, 1233 (1947).
36. Ralston, *Fatty Acids and Their Derivations*, John Wiley & Sons, New York, 1948.
37. Smedley, *Biochem. J.*, 6, 451 (1912).
38. Teresi, J. D., Unpublished. U.S. Naval Radiological Defense Laboratory, San Francisco, Calif.
39. Warth, *The Chemistry and Technology of Waxes*, 2nd ed., Reinhold, New York, 1956.
40. Weitkamp, *J. Am. Chem. Soc.*, 67, 447 (1945).

DENSITIES, SPECIFIC VOLUMES, AND TEMPERATURE COEFFICIENTS OF FATTY ACIDS FROM C_8 TO C_{12}

Acid	Temperature, °C	Density,[a] g/cc	Specific volume, $1/d$	Temp. coeff. per °C
Caprylic	10.0	1.0326	0.9685	0.00098
	15	1.0274	0.9733	—
	20	0.9109	1.0979	0.00046
	20.02	0.9101[b]	—	—
	25	0.9090	1.1002	—
	50.27	0.8862[b]	—	0.00099
Nonanoic	5.0	0.9952	1.0048	0.00074
	10	0.9916	1.0085	—
	15	0.9097	1.0993	0.00104
	15.00	0.9087[b]	—	—
	25	0.9011	1.1097	—
Capric	15.0	1.0266	0.9741	0.00085
	25	1.0176	0.9827	—
	35	0.8927	1.1202	0.00128
	35.05	0.8884[b]	—	—
	40	0.8876	1.1266	—
Hendecanoic	0.12	1.0431	0.9587	0.00054
	10.0	1.0373	0.9640	—
	20	0.9948	1.0052	0.00079
	25	0.9905	1.0096	—
	30	0.8907	1.1227	0.00093
	30.00	0.8889[b]	—	—
	35	0.8871	1.1273	—
	50.15	0.8741[b]	—	0.00095
Lauric	35.0	1.0099	0.9902	0.00087
	40	1.0055	0.9945	—
	45	0.8767	1.1406	0.00142
	45.10	0.8744[b]	—	0.00095
	50	0.8713	1.1477	—
	50.25	0.8707[b]	—	0.00095

[a]By air thermometer method unless specified otherwise.
[b]By pycnometer method.

From Markley, Klare S., *Fatty Acids*, 2nd ed., Part 1, Interscience Publishers, Inc., New York, 1960, 535. With permission of copyright owners.

REFRACTIVE INDICES AND EQUATIONS FOR SOME FATTY ACIDS AND THEIR METHYL ESTERS

Material	Refractive index experimental	Equation R.I.t.[a]
	n_D^{35}	
Methyl oleate	1.44656	1.45968 0.000377t
Methyl eicosenoate	1.44833	1.46134-0.000372t
Methyl erucate	1.44977	1.46288-0.000369t
Oleic acid	1.45442	1.46677 0.000354t
Eicosenoic acid	1.45574	1.46805-0.000351t
Erucic acid	1.45674	1.46892 0.000346t
	$n_D^{60.2}$	
Methyl palmitate	1.42549	1.44830 0.000379t
Methyl stearate	1.42897	1.45149 0.000375t
Methyl arachidate	1.43165	1.45363 0.000366t
Methyl behenate	1.43391	1.45554-0.000358t
	$n_D^{85.6}$	
Palmitic acid	1.42545	1.45589 0.000355t
Stearic acid	1.42830	--
Arachidic acid	1.43066	--
Behenic acid	1.43257	--

[a]R.I.t. = Refractive index at temperature t °C.

From Markley, Klare S., *Fatty Acids*, 2nd ed., Part 1, Interscience Publishers, Inc., New York, 1960, 588. With permission of copyright owners.

REFRACTIVE INDICES[a] OF TWO SERIES OF ALKYL ESTERS AT VARIOUS TEMPERATURES

Substance	20°C	25°C	30°C	35°C	40°C
Ethyl caproate	1.4072	1.4050	1.4029	1.4007	1.3985
Ethyl caprylate	1.4178	1.4157	1.4136	1.4116	1.4095
Ethyl caprate	1.4254	1.4235	1.4215	1.4195	1.4173
Ethyl laurate	1.4315	1.4295	1.4275	1.4255	1.4235
Ethyl myristate	1.4361	1.4340	1.4321	1.4302	1.4282
Ethyl palmitate	--	--	1.4363	1.4343	1.4324
Ethyl stearate	--			1.4375	1.4355
Hexyl ethanoate	1.4091	1.4068	1.4046	1.4023	1.4002
Octyl ethanoate	1.4193	1.4171	1.4150	1.4128	1.4108
Decyl ethanoate	1.4268	1.4247	1.4227	1.4206	1.4186
Dodecyl ethanoate	1.4326	1.4306	1.4286	1.4265	1.4246
Tetradecyl ethanoate	1.4373	1.4352	1.4332	1.4312	1.4293
Hexadecyl ethanoate	—	—	1.4370	1.4350	1.4332
Octadecyl ethanoate	--	-		1.4381	1.4362

[a]Accuracy ±0.0001.

From Markley, Klare S., *Fatty Acids*, 2nd ed., Part 1, Interscience Publishers, Inc., New York, 1960, 588. With permission of copyright owners.

REFRACTIVE INDEX, $n_D^{20°C}$, OF ALKYL MONOESTERS OF CARBOXYLIC AND DIESTERS OF DICARBOXYLIC ACIDS

Material	Methyl	Ethyl	n-Propyl	Iso-Propyl	n-Butyl	Iso-Butyl	n-Amyl	Iso-Amyl
Formate	—	1.35983	1.37693	1.36783	1.38903	1.38546	1.39974	1.39700
Acetate	1.36193	1.37233	1.38442	1.37730	1.39406	1.39018	1.40228	1.40535
Propionate	1.37683	1.38394	1.39319	—	1.40101	—	—	—
n-Butyrate	1.38729	1.39222	1.39950	—	1.40637	—	1.41226	1.41102
Isobutyrate	1.38299	1.38690	1.39552	—	1.40248	—	—	—
Valerate	1.39690	1.40042	1.40672	—	1.41197	—	1.41635	—
Isovalerate	1.39270	1.39621	1.40312	—	1.40875	—	—	—
Caproate	1.40494	1.40712	—	—	—	—	—	—
Heptanoate	1.41152	1.41286	—	—	—	—	—	—
Caprylate	1.41696	1.41803	—	—	—	—	—	—
Caprate	1.42556	1.42556	1.42797	—	1.43048	—	—	—
Laurate	1.43188	1.43108	1.43350	—	1.43620	—	—	—
Oxalate[a]	—	1.41023	1.41646	1.41281	1.42341	—	1.42887	1.42721
Succinate[a]	1.41951	1.41981	1.42521	1.41771	1.42992	1.42666	1.43425	1.43886
Adipate[a]	1.42832	1.42767	1.43143	1.42466	1.43525	—	1.43867	1.43712

[a]Diester.

From Markley, Klare S., *Fatty Acids,* 2nd ed., Part 1, Interscience Publishers, Inc., New York, 1960, 589. With permission of copyright owners.

DIELECTRIC CONSTANTS OF SOME FATS, FATTY ACIDS, AND ESTERS

Compound	Dielectric constant, ε	Temperature °C.	Compound	Dielectric constant, ε	Temperature °C.
Linolenic acid	2.55	−10	Ethyl palmitate	3.07	30
	2.76	20		2.88	69
	2.97	60		2.71	104
	3.01	100		2.57	144
Tripalmitin	2.272	−45		2.46	182
	2.354	−30	Ethyl stearate	2.92	48
	2.402	−6		2.69	100
	2.444	5		2.56	138
	2.544	20		2.48	167
	2.901	55			
	2.954	80	Butyl stearate	3.30	25
	2.924	120	Ethyl oleate	3.17	28
Methyl acetate	6.7	25		3.00	60
Ethyl acetate	6.15	20		2.87	89
Bornyl acetate	4.6	21		2.72	122
Ethyl laurate	3.44	20		2.63	150
	3.16	60	Butyl oleate	4.0	25
	2.91	101	Glyceryl triacetate	9.4	24
	2.73	143			

From Markley, Klare S., *Fatty Acids,* 2nd ed., Part 1, Interscience Publishers, Inc., New York, 1960, 600, 601. With permission of copyright owners.

SOLUBILITIES OF FATTY ACIDS IN WATER

Acid	Grams acid per 100 g water				
	0°C	20°C	30°C	45°C	60°C
Caproic	0.864	0.968	1.019	1.095	1.171
Heptanoic	0.190	0.244	0.271	0.311	0.353
Caprylic	0.044	0.068	0.079	0.095	0.113
Nonanoic	0.014	0.026	0.032	0.041	0.051
Capric	0.0095	0.015	0.018	0.023	0.027
Hendecanoic	0.0063	0.0093	0.011	0.013	0.015
Lauric	0.0037	0.0055	0.0063	0.0075	0.0087
Tridecanoic	0.0021	0.0033	0.0038	0.0044	0.0054
Myristic	0.0013	0.0020	0.0024	0.0029	0.0034
Pentadecanoic	0.00076	0.0012	0.0014	0.0017	0.0020
Palmitic	0.00046	0.00072	0.00083	0.0010	0.0012
Heptadecanoic	0.00028	0.00042	0.00055	0.00069	0.00081
Stearic	0.00018	0.00029	0.00034	0.00042	0.00050

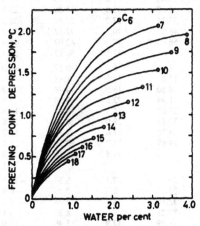

Effect of addition of water on the freezing point of the fatty
acids from C_6 to C_{18}

From Markley, Klare S., *Fatty Acids*, 2nd ed., Part 1,
Interscience Publishers, Inc., New York, 1960, 616. With
permission of copyright owners.

APPROXIMATE SOLUBILITIES OF WATER IN SATURATED FATTY ACIDS AT VARIOUS TEMPERATURES

Acid	Temperature. °C.	Water. %	Acid	Temperature. °C.	Water. %
Caproic	−5.4	2.21	Lauric	42.7	2.35
	12.3	4.73		75.0	2.70
	31.7	7.57		90.5	2.85
	46.3	9.70	Tridecanoic	40.8	2.00
Heptanoic	−8.3	2.98	Myristic	53.2	1.70
	42.5	9.98	Pentadecanoic	51.8	1.46
Caprylic	14.4	3.88	Palmitic	61.8	1.25
Nonanoic	10.5	3.45	Heptadecanoic	60.4	1.06
Capric	29.4	3.12	Stearic	68.7	0.92
Hendecanoic	26.8	2.72		92.4	1.02
	57.5	4.21			

From Markley, Klare S., *Fatty Acids*, 2nd ed., Part 1, Interscience Publishers, Inc., New York, 1960, 617. With permission of copyright owners.

SOLUBILITY[a] OF SIMPLE SATURATED TRIGLYCERIDES

Glyceride	Benzene		Diethyl ether		Chloroform		Ethanol	
	°C	Sol.	°C	Sol.	°C	Sol.	°C	Sol.
Tristearin	14.5	0.45	25.5	0.51	−3.4	0.46	59.8	0.074
	24.0	2.64	27.4	0.98	6.0	1.94	60.8	0.15
	26.7	5.07	31.2	2.11	11.9	4.52	62.4	0.22
	33.6	10.57	34.0	4.80	20.3	10.85	66.8	0.87
	38.1	18.91	40.3	14.25	25.8	15.71	66.9	1.55
	39.6	22.23	44.6	26.20	33.8	25.11		
	41.8	29.10	48.9	39.00	40.4	34.66		
	47.8	44.58	65.1	83.54	49.7	49.31		
	60.4	75.72			61.0	74.15		
Tripalmitin	13.7	7.74	19.0	0.75	2.5	3.08		
	18.3	4.61	24.8	2.12	8.8	7.38		
	22.8	9.69	28.0	4.49	13.5	12.13		
	26.4	16.43	31.0	8.10	18.6	18.40		
	29.5	25.30	33.8	14.06	23.3	24.24		
	34.3	37.11	37.2	21.86	28.3	31.60		
	38.4	48.07	40.3	32.62	32.3	37.67		
	48.0	56.43	43.2	42.07	41.9	52.38		
			47.5	58.12	52.4	71.08		
Trimyristin	11.3	7.56	6.7	0.57	−8.0	3.98		
	14.1	12.03	13.3	1.88	−4.7	6.12		
	15.5	14.50	18.0	4.76	0.9	10.79		
	19.1	21.94	22.2	9.54	5.5	15.04		
	21.2	27.02	25.3	15.12	10.6	21.46		
	24.9	35.85	28.0	24.46	14.8	26.36		
	30.9	49.76	31.0	34.73	19.2	32.25		
	37.2	64.69	35.7	50.53	22.6	38.04		
			40.3	65.16	24.3	40.29		
					38.1	62.90		
Trilaurin	9.0	23.50	−7.2	0.57	−12.5	13.09		
	11.6	28.25	0.8	2.25	−6.9	18.17		
	12.0	32.19	5.1	4.44	0.0	25.29		
	14.3	37.21	9.0	8.36	5.1	30.90		
	16.0	41.29	12.9	15.49	11.0	38.00		
	21.0	52.44	16.0	24.24	19.3	49.41		
	29.5	69.71	19.9	34.42	31.4	69.65		
			24.4	49.78				
			28.0	60.28				
Tricaprin	2.2	45.29	−14.2	3.46			9.5	0.44
	7.2	56.00	−9.5	6.67			13.8	0.99
	9.4	60.39	−3.7	14.64			17.6	2.01
	11.6	64.58	−0.3	21.57			23.4	5.81
			1.2	25.36			25.1	9.87
			3.0	30.40			25.2	14.36
			4.6	36.03			58.5	29.32
			8.5	48.43				
			15.9	69.20				

[a]All solubilities expressed in grams of triglyceride per 100 g solution.

From Markley, Klare S., *Fatty Acids,* 2nd ed., Part 1, Interscience Publishers, Inc., New York, 1960, 644.

SOLUBILITIES[a] OF MIXED TRIACID TRIGLYCERIDES AT 25°C

Material	2-Acyl equals	M.p., °C	Diethyl ether	Petroleum ether	Acetone	Ethanol
1-Stearyl-2-acyl-3-palmitin	Myristyl	59.5	10.97	7.59	0.18	0.03
	Lauryl	57.5	16.49	9.49	0.31	0.03
	Capryl	55.0	22.87	10.60	0.59	0.03
1-Stearyl-2-acyl-3-myristin	Palmityl	58.5	11.03	5.46	0.18	0.03
	Lauryl	55.0	30.68	16.26	0.68	0.04
	Capryl	52.5	53.75	37.03	1.96	0.08
1-Stearyl-2-acyl-3-Laurin	Palmityl	52.0	72.63	58.88	1.47	0.06
	Myristyl	49.5	112.59	81.44	2.53	0.07
	Capryl	41.8	192.13	179.56	13.49	0.39
1-Stearyl-2-acyl-3-caprin	Palmityl	50.0	--	89.97	2.38	0.09
	Myristyl	45.0	—	116.35	9.03	0.31
	Lauryl	44.0	—	148.42	26.04	0.36

[a]All solubilities expressed in grams of triglyceride per 100 g solution.

From Markley, Klare S., *Fatty Acids*, 2nd ed., Part 1, Interscience Publishers, Inc., New York, 1960, 664. With permission of copyright owners.

FORCE-AREA AND RELATED DATA FROM MONOMOLECULAR FILM MEASUREMENTS OF LINSEED OIL ACIDS AND ESTERS

Compound	Refractive index	Mol wt	Area, cm² × 10⁻¹⁶ cm	Molecule length, cm × 10⁻⁸	Area per mol. at point of collapse, cm² × cm 10⁻¹⁶	Force at point of collapse, dynes/cm
Stearic acid	--	284.3	22.5	21.9	18	60
Oleic acid	1.4606	282.3	52	10.2	28	28
Mixed acids[a]	1.4728	280	67	8.2	28	28
Oleic monoglyceride	1.4605	356	47	12.8	25	29
Oleic diglyceride	1.4661	621	86	12.7	63	16.7
Oleic triglyceride	1.4709	885	127	12.3	100	12.3
Stearic monoglyceride		358	27	20.6	20	55
Stearic diglyceride	....	625	49	21.3	41	56
Stearic triglyceride	--	891	72	21.5	—	—
Mixed monoglyceride	1.4788	354	61	10.3	35	25
Mixed diglyceride	1.4811	617	103	10.3	73	15
Mixed triglyceride	1.4832	879	143	10.7	110	12
Lead oleate	.	767	100	10.5	47	27
Manganese linoleate	--	615	125	7.46	57	26.5
Ethylene glycol ester[a]	1.4779	586	98	10.9	72	14
Dimannitol ester[a]	1.4880	706	105	11.5	75	15
Diethylene glycol ester[a]	1.4777	630	110	10.2	73	18.4
Tetramannitol ester[a]	1.4880	1230	176	12.1	147	8.2

[a]Chilled, filtered, and distilled fatty acids of linseed oil.

From Markley, Klare S., *Fatty Acids*, 2nd ed., Part 1, Interscience Publishers, Inc., New York, 1960, 629. With permission of copyright owners.

MOLECULAR DIMENSIONS OF LONG-CHAIN ALIPHATIC ACIDS AND RELATED COMPOUNDS CALCULATED FROM MONOMOLECULAR FILM MEASUREMENTS

Substance	Number of carbon atoms	Head Group	Cross sections, A. (as packed in films)		Approx. length. A.
			Chain	Head	
Myristic acid	14	$-CH_2-CH_2-COOH$	21.0	25.1	21.1
Pentadecanoic acid	15	$-CH_2-CH_2-COOH$	21.0	25.1	22.4
Stearic acid	18	$-CH_2-CH_2-COOH$	21.0	25.1	26.2
Behenic acid	22	$-CH_2-CH_2-COOH$	21.0	25.1	31.4
Iso-oleic acid	18	$-CH=CH-COOH$	21.0	28.7	26.2
Octadecyl urea	19	$-NH-CO-NH_2$	21.0	26.3	28.8
Stearic amide	18	$-CONH_2$	21.0	21.5	26.1
Ethyl palmitate	18	$-COOC_2H_5$	21.0	22.3	26.1
Ethyl behenate	24	$-COOC_2H_5$	21.0	22.3	34.0
Cetyl alcohol	16	$-CH_2OH$	21.0	21.7	22.4
Stearic nitrile	18	$-CH_2CN$	21.0	27.5	—

From Markley, Klare S., *Fatty Acids*, 2nd ed., Part 1, Interscience Publishers, Inc., New York, 1960, 628. With permission of copyright owners.

NMR SPECTRA OF SOME UNSATURATED METHYL ESTERS

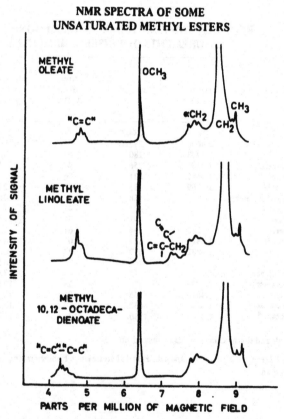

N.M.R. spectra of some unsaturated methyl esters. (Hopkins, *J. Amer. Oil Chem. Soc.*, 38, 664, 1961.)

From Chapman, D., *The Structure of Lipids*, John Wiley & Sons, New York, 1965, 193. With permission of copyright owners.

PROTON CHEMICAL SHIFTS (τ)

Group	Resonance lines of the "bold faced" protons, τ	Group	Resonance lines of the "bold faced" protons, τ
Alkane		or $-CH_2-O-Ar$	5.71–6.08
		$-CH_2-Cl$	6.43–6.65
$\triangle CH_2$	9.78	$-CH_2-Br$	6.42–6.75
$-CH_2-$	8.52–8.75	$-CH_2-I$	6.80–6.97
		CH_3-SO-R	7.50
β-functional groups		$-CH_2-SO_2-R$	7.08
$-CH_2-C-N$	8.38–8.80	CH_3-SO_2-Cl	6.36
$-CH_2-C-CO-R$	8.10–8.37	$-CH_2-SO_2F$	6.72
CH_3-C-N	8.92–9.12	$CH_3-O-SO-OR$	6.42
$CH_3-C-N-CO-R$	8.80	CH_3-O-SO_2-OR	6.06
$CH_3-C-CO-R$	8.88–9.07	$CH_3-S-C\equiv N$	7.37
$-CH_2-C-C=C-$	8.40–8.82	$-CH_2-N=C=S$	6.39
$-CH_2-C-Ar$	8.22–8.40	$-CH_2-NO_2$	5.62
$-CH_2-C-O-R$	8.19–8.79	$-CH_2(C=C-)_2$	6.95–7.10
$-CH_2-C-O-COR$ and $-CH_2-C-O-Ar$	8.50	$Ar-CH_2-C=C-$	6.62
$-CH_2-C-Cl$	8.04–8.40	**Alkyl Groups α to Two or More Functional Groups**	
$-CH_2-C-Br$	7.97–8.32	$Ar-CH_2-Ar$	6.08–6.19
$-CH_2-C-I$	8.14–8.35	$Ar-CH_2-N$	6.68
$-CH_2-C-SO_2-R$	7.84	$Ar-CH_3-OR$	5.51–5.64
$-CH_2-C-NO_2$	7.93	$Ar-CH_2-Cl$	5.50
		$Ar-CH_2-Br$	5.57–5.59
α-functional groups		$Ar-CH_2-O-CO-R$	4.74
$-CH_2-\overset{\vert}{C}=\overset{\vert}{C}-$	7.69–8.17	$-C=C-CH_2-O-R$	6.03–6.10
		$-C=C-CH_2-Cl$	5.96–6.04
$CH_3-\overset{\vert}{C}=\overset{\vert}{C}-CO-R$	7.94–8.07	$-C=C-CH_2-OR$	5.82
$-CH_2-\overset{\vert}{C}=\overset{\vert}{C}-O-R$	8.07	$-C\equiv C-CH_2-Cl$	5.84–5.91
		$-C\equiv C-CH_2-Br$	6.18
$CH_3-\overset{\vert}{C}=\overset{\vert}{C}-$ $\overset{\vert}{COOR}$ or CN	7.97–8.06	$Cl-CH_2-C\equiv N$	5.93
		$Br-CH_2-C\equiv N$	6.30
$CH_3-\overset{\vert}{C}=\overset{\vert}{C}-$ $\overset{\vert}{O-CO-R}$	8.09–8.13	$-CH(OR)_2$	4.80–5.20
$CH_3-\overset{\vert}{C}=\overset{\vert}{C}-$ $-C=C-$	8.17	**Acetylenic and Olefinic Protons**	
$-CH_2-Ar$	6.94–7.47	$-C\equiv C-H$	7.07–7.67
$-CH_2-C\equiv N$	7.42	$-C=C-C\equiv C-H$	7.13
$CH_3-C=NOH$	8.19	$Ar-C\equiv C-H$	6.95
$-CH_2-CO-R$	7.61–7.98	$-C=CH-$	4.87
(R=H, Alkyl, Aryl, OH, OR or NH₂)		$-C=CH_2$	5.37
$CH_3-CO-Cl$ (or Br)	7.19–7.34	$-C=CH-CO-R$	3.95–4.32
$CH_3-CO-C=C-$ or $CH_3-CO-Ar$	7.32–8.17	$-CH=C-CO-R$	2.96–4.53
$CH_3-CO-SR$	7.46–7.67	$-C=CH-O-R$	3.55–3.78
$-CH_3-S-R$	7.47–7.61	$-CH=C-O-R$	4.45–5.46
$-\overset{\vert}{N}-\overset{\vert}{C}-$ $\overset{\vert}{CH_2}$	8.52	$C=CH-O-CO-CH_3$	2.75
		$H_2C=C-O-CH_2-C=C$	5.87–6.17
$-CH_2-N$	6.88–7.72	$R-CO-CH=C-CO-R$	3.87–3.97
$-CH_2-N-CO-R$ (or $N-SO_2R$ or $N-Ar$)	6.63–6.72	$Br-CH=C-$	3.00–3.38
$-CH_2-N^+-$	6.60	$-CH=C-C\equiv N$	4.25
CH_3-N-N-	7.67	$Ar-C=CH-$	4.60–4.72
$-\overset{\vert}{C}-O$ $\overset{\vert}{CH_2}$	7.71	$Ar-CH=C-$	3.72–3.77
		$\overset{H-C=C-}{\underset{H \quad CO-R}{}}$	3.60–3.70
$-CH_2-O-R$	6.42–7.69	$Ar-CH-C-CO-R$	2.28–2.62
$-CH_3-O-CO-R$		**Aldehydes**	
		$R-CHO$	0.20–0.43
		$>C=C-CHO$	0.32–0.57
		$Ar-CHO$	−0.08 to +0.35
		Carboxylic Acids	
		$R-COOH$	−0.97 to −1.52
		$>C=C-COOH$	−1.57 to −2.18

PROTON CHEMICAL SHIFTS (τ) (continued)

Hydroxyl Groups. The position of the hydroxyl proton is very dependent on concentration, temperature, and the presence of other easily exchanged protons (H_2O!). It is displaced strongly to lower τ values by intramolecular hydrogen bonding (in some stable planar systems to $\tau = -5.0$) and to higher values by increased shielding.

Amine Protons. The position of $-NH_2$ and $-NH$ protons is dependent above all on the basicity of the nitrogen atom. Strongly basic amines show $NH-$ absorption in the C-methyl region.

R$-$NH$_2$ and R$-$NH$-$	7.88–8.90
R$-$CO$-$NH$-$	2.3 –3.9
	2.6 –2.7

2.68 τ is due to the symmetrically placed aromatic protons; this assignment is justified on the basis of the chemical shift as well as the known patterns for *p*-disubstituted benzene derivatives. Area measurements indicate that the quartet around 5.58 τ is a one proton signal. The multiplet centered at 6.75 τ must account for the remaining two protons. The first degree approximation of the $n + 1$ rule is not applicable here. The three protons on the heterocyclic ring constitute a special grouping (ABX) and lead to a characteristic pattern.

From *Interpretive Spectroscopy,* Freeman, Stanley K., ed. Copyright © 1965 by Reinhold Publishing Corporation, by permission of Van Nostrand Reinhold Company.

MASS SPECTRA OF METHYL OLEATE, METHYL LINOLEATE AND METHYL LINOLENATE

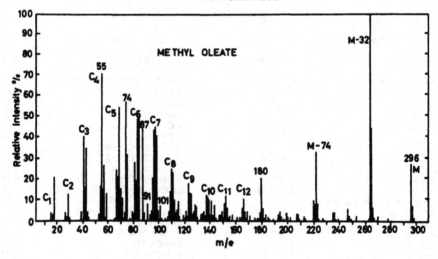

MASS SPECTRA OF METHYL OLEATE, METHYL LINOLEATE AND
METHYL LINOLENATE (continued)

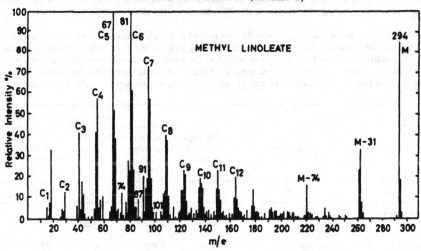

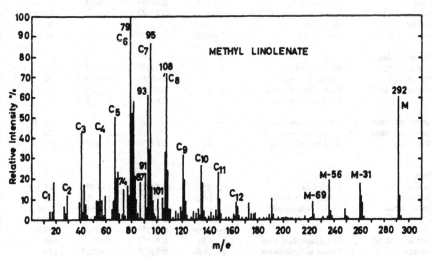

Mass spectra of: (*top*) methyl oleate (methyl $\Delta^{9:10}$-octadecenoate) (M = 296): (*middle*) methyl linoleate (methyl $\Delta^{9:10,12:13}$-octadecdienoate) (M = 294): (*bottom*) methyl linolenate (methyl $\Delta^{9:10,12:13,15:16}$-octadec-trienoate) ($M$ = 292). (Hallgren, Rvhage and Stenhagen *Acta Chem Scand* 13, 845, 1959.)

PROPERTIES AND FATTY ACID COMPOSITION OF FATS AND OILS

These data were compiled originally for Harwood, H. J. and Geyer, R. P., *Biology Data Book,* the Federation of American Societies for Experimental Biology, Washington, D.C., 1964, 380. By permission of the copyright owners.

Values are typical rather than average and frequently were derived from specific analyses for particular samples (especially the constituent fatty acids). Extreme variations may occur, depending on a number of variables such as source, treatment, and age of a fat or oil. Specific Gravity (column D) was calculated at the specified temperature (degrees centigrade) and referred to water at the same temperature, unless otherwise specified. Density, shown in parentheses (column D), was measured at the specified temperature (degrees centigrade). Refractive Index (column E) was measured at 50°C, unless otherwise specified.

			Constants			
Fat or Oil	Source	Melting (or solidi-fication) point, °C	Specific gravity (or density)	Refractive index $n_D^{40\,°C}$	Iodine value	Saponi-fication value
No (A)	(B)	(C)	(D)	(E)	(F)	(G)
Land Animals						
1 Butterfat	*Bos taurus*	32.2	$0.911^{40/15'}$	1.4548	36.1	227
2 Depot fat	*Homo sapiens*	(15)	$0.918^{15'}$	1.4602	67.6	196.2
3 Lard oil	*Sus scrofa*	(30.5)	$0.919^{15'}$	1.4615	58.6	194.6
4 Neat's-foot oil	*B.taurus*	—	$0.910^{25'}$	1.464^{25}	69–76	190–199
5 Tallow, beef	*B. taurus*	—	—	—	49.5	197
6 Tallow, mutton	*Ovis aries*	(42.0)	$0.945^{15'}$	1.4565	40	194
Marine Animals						
7 Cod-liver oil	*Gadus morhua*	—	$0.925^{25'}$	$1.481^{25'}$	165	186
8 Herring oil	*Clupea harengus*	—	0.900^{60}	$1.4610^{60'}$	140	192
9 Menhaden oil	*Brevoortia tyrannus*	—	$0.903^{60'}$	1.4645^{60}	170	191
10 Sardine oil	*Sardinops caerulea*	—	0.905^{60}	1.4660^{60}	185	191
11 Sperm oil, body	*Physeter macrocephalus*	—	—	—	76–88	122–130
12 Sperm oil, head	*P. macrocephalus*	—	—	—	70	140–144
13 Whale oil	*Balaena mysticetus*	—	$0.892^{60'}$	$1.460^{60'}$	120	195
Plants						
14 Babassu oil	*Attalea funifera*	22–26	$(0.893^{60'})$	1.443^{60}	15.5	247
15 Castor oil	*Ricinus communis*	(−18.0)	$0.961^{15'}$	1.4770	85.5	180.3
16 Cocoa butter	*Theobroma cacaô*	34.1	$0.964^{15'}$	1.4568	36.5	193.8
17 Coconut oil	*Cocos nucifera*	25.1	$0.924^{15'}$	1.4493	10.4	268
18 Corn oil	*Zea mays*	(−20.0)	$0.922^{15'}$	1.4734	122.6	192.0
19 Cotton seed oil	*Gossypium hirsutum*	(−1.0)	0.917^{25}	1.4735	105.7	194.3
20 Linseed oil	*Linum usitatissimum*	(−24.0)	$0.938^{15'}$	$1.4782^{25'}$	178.7	190.3
21 Mustard oil	*Brassica hirta*	—	$0.9145^{15'}$	1.475	102	174
22 Neem oil	*Melia azadirachta*	−3	$0.917^{15'}$	1.4615	71	194.5
23 Niger-seed oil	*Guizotia abyssinica*	—	$0.925^{15'}$	1.471	128.5	190
24 Oiticica oil	*Licania rigida*	—	$0.974^{25'}$	—	140–180	—
25 Olive oil	*Olea europaea sativa*	(−6.0)	$0.918^{15'}$	1.4679	81.1	189.7
26 Palm oil	*Elaeis guineensis*	35.0	$0.915^{15'}$	1.4578	54.2	199.1
27 Palm-kernel oil	*E. guineensis*	24.1	$0.923^{15'}$	1.4569	37.0	219.9
28 Peanut oil	*Arachis hypogaea*	(3.0)	$0.914^{15'}$	1.4691	93.4	192.1
29 Perilla oil	*Perilla frutescens*	—	$(0.935^{15'})$	$1.481^{25'}$	195	192
30 Poppy-seed oil	*Papaver somniferum*	(−15)	$0.925^{15'}$	1.4685	135	194
31 Rapeseed oil	*Brassica campestris*	(−10)	$0.915^{15'}$	1.4706	98.6	174.7
32 Safflower oil	*Carthamus tinctorius*	—	$(0.900^{60'})$	$1.462^{60'}$	145	192
33 Sesame oil	*Sesamum indicum*	(−6.0)	$0.919^{25'}$	1.4646	106.6	187.9
34 Soybean oil	*Glycine soja*	(−16.0)	$0.927^{15'}$	1.4729	130.0	190.6
35 Sunflower-seed oil	*Helianthus annuus*	(−17.0)	$0.923^{15'}$	1.4694	125.5	188.7
36 Tung oil	*Aleurites fordi*	(−2.5)	$0.934^{15'}$	$1.5174^{25'}$	168.2	193.1
37 Wheat-germ oil	*Triticum aestivum*	—	—	—	125	—

PROPERTIES AND FATTY ACID COMPOSITION OF FATS AND OILS (continued)

Constituent fatty acids, g 100 g total fatty acids

	Saturated						Unsaturated					
	Lauric	Myristic	Palmitic	Stearic	Arachidic	Other	Palmitoleic	Oleic	Linoleic	Linolenic	Other	
No	(H)	(I)	(J)	(K)	(L)	(M)	(N)	(O)	(P)	(Q)	(R)	No
1	2.5	11.1	29.0	9.2	2.4	2.0^a; 0.5^b; 2.3^c	4.6	26.7	3.6	—	3.6^d; 0.1^e; 0.1^f; 0.9^g; 1.4^h; 1.0^i; 1.0^j; 0.4^k	1
2	—	2.7	24.0	8.4	—	—	5	46.9	10.2	—	2.5	2
3	—	1.3	28.3	11.9	—	—	2.7	47.5	6	--	0.2^g; 2.1^h	3
4	—	—	17–18	2–3	—	—	—	74–76	—	—		4
5	—	6.3	27.4	14.1	—	—	—	49.6	2.5	-.-	—	5
6	—	4.6	24.6	30.5	—	—	—	36.0	4.3	-	—	6
7	—	5.8	8.4	0.6	--	—	20.0	←——29.1——→		—	25.4^l; 9.6^m	7
8	—	7.3	13.0	Trace	—	—	4.9	—	--	<1%	30.1^l; 23.2^m	8
9	—	5.9	16.3	0 6	0.6	—	15.5	—	—	<1%	19.0^l; 11.7^m; 0.8^n	9
10	—	5.1	14.6	3.2	---	—	11.8	←——17.8——→		--	18.1^l; 14.0^m; trace^g; 15.4	10
11	1	5	6.5	—	—	—	26.5	37	19	—	1^m; 4^g; 19^p	11
12	16	14	8	2	—	3.5^c	15	17	6.5	—	4^f; 14^g; 6.5^p	12
13	0.2	9.3	15.6	2.8	---	—	14.4	35.2	—	--	13.6^l; 5.9^m; 2.5^g; 0.2^q	13
14	44.1	15.4	8.5	2.7	0.2	0.2^a; 4.8^b; 6.6^c	—	16.1	1.4	—	—	14
15	←———2.4———→				--	.	--	7.4	3.1	---	87^r	15
16	—	—	24.4	35.4	—	—	—	38.1	2.1	—	—	16
17	45.4	18.0	10.5	2.3	0.4^s	0.8^a; 5.4^b; 8.4^c	0.4	7.5	Trace	---	---	17
18	—	1.4	10.2	3.0	--	—	1.5	49.6	34.3	—	---	18
19	—	1.4	23.4	1.1	1.3	—	2.0	22.9	47.8	—	--	19
20	—	—	6.3	2.5	0.5	—	-.-	19.0	24.1	47.4	0.2^n	20
21	—	1.3^t	—	—	—	—	—	27.2^t	16.6^t	1.8^t	1.1^n; 1.0^u; 51.0^v	21
22	—	2.6^t	14.1^t	24.0^t	0.8^t	--	—	58.5^t	—	—	—	22
23	—	3.3^t	8.2^t	4.8^t	0.5^t	—	—	30.3^t	57.3^t	—	—	23
24	←———11.3^w———→					—	--	6.2	—	—	82.5^x	24
25	—	Trace	6.9	2.3	0.1	—	--	84.4	4.6	—	—	25
26	—	1.4	40.1	5.5	—	—	—	42.7	10.3	—	—	26
27	46.9	14.1	8.8	1.3	—	2.7^b; 7.0^c	—	18.5	0.7	—	—	27
28	—	—	8.3	3.1	2.4	—	—	56.0	26.0	—	3.1^n; 1.1^u	28
29	←———9.6^w———→					—	—	17.8	—	17.5	—	29
30	—	—	4.8^t	2.9^t	—	—	—	30.1^t	62.2^t	—	—	30
31	—	—	1	—	—	--	—	32	15	1	50^v	31
32	←———6.8^w———→					—	—	18.6	70.1	3.4	--	32
33	—	—	9.1	4.3	0.8	—	—	45.4	40.4	—	--	33
34	0.2	0.1	9.8	2.4	0.9	—	0.4	28.9	50.7	6.5	0.1^g	34
35	—	—	5.6	2.2	0.9	—	—	25.1	66.2	—	—	35
36	←———4.6^w———→					—	—	4.1	0.6	—	90.7^y	36
37	←———16.0^w———→					—	—	28.1	52.3	3.6	—	37

[a] Caproic.
[b] Caprylo.
[c] Capric.
[d] Butyric.
[e] Decenoic.
[f] C_{12} monoethenoic.
[g] C_{14} monoethenoic.
[h] Gadoleic plus erucic.
[i] C_{12} n-pentadecanoic.
[j] C_{17} margaric.

[k] 12-Methyl tetradecanoic.
[l] C_{20} polyethenoic.
[m] C_{22} polyethenoic.
[n] Behenic.
[o] C_{14} polyethenoic.
[p] Gadoleic.
[q] C_{24} polyethenoic.
[r] Ricinoleic.
[s] Includes behenic and lignoceric.
[t] Percent by weight.

[u] Lignoceric.
[v] Erucic.
[w] Includes behenic.
[x] Licanic.
[y] Eleostearic.

COMPOSITION OF ACIDS OF BEESWAX FRACTIONS

Chain length	Whole wax	Free acids	Monoesters	Diesters	Triesters	Hydroxy monoesters	Hydroxy polyesters	Acid esters	Acid polyesters	Unidentified
16	59.8		85.1	85.0	92.7	91.4	92.8	86.4	69.4	70.4
18:0	2.6		3.0	3.6	4.8	5.5	3.9	6.9	4.8	8.2
18:1[a]	4.1		10.9	10.6	1.3	2.4	—	6.7	11.1	8.3
20	1.5		1.0	0.4	0.4	0.3	0.1	—	0.2	2.4
22	1.3	3.3	—	—	0.3	—	0.2	—	1.4	1.5
24	11.9	46.8	—	0.4	0.5	0.4	1.5	—	6.5	3.5
26	4.2	12.3	—	—	—	—	0.3	—	1.2	0.9
28	4.3	12.1	—	—	—	—	0.3	—	1.1	0.8
30	3.8	8.4	—	—	—	—	0.3	—	1.2	0.7
32	3.2	7.8	—	—	—	—	0.3	—	1.2	0.7
34	3.1	8.3	—	—	—	—	0.3	—	1.7	1.1
36	0.2	10	—	—	—	—	—	—	0.2	0.1
Unidentified	—	—	—	—	—	—	—	—	—	1.4

[a]Shown to be oleic acid.

From Tulloch, *Chem. Phys. Lipids*, 6, 245 (1971). With permission.

ECL[a] OF METHYL OCTADECADIENOATES AND OCTADECATRIENOATES

			ECL			
Ester	Apiezon L	PPE	DEGS	XF1150	110% CN	TCPE
cis-5,cis-12		18.04				
cis-6,cis-10		18.06				
cis-6,cis-11		18.01				
cis-6,cis-12		18.10				
cis-7,cis-12		18.05				
cis-8,cis-12		18.15				
cis-9,cis-12	17.50	18.19	19.06	19.08	19.16	19.49
cis-9,trans-12	17.59	18.35		18.95	18.96	19.36
trans-9,cis-12		18.43				19.42
trans-9,trans-12	17.65	18.41	19.00	18.67	18.69	19.14
cis 9,cis-15	17.66	18.32	19.24	19.22	19.29	19.59
cis-9,trans-15	17.60	18.30	19.04	18.89		19.32
trans-9,cis-15	17.75	18.45	19.18	19.05		19.46
trans-9,trans-15	17.68	18.40	18.98	18.68		19.13
cis-12,cis-15	17.83	18.46	19.45	19.41	19.48	19.82
cis-12,trans-15		18.51	19.30			19.56
trans-12,cis15		18.61	19.38			19.68
trans-12,trans-15	17.85	18.55	19.23			19.34
cis-9,cis-12,cis-15		18.52	19.91	19.90	20.00	20.49
cis-9,trans-12cis-15		18.55		19.91	19.80	
trans-9,cis-12,trans-15		18.79		19.50	19.52	20.15
trans-9,trans-12,trans-15		18.83	19.75	19.14	19.12	19.91

[a]Abbreviations: ECL, equivalent chain length; PPE, polyphenyl ether; DEGS, diethylene glycol succinate; 100% CN, 100% cyanoethyl silicone; TCPE, tetracyanoethylated pentaerythritol.

From Scholfield and Dutton, *J. Am. Oil Chem. Soc.*, 48, 228, (1971). With permission.

COLUMNS USED FOR DETERMINATION
OF ECL[a] VALUES

Coating	Temperature °C	Pressure psi	Length ft
Apiezon L	200	45–55	200
PPE 6 ring	190	40	150
DEGS	165	45	200
GE X F1150	170	30	200
100% CN	200	20	200
TCPE	160	45	200

[a]Abbreviations: ECL, equivalent chain length; PPE, polyphenyl ether; DEGS, diethylene glycol succinate; 100% cyanoethyl silicone; TCPE, tetracyanoethylated pentaerythritol.

From Scholfield and Dutton, *J. Am. Oil Chem. Soc.*, 48,228 (1971). With permission.

KEY FRAGMENTS IN THE SPECTRA OF PYRROLIDIDES OF MONOUNSATURATED FATTY ACIDS

Pyrrolidide	m/e	Relative intensity	m/e	Relative intensity	m/e	Relative intensity	m/e	Relative intensity	m/e	Relative intensity	m/e	Relative intensity	Molecular peak m/e	Relative intensity
cis-4-18:1	124	1.8	126	10.8	138	2.9	139	4.2	152	13.9	166	57.0	335	17.2
cis-5-18:1	126	6.3	138	0.3	140	0.6	152	0.5	166	1.6	180	2.5	335	5.3
cis-6-18:1	140	7.7	152	1.5	154	1.7	166	5.6	168	1.5	180	8.1	335	14.3
cis-7-18:1	154	9.8	166	2.5	168	4.4	180	6.5	182	2.5	194	7.2	335	16.6
cis-8-18:1	168	13.2	180	2.0	182	4.5	194	2.4	196	0.9	208	4.2	335	18.1
cis-9-18:1	182	11.4	194	1.0	196	2.5	208	2.3	210	0.7	222	3.6	335	24.8
trans-9-18:1	182	11.0	194	1.2	196	2.4	208	2.2	210	0.8	222	3.6	335	24.0
cis-10-18:1	196	7.4	208	1.0	210	2.0	222	1.8	224	0.7	236	3.3	335	29.8
cis-11-18:1	210	4.9	222	1.1	224	1.6	236	1.5	238	0.7	250	2.7	335	29.0
cis-12-18:1	224	4.8	236	0.7	238	1.5	250	1.2	252	0.8	264	3.0	335	33.8
cis-13-18:1	238	4.5	250	0.6	252	1.3	264	1.1	266	0.5	278	2.9	335	33.0
cis-14-18:1	252	3.9	264	0.4	266	0.9	278	1.2	280	0.5	292	2.6	335	28.8
cis-15-18:1	266	3.1	278	0.5	280	1.0	292	1.3	306	2.4	320	2.9	335	28.4
cis-16-18:1	266	2.3	278	0.6	280	3.3	292	1.1	294	0.7	306	1.2	335	26.0
cis-17-18:1	280	0.9	292	0.6	294	1.6	306	0.4	308	0.2	320	0.4	335	8.1
cis-4-10:1	124	3.5	126	6.9	138	6.0	139	6.1	152	26.0	166	99.0	223	33.5
cis-9-14:1	182	12.0	194	1.4	196	2.7	208	2.6	210	1.0	222	4.0	279	28.0
cis-9-16:1	182	11.0	194	1.4	196	2.2	208	3.3	210	0.8	222	3.8	307	26.0
cis-11-20:1	210	4.4	222	0.9	224	1.8	236	1.4	238	0.9	250	2.7	363	28.0
cis-13-22:1	238	4.4	250	2.1	252	2.8	264	2.0	266	1.2	278	4.2	391	37.0
cis-15-24:1	266	2.3	278	0.6	280	1.1	292	1.0	294	0.6	306	2.9	419	34.3

From Andersson and Holman, *Lipids*, 9, 185 (1974). With permission.

THE LIPID COMPOSITION OF VARIOUS PARTS OF ADULT HUMAN SKIN

Component	Sebum[a] %	Epidermis[b] %	Surface lipids[c] %
Squalene	12	<0.5	10
Sterol esters	<1	10	2.5
Sterols (unesterified)	0	20	1.5
Wax esters	23	0	22
Triacyl glycerols	60[d]	10	25
Di- and monoacyl glycerols	0	10	10
Unesterified fatty acids	0	10	25
Glyco- and phospholipids	0	30	0
Unidentified	5	10	4

[a]Computed from thin-layer chromatography data of sebaceous gland lipids (1) and unpublished data (2).
[b]Computed from Miettinen and Luukkäinen (3) and Nicolaides (1).
[c]Computed from Nicolaides (1).
[d]Note that the sum of the tri-, di-, and monoacyl glycerols plus the unesterified fatty acids constitute 60% of the lipids for both sebum and surface lipids.

From Nicolaides, *Science*, 186, 19 (1974). Copyright 1974 by the American Association for the Advancement of Science. With permission.

REFERENCES

1. Nicolaides, *J. Am. Oil Chem. Soc.*, 42, 691 (1965).
2. Nicolaides and Wells, *J. Invest. Dermatol.*, 29, 423 (1957).
3. Miettnen and Luukkäinen, *Acta Chem. Scand.*, 22, 2603 (1968).

TWENTY-ONE OF THE FATTY ACIDS OF HUMAN SKIN SURFACE LIPIDS

Each of the Fatty Acids Listed Constitutes at Least 0.5% of the Total

Name	Abbreviated formula	Amount %
Palmitic[a]	$n\text{-}C_{16}$	25.33
cis-Hexadec-6-enoic	$C_{16:1}\Delta6$	21.70
cis-Octadec-8-enoic	$C_{18:1}\Delta8$	8.75
Myristic[a]	$n\text{-}C_{14}$	6.88
cis-15-Methylpentadec-6-enoic	iso-$C_{16:1}\Delta6$	3.96
Pentadecanoic	$n\text{-}C_{15}$	3.95
Stearic[a]	$n\text{-}C_{18}$	2.89
cis-Octadec-6-enoic (petroselenic)	$C_{18:1}\Delta6$	1.87
Oleic[a]	$C_{18:1}\Delta9$	1.87
cis-Heptadec-6-enoic	$C_{17:1}\Delta6$	1.31
12-Methyltetradecanoic	anteiso-C_{15}	1.13
Octadeca-5,8-dienoic (sebaleic)	$C_{18:2}\Delta5,8$	1.12
cis-Tetradec-6-enoic	$C_{14:1}\Delta6$	1.06
Heptadecanoic	$n\text{-}C_{17}$	1.06
cis-Heptadec-8-enoic	$C_{17:1}\Delta8$	0.82
cis-14-Methylhexadec-6-enoic	anteiso-$C_{17:1}\Delta6$	0.81
cis-16-Methylheptadec-8-enoic	iso-$C_{18:1}\Delta8$	0.78
4-Methyltetradecanoic	4-Me-C_{14}	0.70
Linoleic[a]	$C_{18:2}\Delta9,12$	0.53
cis-Eicos-10-enoic	$C_{20:1}\Delta10$	0.52
cis-Eicos-7,10-dienoic	$C_{20:2}\Delta7,10$	0.51
Total[b]		87.55

[a]"Biologically valuable" acids (total, 37%).
[b]Some 200 additional acids make up the remaining 12.45%.

From Nicolaides, *Science,* 186, 19 (1974). Copyright 1974 by the American Association for the Advancement of Science. With permission.

FATTY ACIDS OF WAX ESTERS AND STEROL ESTERS FROM VERNIX CASEOSA AND FROM HUMAN SKIN SURFACE LIPID[a]

	Wax esters				Sterol esters			
	Saturates		Hydrogenated monoenes		Saturates		Hydrogenated monoenes	
ECL[c]	VC[b] %	HSL %	VC %	HSL %	VC %	HSL %	VC %	HSL %
11.22	0.02	Trace						
11.50	0.43					Trace		
11.65	Trace	0.17			Trace	0.21		
12	0.77	0.96	Trace	Trace	Trace	0.64		
12.12	Trace	0.30				Trace		
12.48	2.01	1.24				0.54		
12.68	0.87	0.12			Trace	Trace		
13	0.76	0.37	0.04	0.04	Trace	0.37		
13.15	Trace	Trace				Trace		
13.20	0.44	0.24			Trace			
13.3						Trace		
13.48	0.15	Trace			Trace	0.06		
13.66	9.28	5.99	0.03	Trace	2.25	3.18	Trace	Trace
14	8.13	13.04	7.62	6.76	1.25	13.69	0.60	5.25
14.2	Trace	Trace	Some ?	Trace ?	Some ?	Some ?		
14.48	2.85	2.78			Trace	2.49		
14.69	16.60	5.32	0.63	2.23	6.41	4.75	Trace	1.05
15	5.22	6.85	6.86	5.06	1.02	7.12	0.70	3.54
15.2	Trace	Trace	Some ?			Some ?		
15.49	Trace	0.07			Trace	0.20		
15.65	14.63	5.04	8.78	21.56	15.24	4.62	2.02	10.09
16	20.50	40.13	48.39	47.01	5.02	32.25	11.61	45.83
16.2	Trace	Trace	Some	Some ?		Some ?		
16.50	2.17	3.99	Some	Some ?	Trace	3.09	Trace	
16.72	5.76	0.75	6.92	3.84	3.45	1.31	1.21	2.22
17	0.96	2.02	5.13	2.07	0.24	2.32	1.93	3.34
17.22	0.08	Trace	Some ?		0.05	0.07		
17.52	Trace	0.04		Some		0.07		
17.65	0.84	0.38	0.98	1.49	3.65	0.60	3.32	2.49
18	3.78	4.83	13.18	8.60	1.29	6.05	32.24	20.76
18.2	Trace	Trace	Some ?			0.05		
18.49	Trace	Trace	0.02		0.15	0.05		
18.6						0.07		
18.72	0.69	Trace	0.04	0.14	1.32	0.21	0.40	0.22

[a]VC = vernix caseosa, HSL = human surface lipid. Percentage figures are given to two decimal places simply to round out the data and show relative amounts of the minor components. Accuracy is estimated at ± 5%.

[b]Traces of material to ECL's of 10.50 were seen for this sample.

[c]ECL = equivalent chain length (1). The ECL's listed are an average of all eight samples. Where only one decimal is listed the error is estimated at ± 0.05 for all samples: Where two decimals are given maximum error for all samples is ± 0.04 and usually ± 0.02 or less.

FATTY ACIDS OF WAX ESTERS AND STEROL ESTERS FROM VERNIX CASEOSA AND FROM HUMAN SKIN SURFACE LIPID[a] (continued)

| | Wax esters | | | | Sterol esters | | | |
| | Saturates | | Hydrogenated monoenes | | Saturates | | Hydrogenated monoenes | |
ECL[c]	VC[b] %	HSL %	VC %	HSL %	VC %	HSL %	VC %	HSL %
19	0.07	0.26	0.19	0.21	0.06	0.58	0.66	0.58
19.66	0.76	0.24	0.09	0.09	12.90	1.23	3.38	0.52
20	0.25	0.70	0.64	0.53	0.84	1.68	9.55	1.53
20.4		Trace			0.60	0.01		
20.5	Trace	Trace				0.04	Trace ?	
20.72	0.25	0.09	0.02	0.01	6.80	0.55	0.39	0.06
21	Trace	0.05	0.03	0.01	Trace	0.32	0.49	0.06
21.47			0.02	0.03	Some			
21.65	0.30	0.21	0.03	0.01	12.43	1.25	1.59	0.14
22	0.12	0.47	0.11	0.07	0.64	1.23	12.47	0.06
22.2			0.02			Some ?		
22.5					0.60	0.20		
22.74	0.15	0.15	0.01	Trace	4.69	0.49	0.18	0.05
23	0.02	0.16	0.02	0.01	0.20	0.26	0.35	0.06
23.2		Trace						
23.3	Trace							
23.4	Trace		Trace			Trace		
23.5				Trace	Some			
23.64	0.35	0.52	0.01	0.04	7.76	1.57	1.88	0.27
24	0.30	1.11	0.07	0.05	0.95	2.90	9.04	0.75
24.2						0.07		
24.5	Trace	Some ?	0.01		0.60	0.05		
24.75	0.25	0.43	0.01	Trace ?	3.96	1.00	0.16	0.07
25	0.02	0.28	0.01	Trace	Trace	0.54	0.14	0.07
25.4					Some ?			
25.6	0.15	0.33	0.01	0.04	3.38	0.88	0.64	0.26
26	0.03	0.37	0.04	0.04	0.40	0.94	1.43	0.19
26.4						0.03		
26.7	0.02	Trace	Trace	0.02	1.11	0.07	Trace	Trace
27	Trace	Trace	Trace	0.02	Trace	0.04	Trace	Trace
27.6	0.02	Trace	0.01	0.01	0.60	0.03	Trace	Trace
28	Trace	Trace	0.02	0.01	Trace	0.03	0.50	Trace
28.4					Trace			
28.7					0.14			Trace
29			Trace			0.03	Trace	Trace
29.5					Trace			
29.6								Trace
30		Trace	0.02				0.21	
	100.00	100.00	100.00	100.00	100.00	100.00	100.00	100.00

REFERENCE

1.   Miwa, Mikolajczak, Earle, and Wolff, *Anal. Chem.*, 32, 1739 (1960).

From Nicolaides, Fu, Hwei, Ansari, and Rice, *Lipids*, 7, 506 (1972). With permission.

THE ANALYSIS OF FATTY ACIDS

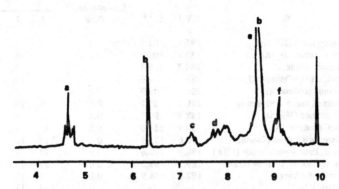

NMR spectrum of methyl linoleate in carbon tetrachloride solution (15% w/v) at 60 MHz tetramethylsilane as internal standard).

From Christie, *Lipid Analysis*, Pergamon Press, Oxford, 1973. With permission.

SUNFLOWER HULL COMPOSITION

Wax Fatty Acids Composition

Fatty acids	%[a]
Myristic	1.94
Pentadecanoic	0.4
Palmitic	6.8
Heptadecanoic	0.2
Iso-stearic	0.35
Stearic	5.6
Oleic	4.72
Nonadecylic	3.07
Linoleic	0.78
Iso-arachidic	1.3
Arachidic	46.5
Iso-medullic	0.9
Medullic	0.7
Behenic	16.3
Tricosanoic	0.53
Lignoceric	4.5
Pentacosanoic	0.23
Montanic	2.2

[a]Unknown peaks account for the difference between the total and 100%.

From Cancalon, *J. Am. Oil Chem. Soc.*, 48, 629 (1971). With permission.

CONTENT OF UNSAPONIFIABLES IN VEGETABLE OILS AND YIELD OF FOUR FRACTIONS FROM UNSAPONIFIABLES BY THIN LAYER CHROMATOGRAPHY

Oil	S.V.[a]	I.V.[b]	Unsaponifiables % oil	Fraction[c] % unsaponifiables			
				1	2	3	4
Corn, soap stock (Mexico)	195.9	105.3	1.3	8	1	1	90
Rice bran, crude (Japan)	180.1	103.9	4.2	19	28	10	43
Wheat germ, crude	184.7	134.4	3.2	7	7	5	81
Coconut, crude (Philippine)	256.4	9.9	0.4	22	17	4	57
Palm, crude (Indonesia)	200.0	56.9	0.4	19	8	9	64
Palm kernel, crude (Indonesia)	246.4	20.7	0.4	48	18	1	33
Peanut, refined (Nigeria)	188.8	90.7	0.4	27	9	4	60
Soybean, crude (USA)	190.7	134.6	0.6	15	14	11	60
Sunflower, winterized (Canada)	190.6	135.4	0.7	18	10	16	56
Safflower, linoleic-rich, crude (USA)	190.3	143.6	0.6	27	11	4	58
Safflower, oleic-rich, crude (USA)	189.3	93.2	0.6	21	10	5	64
Olive, refined (France)	192.0	84.9	0.8	62	18	2	18
Olive (Italy)	–	–	–	68	17	1	14
Castor, crude (Pakistan)	181.1	87.4	0.5	27	9	4	57
Kapok, deodorized (Indonesia)	192.6	105.0	0.5	19	19	5	57
Cottonseed, crude (Sudan)	195.2	105.0	0.6	14	8	7	71
Linseed, crude (Canada)	189.6	188.0	0.7	11	22	7	60
Rapeseed, crude (Canada)	179.0	109.9	0.9	23	6	3	68
Sesame, crude (Ethiopia)	188.0	109.2	1.4	14	13	29	44
Cocoa butter, crude (Ghana)	190.3	34.6	0.4	9	13	4	74
Coffee seed, crude (Brazil)	183.7	100.0	3.4	16	13	17	54

[a]Saponification value.
[b]Iodine value, Wijs' method.
[c]Fraction 1: Less polar compounds (hydrocarbon, aliphatic alcohols, etc.); Fraction 2: Triterpene alcohols; Fraction 3: 4-Methylsterols; Fraction 4: Sterols.

From Itoh, Tamura, and Matsumoto, *J. Am. Oil Chem. Soc.*, 50, 122 (1973). With permission.

SOLUBILITY OF SELECTED LIPIDS IN ORGANIC SOLVENTS (mg/ml)

	Hexane 1.89	Chloroform 4.80	Chloroform methanol 2:1	Acetone 20.7	Methanol 33.6
Sodium octanoate	<0.001	0.12	16.15	0.08	>40.0
Lauric acid	>40.0	>40.0	>40.0	>40.0	>40.0
Sodium laurate	<0.001	0.08	7.86	0.06	>40.0
Palmitic acid	>40.0	>40.0	>40.0	>40.0	>40.0
Stearic acid	15.14	>40.0	>40.0	23.08	10.48
Behenic acid	1.13	18.16	>40.0	2.92	0.84
Heptacosanoic acid	0.19	3.92	6.77	0.16	0.02
2-Hydroxystearic acid	0.14	6.98	14.49	4.69	9.71
3-Hydroxypalmitic acid	0.10	>40.0	>40.0	32.96	>40.0
9,10,16-Trihydroxypalmitic	<0.001	0.24	>40.0	2.96	>40.0
Dodecylstearate	>40.0	>40.0	>40.0	22.01	0.52
Cholesterol	6.50	>40.0	>40.0	23.96	5.82
Trimyristin	>40.0	>40.0	>40.0	4.01	0.04
Tripalmitin	5.84	>40.0	>40.0	0.22	0.01
Tristearin	1.04	>40.0	12.89	<0.001	0.11
1,3-Distearin	0.25	>40.0	>40.0	0.52	0.27
Monostearin	0.09	>40.0	>40.0	7.79	9.60

From Schmid and Hunter, *Physiol. Chem. Phys.*, 3, 98 (1971). With permission.

ISOMERS IN RAT CARDIAC LIPIDS

Monoethylenic Isomers in Partially Hydrogenated Herring Oil and Cardiac Lipids of Experimental Rats at 1 and 16 Weeks

Chain length	Lipid source	Composition of aldehyde-esters, mol%										
		5	6	7	8	9	10	11	12	13	14	15
16	HHO[a] (7.5%)[b]											
	trans (37%)[c,d]	1	12	4	14	45	14	6	3	1	–	–
	cis (63%)	–	2	3	5	80	5	4	1	–	–	–
	1W (1.0%)											
	trans (53%)	22	11	5	20	26	7	6	2	1	–	–
	cis (47%)	–	6	12	8	61	5	4	2	2	–	–
	16W (2.7%)											
	trans (55%)	14	9	6	13	34	12	6	4	2	–	–
	cis (45%)	3	3	11	5	66	5	4	2	1	–	–
18	HHO (13.1%)											
	trans (35%)	–	–	5	11	40	17	17	7	3	–	–
	cis (65%)	–	–	6	3	66	3	16	3	3	–	–
	1W (15.1%)											
	trans (23%)	6	3	11	10	39	7	12	6	3	3	–
	cis (77%)	–	–	11	4	63	2	18	1	1	–	–
	16W (16.7%)											
	trans (34%)	4	3	14	8	41	5	10	8	3	4	–
	cis (66%)	–	–	13	2	57	1	25	1	1	–	–
20	HHO (19.9%)											
	trans (33%)	–	–	–	3	9	15	50	15	5	2	1
	cis (67%)	–	–	–	1	10	4	75	5	5	–	–
	1W (13.5%)											
	trans (20%)	–	–	4	4	25	16	32	10	6	3	–
	cis (80%)	–	–	1	2	25	4	56	4	7	–	–
	16W (5.3%)											
	trans (19%)	–	–	2	3	14	14	40	16	7	4	–
	cis (81%)	–	–	–	2	28	3	56	4	8	–	–
22	HHO (29.0%)											
	trans (32%)	–	–	–	–	2	15	57	17	6	2	1
	cis (68%)	–	–	–	–	2	3	82	4	9	–	–
	1W (15.7%)											
	trans (27%)	–	–	–	–	6	12	56	15	9	2	–
	cis (73%)	–	–	–	–	3	4	83	4	6	–	–
	16W (3.1%)											
	trans (26%)	–	–	–	–	5	15	52	16	10	2	–
	cis (74%)	–	–	–	–	3	5	80	4	8	–	–

[a]HHO refers to partially hydrogenated herring oil; 1W and 16W refer to cardiac lipids at 1 and 16 weeks, respectively.

[b]Figures in parentheses after HHO, 1W and 16W refer to percentage of monoene in total methyl esters.

[c]Figures in parentheses after cis and trans refer to percent within monoene.

[d]All silver ion thin layer chromatography separation and ozonolysis reactions were carried out in duplicate, except with fraction 16 where insufficient material was available.

From Conacher, Page, and Beare-Rogers, *Lipids*, 8,256, (1973.) With permission.

SOLUBILITY OF SELECTED LIPIDS IN CHLORINATED
HYDROCARBON SOLVENTS (mg/ml)

	Solubility (mg/ml)		
	Carbon tetrachloride δ 8.55	Chloroform δ 9.16	Tetrachloroethylene δ 9.28
Dodecylstearate	>40.0	>40.0	–
Tristearin	>40.0	>40.0	>23.0
Distearin	8.2	>40.0	5.7
Monostearin	1.4	>40.0	4.6
Stearic acid	>40.0	>40.0	>40.0
Heptacosanoic acid	3.2	3.9	1.6
α-Hydroxystearic acid	–	6.98	1.44
Trihydroxypalmitic acid	1.5	0.24	0.04

From Schmid, *Physiol. Chem. Phys.*, 5, 141 (1973). With permission.

SOLUBILITY OF SELECTED LIPIDS IN CHLORINATED HYDROCARBON
MIXTURES WITH 33% METHANOL (mg/ml)

	Carbon tetrachloride δ 10.53	Chloroform δ 10.94	Tetrachloroethylene δ 11.02
Dodecylsterate	>40.0	>40.0	–
Tristearin	9.4	12.9	–
Distearin	>20.0	>40.0	–
Monostearin	>40.0	>40.0	>40.0
Stearic acid	–	>50.0	>40.0
Heptacosanoic acid	16.0	–	18.5
α-Hydroxystearic acid	–	>40.0	–
Trihydroxypalmitic acid	>40.0	>40.0	20.0
Phosphatidyl ethanolamine	15.0	6.9	–
Phosphatidyl serine	30.0	>32.0	–

From Schmid, *Physiol. Chem. Phys.*, 5, 141, (1973). With permission.

SURFACE AREAS FOR PURE METHYL ESTERS AND TRIGLYCERIDES MEASURED AT CONSTANT SURFACE PRESSURE USING TTP AS THE PISTON OIL

Lipid	Surface area	
	Molecule	Hydrocarbon chain
	A^2	
Palmitic acid[a]	22.8 ± 0.4[b]	22.8
Methyl oleate (3)[c]	39.0 ± 0.4	39.0
Methyl linoleate (2)	39.7	39.7
Methyl linolenate (4)	39.2 ± 0.6	39.2
Methyl arachidonate (3)	39.8 ± 0.8	39.8
Tripalmitin (1)	62.0	20.7
Triolein (4)	102.2 ± 1.6	34.1
Trilinolein (5)	108.9 ± 0.6	36.3
Trilinolenin (2)	108.2	36.1

[a]Data from Heikkila, Kwong, and Cornwell, *J. Lipid Res.*, 11, 190 (1970), at 10 dynes/cm.
[b]Means ± sD.
[c]Number of lipid samples weighed is in parentheses. Surface area of each sample was measured at least three times.

From Burke, Patil, Panganamala, Geer, and Cornwell, *J. Lipid Res.*, 14, 9 (1973). With permission.

PROPERTIES OF POLYOL ESTERS

Polyol esters	Acid value	Density, g/cm³	Hydroxyl value	
			Calculated	Found
Glycerol				
Acetate	0.10	1.205	835	741
Butyrate	0.10	1.110	691	606
Caproate	0.10	1.045	589	525
Benzoate	0.02	1.223	572	514
Caprylate	0.05	1.008	514	415
Pelargonate	0.08	0.990	482	362
Caprate	0.12	0.979	456	320
Laurate	0.36	–	409	215
Triglycerol				
Acetate	0.25	1.255	793	792
Butyrate	0.26	1.200	722	743
Caproate	0.31	1.158	663	718
Benzoate	0.30	1.261	652	612
Caprylate	0.48	1.112	612	603
Pelargonate	0.40	1.100	589	613
Caprate	0.40	1.081	569	560
Laurate	0.14	1.059	532	508
Hexaglycerol				
Acetate	0.39	1.266	779	764
Butyrate	0.15	1.245	737	752
Caproate	0.13	1.212	701	701
Benzoate	0.39	1.275	693	629
Caprylate	0.18	1.184	667	680
Pelargonate	0.30	1.176	652	647
Caprate	0.28	1.157	636	623
Laurate	0.20	1.139	610	604
Decaglycerol				
Acetate	0.21	1.288	771	729
Butyrate	0.16	1.263	745	702
Caproate	0.19	1.236	720	673
Benzoate	0.38	1.297	715	659
Caprylate	0.39	1.219	697	659
Pelargonate	0.22	1.216	687	642
Caprate	0.30	1.204	676	631
Laurate	0.45	1.189	656	615

From Babayan and McIntryre, *J. Am. Oil Chem. Soc.*, 48, 307 (1971). With permission.

PHYSICAL CONSTANTS OF THE METHYL ESTERS OF SOME SYNTHETIC ALKENYL- AND ALKYL SUBSTITUTED FATTY ACID METHYL ESTERS

No.		m	n	R	N_D^{20} °C	Mp °C [a] (acid)	Yield %	Analysis			
								Calculated		Found	
								%C	%H	%C	%H
II	Methyl 10-n-hexylpentadec-10-enoate	8	5	C_6H_{13}	1.4569	—	67.0	78.05	12.50	78.11	12.46
III	Methyl 12-n-hexyltridec-12-enoate	10	5	H	1.4547	—	79.5	77.36	12.34	77.43	12.27
IV	Methyl 12-n-hexyltetradec-12-enoate	10	5	CH_3	1.4570	—	72.0	77.72	12.42	77.75	12.39
V	Methyl 12-n-hexylhexadec-12-enoate	10	5	C_3H_7	1.4579	—	70.3	78.35	12.57	78.26	12.53
VI	Methyl 12-n-hexylnonadec-12-enoate	10	5	C_6H_{13}	1.4588	—	68.0	79.12	12.77	79.16	12.76
VII	Methyl 12-n-hexyldocos-12-enoate	10	5	C_9H_{19}	1.4600	—	73.5	79.75	12.92	79.81	12.87
VIII	Methyl 12-n-hexyltetracos-12-enoate	10	5	$C_{11}H_{23}$	1.4619	—	66.5	80.10	13.01	80.14	13.04
IX	Methyl 12-n-hexylhexacos-12-enoate	10	5	$C_{13}H_{27}$	1.4623	—	47.4	80.42	13.09	80.62	12.99
X	Methyl 12-n-hexyltriacont-12-enoate	10	5	$C_{17}H_{35}$	1.4615	—	68.6	80.95	13.22	80.98	13.23

No.		m	n	R	N_D^{20} °C	Mp °C (acid)	Yield[b] %	Analysis[c]			
								Calculated		Found	
								%C	%H	%C	%H
XII	Methyl 10-n-Pentylhexadecanoate	8	5	C_6H_{13}	1.4501	<0	—	—	—	—	—
XIII	Methyl 12-methyloctadecanoate	10	5	H	1.4469	36.5–38.0	—	—	—	—	—
XIV	Methyl 12-ethyloctadecanoate	10	5	CH_3	1.4492	<15	—	—	—	—	—
XV	Methyl 12-n-butyloctadecanoate	10	5	C_3H_7	1.4508	23.0–24.5	—	—	—	—	—
XVI	Methyl 12-n-hexylnonadecanoate	10	5	C_6H_{13}	1.4537	28.0–29.5	—	—	—	—	—
XVII	Methyl 12-n-hexyldocosanoate	10	5	C_9H_{19}	1.4562	<15	—	—	—	—	—
XVIII	Methyl 12-n-hexyltetracosanoate	10	5	$C_{11}H_{23}$	1.4579	15.5–18.0	—	—	—	—	—
XIX	Methyl 12-n-hexylhexacosanoate	10	5	$C_{13}H_{27}$	1.4588	61.0–63.0	—	—	—	—	—
XX	Methyl 12-n-hexyltriacontanoate	10	5	$C_{17}H_{35}$	1.4611	73.5–74.5	—	—	—	—	—

[a] All samples of monoenoic acids were liquid.
[b] Yields were virtually all 100% since these compounds originated by simple hydrogenation of the monoenes.
[c] C,H, analysis of the hydrogenated compounds were not carried out.

From Chasin and Perkins, *Chem. Phys. Lipids*, 6, 8 (1971). With permission.

NORMALIZED INTENSITIES OF KEY FRAGMENTS IN THE MASS SPECTRA OF METHYL ESTERS OF ALKENYL BRANCHED CHAIN ACIDS

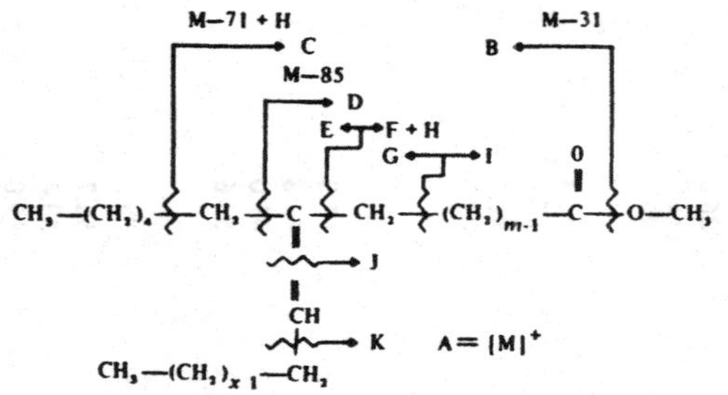

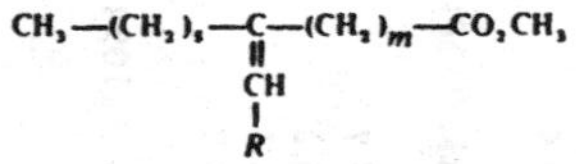

Fragmentation scheme:

$M-71+H \rightarrow C$
$M-31 \rightarrow B$
$M-85 \rightarrow D$

$CH_3-(CH_2)_x-\overset{\underset{|}{CH}-R}{C}-(CH_2)_{m-1}-\overset{O}{\overset{||}{C}}-O-CH_3$

Labels: E, F+H, G, I, J, K, $A = [M]^+$

$R = (CH_2)_{x-1}-CH_3$

$CH_3-(CH_2)_x-\overset{\underset{|}{\underset{R}{CH}}}{C}-(CH_2)_m-CO_2CH_3$

Fragment: m/e/relative intensity (%)

m	(R)	(x)	A	B	C	D	E	F	G	I	J	K
8	C_4H_9	4	338/61	307/20	268/17	253/9	167/12	171/11	182/48	157/56	267/10	282/11
10	H	0	310/20	279/51	240/18	225/31	111/87	199/6	126/92	185/94	295/0.6	310/A
10	CH_3	1	324/37	293/28	254/13	239/10	125/27	199/9	140/61	185/61	295/12	310/0.6
10	C_3H_7	3	352/75	321/47	282/26	267/17	153/71	199/18	168/80	185/88	295/17	310/18
10	C_6H_{13}	6	394/47	363/41	324/30	309/26	195/21	199/21	210/94	185/91	295/24	310/35
10	C_9H_{19}	9	436/48	405/20	366/11	351/12	237/9	199/13	252/41	185/73	295/13	310/15
10	$C_{11}H_{23}$	11	464/37	433/20	394/10	379/11	265/13	199/15	280/39	185/80	295/15	310/18
10	$C_{13}H_{27}$	13	492/33	461/22	424/11	409/14	293/10	199/13	308/34	185/79	295/22	310/21
10	$C_{17}H_{35}$	17	548/15	517/19	478/9	463/13	349/6	199/13	364/28	185/83	295/29	310/29

From Chasin and Perkins, *Chem. Phys. Lipids*, 6, 8 (1971). With permission.

COMPARISON OF SURFACE PRESSURES AT TRANSITION AND COLLAPSE OF VARIOUS *n*-SATURATED FATTY ACID MONOLAYERS

Compression rate A^2 /molecule /min	Transition pressure dynes/cm π_T	Collapse pressure dynes/cm π_C
Pentadecanoic Acid (C-15)		
2.4	20.3	36.5
1.2	20.3	35.3
0.60	20.7	33.6
0.24	20.3	30.9
Palmitic Acid (C-16)		
2.4	21.3	34.2
1.2	21.9	32.0
0.60	21.1	30.8
0.24	20.9	26.5
Heptadecanoic Acid (C-17)		
2.4	22.7	53.2
1.2	22.8	50.4
0.60	23.2	43.7
0.24	21.7	37.3
Stearic Acid (C-18)		
2.4	23.8	51.3
1.2	23.8	49.8
0.60	24.1	41.0
0.24	23.8	34.6
Nonadecanoic Acid (C-19)		
2.4	24.5	55.7
1.2	24.3	53.4
0.60	25.3	49.0
0.24	23.4	47.3
Eicosanoic Acid (C-20)		
2.4	25.7	52.4
1.2	25.2	50.9
0.60	25.3	46.9
0.24	24.9	45.2

From Sims and Zografi, *Chem. Phys. Lipids*, 6, 109 (1971). With permission.

CONTENT OF TOTAL LIPIDS, CHOLESTERYL ESTERS, AND PHOSPHOLIPIDS IN THE DIFFERENT TISSUES

	Corn oil	Milk fat	Beef tallow	Hydrogenated soybean fat	Fat-free diet
		15-week Feeding			
Liver[a]					
Total lipids[b]	45.0 ± 1.8	46.1 ± 1.4	48.0 ± 1.6	46.0 ± 1.7	35.2 ± 0.7
Cholesteryl esters	4.7 ± 0.5	4.7 ± 0.6	7.5 ± 0.6	5.3 ± 0.2	5.1 ± 0.5
Phospholipids	33.0 ± 0.9	31.0 ± 0.8	31.8 ± 1.0	35.0 ± 1.2	25.8 ± 1.1
Heart[a]					
Total lipids[b]	48.7 ± 2.1	40.6 ± 0.5	42.0 ± 1.6	62.6 ± 1.8	58.8 ± 0.8
Cholesteryl esters	4.0 ± 0.6	4.0 ± 0.7	2.5 ± 0.2	5.3 ± 0.5	2.0 ± 0.1
Phospholipids	33.0 ± 0.9	26.0 ± 0.7	22.0 ± 0.6	18.0 ± 0.6	22.0 ± 1.1
Adrenals[c]					
Total lipids[b]	13.0	13.3	14.0	15.0	14.5
Cholesteryl esters	9.4	15.6	9.4	13.1	8.3
Phospholipids	4.0	4.2	4.8	4.5	1.5
VLDL[d]					
Total lipids[b]	70.5	65.8	87.1	48.0	85.1
Cholesteryl esters	10.7	11.3	12.5	11.0	36.7
Phospholipids	13.3	12.5	17.9	16.0	42.0
LDL[d]					
Total lipids[b]	50.5	61.2	51.5	88.2	67.2
Cholesteryl esters	36.7	35.0	23.2	28.7	20.5
Phospholipids	36.0	38.8	34.0	37.5	35.5
HDL[d]					
Total lipids[b]	42.8	40.2	65.0	41.3	39.5
Cholesteryl esters	20.3	19.0	25.4	13.0	15.0
Phospholipids	22.3	16.3	22.9	9.7	16.1

[a]Results for liver and heart are expressed as mg/g wet tissue and are means ± SD for four animals.

[b]Includes primarily triglycerides, but also free cholesterol and free fatty acids. In the interest of simplicity and clarity, the values for the individual classes of lipids are not included in the table.

[c]Results are expressed as percentage of wet weight of tissue, and each is the mean of two samples (two pairs of adrenals per sample), with duplicate determinations on each sample.

[d]Values are expressed as mg/100 ml of plasma, and each represents the mean for triplicate determinations on a plasma sample pooled from four rats.

CONTENT OF TOTAL LIPIDS, CHOLESTERYL ESTERS, AND PHOSPHOLIPIDS IN THE DIFFERENT TISSUES (continued)

	Corn oil	Milk fat	Beef tallow	Hydrogenated soybean fat	Fat-free diet
			20-week Feeding		
Liver[a]					
Total lipids[b]	58.1 ± 2.2	48.7 ± 2.0	52.3 ± 2.1	45.8 ± 1.1	37.2 ± 1.0
Cholesteryl esters	3.9 ± 0.4	2.9 ± 0.1	3.5 ± 0.3	2.8 ± 0.1	2.5 ± 0.2
Phospholipids	30.8 ± 1.4	27.5 ± 1.0	30.7 ± 0.9	31.5 ± 0.8	25.2 ± 0.7
Heart[a]					
Total lipids[b]	52.0 ± 2.1	42.1 ± 1.6	24.0 ± 1.3	30.9 ± 1.1	32.6 ± 1.2
Cholesteryl esters	1.5 ± 0.1	3.3 ± 0.2	2.6 ± 0.2	2.9 ± 0.2	2.7 ± 0.1
Phospholipids	30.8 ± 1.4	18.9 ± 1.1	18.4 ± 0.6	23.1 ± 1.3	20.7 ± 1.4
Adrenals[c]					
Total lipids[b]	13.3	13.6	13.8	36.0	15.7
Cholesteryl esters	20.0	19.5	20.2	25.5	18.7
Phospholipids	6.5	6.2	5.2	5.0	3.6
VLDL[d]					
Total lipids[b]	220.5	150.0	295.0	220.5	145.1
Cholesteryl esters	23.0	27.3	17.7	19.3	18.3
Phospholipids	39.7	31.8	17.9	24.4	40.8
LDL[d]					
Total lipids[b]	151.2	131.2	239.1	151.2	121.2
Cholesteryl esters	35.8	37.8	18.7	17.5	18.8
Phospholipids	40.0	38.2	33.9	33.7	38.2
HDL[d]					
Total lipids[b]	113.2	61.8	174.1	113.2	66.3
Cholesteryl esters	25.1	20.5	30.3	15.4	17.8
Phospholipids	29.3	17.5	28.3	20.3	20.0

From Egwim and Kummerow, *J. Lipid Res.*, 13, 500 (1972). With permission.

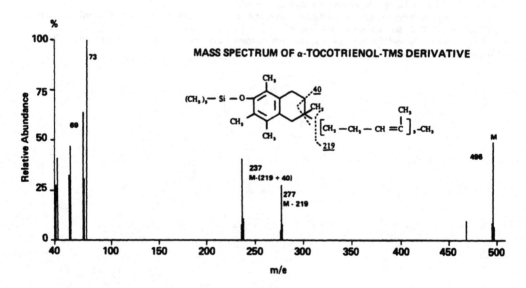

From Rao and Perkins, *J. Agric. Food Chem.*, 20, 240 (1972).

INDIVIDUAL TOCOPHEROL CONTENTS OF VEGETABLE OILS (AVERAGE OF THREE DETERMINATIONS)

Oil	Total tocopherol mg/100 g oil	Individual tocopherol, %						
		α-	β-	γ-	δ-	α_3-	β_3-	γ_3-
Oats	1.68	17.9[a] (17.3–18.6)	6.0 (5.3–6.6)			58.3 (57.6–59.1)	17.3 (17.4–18.4)	
Wheat germ	212.00	51.9 (51.1–52.8)	38.1 (37.9–38.6)			4.0 (3.3–4.6)	6.0 (5.4–6.8)	
Barley	2.10	14.3 (12.9–15.3)	2.4 (1.9–3.0)	2.4 (1.5–3.3)	1.9 (1.9–2.7)	57.1 (55.4–58.5)	14.2 (13.7–14.6)	7.6 (6.9–8.5)
Soybean	89.70	11.5 (10.4–12.3)		61.9 (60.7–62.6)	26.6 (25.8–27.3)			
Coconut	2.80	14.3 (13.2–15.1)		16.1 (15.8–16.4)		10.7 (9.9–11.4)	5.3 (4.8–5.7)	53.6 (53.0–54.2)

[a]Figures on top are mean of three determinations. Figures in parentheses are minimum and maximum values.

Reprinted with permission from Rao and Perkins, *J. Agric. Food Chem.*, 20, 240 (1972). Copyright by the American Chemical Society.

EFFECT OF DIETARY FAT ON FATTY ACID COMPOSITION IN PLASMA AND ERYTHROCYTE LIPIDS [a]

Fatty acid[b]	Plasma			Erythrocyte		
	Corn oil	Basal	Hydrogenated fat	Corn oil	Basal	Hydrogenated fat
14:0	0.3 ± 0.0[c]	0.6 ± 0.1	0.6 ± 0.0	0.4 ± 0.1	1.3 ± 0.4	2.3 ± 1.9
16:0	17.2 ± 0.5	22.4 ± 1.6	17.8 ± 0.1	30.6 ± 0.8	35.5 ± 2.9	30.6 ± 0.6
16:1	1.5 ± 0.1	2.7 ± 0.1	2.8 ± 0.2	Trace	Trace	Trace
18:0	12.7 ± 0.8	12.4 ± 0.3	11.4 ± 0.3	15.0 ± 0.3	12.9 ± 0.2	12.0 ± 0.7
18:1	14.3 ± 0.6	21.7 ± 0.6	35.0 ± 1.0	24.5 ± 0.1	26.6 ± 1.9	35.4 ± 1.1
18:2	47.0 ± 1.2	33.1 ± 0.5	26.6 ± 1.0	26.0 ± 1.0	19.6 ± 0.2	16.5 ± 0.6
20:4	7.0 ± 0.3	7.1 ± 0.3	5.7 ± 0.1	3.5 ± 0.2	4.2 ± 0.5	3.0 ± 0.5

[a]Expressed as a percentage of the total fatty acids.
[b]Numbers before and after colon represent carbon chain length and number of double bonds, respectively.
[c]Mean for three samples ± SEM, each containing pooled blood from four swine.

From Yeh, Mizuguchi, and Kummerow, *Proc. Soc. Exp. Biol. Med.*, 146, 236 (1974). With permission.

Table 1

PROPERTIES OF SOME ATLANTIC HERRING AND TWO OTHER OILS WITH WEIGHT PERCENT COMPOSITIONS OF THE FATTY ACID METHYL ESTERS DERIVED FROM THE OILS

		Atlantic herring oils												Pacific herring oil (this study)	Pacific pilchard oil[1]
Sample no:		1	2	3	4	5	6	7	8	9	10	11	12		
Oil iodine value (Wijs):		111.6	121.4	124.8	124.6	128.0	123.6	129.8	131.6	129.8	130.8	138.3	139.2	129.8	192
Percent nonsaponifiables:		0.85	0.74	1.17	0.74	0.80	1.74	1.74	0.91	1.35	1.09	1.19	0.78	0.60	0.69
Refractive index (n_D25):		1.47107	1.47211	1.47225	1.47307	1.47273	1.47220	1.47314	1.47284	1.47303	1.47275	1.47425	1.47389	1.47282	–
Fatty acid[a]	Double bond positions[b]	Wt % fatty acid methyl ester compositions[e,f]													
12:0	–	0.07	0.09	0.13	0.06	0.10	0.10	0.11	0.05	0.11	0.13	0.09	0.11	0.08	–[d]
14:0	–	5.11	6.01	8.36	4.60	6.90	5.90	7.91	6.42	5.07	4.87	7.58	8.15	5.66	7.6
14:1	9c	0.34	0.27	0.30	0.24	0.45	0.44	0.28	0.23	0.39	0.46	0.20	0.33	0.20	TRA
15:0	–	0.32	0.39	0.40	0.28	0.28	0.52	0.39	0.30	0.36	0.42	0.23	0.39	0.25	0.6
15:1	9c	0.04	0.09	0.05	0.05	0.04	0.10	0.05	0.07	0.15	0.14	0.06	0.09	0.08	TRA
16:0	–	10.10	11.84	11.88	10.55	11.59	12.79	12.22	12.72	10.89	10.26	15.00	12.50	16.64	16.2
16:1	9c	10.19	9.32	6.30	11.56	7.87	7.00	6.30	8.80	12.01	11.63	8.94	8.50	7.63	9.2
16:2	9,12	0.68	0.48	1.02	0.78	0.93	0.41	0.80	0.68	0.70	0.85	0.73	0.72	0.79	1.3
16:3	6,9,12	0.27	0.27	0.59	0.47	0.44	0.20	0.53	0.48	0.58	0.52	0.62	0.67	0.39	1.0
16:4	6,9,12,15	0.62	0.89	0.29	0.89	0.78	0.21	0.37	0.50	1.15	1.12	0.59	0.81	0.54	1.2
17:0	–	0.11	0.22	0.20	0.21	0.13	0.22	0.29	0.19	0.21	0.29	0.20	0.18	0.27	0.7
17:1	9c	0.24	0.13	0.18	0.12	0.14	0.30	0.28	0.12	0.12	0.30	0.14	0.15	0.29	0.2
18:0	–	0.68	1.00	0.73	0.82	1.07	2.13	1.20	0.94	1.16	1.12	1.30	0.77	1.79	3.5
18:1	9c	9.31	13.01	11.09	10.18	12.07	21.36	11.86	12.74	12.63	12.53	13.60	9.86	22.69	11.4
18:2	9,12	0.59	0.98	1.35	0.58	1.32	2.88	1.47	1.14	0.74	0.58	1.15	1.08	0.55	1.3
18:3	6,9,12	0.05	0.06	0.04	0.14	0.04	0.09	0.04	0.07	0.09	0.10	0.15	0.11	0.08	TRA
18:3	9,12,15	0.37	0.60	0.76	0.16	0.79	0.80	1.08	0.55	0.28	0.36	0.67	0.58	0.43	0.9

[a] Shorthand notation for chain length: number of double bonds.
[b] From carboxyl group.
[c] Other isomers may be present.
[d] Analysis for these materials not carried out.
[e] NSA = no significant amount present; TRA = trace.
[f] Branched chain fatty acids included in major components.

Table 1 (continued)
PROPERTIES OF SOME ATLANTIC HERRING AND TWO OTHER OILS WITH WEIGHT PERCENT COMPOSITIONS OF THE FATTY ACID METHYL ESTERS DERIVED FROM THE OILS

Fatty acid[a]	Double bond positions[b]	Atlantic herring oils — Wt % fatty acid methyl ester compositions[e,f]												Pacific herring oil (this study)	Pacific pilchard oil[1]
Sample no:		1	2	3	4	5	6	7	8	9	10	11	12		
18:4	6,9,12,15	1.24	1.71	2.38	1.14	2.19	1.10	2.54	1.69	1.53	1.47	2.30	2.50	1.63	2.0
19:0	—	NSA	NSA	NSA	NSA	NSA	TRA	NSA	NSA	NSA	NSA	NSA	NSA	TRA	0.02
19:1	9[c]	0.05	0.09	0.11	0.10	0.06	0.05	0.08	0.05	0.06	0.12	0.07	0.04	0.10	TRA
19:4	?	TRA	TRA	TRA	TRA	TRA	TRA	TRA	NSA	NSA	NSA	TRA	TRA	NSA	—[d]
20:0	—	NSA	NSA	NSA	NSA	NSA	TRA	NSA	NSA	NSA	TRA	NSA	NSA	TRA	TRA
20:1	11[c]	19.94	17.08	13.49	16.78	15.16	13.00	15.07	14.10	16.12	15.91	10.99	14.93	10.68	3.2
20:2	11,14	0.18	0.20	0.25	0.13	0.17	0.31	0.25	0.18	0.14	0.16	0.16	0.14	0.16	TRA
20:3	5,8,11	NSA	NSA	NSA	NSA	NSA	NSA	NSA	NSA	NSA	NSA	NSA	NSA	NSA	TRA
20:3	8,11,14	0.21	0.17	0.14	0.09	0.14	0.26	0.18	0.16	0.08	0.12	0.11	0.11	0.12	0.1
20:4	5,8,11,14	0.18	0.35	0.23	0.15	0.32	0.53	0.42	0.33	0.40	0.46	0.34	0.20	0.38	1.1
20:4	8,11,14,17	0.26	0.33	0.52	0.39	0.47	0.70	0.65	0.53	0.42	0.36	0.72	0.76	0.60	0.5
20:5	5,8,11,14,17	3.89	5.70	5.56	8.19	5.86	5.13	5.22	8.42	7.39	8.34	8.83	8.53	8.14	16.9
21:5	?	0.26	0.25	0.46	0.28	0.50	0.32	0.43	0.54	0.33	0.38	0.55	0.59	0.61	0.6
22:1	11[c]	30.57	22.18	25.95	25.62	23.41	14.75	21.61	20.84	19.82	20.58	16.93	19.29	11.96	3.8
22:4	7,10,13,16	NSA	NSA	TRA	NSA	TRA	NSA	TRA	TRA	NSA	NSA	TRA	TRA	TRA	0.1
22:5	4,7,10,13,16	0.12	0.14	0.19	0.16	0.30	0.28	0.23	0.18	0.41	0.36	0.22	0.23	0.17	0.2
22:5	7,10,13,16,19	0.60	0.47	0.60	0.49	0.72	1.30	0.56	0.77	1.13	1.21	0.76	0.77	0.75	2.3
22:6	4,7,10,13,16,19	2.02	4.81	5.15	3.58	4.50	5.27	6.20	4.86	3.87	4.55	4.95	5.32	4.83	12.9
24:1	?	0.83	0.86	0.75	0.72	0.80	0.91	0.79	0.76	0.36	0.24	1.21	0.88	0.94	0.5
24:5	?	0.42	0.24	0.43	0.35	0.52	0.41	0.48	0.40	0.47	—[d]	0.37	0.54	0.34	0.2
24:6	?	0.05	0.09	0.09	0.11	0.21	0.16	0.12	0.13	0.29	—[d]	0.14	0.13	0.14	0.1
Iodine value calcd from composition:		99.2	116.1	117.4	119.7	119.9	120.7	122.5	126.1	126.5	127.9	128.3	131.0	121.9	190

REFERENCE

1. Ackman and Sipos, J. Fish Res. Board Can., 21(4), 841 (1964).

From Ackman and Eaton, J. Fish Res. Board Can., 23(7), 994 (1966). With permission.

Table 2
CHAIN LENGTH COMPOSITIONS OF SOME ATLANTIC HERRING OILS, OF SOME OTHER HERRING OILS, AND OF PILCHARD OIL

Sample no.	Averages nos. 1–12 only	Atlantic herring oils												Other herring oils			Pacific pilchard oil
														Pacific		European	
		1	2	3	4	5	6	7	8	9	10	11	12	This study	Gruger et al.[1]	Klenk and Eberhagen[2]	Ackman and Sipos[3]
Fatty acid chain length					Wt % different chain lengths[c]												
C_{13}	0.10	0.07	0.09	0.13	0.06	0.10	0.10	0.11	0.05	0.11	0.13	0.09	0.11	0.08	–	–	–
C_{14}	6.73	5.45	6.28	8.66	4.48	7.35	6.34	8.19	6.65	5.46	5.33	7.78	8.48	5.86	7.6	6	7.6
C_{15}	0.43	0.36	0.48	0.45	0.33	0.32	0.62	0.44	0.37	0.56	0.51	0.29	0.48	0.33	0.4	+	0.6
C_{16}	22.78	21.86	22.80	20.08	24.25	21.61	20.62	20.22	23.18	25.33	24.38	25.88	23.20	25.99	27.6	19	28.9
C_{17}	0.39	0.35	0.35	0.38	0.33	0.27	0.52	0.57	0.31	0.33	0.59	0.34	0.33	0.56	0.5	+	0.9
C_{18}	17.23	12.24	17.36	16.35	13.02	17.48	28.36	18.19	17.13	16.43	16.16	19.17	14.90	27.17	24.1	26	19.1
C_{19}	–	+	+	+	+	+	+	+	+	+	+	+	+	+	+	+	+
C_{20}	23.19	24.66	23.83	20.19	25.73	22.12	19.93	21.79	23.72	25.09	25.35	21.15	24.67	20.08	18.4	21	21.8
C_{21}	0.41	0.26	0.25	0.46	0.28	0.50	0.32	0.43	0.54	0.33	0.38	0.55	0.59	0.61	–	+	+
C_{22}	27.40	33.31	27.60	31.89	29.85	28.93	21.60	28.60	26.65	25.23	26.70[b]	22.86	25.61	17.71	20.5	24	19.3
C_{23}	1.36[a]	1.30	1.19	1.27	1.18	1.53	1.48	1.39	1.29	1.12	0.24[b]	1.72	1.55	1.42	0.9	1	0.8

[a]For all samples.
[b]Polyunsaturated omitted.
[c]+ signifies present in small amounts.

REFERENCES

1. Gruger, Nelson, and Stansby, *J. Am. Oil Chem. Soc.*, 41, 662 (1964).
2. Klenk and Eberhagen, *Hoppe-Seyler's Z. Physiol. Chem.*, 328, 180 (1962).
3. Ackman and Sipos, *J. Fish. Res. Board Can.*, 21(4), 841 (1964).

From Ackman and Eaton, *J. Fish. Res. Board Can.*, 23(7), 994 (1966). With permission.

Table 3

COMPARISONS OF PROPERTIES OF INTEREST OF SOME ATLANTIC HERRING OILS, FOR SOME OTHER HERRING OILS, AND FOR PILCHARD OIL

Property compared	Averages nos. 1–12 only	Atlantic herring oils Sample no.											
		1	2	3	4	5	6	7	8	9	10	11	12
Wt % saturated	20.0	16.4	19.6	21.7	16.5	20.1	21.7	22.1	20.6	17.8	17.1	24.4	22.1
Wt % monounsaturated	60.0	71.5	63.0	58.2	65.4	60.0	57.9	56.3	57.7	61.7	61.9	52.1	54.1
Total wt % saturated + monounsaturated	80.0	87.9	82.6	79.9	81.9	80.1	79.6	76.4	78.3	79.5	79.0	76.5	76.2
Total wt % dienoic	2.1	1.4	1.7	2.6	1.5	2.4	3.6	2.5	2.0	1.6	1.6	2.0	1.9
Total wt % trienoic	1.3	0.9	1.1	1.5	0.9	1.4	1.4	1.8	1.3	1.0	1.1	1.6	1.5
Total wt % tetraenoic	3.3	2.3	3.2	3.4	2.6	3.8	2.6	4.0	3.1	3.5	3.4	4.0	4.3
Total wt % pentaenoic	8.6	5.3	6.8	7.3	9.5	7.9	7.4	5.9	10.1	9.7	10.3	10.7	10.7
Total wt % hexaenoic	4.7	2.1	4.9	5.2	3.7	4.7	5.4	6.3	5.0	4.2	4.5	5.1	5.5
Total wt % polyunsaturated	20.0	12.0	17.7	20.1	18.1	20.2	20.4	21.6	21.6	20.0	20.9	23.4	23.8
Hexadecanoic as percent of saturated	59.5	61.6	60.5	54.7	62.9	57.6	59.0	55.3	61.8	61.0	60.0	61.4	56.6
Ratio 16:0/16:1	1.4	1.0	1.3	1.9	0.9	1.5	1.8	1.9	1.5	0.9	0.9	1.7	1.5
Ratio 16:0/(16:1 + 18:1)	0.56	0.52	0.53	0.68	0.49	0.58	0.45	0.67	0.59	0.44	0.43	0.66	0.68
Ratio 16:1/18:1	0.8	1.1	0.7	0.6	1.1	0.7	0.3	0.5	0.7	0.9	0.9	0.7	0.9
Ratio $(20{:}x\omega6 + 22{:}x\omega6)/(18{:}2\omega6 + 18{:}3\omega6)$	0.82	1.07	0.83	0.58	0.73	0.68	0.46	0.71	0.70	1.24	1.61	0.64	0.57
Ratio $20{:}x\omega3/18{:}x\omega3$	3.3	2.6	2.6	1.9	6.6	2.2	3.1	1.6	4.0	4.8	4.8	3.2	3.0
Ratio $22{:}x\omega3/18{:}x\omega3$	2.4	1.6	2.3	1.8	3.1	1.8	3.5	1.9	2.5	2.8	3.4	1.9	2.0
Ratio $22{:}x\omega3/20{:}x\omega3$	0.78	0.63	0.89	0.95	0.48	0.82	1.12	1.15	0.68	0.61	0.65	0.60	0.66
Ratio $\Sigma\omega3/\Sigma\omega6$	7.5	6.3	7.2	6.8	11.2	6.3	3.3	6.3	7.4	7.7	9.2	8.6	9.9
Ratio $\Sigma n{:}x\omega3/\Sigma n{:}x{-}1\omega3$	7.4	5.8	8.7	7.0	12.4	6.3	4.1	6.1	8.1	7.3	7.5	7.5	7.7

[a]From alkali isomerization data.
[b]European origin assumed.

Table 3 (continued)
COMPARISONS OF PROPERTIES OF INTEREST OF SOME ATLANTIC HERRING OILS, FOR SOME OTHER HERRING OILS, AND FOR PILCHARD OIL

Property compared	Pacific herring oils				European herring oils					Pacific pilchard oil Ackman and Sipos[5]
	This study	Gruger et al.[1]	Lambertson and Braektan[2]	Klenk and Eberhagen[3]	Dunn and Robson[4],[b]					
					Average nos. 1—4	Replicate analyses				
						1	2	3	4	
Wt % saturated	24.7	29.0	26.1	20	25.9	24.2	27.1	26.4	25.7	28.8
Wt % monounsaturated	54.6	46.2	50.4	59	58.7	60.2	58.6	58.1	57.9	28.3
Total wt % saturated + monounsaturated	79.3	75.2	76.5	79	85.6	84.4	85.7	84.5	83.6	57.1
Total wt % dienoic	1.5	—	—	1.8[a]	3.6	2.5	4.7	4.0	3.1	2.6
Total wt % trienoic	1.0	—	—	2.0[a]						2.0
Total wt % tetraenoic	3.1	—	—	4.2[a]	11.8	13.1	9.4	11.5	13.3	4.9
Total wt % pentaenoic	10.0	—	—	4.6[a]						19.4
Total wt % hexaenoic	5.0	—	—	5.2[a]						12.9
Total wt % polyunsaturated	20.6	24.8	23.5	21	15.4	15.6	14.1	15.5	16.4	41.8
Hexadecanoic as percent of saturated	67.4	63.1	57	65	—	—	—	—	—	56.3
Ratio 16:0/16:1	2.2	2.2	1.6	2.2	—	—	—	—	—	1.8
Ratio 16:0/(16:1 + 18:1)	0.55	0.73	0.70	0.46	—	—	—	—	—	0.79
Ratio 16:1/18:1	0.3	0.5	0.7	0.3	—	—	—	—	—	0.8
Ratio (20:xω6 + 22:xω6)/(18:2ω6 + 18:3ω6)	1.31	—	—	—	—	—	—	—	—	1.15
Ratio 20:xω3/18:xω3	4.2	—	—	—	—	—	—	—	—	6.0
Ratio 22:xω3/18:xω3	2.7	—	—	—	—	—	—	—	—	5.2
Ratio 22:xω3/20:xω3	0.64	—	—	—	—	—	—	—	—	0.87
Ratio Σω3/Σω6	11.2	—	—	—	—	—	—	—	—	12.7
Ratio Σn:xω3/Σn:x−1ω3	8.2	—	—	—	—	—	—	—	—	6.4

REFERENCES

1. Gruger, Nelson, and Stansby, J. Am. Oil Chem. Soc., 41, 662 (1964).
2. Lambertson and Braektan, Fiskeridir. Skr. Ser. Teknol. Unders., 4(13), 15 (1965).
3. Klenk and Eberhagen, Hoppe-Seyler's Z. Physiol. Chem., 328, 180 (1962).
4. Dunn and Robson, J. Chromatogr., 17, 501 (1965).
5. Ackman and Sipos, J. Fish Res. Board Can., 21(4), 841 (1964).

From Ackman and Eaton, J. Fish. Res. Board Can., 23(7), 994 (1966). With permission.

Steroids

Table 2 (continued)
BILE ACIDS

No.	Substance[a]	Structure	Formula (mol wt)	Melting point °C	Spectral data[b]						$[\alpha]_D^c$	Potency
					IR	NMR	λ_{max}	ϵ	$E_{1cm}^{1\%}$			
13	3α,6α-dihydroxy-cholanic acid HYODESOXYCHOLIC ACID	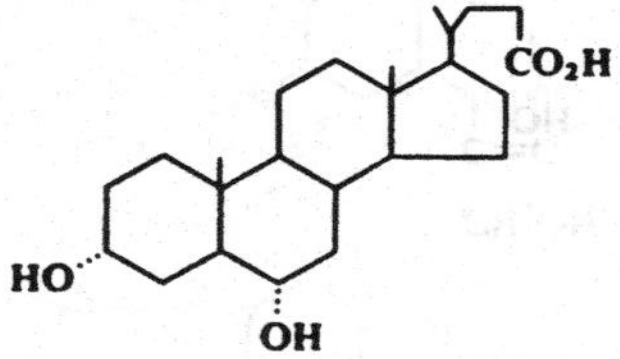	$C_{24}H_{40}O_4$ (392)	197	Ester (9)	—	—	—	—		+8(U)	—
14	3α,7β-dihydroxy-cholanic acid URSODESOXYCHOLIC ACID	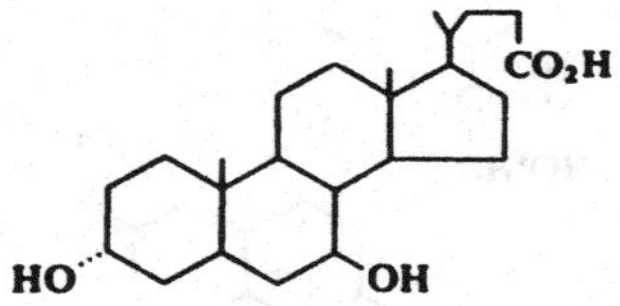	$C_{24}H_{40}O_4$ (392)	203	—	—	—	—	—		+57(U)	—
15	3α-hydroxy-cholanic acid LITHOCHOLIC ACID	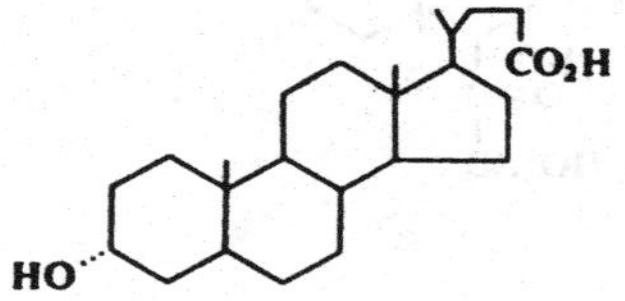	$C_{24}H_{40}O_3$ (376)	186	Ester (9)	—	—	—	—		+35(E)	—

Compiled by F. Edward Roberts and T. Windholz.

Table 3
CORTICOIDS

No.	Substance[a]	Structure	Formula (mol wt)	Melting point °C	Spectral data[b]		Ultraviolet			$[\alpha]_D^c$	Potency[d]
					IR	NMR	λ_{max}	ϵ	$E_{1cm}^{1\%}$		
16	Pregn-4-ene-17α,21-diol-3,11,20-trione CORTISONE	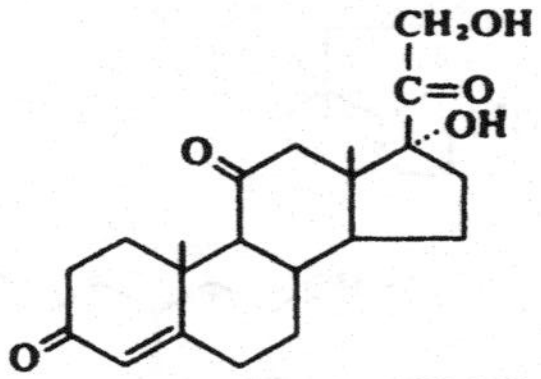	$C_{21}H_{28}O_5$ (360.4)	220–224	(1)	(6)	238	15,400	441	+209(E)	0.4
17	Pregn-4-ene-11β,17α,21-triol-3,20-dione HYDROCORTISONE	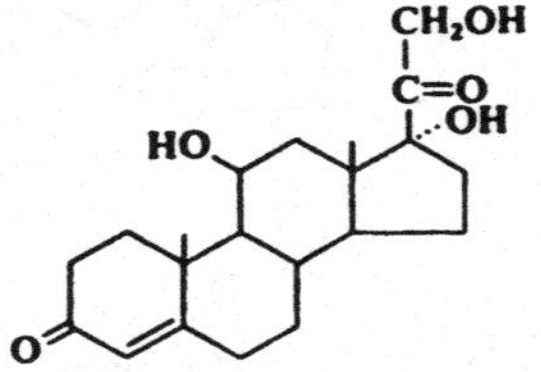	$C_{21}H_{30}O_5$ (362.4)	217–220	(1)	(5)	24	16,300	450	+167(E)	1.0
18	Pregn-1,4-diene-11β,17α,21-triol-3,20-dione PREDNISOLONE	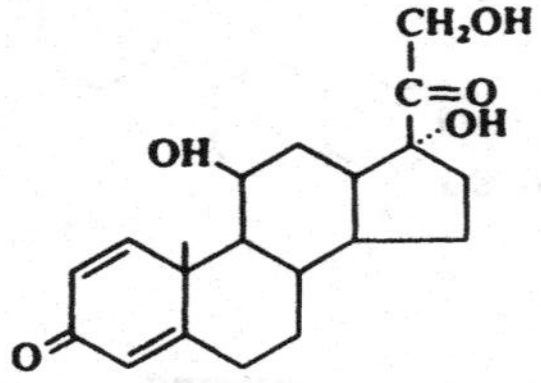	$C_{21}H_{28}O_5$ (360.4)	Mod. A 223–227 Mod. B 232	(1)	(5)	242	15,200	422	Mod. A +112(M) Mod. B +97(D)	3.1

[a] Systematic nomenclature. Numbers after the symbol "Δ" indicate the position of double bonds in the basic cyclopentano perhydrophenanthrene ring. Trivial names are included when available.

[b] Spectral data for infrared (IR) and nuclear magnetic resonance (NMR) can be found in references indicated in ( ). ϵ is molar extinction and $E_{1cm}^{1\%}$ is extinction of 1% solutions in methanol with 1 cm light path.

[c] Specific rotation at the sodium D line unless given in brackets, [ ], when the rotation was obtained at the 546.1 Hg line. Solvents are (A) for acetone, (C) for chloroform, (D) for dioxane, (E) for ethanol, (M) for methanol, (P) for pyridine, and (U) when unspecified.

[d] Relative potency by anti-inflammaotry response.[1] Cortisol = 1.

Table 3 (continued)
CORTICOIDS

No.	Substance[a]	Structure	Formula (mol wt)	Melting point °C	IR	NMR	λ_{max}	ϵ	$E_{1cm}^{1\%}$	$[\alpha]_D^c$	Potency[d]
							Ultraviolet				
19	Pregn-4-ene-9α-fluoro-11β,17α-21-triol-3,20-dione FLUOROHYDROCORTISONE	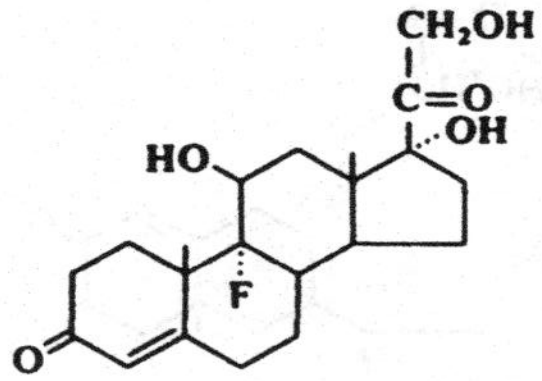	$C_{21}H_{29}O_5F$ (380.4)	253–255	(1)	—	238	17,100	449	+137(E)	8.0[e]
20	Pregn-1,4-diene-9α-fluoro-11β,17α,21-triol-3,20-dione acetate 9α-FLUOROPREDNISOLONE ACETATE	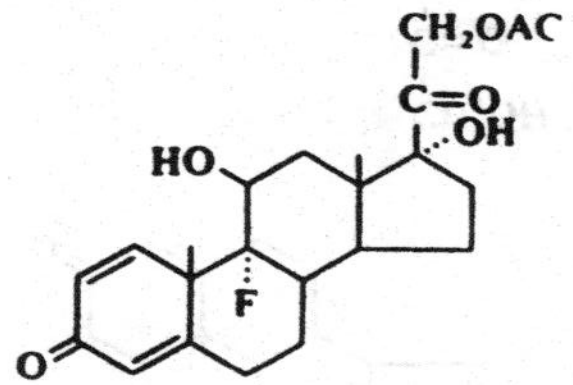	$C_{23}H_{29}O_6F$ (420.4)	237	(8)	—	(8)	(8)	(8)	+110.9(A)	16.5
21	Pregn-1,4-diene-9α-fluoro-16α-methyl-11β,17α, 21-triol-3,20-dione DEXAMETHASONE	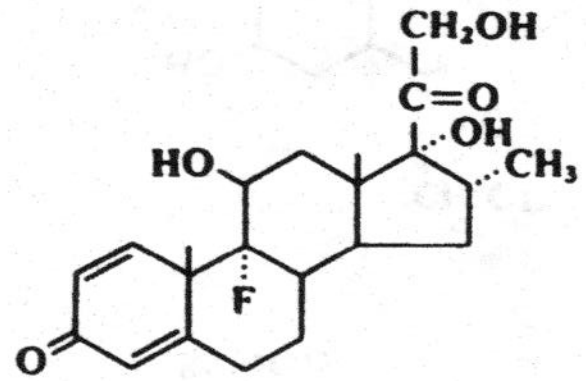	$C_{22}H_{29}O_5F$ (392.4)	256–258	(1)	—	238	15,400	392	+86(D)	164.0[e]

[e]As acetate.

Table 3 (continued)
CORTICOIDS

No.	Substance[a]	Structure	Formula (mol wt)	Melting point °C	Spectral data[b]							$[\alpha]_D$[c]	Potency[d]
					IR	NMR	Ultraviolet						
							λ_{max}	ϵ	$E_{1cm}^{1\%}$				
22	Pregn-4-ene-11β,21-diol-3,20-dione CORTICOSTERONE	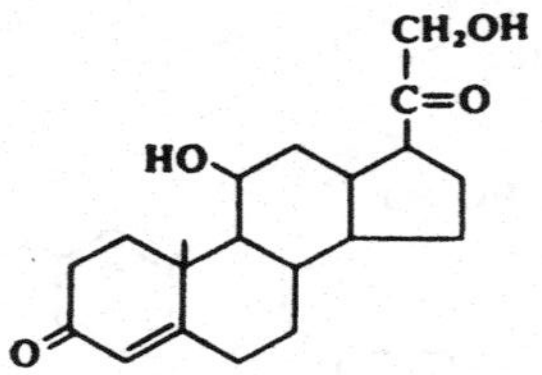	$C_{21}H_{30}O_4$ (346.4)	180–182	(1)	(5)	240	16,700	482			+262(E) +224(E)	0.32
23	Pregn-4-ene-21-ol-3,11,20-trione DEHYDROCORTICOSTERONE	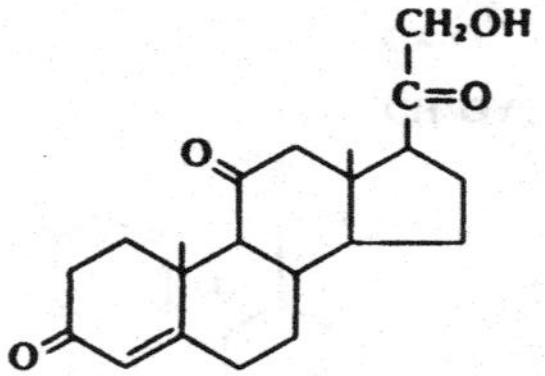	$C_{21}H_{28}O_4$ (344.4)	178–180	(8)	—	—	—	—			+258(U)	—
24	Pregn-4-ene-21-ol-3,20-dione DEOXYCORTICOSTERONE	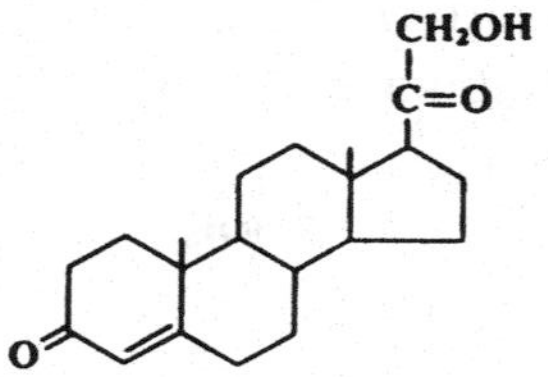	$C_{21}H_{30}O_3$ (330)	141–142	(1)	(1)	240	17,200	520			+178(E) +184(C)	—

Compiled by F. Edward Roberts and T. Windholz.

Table 4
ESTROGENS

No.	Substance[a]	Structure	Formula (mol wt)	Melting point °C	Spectral data[b]					[α]$_D$[c]	Potency[d]
					IR	NMR	Ultraviolet				
							λ_{max}	ϵ	$E_{1cm}^{1\%}$		
25	Estr-1,3,5(10),6,8-pentaene-3α-ol-17-one EQUILENIN	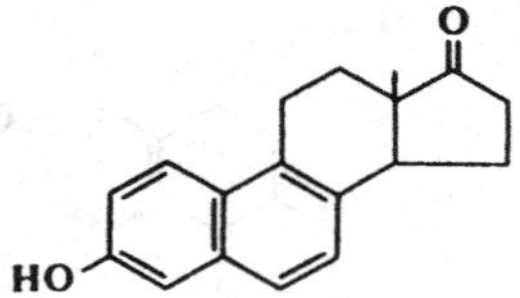	$C_{18}H_{18}O_2$ (266.4)	258–259	(10)	—	(11)	(11)	(11)	+89(D)	0.625
26	Estr-1,3,5(10),7-tetraene-3-ol-17-one EQUILIN	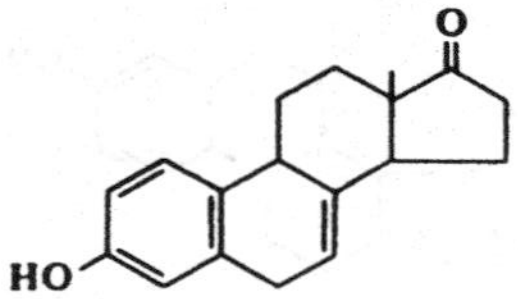	$C_{18}H_{20}O_2$ (268.4)	238–240	(10)	—	—	—	—	+308(U)	1.250
27	Estr-1,3,5(10)-triene-3-ol-17-one ESTRONE	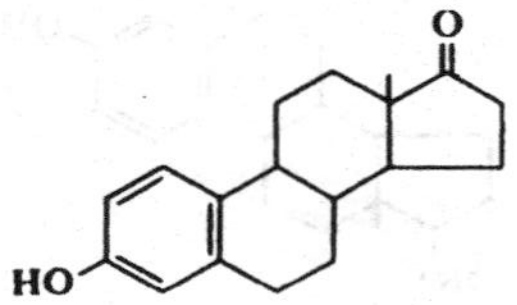	$C_{18}H_{22}O_2$ (270.4)	255	(1)	(12)	280	2,080	77	+170(D) +156(C)	1.250

[a] Systematic nomenclature. Numbers after the symbol "Δ" indicate the position of double bonds in the basic cyclopentano perhydrophenanthrene ring. Trivial names are included when available.

[b] Spectral data for infrared (IR) and nuclear magnetic resonance (NMR) can be found in references indicated in ( ). ϵ is molar extinction and $E_{1cm}^{1\%}$ is extinction of 1% solutions in methanol with 1 cm light path.

[c] Specific rotation at the sodium D line unless given in brackets, [ ], when the rotation was obtained at the 546.1 Hg line. Solvents are (A) for acetone, (C) for chloroform, (D) for dioxane, (E) for ethanol, (M) for methanol, (P) for pyridine, and (U) when unspecified.

[d] Minimum dose in micrograms to produce 70% increase in uterine weight in 6 hr when applied subcutaneously to rats.[19]

Table 4 (continued)
ESTROGENS

No.	Substance[a]	Structure	Formula (mol wt)	Melting point °C	Spectral data[b]						$[\alpha]^c_D$	Potency[d]
					IR	NMR	λ_{max}	Ultraviolet ϵ	$E^{1\%}_{1cm}$			
28	Estr-1,3,5(10)-triene-3,17β-diol 17β-ESTRADIOL	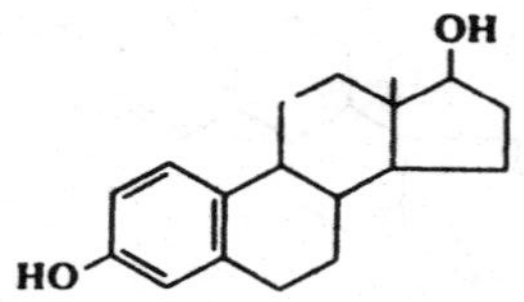	$C_{18}H_{24}O_2$ (272.4)	174–176	(1)	(5)	281	2,120	78	+76(D)	0.100
29	Estr-1,3,5(10)-triene-3,16α,17β-triol ESTRIOL	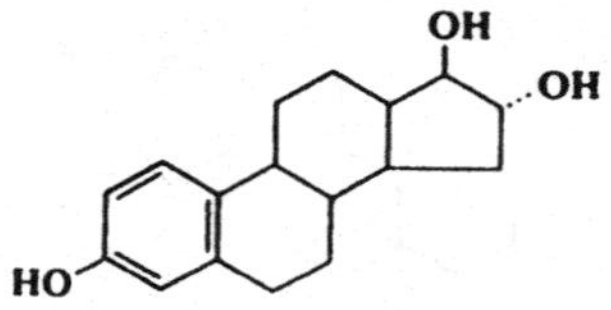	$C_{18}H_{24}O_3$ (288)	282	(1)	—	280	2,150	75	+61(E) +35(P)	0.078
30	Estr-1,3,5(10)-triene-17α-ethinyl-3,17-diol ETHINYL ESTRADIOL	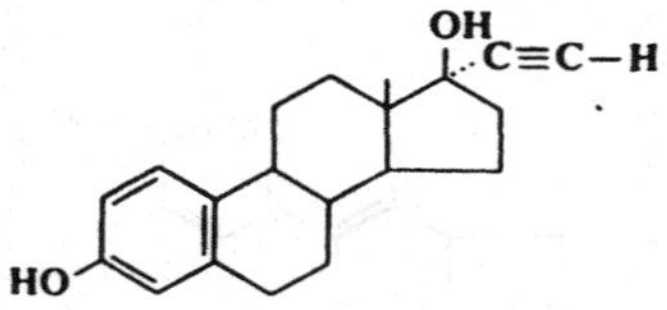	$C_{20}H_{24}O_2$ (296.4)	180–182	(1)	(13)	280	2,130	72	+4(C) +0(D) [+5](C)	8[e]
31	Estr-1,3,5(10)-triene-17α-ethinyl-3-methoxy-17β-ol ETHINYL ESTRADIOL METHYL ETHER	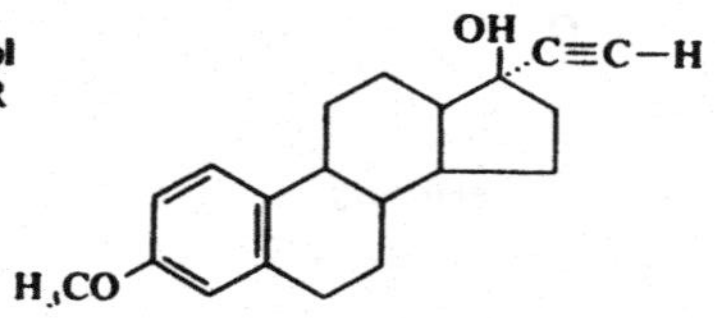	$C_{21}H_{26}O_2$ (310.4)	149-150	(1)	—	278	1,050	66	+3(C) [+8](C)	·

Compiled by F. Edward Roberts and T. Windholz.

[e]About eight times the effect of estrone.[10]

Table 5
PROGESTAGENS

No.	Substance[a]	Structure	Formula (mol wt)	Melting point °C	Spectral data[b] IR	NMR	Ultraviolet λ_{max}	ϵ	$E_{1cm}^{1\%}$	$[\alpha]_D^c$	Potency[d]
32	Estr-4-ene-17α-ethinyl-17β-hydroxy-3-one NORETHINDRONE (ENT)	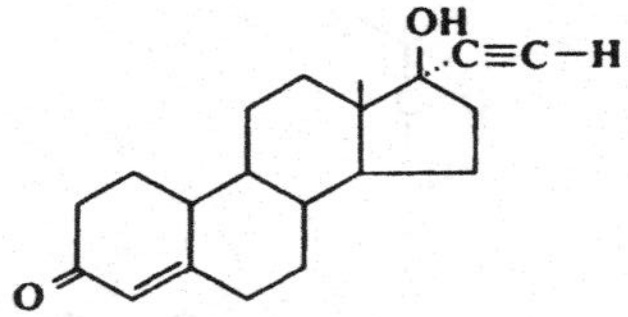	$C_{20}H_{26}O_2$ (298.4)	203–204	(1)	—	240	17,600	590	−24(C)	1
33	Estr-5(10)-ene-17α-ethinyl-17β-hydroxy-3-one NORETHYNODREL	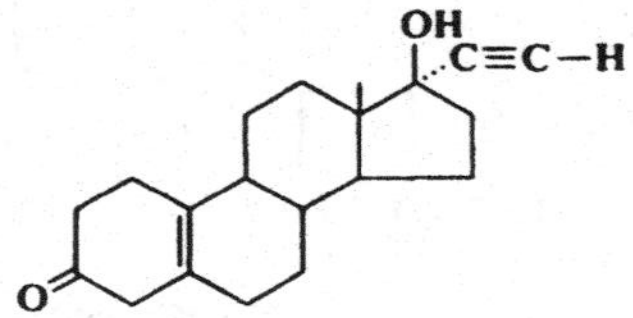	$C_{20}H_{26}O_2$ (298.4)	169–170	—	—	—	—	—	+108(C)	0.25
34	Androst-4-ene-17α-ethinyl-17β-hydroxy-3-one ETHISTERONE	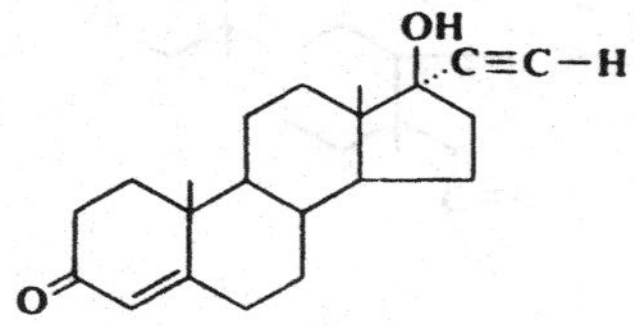	$C_{21}H_{28}O_2$ (312.4)	264–268	(1)	—	241	16,900	541	+31(P) +22(D)	0.06

[a]Systematic nomenclature. Numbers after the symbol "Δ" indicate the position of double bonds in the basic cyclopentano perhydrophenanthrene ring. Trivial names are included when available.

[b]Spectral data for infrared (IR) and nuclear magnetic resonance (NMR) can be found in references indicated in ( ). ϵ is molar extinction and $E_{1cm}^{1\%}$ is extinction of 1% solutions in methanol with 1 cm light path.

[c]Specific rotation at the sodium D line unless given in brackets, [ ], when the rotation was obtained at the 546.1 Hg line. Solvents are (A) for acetone, (C) for chloroform, (D) for dioxane, (E) for ethanol, (M) for methanol, (P) for pyridine, and (U) when unspecified.

[d]Relative potency by oral Clauberg test in rabbits.[21] Norethindrone = 1.

Table 5 (continued)
PROGESTAGENS

No.	Substance[a]	Structure	Formula (mol wt)	Melting point °C	Spectral data[b]			Ultraviolet			$[\alpha]_D^c$	Potency[d]
					IR	NMR		λ_{max}	ϵ	$E_{1cm}^{1\%}$		
35	Pregn-4-ene-3,20-dione PROGESTERONE	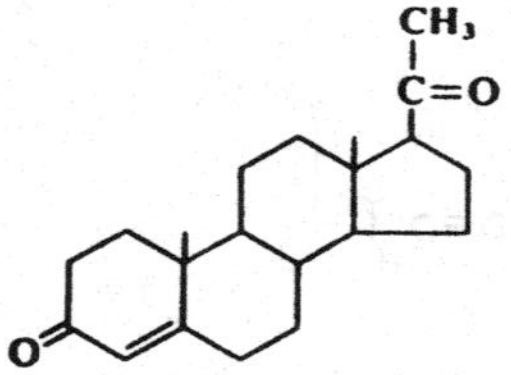	$C_{21}H_{30}O_2$ (314.4)	128–129	(1)	(2,3)		240	17,000	541	+201(C) +181(D) +191(M)	1
36	Estr-4-en-17α-ethinyl-17β-hydroxy-3-one acetate NORETHINDRONE ACETATE	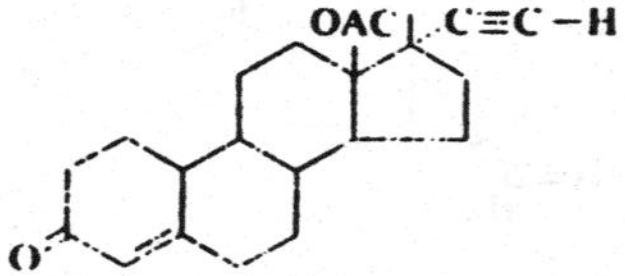	$C_{22}H_{28}O_2$ (340.4)	161–162	(1)	(1)		239	17,700	520	−29(C) [−37](U)	3
37	Pregn-4,6-diene-5-chloro-17β-hydroxy-3,20-dione acetate CHLORMADINONE		$C_{23}H_{29}ClO_3$ (404.9)	212–214	(1)			284	22,700	561	+8(C)	35–50

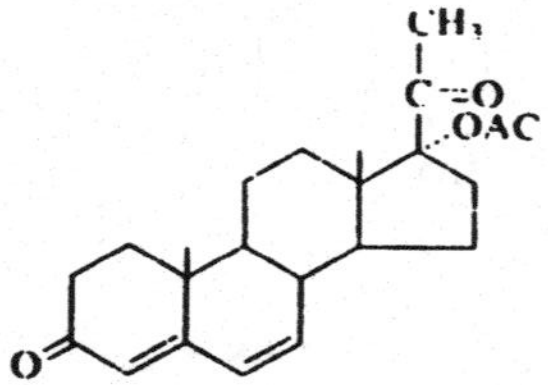

Table 5 (continued)
PROGESTAGENS

No.	Substance[a]	Structure	Formula (mol wt)	Melting point °C	Spectral data[b]					[α]$_D^c$	Potency[d]
					IR	NMR	Ultraviolet λ_{max}	ε	$E^{1\%}_{1cm}$		
38	Pregn-4,6-diene-6-methyl-17α-hydroxy-3,20-dione acetate MEGESTROL ACETATE	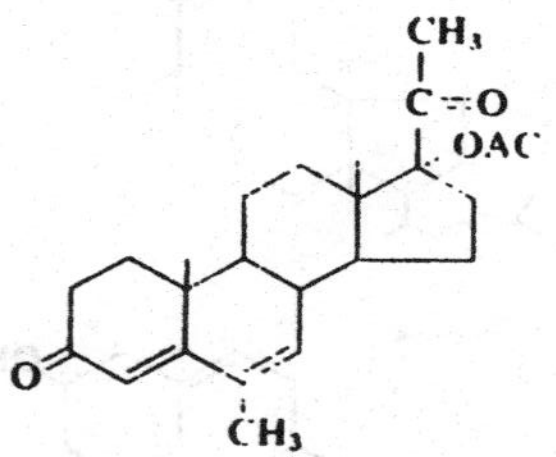	$C_{23}H_{32}O_4$ (384.5)	218-220	(1)	---	289	24,000	590	+11(U)	12
39	Pregn-4-en-6α-methyl-17α-hydroxy-3,20-dione acetate MEDROXYPROGESTERONE ACETATE	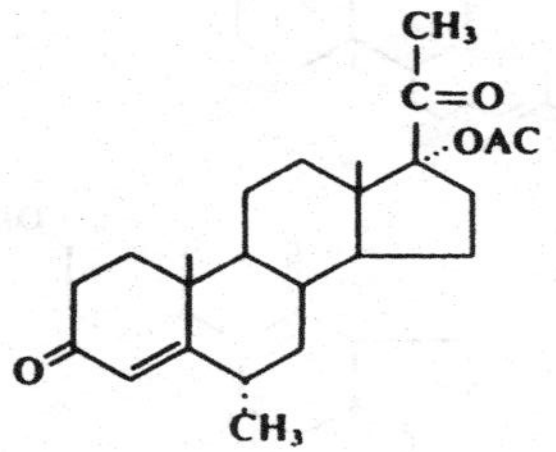	$C_{24}H_{34}O_4$ (386.5)	203-205	—	—	240	16,000	—	+58(C)	10
40	Pregn-4,6-diene-6-methyl-16-methylene-17α-hydroxy 3,20-dione acetate MELENGESTROL ACETATE	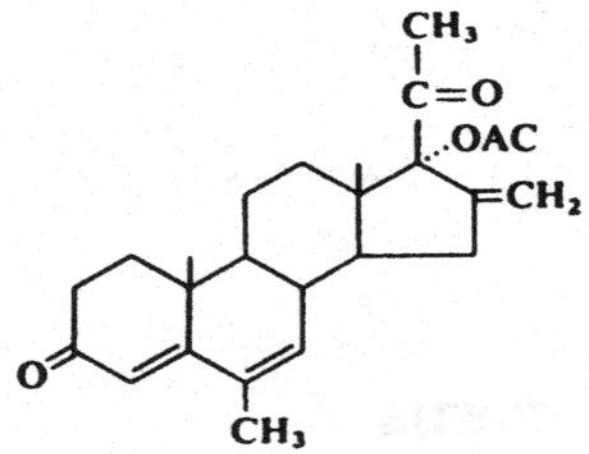	$C_{25}H_{32}O_4$ (396.5)	224-226	—	—	287	22,400	—	−127(U)	72

Compiled by F. Edward Roberts and T. Windholz.

Table 6
STEROLS

No.	Substance[a]	Structure	Formula (mol wt)	Melting point °C	Spectral data[b]		Ultraviolet			$[\alpha]_D^c$
					IR	NMR	λ_{max}	ϵ	$E_{1cm}^{1\%}$	
41	Cholest-5,7,-diene-3β-ol 7-DEHYDROCHOLESTEROL	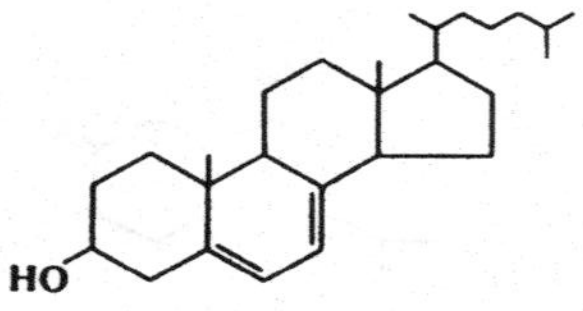	$C_{27}H_{44}O$ (384.6)	150	(9)	(3)	—	—	—	−114(C)
42	Cholest-5,24(25)-diene-3β-ol 24-DEHYDROCHOLESTADIONE-3β-OL	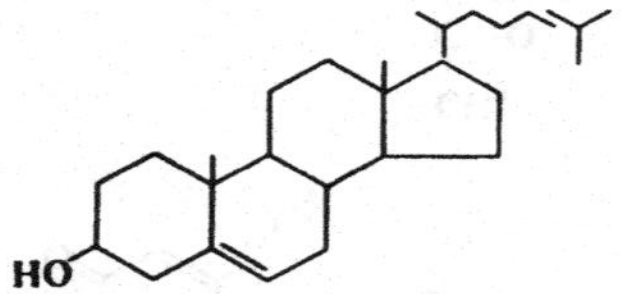	$C_{27}H_{44}O$ (384.6)	117	—	—	—	—	—	−38(C)
43	Cholest-5-ene-3β-ol CHOLESTEROL	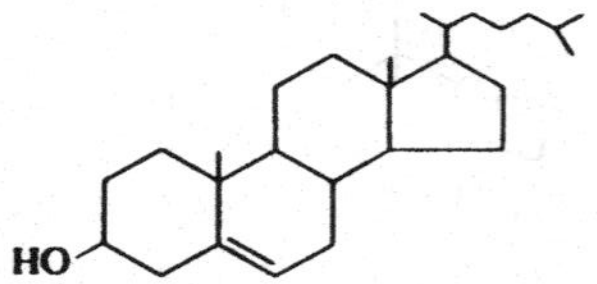	$C_{27}H_{46}O$ (386.6)	149	(1)	(13)	—	—	—	−39(C)

[a]Systematic nomenclature. Numbers after the symbol "Δ" indicate the position of double bonds in the basic cyclopentano perhydrophenanthrene ring. Trivial names are included when available. Data selected from *Biology Data Book*.[23]

[b]Spectral data for infrared (IR) and nuclear magnetic resonance (NMR) can be found in references indicated in ( ). ε is molar extinction and $E_{1cm}^{1\%}$ is extinction of 1% solutions in methanol with 1 cm light path.

[c]Specific rotation at the sodium D line unless given in brackets, [ ], when the rotation was obtained at the 546.1 Hg line. Solvents are (A) for acetone, (C) for chloroform, (D) for dioxane, (E) for ethanol, (M) for methanol, (P) for pyridine, and (U) when unspecified.

Table 6 (continued)
STEROLS

No.	Substance[a]	Structure	Formula (mol wt)	Melting point °C	Spectral data[b]						[α]$_D$[c]
					IR	NMR	Ultraviolet				
							λ$_{max}$	ε	E$^{1\%}_{1cm}$		
44	Coprostan-3β-ol COPROSTANOL	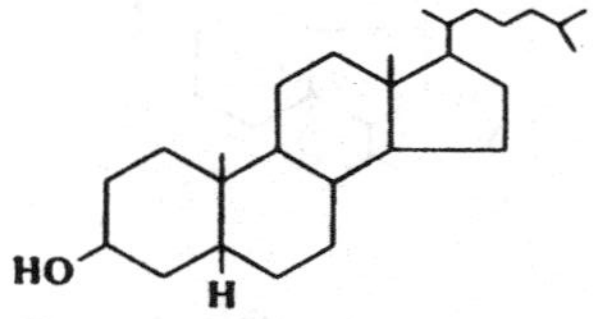	C$_{27}$H$_{48}$O (388.4)	101	(9)	—	—	—	—		+28(C)
45	Cholestan-3β-ol CHOLESTANOL	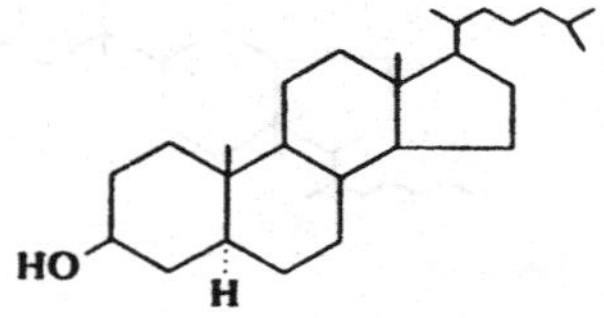	C$_{27}$H$_{48}$O (388.4)	140–142	(1)	(14)	—	—	—		+23(C)
46	Ergosta-5,7,22-trien-3β-ol ERGOSTEROL	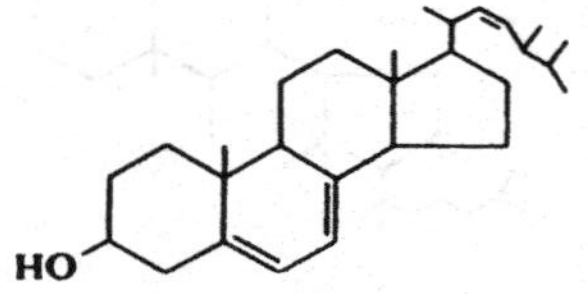	C$_{28}$H$_{44}$O (396)	165	(9)	—	282	11,900	—		−130(C)
47	Stigmasta-5,22-dien-3β-ol STIGMASTEROL	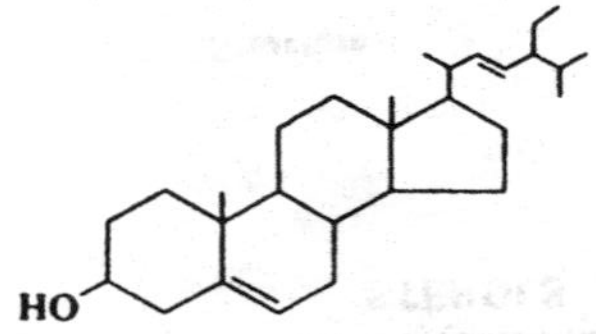	C$_{29}$H$_{48}$O (412)	170	—	—	—	—	—		−49(C)

Table 6 (continued)
STEROLS

No.	Substance[a]	Structure	Formula (mol wt)	Melting point °C	Spectral data[b] IR	Spectral data[b] NMR	Ultraviolet λ_{max}	Ultraviolet ϵ	Ultraviolet $E_{1cm}^{1\%}$	$[\alpha]_D^c$
48	Stigmast-5-ene-3β-ol β-SITOSTEROL	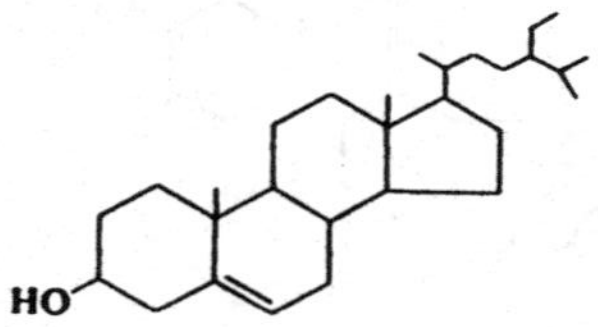	$C_{29}H_{50}O$ (414)	140	(9)	(15)	—	—	—	−36(C)
49	Δ³,⁵-Cholestadien-7-one	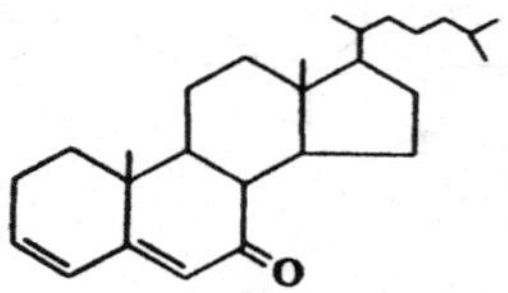	$C_{27}H_{42}O$ (382.6)	112	—	—	—	—	—	−305(C)
50	Δ⁴,⁶-Cholestadien-3-one	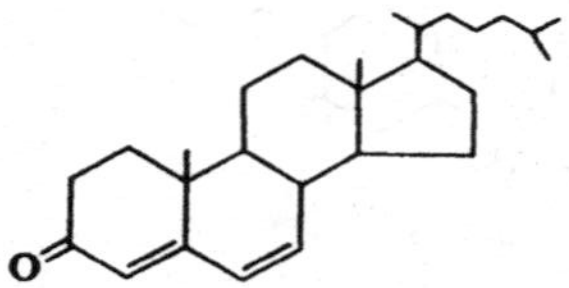	$C_{27}H_{42}O$ (382.6)	80	—	—	—	—	—	+35(C)
51	Δ⁵,⁷,²²-Cholestatrien-3β-ol	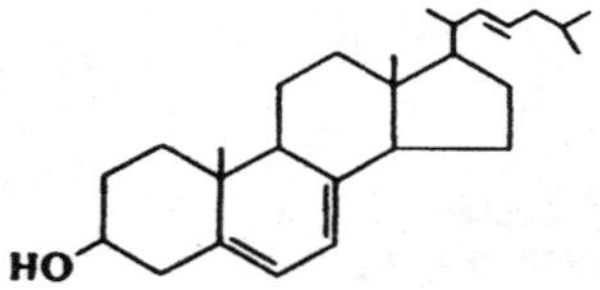	$C_{27}H_{42}O$ (382.6)	—	—	—	—	—	—	—

Table 6 (continued)
STEROLS

No.	Substance[a]	Structure	Formula (mol wt)	Melting point °C	Spectral data[b]					$[\alpha]_D^c$
					IR	NMR	λ_{max}	ϵ	$E_{1cm}^{1\%}$	
52	Δ^4-Cholesten-3-one	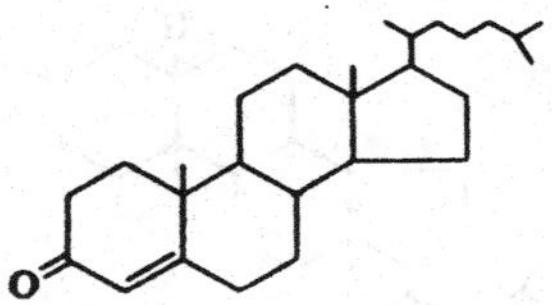	$C_{27}H_{44}O$ (384.6)	81	---	---	---	---	---	+89(C)
53	$\Delta^{5,22}$-Cholestadien-3β-ol 22-DEHYDROCHOLESTEROL	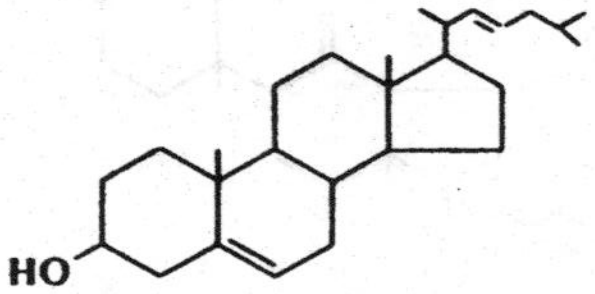	$C_{27}H_{44}O$ (384.6)	135	---	---	---	---	---	−57(C)
54	$\Delta^{8,24}$-Cholestadien-3β-ol ZYMOSTEROL	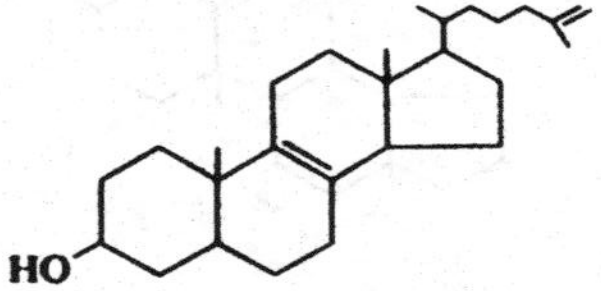	$C_{27}H_{44}O$ (384.6)	108	---	---	---	---	---	+47(C)
55	Cholestane-3,6-dione	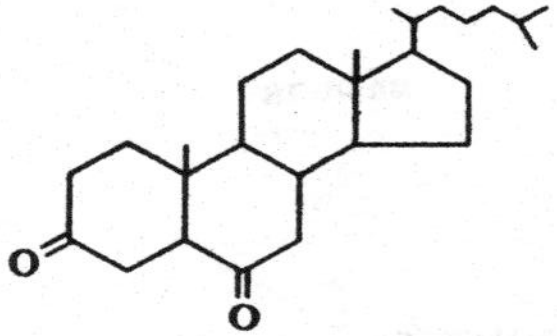	$C_{27}H_{44}O_2$ (400.6)	175	---	---	---	---	---	---

Table 6 (continued)
STEROLS

No.	Substance[a]	Structure	Formula (mol wt)	Melting point °C	Spectral data[b]					[α]$_D^c$
					IR	NMR	Ultraviolet			
							λ_{max}	ϵ	$E_{1cm}^{1\%}$	
56	Δ⁵-Cholesten-3β-ol-7-one 7-KETOCHOLESTEROL	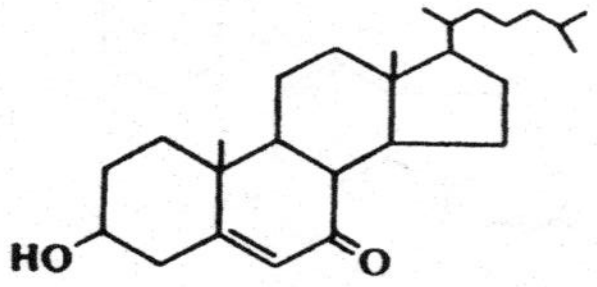	$C_{27}H_{44}O_2$ (400.6)	170	—	—	—	—	—	−104(C)
57	Δ⁷-Cholesten-3β-ol LATHOSTEROL	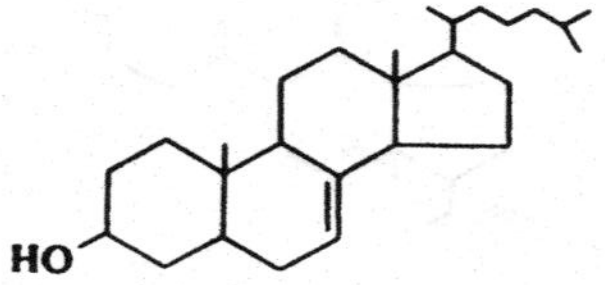	$C_{27}H_{46}O$ (386.6)	122	—	—	—	—	—	+5.7(C)
58	Coprostan-3-one	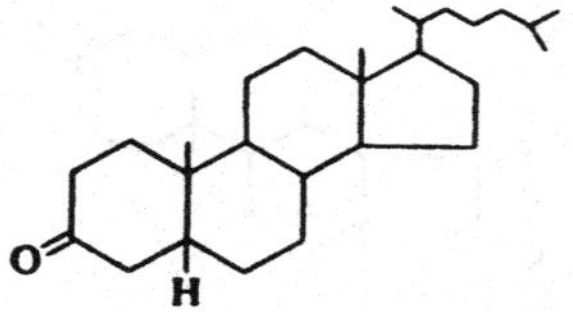	$C_{27}H_{46}O$ (386.6)	63	—	—	—	—	—	+36(C)
59	Δ⁴-Cholesten-3β,6β-diol	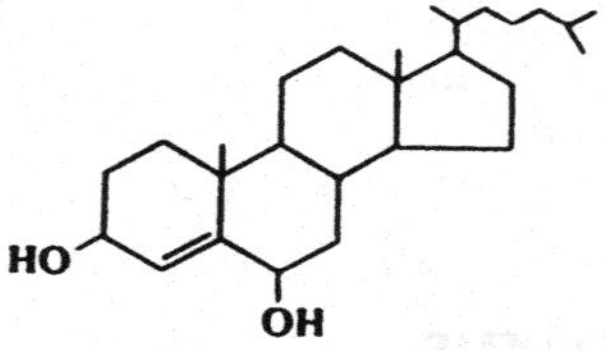	$C_{27}H_{46}O_2$ (402.6)	258	—	—	—	—	—	+9(C)

Table 6 (continued)
STEROLS

No.	Substance[a]	Structure	Formula (mol wt)	Melting point °C	IR	NMR	λ_{max}	ϵ	$E_{1cm}^{1\%}$	$[\alpha]_D^c$
								Ultraviolet		
								Spectral data[b]		
60	Δ⁵-Cholestene-3β,7α-diol 7α-HYDROXYCHOLESTEROL	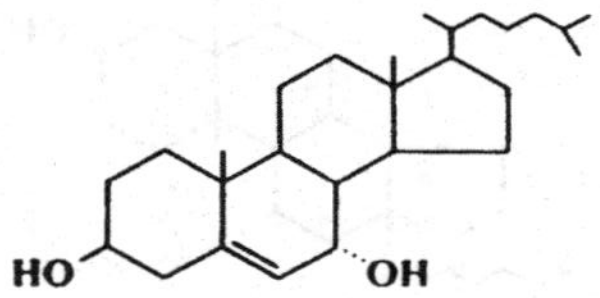	$C_{27}H_{46}O_2$ (402.6)	184	—	—	—	—	—	−93(C)
61	Δ⁵-Cholestene-3β,7β-diol 7β-HYDROXYCHOLESTEROL	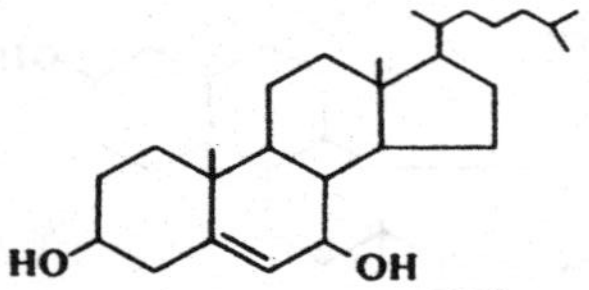	$C_{27}H_{46}O_2$ (402.6)	178	—	—	—	—	—	+7(C)
62	Δ⁵-Cholestene-3β,20α-diol 22-HYDROXYCHOLESTEROL	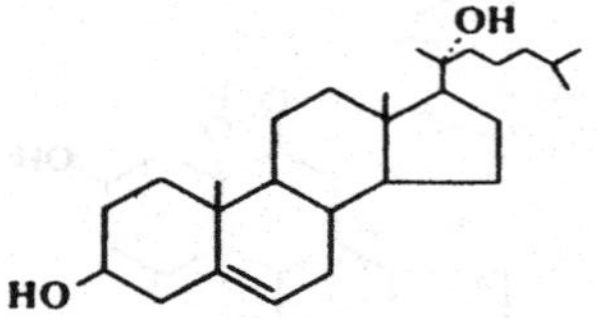	$C_{27}H_{46}O_2$ (402.6)	186	—	—	—	—	—	−39(C)
63	Cholestan-3β-ol-6-one	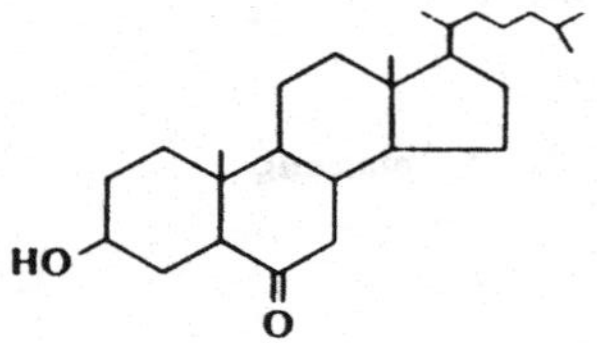	$C_{27}H_{46}O_2$ (402.6)	143						

Table 6 (continued)
STEROLS

No.	Substance[a]	Structure	Formula (mol wt)	Melting point °C	IR	NMR	Ultraviolet λmax	ε	E$_{1cm}^{1\%}$	[α]$_D^c$
64	Cholestane-3β,5α-diol-6-one	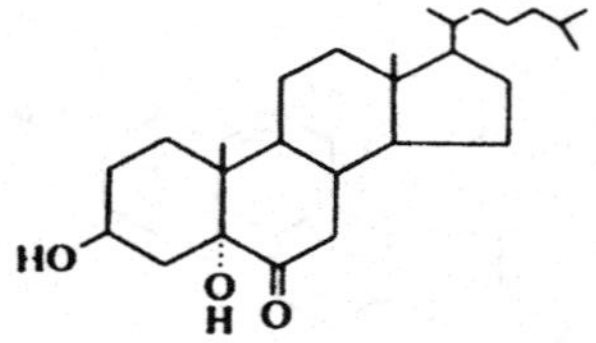	$C_{27}H_{46}O_3$ (418.6)	236	—	—	—	—	—	—
65	Cholestan-3β-ol CHOLESTANOL	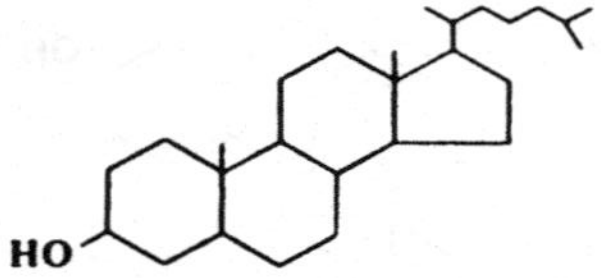	$C_{27}H_{48}O$ (388.6)	142	—	—	—	—	...	+24(C)
66	Coprostan-3β-ol COPROSTANOL	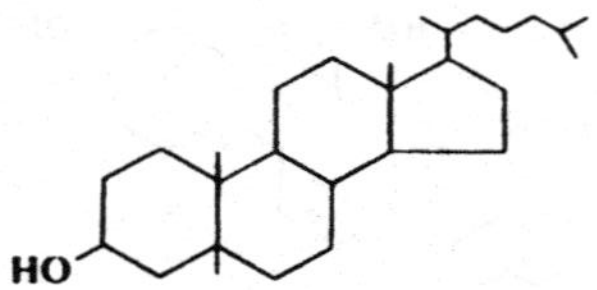	$C_{27}H_{48}O$ (388.6)	101	—	—	—	—	—	+28(C)
67	Coprostan-3α-ol EPICOPROSTANOL	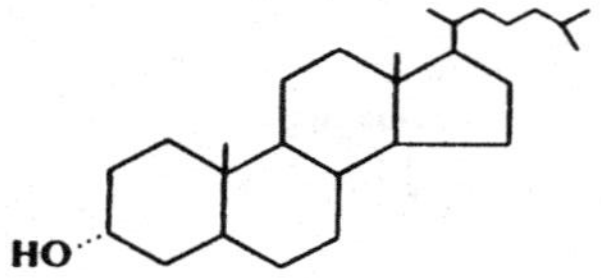	$C_{27}H_{48}O$ (388.6)	117	—	—	—	—	—	+32(C)

Table 6 (continued)
STEROLS

No.	Substance[a]	Structure	Formula (mol wt)	Melting point °C	Spectral data[b]						[α]$_D^c$
					IR	NMR	Ultraviolet				
							λ$_{max}$	ε	E$_{1cm}^{1\%}$		
68	Cholestane-3β,5,6β-triol	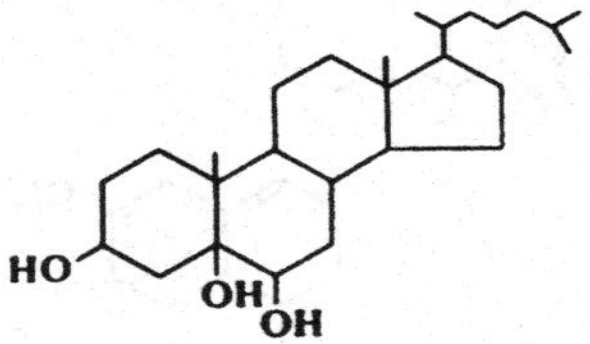	C$_{27}$H$_{48}$O$_3$ (420.6)	239	—	—	—	—	—		+3(C)
69	Δ$^{5,7,9(11),22}$-Ergostatetraen-3β-ol DEHYDROERGOSTEROL	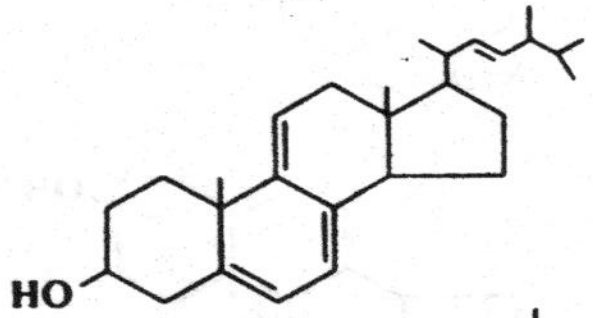	C$_{28}$H$_{42}$O (394.6)	146	—	—	—	—	—		+149(C)
70	Δ^{5,7,14,22}-Ergostatetraen-3β-ol 14-DEHYDROERGOSTEROL	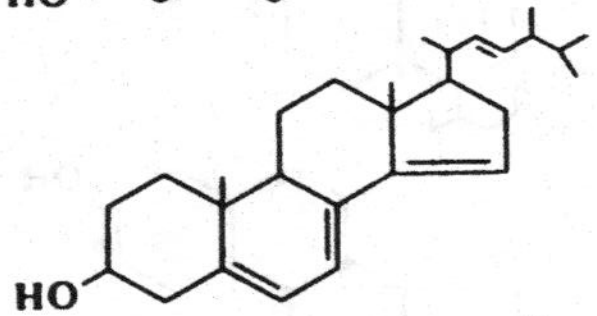	C$_{28}$H$_{42}$O (394.6)	198	—	—	—	—	—		−396(C)
71	Δ$^{5,7,22,24(28)}$-Ergostatetraen-3β-ol 24-DEHYDROERGOSTEROL	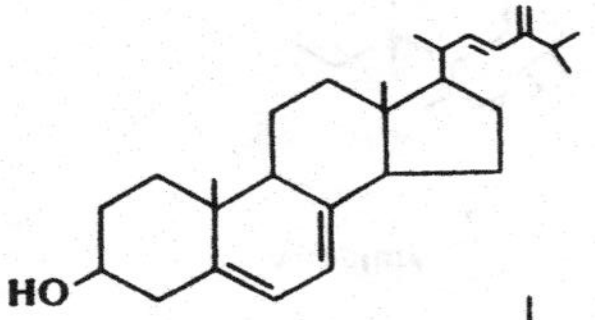	C$_{28}$H$_{42}$O (394.6)	118	—	—	—	—	—		−78(C)
72	Δ^7-Ergosten-3β-ol FUNGISTEROL	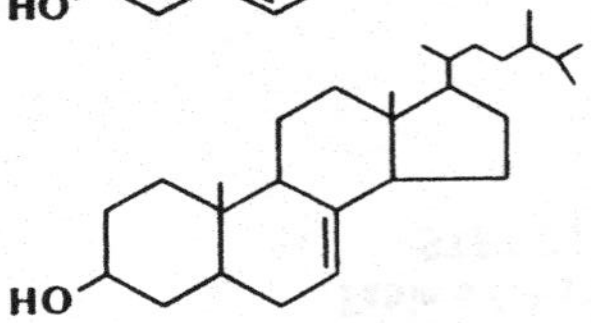	C$_{28}$H$_{44}$O (396.6)	148	—	—	—	—	—		−0.2(C)

Table 6 (continued)
STEROLS

No.	Substance[a]	Structure	Formula (mol wt)	Melting point °C	Spectral data[b]						$[\alpha]_D^c$
					IR	NMR	Ultraviolet				
							λ_{max}	ϵ	$E_{1cm}^{1\%}$		
73	$\Delta^{5,7,22}$-Ergostatrie-3β-ol ERGOSTEROL	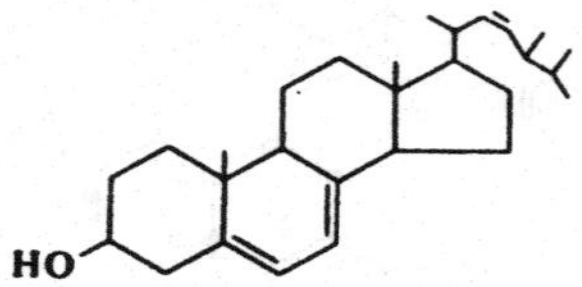	$C_{28}H_{44}O$ (396.6)	165	⋮	⋮	⋮	⋮	⋮		$-130(C)$
74	$\Delta^{5,7}$-Ergosta-dien-3β-ol 22-DIHYDROERGOSTEROL	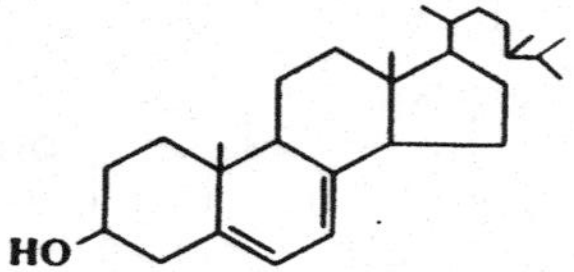	$C_{28}H_{46}O$ (398.6)	153	⋮	⋮	⋮	⋮	⋮		$-109(C)$
75	$\Delta^{5,22}$-Ergostadien-3β-ol BRASSICASTEROL	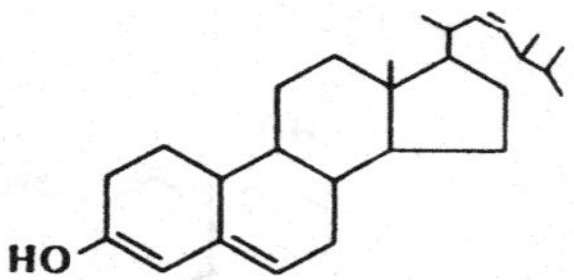	$C_{28}H_{46}O$ (398.6)	148	⋮	⋮	⋮	⋮	⋮		$-64(C)$
76	$\Delta^{5,24(28)}$-Ergostadien-3β-ol 24-METHYLENECHOLESTEROL	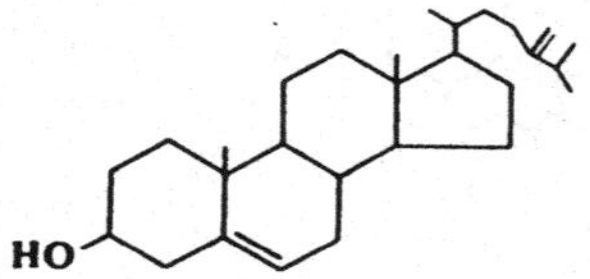	$C_{28}H_{46}O$ (398.6)	144	⋮	⋮	⋮	⋮	⋮		$-42(C)$
77	$\Delta^{7,22}$-Ergosta-dien-3β-ol 5-DIHYDROERGOSTEROL	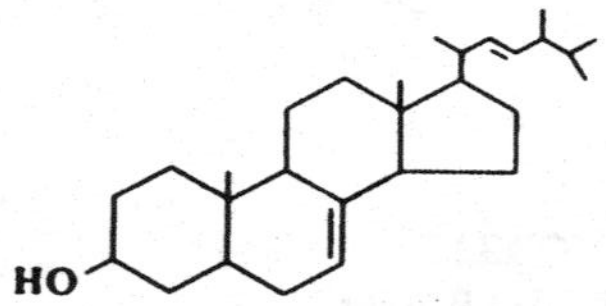	$C_{28}H_{46}O$ (398.6)	174	⋮	⋮	⋮	⋮	⋮		$-20(C)$

Table 6 (continued)
STEROLS

No.	Substance[a]	Structure	Formula (mol wt)	Melting point °C	Spectral data[b]						$[\alpha]_D^c$
					IR	NMR	Ultraviolet				
							λ_{max}	ϵ	$E_{1cm}^{1\%}$		
78	$\Delta^{7,24(28)}$-Ergostadien-3β-ol	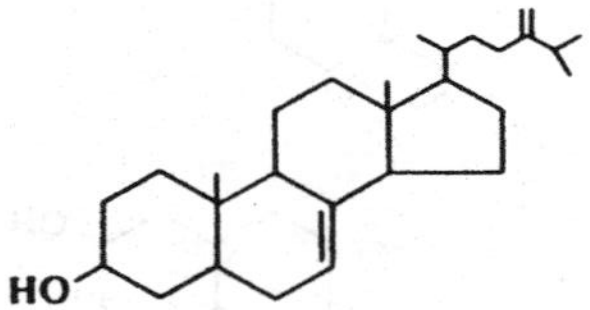	$C_{28}H_{46}O$ (398.6)	130	—	—	—	—	—		+6.0(C)
79	$\Delta^{7,24(28)}$-Ergostadien-3β-ol EPISTEROL	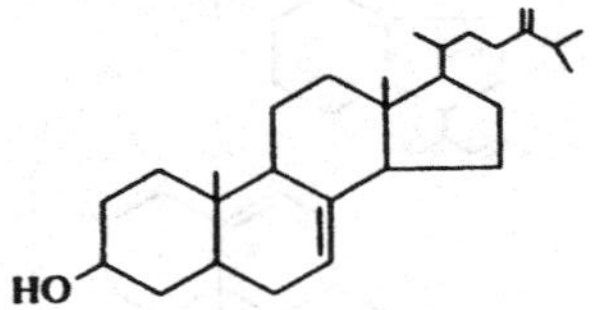	$C_{28}H_{46}O$ (398.6)	151	—	—	—	—	—		−5(C)
80	$\Delta^{8,24(?)}$-Ergostadien-3β-ol ASCOSTEROL	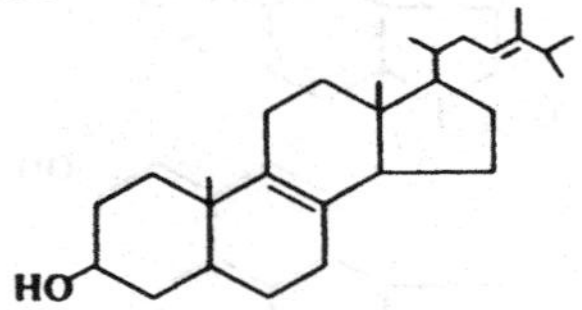	$C_{28}H_{46}O$ (398.6)	147	—	—	—	—	—		+45(C)
81	$\Delta^{8,24(28)}$-Ergostadien-3β-ol FECOSTEROL	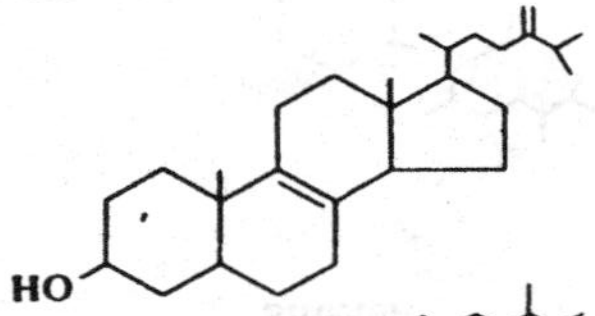	$C_{28}H_{46}O$ (398.6)	162	—	—	—	—	—		+42(C)
82	$\Delta^{7,22}$-Ergostadiene-3β,5α,6β-triol CEREVISTEROL	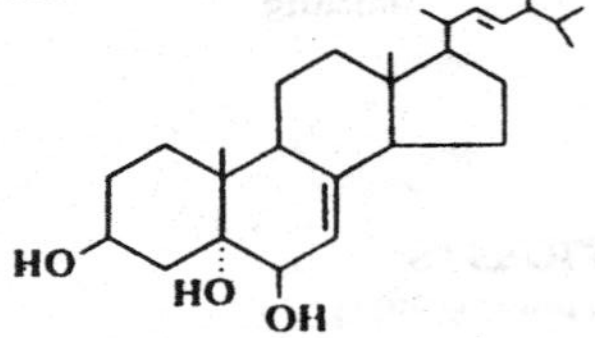	$C_{28}H_{46}O_3$ (430.6)	265	—	—	—	—	—		−79(C)

Table 6 (continued)
STEROLS

No.	Substance[a]	Structure	Formula (mol wt)	Melting point °C	Spectral data[b]					$[\alpha]_D^c$
					IR	NMR	λ_{max}	ϵ	$E_{1cm}^{1\%}$	
83	HALICLONASTEROL	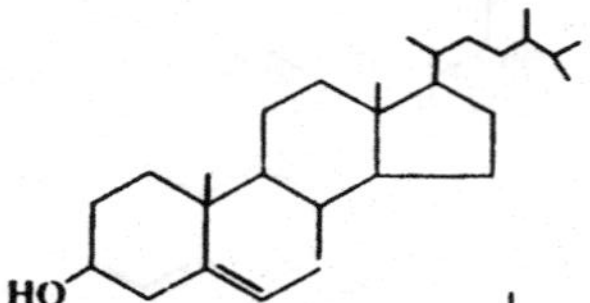	$C_{28}H_{48}O$ (398.6)	141	—	—	—			−41.5(C)
84	Δ^5-24-Isoergosten-3β-ol CAMPESTEROL	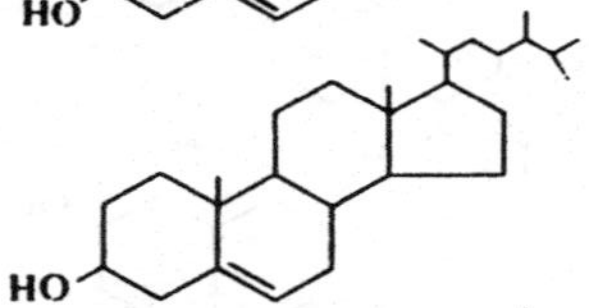	$C_{28}H_{48}O$ (398.6)	158	—	—	—			−33(C)
85	Δ^{22}-24-Isoergosten-3β-ol NEOSPONGOSTEROL	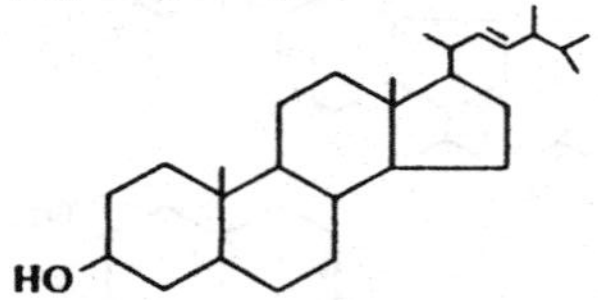	$C_{28}H_{48}O$ (398.6)	153	—	—	—			+10(C)
86	$\Delta^{5,24(28)}$-Stigmastadien-3β-ol FUCOSTEROL	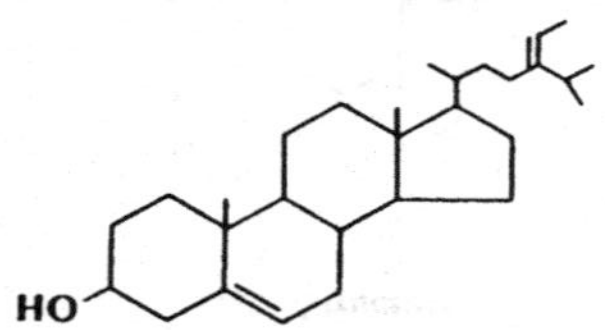	$C_{29}H_{48}O$ (410.6)	124	—	—	—			−38(C)
87	APTOSTANOL	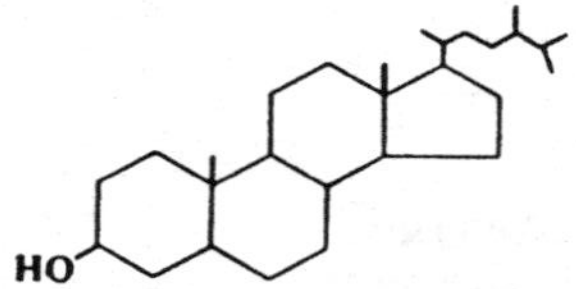	$C_{28}H_{40}O$ (400.6)	135	—	—	—			+22(C)

555

Table 6 (continued)
STEROLS

No.	Substance[a]	Structure	Formula (mol wt)	Melting point °C	IR	NMR	Ultraviolet λ_{max}	ϵ	$E_{1cm}^{1\%}$	$[\alpha]_D^c$
							Spectral data[b]			
88	Ergostan-3β-ol ERGOSTANOL	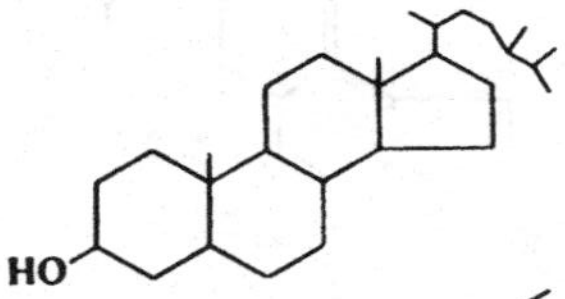	$C_{28}H_{50}O$ (402.4)	143	—	—	—	—	—	+16(C)
89	Δ5-Stigmasten-3β-ol β-SITOSTEROL	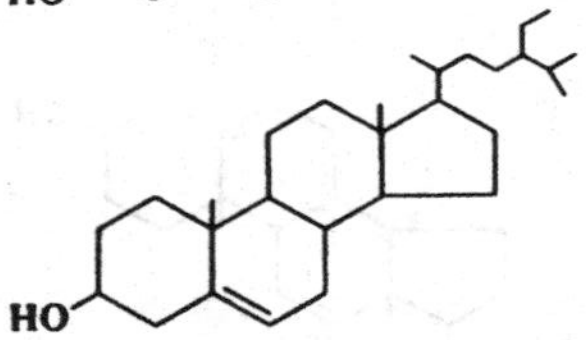	$C_{29}H_{50}O$ (414.4)	140	—	—	—	—	—	−36(C)
90	Δ5,7,22-Stigmastadien-3β-ol CORBISTEROL	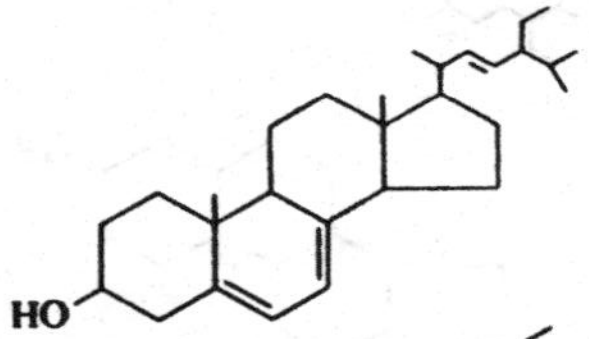	$C_{29}H_{46}O$ (410.4)	154	—	—	—	—	—	−114(C)
91	Δ7,22-24-Isoergostadien-3β-ol CHONDRILLASTEROL	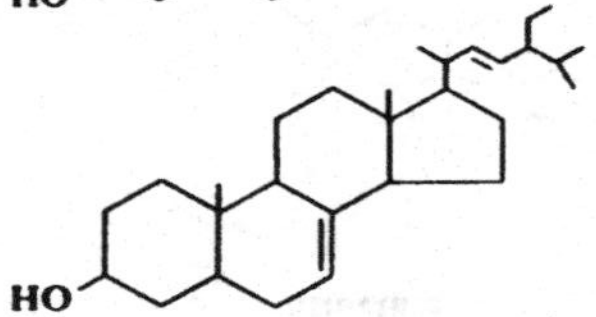	$C_{29}H_{48}O$ (410.6)	164	—	—	—	—	—	−2(C)
92	Δ5,22-24-Isostigmastadien-3β-ol PORIFERASTEROL	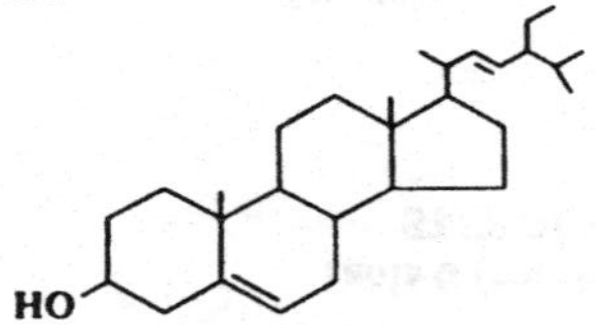	$C_{29}H_{48}O$ (410.6)	156	—	—	—	—	—	−49(C)

Table 6 (continued)
STEROLS

No.	Substance[a]	Structure	Formula (mol wt)	Melting point °C	Spectral data[b]						$[\alpha]_D^c$
					IR	NMR	Ultraviolet				
							λ_{max}	ϵ	$E_{1cm}^{1\%}$		
93	$\Delta^{5,24(28)}$-20-Isostigmastadien-3β-ol SARGASTEROL	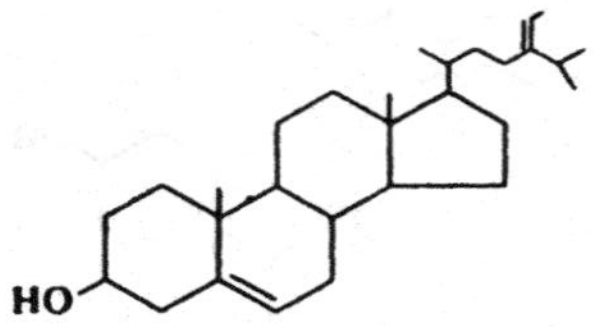	$C_{29}H_{48}O$ (410.6)	133.5	—	—	—	—	—		−47.5(C)
94	$\Delta^{5,11(12)}$-Stigmastadien-3β-ol Δ⁵-AVENASTEROL	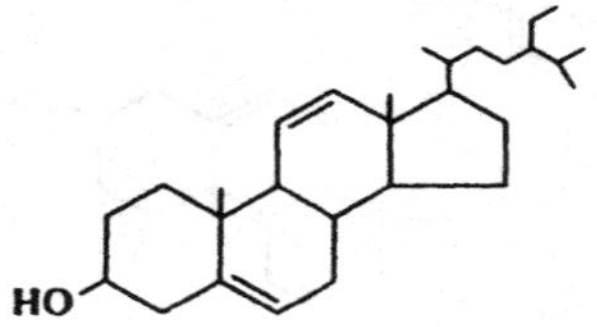	$C_{29}H_{48}O$ (410.6)	137	—	—	—	—	—		−37(C)
95	$\Delta^{7,11(12)}$-Stigmastadien-3β-ol Δ⁷-AVENASTEROL	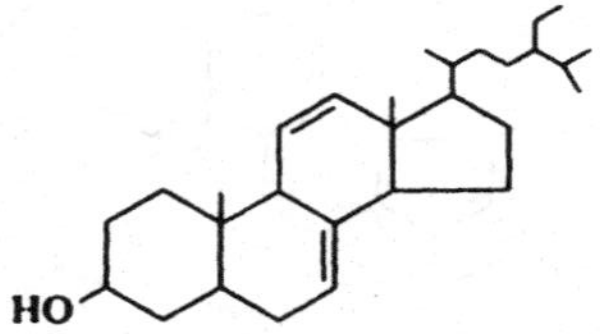	$C_{29}H_{48}O$ (410.6)	145	—	—	—	—	—		+8.8(C)
96	$\Delta^{5,22}$-Stigmastadien-3β-ol STIGMASTEROL	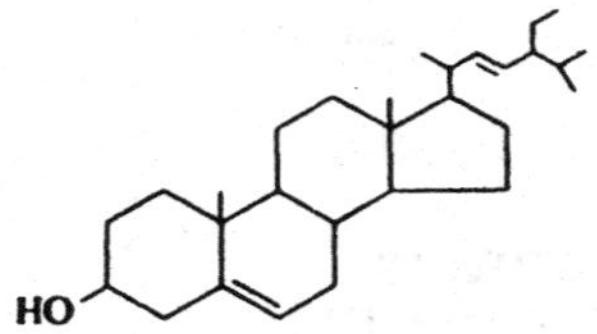	$C_{29}H_{48}O$ (410.6)	170	—	—	—	—	—		−49(C)

Table 6 (continued)
STEROLS

No.	Substance[a]	Structure	Formula (mol wt)	Melting point °C	Spectral data[b] IR	NMR	Ultraviolet [α]max	ε	$E_{1cm}^{1\%}$	$[\alpha]_D^c$
97	Δ7,22-Stigmastadien-3β-ol α-SPINASTEROL	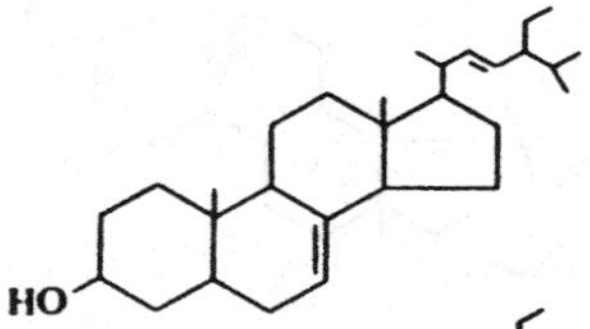 (structure)	C29H48O (410.6)	175	—	—	—	—	—	−2.7(C)
98	PALYSTEROL	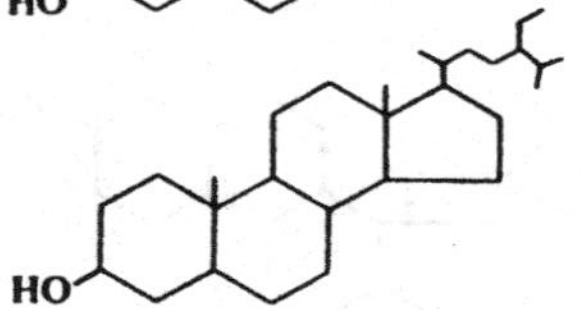 (structure)	C29H50O (412.6)	140	—	—	—	—	—	−47(C)
99	Δ5-24-Isostigmasten-3β-ol? CLIONASTEROL	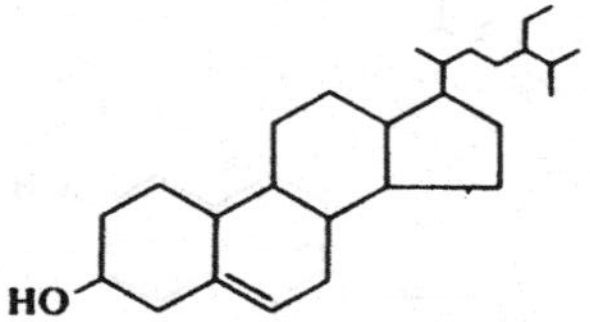 (structure)	C29H50O (412.6)	138	—	—	—	—	—	−37(C)
100	Δ5-24-Isostigmasten-3β-ol γ-SITOSTEROL	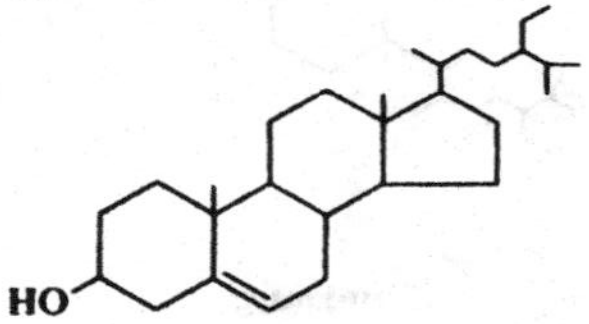 (structure)	C29H50O (412.6)	148	—	—	—	—	—	−43(C)
101	Δ7-Stigmasten-3β-ol	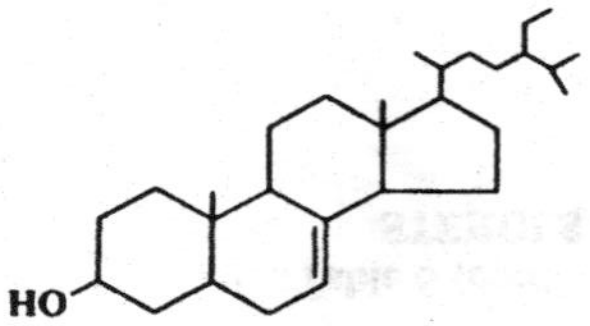 (structure)	C29H50O (412.6)	145	—	—	—	—	—	+9(C)

Table 6 (continued)
STEROLS

No.	Substance[a]	Structure	Formula (mol wt)	Melting point °C	Spectral data[b]						[α]$_D^c$
					IR	NMR	Ultraviolet				
							λ_{max}	ϵ	$E_{1cm}^{1\%}$		
102	Stigmastan-3β-ol DIHYDROSITOSTEROL	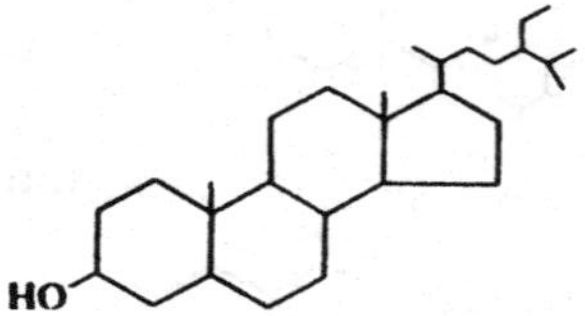	C$_{29}$H$_{52}$O (414.6)	140	—	—	—	—	—		+25(C)
103	22-Stigmasten-3β-ol	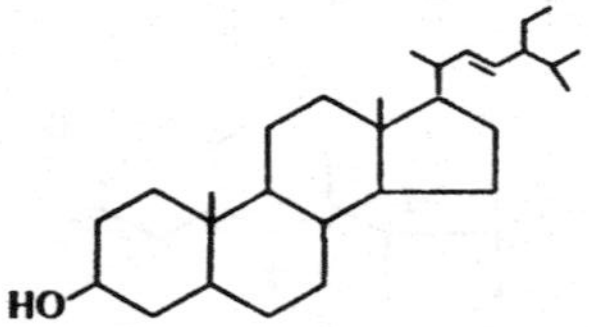	C$_{29}$H$_{50}$O (414.6)	159	—	—	—	—	—		+3.3(C)
104	DICHOLESTERYLETHER	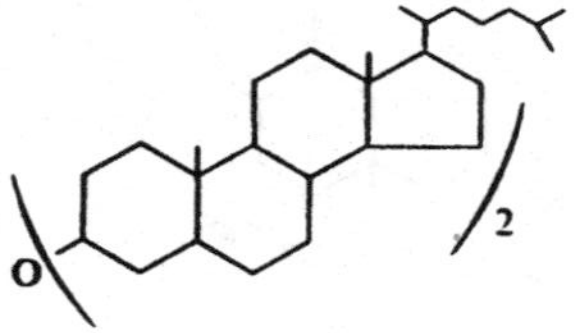	C$_{54}$H$_{90}$O (754)	196	—	—	—	—	—		-38(C)

Compiled by F. Edward Roberts and T. Windholz.

REFERENCES

1. Neudert and Ropke, *Atlas of Steroid Spectra*, Springer-Verlag, New York, 1965.
2. Tsuda, Okamoto, Kawazoe, Sato, Natsume, and Hasegawa, *Chem. Pharm. Bull.*, 10, 338 (1962).
3. Zurcher, *Helv. Chim. Acta*, 44, 1380 (1961).
4. Caspi, Grover, Grover, Lynde, and Nussbaumer, *J. Chem. Soc.* (Lond.), p. 1711 (1962).
5. Hampel and Kramer, *Chem. Ber.*, 98, 3255 (1965).
6. Cross, Landis, and Murphy, *Steroids*, 5, 655 (1965).
7. Zurcher, *Helv. Chim. Acta*, 46, 2054 (1963).
8. Herschman, Miller, Beyler, Sarett, and Tishler, *J. Am. Chem. Soc.*, 77, 3166 (1955).
9. Dobriner, Katzenellenbogen, and Jones, *Infrared Absorption Spectra of Steroids – An Atlas*, Interscience, New York, 1953.
10. Carol, *J. Assoc. Off. Agric. Chem.*, 40, 837 (1957).
11. Patton, *J. Org. Chem.*, 26, 1677 (1961).
12. Caspi, *Chem. Ind.* (Lond.), p. 1716 (1962).
13. Varian Associates Catalog High Resolution Spectra, 1963.
14. Tori, Komena, and Nakagawa, *J. Org. Chem.*, 29, 1136 (1964).
15. Slomp and MacKellar, *J. Am. Chem. Soc.*, 84, 204 (1962).
16. Samuels, Brannon, and Hayden, *J. Assoc. Off. Agric. Chem.*, 47, 918 (1964).
17. Dorfman, in *Encyclopedia of Chemical Technology*, Kirk and Othmer, Eds., J. Wiley & Sons, New York, 1966.
18. Ringler, *Meth. Horm. Res.*, 3A, 227 (1964).
19. Emmons and Martin, *Meth. Horm. Res.*, 3A, 1 (1964).
20. Fieser and Fieser, *Steroids*, Rheinhold, 1957, 477.
21. Miyaki and Rooks, *Meth. Horm. Res.*, 5, 59 (1966).
22. Pincus, *The Control of Fertility*, Academic, New York, 1965, 165.
23. Altman and Dittmer, Eds., *Biology Data Book*, Federation of American Societies for Experimental Biology, Washington, D.C., 1964, 385.

These tables originally appeared in Sober, Ed., *Handbook of Biochemistry and selected data for Molecular Biology*, 2nd ed., Chemical Rubber Co., Cleveland, 1970.

Index

INDEX

A

Printed in the United States
by Baker & Taylor Publisher Services